Skin Necrosis

Luc Téot • Sylvie Meaume
Sadanori Akita
Véronique Del Marmol
Sebastian Probst
Editors

Skin Necrosis

Second Edition

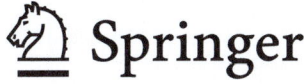

Editors
Luc Téot
Department of Plastic Surgery, Burns
and Wound Healing
Montpellier University Hospital,
Hôpital La Colombière, CICAT
Occitanie
Montpellier Cedex 5, France

Sadanori Akita
Department of Plastic and
Reconstructive Surgery
Tamaki Aozora Hospital, Fukushima
Medical University
Tokushima, Tokushima, Japan

Sebastian Probst
Geneva School of Health Sciences,
HES-SO University of Applied Sciences
and Arts Western Switzerland
Geneva, Switzerland

Sylvie Meaume
Department of Dermatology, Wound
Healing and Geriatrics
Hôpital Rothschild – Hôpitaux
Universitaires Est Parisien
Paris, France

Véronique Del Marmol
Department of Dermatology
Hôpital Erasme-Université Libre de
Bruxelles
Bruxelles, Belgium

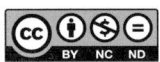

ISBN 978-3-031-60953-4   ISBN 978-3-031-60954-1   (eBook)
https://doi.org/10.1007/978-3-031-60954-1

Previously published with Springer-Verlag Wien 2015

This book is an open access publication.

Université de Genève Fukuoka University Société Francaise et Francophone des Plaies et Cicatrisations (SFFPC)

© The Editor(s) (if applicable) and The Author(s) 2024

Open Access This book is licensed under the terms of the Creative Commons Attribution-NonCommercial-NoDerivatives 4.0 International License (http://creativecommons.org/licenses/by-nc-nd/4.0/), which permits any noncommercial use, sharing, distribution and reproduction in any medium or format, as long as you give appropriate credit to the original author(s) and the source, provide a link to the Creative Commons license and indicate if you modified the licensed material. You do not have permission under this license to share adapted material derived from this book or parts of it.

The images or other third party material in this book are included in the book's Creative Commons license, unless indicated otherwise in a credit line to the material. If material is not included in the book's Creative Commons license and your intended use is not permitted by statutory regulation or exceeds the permitted use, you will need to obtain permission directly from the copyright holder.

The use of general descriptive names, registered names, trademarks, service marks, etc. in this publication does not imply, even in the absence of a specific statement, that such names are exempt from the relevant protective laws and regulations and therefore free for general use.

The publisher, the authors and the editors are safe to assume that the advice and information in this book are believed to be true and accurate at the date of publication. Neither the publisher nor the authors or the editors give a warranty, expressed or implied, with respect to the material contained herein or for any errors or omissions that may have been made. The publisher remains neutral with regard to jurisdictional claims in published maps and institutional affiliations.

This Springer imprint is published by the registered company Springer Nature Switzerland AG
The registered company address is: Gewerbestrasse 11, 6330 Cham, Switzerland

If disposing of this product, please recycle the paper.

Contents

Part I Definitions, Physiopathology, Vascular and Imaging Investigations in Skin Necrosis

1 Introduction to Physiopathology, Vascular, and Imaging Investigations in Skin Necrosis 3
Luc Téot

2 Dry Necrosis, Wet Necrosis: When to Debride, When Not to Debride 7
Luc Téot and Sergiu Fluieraru
2.1 Introduction 7
2.2 Dry Necrosis 7
2.3 Wet Necrosis 8
2.4 Debridement 8
    2.4.1 Algorithm of Debridement 9
    2.4.2 Dissecting Haematomas 9
2.5 How to Manage Skin Necrosis 11
2.6 Conclusion 13
References 13

3 Ischemia/Reperfusion: A Potential Cause of Tissue Necrosis 15
Poon Apichartpiyakul, Raj Mani, Supapong Arworn, and Kittipan Rerkasem
3.1 Introduction 15
3.2 Pathophysiology 15
3.3 Clinical Manifestations 17
3.4 Treatment and Prevention 18
3.5 Conclusion and Future Research 19
References 19

4 Imaging, Vascular Assessment: Extension in Depth and Vascular Anomalies 23
Sadanori Akita, Hideki Ishimaru, and Miho Noguchi
4.1 Introduction 23
4.2 Assessment and Imaging Tools 24
    4.2.1 Conventional X-Rays 24
    4.2.2 Duplex Ultrasonography 24

		4.2.3	Computed Tomography (CT)...............	25
		4.2.4	Magnetic Resonance Imaging (MRI).........	25
		4.2.5	Vascular Imaging........................	25
	4.3	Treatment......................................		26
		4.3.1	AVM..................................	26
	References..			32

5 Imaging of Hypodermal Fat Necrosis 33
Ximena Wortsman

	5.1	Introduction	33
	5.2	Imaging Methods..................................	33
		5.2.1 X-Ray Mammography......................	33
		5.2.2 Ultrasound	34
		5.2.3 Magnetic Resonance Imaging	36
		5.2.4 Computed Tomography and Positron Emission Tomography...............................	37
	5.3	Conclusion	38
	References..		38

6 Skin Necrosis and the Need for Vascular Assessments 41
Saritphat Orrapin, Kittipan Rerkasem, and Rajgopal Mani

	6.1	Introduction	41
	6.2	Epidemiology of Peripheral Arterial Disease	41
	6.3	Pathophysiology of Peripheral Arterial Disease	43
	6.4	Atherosclerosis and Symptomatology	43
	6.5	The Effects of Diabetes on PAD and the Diabetic Foot......	45
	6.6	Macrovascular and Microvascular Assessment Tools	46
	6.7	Macrovascular Assessments of Tissue Viability	46
	6.8	Microvascular Assessments of Tissue Viability...........	51
	6.9	Treatment Strategy for Limb Salvage	53
	6.10	Revascularization Procedure	54
	6.11	Wound Care and Biological Therapy...................	54
	6.12	Nonoperative Treatment............................	55
	6.13	Conclusion	55
	References..		56

7 Arterial and Mixed Leg Ulcer 61
Monira Nou Howaldt

	7.1	Introduction	61
	7.2	Metabolic Origin	61
	7.3	Pathophysiology...................................	61
	7.4	Clinical Diagnosis	63
	7.5	Vascular Explorations	64
	7.6	Treatment..	65
	7.7	Conclusion	65
	References..		66

Part II Different Clinical Context of Skin Necrosis Physical Injuries

8 Introduction to Physical Injuries in Skin Necrosis 71
Sebastian Probst
Reference 71

9 Skin Mechanobiology: From Basic Science to Clinical Applications 73
Aleksei Orlov and Amit Gefen
9.1 Introduction 73
9.2 Skin Biomechanics on a Tissue Scale 74
9.3 The Mechanobiology of Skin at a Cell Scale: Focus on Fibroblasts 77
9.4 Conclusion 79
References.. 79

10 Necrosis in Burns 81
Christoph Hirche, Holger Engel, Thomas Kremer, and Ulrich Kneser
10.1 Pathophysiology of Burns with Respect to Necrosis....... 81
10.2 Apoptosis and Oncosis in Burn Wounds 83
10.3 Inflammation as a Key Step in Burns................. 83
10.4 How to Prevent Necrotic Burns 83
   10.4.1 Primary Necrosis 83
   10.4.2 Secondary Necrosis 84
   10.4.3 Tertiary Necrosis 84
References.. 85

11 Electrical Burns....................................... 87
Christian Herlin
11.1 Introduction 87
11.2 Tissue Injury 88
   11.2.1 Entry and Exit Skin Points................... 88
   11.2.2 Muscle Injury.............................. 88
   11.2.3 Myocardial Damage......................... 89
   11.2.4 Buccal Mucosa Damage 89
   11.2.5 Nerve Damage............................. 89
   11.2.6 Deep Damage (Except Viscera)............... 89
   11.2.7 Other Damages 89
11.3 Medical Management............................... 89
   11.3.1 Monitoring................................ 89
   11.3.2 Assessment of the Lesions................... 90
11.4 Surgical Management 90
   11.4.1 First Surgery 90
   11.4.2 Second Look 90
11.5 Global Management................................ 91
11.6 Prevention 91
11.7 Conclusion.. 92
References.. 92

12 Gunshot Wounds ... 93
Supaporn Opasanon and Apirag Chuangsuwanich
- 12.1 Introduction ... 93
- 12.2 Etiopathogeny ... 93
- 12.3 Clinical Detailing ... 93
  - 12.3.1 Characteristics of GSWs ... 93
- 12.4 General Principles of GSW Management ... 95
  - 12.4.1 Save Life ... 95
  - 12.4.2 Local Wound Care to Prevent Infection ... 95
- 12.5 Gunshot Wound Management ... 95
  - 12.5.1 Initial Dressing ... 95
  - 12.5.2 Wound Surgery ... 95
  - 12.5.3 Irrigation and Debridement ... 95
  - 12.5.4 Dressing and Closure ... 96
  - 12.5.5 Instructions for Special Areas ... 96
- 12.6 Conclusion ... 96
- References ... 96

13 Frostbite ... 99
Marc-James Hallam, Steven J. Lo, and Christopher Imray
- 13.1 Aetiology ... 99
- 13.2 Classification of Frostbite ... 99
- 13.3 Pathology ... 100
  - 13.3.1 Intracellular Effects ... 100
  - 13.3.2 Extracellular Effects: The Freeze-Thaw-Refreeze Injury ... 101
  - 13.3.3 Long-Term Sequelae ... 101
- 13.4 Clinical Evaluation of Frostbitten Patients ... 101
  - 13.4.1 History ... 101
  - 13.4.2 Examination ... 101
  - 13.4.3 Radiological Investigations in Frostbite ... 102
- 13.5 Acute Frostbite Management ... 102
  - 13.5.1 Prioritisation of Life-Threatening Injuries and Specialist Referral ... 102
  - 13.5.2 Prevention of Refreezing and Differential Approach to Rewarming ... 102
  - 13.5.3 Pharmacological Support During Rewarming ... 103
- 13.6 Post-thaw Frostbite Care ... 104
  - 13.6.1 Management of Blisters ... 104
  - 13.6.2 Physiotherapy Protocols ... 105
  - 13.6.3 Surgery ... 105
- 13.7 Summary Points ... 107
- References ... 107

14 How to Manage Radiation Injuries ... 109
Chikako Senju, Masaki Fujioka, Katsumi Tanaka, and Sadanori Akita
- 14.1 Introduction ... 109
- 14.2 Ionizing Radiation ... 109

		14.3	Radiation Ulcers	110
		14.4	Management of Radiation Ulcers	110
			14.4.1 Debridement	110
			14.4.2 Methods of Wound Closure	110
		14.5	Case Reports	111
			14.5.1 Case 1	111
			14.5.2 Case 2	111
			14.5.3 Case 3	111
			14.5.4 Case 4	112
		14.6	Conclusion	114
		References		114

15 Excessive Internal Pressure (Dissecting Hematoma, Abdominal Hyperpressure, Abscesses, etc.) Leading to Skin Necrosis 117
Luc Téot
- 15.1 Introduction 117
- 15.2 Gastroschisis 117
- 15.3 Dissecting Hematoma 117
- 15.4 Foreign Bodies and Paraosteoarthropathy 118
- 15.5 Diabetic Foot Abscesses 118
- References 119

16 Telemedicine and Skin Necrosis 121
Anne Dompmartin and Véronique Hyppolite
- 16.1 Introduction 121
- 16.2 Diagnosis of Skin Necrosis 121
- 16.3 Tele-Assistance 122
- 16.4 Technology 122
- 16.5 Telemedicine and Skin Necrosis 122
- 16.6 Conclusion 123
- References 123

Part III Skin Necrosis of Toxic Origin

17 Introduction to Skin Necrosis of Toxic Origin 127
Sadanori Akita

18 Resuscitation Foot Necrosis: A New Entity for a Complex Management? 129
Franck Duteille
- 18.1 Introduction 129
- 18.2 Clinical Presentation 129
- 18.3 The Therapeutic Decision 129
  - 18.3.1 Evolution 129
  - 18.3.2 The Strategy Concerning the Therapeutic Attitude 131
  - 18.3.3 Surgical Intervention 132
  - 18.3.4 Follow-Up 133
- 18.4 Conclusion 134
- Bibliography 134

19	**Skin Necrosis and Ulcers Induced by Medications** 135

Joachim Dissemond

- 19.1 Introduction 135
- 19.2 Medications 135
  - 19.2.1 Hydroxyurea 135
  - 19.2.2 Anagrelide 137
  - 19.2.3 Coumarins 137
  - 19.2.4 Heparin 138
  - 19.2.5 Methotrexate 138
  - 19.2.6 Leflunomide 139
  - 19.2.7 Hydralazine 139
  - 19.2.8 Amezinium Methylsulfate 139
  - 19.2.9 Diltiazem 140
  - 19.2.10 Propylthiouracil 140
  - 19.2.11 Nicorandil 140
  - 19.2.12 Levamisole 140
  - 19.2.13 Pentazocine 141
  - 19.2.14 Tyrosine Kinase Inhibitors 141
- 19.3 Therapy 142
- 19.4 Conclusion 142
- References 142

20	**Toxic Syndromes** 145

Shota Suda, Sho Yamakawa, and Kenji Hayashida

- 20.1 Epidemiology and Clinical Features 145
  - 20.1.1 Staphylococcal Toxic Shock Syndrome 145
  - 20.1.2 Skin Manifestation 146
- 20.2 Pathophysiology 148
- 20.3 Treatment 148
  - 20.3.1 Antibiotic Therapy 148
  - 20.3.2 Intravenous Immune Globulin 149
  - 20.3.3 Surgical Therapy 149
- References 149

21	**Skin Necrosis Due to Snakebites** 151

Masaki Fujioka

- 21.1 Introduction 151
- 21.2 Systemic and Local Complications After Envenomation . . . 151
- 21.3 Dry Bite 152
- 21.4 First Aid 153
- 21.5 Antivenom Treatment 153
- 21.6 Allergic Reactions to Antivenom 153
- 21.7 Surgical Treatment 153
- 21.8 Immediate Debridement of Fang Marks 154
- 21.9 Case Reports 154
  - 21.9.1 Case 1 154
  - 21.9.2 Case 2 155
  - 21.9.3 Case 3 155
- 21.10 Conclusion 157
- References 157

22	**Stonefish Necrosis**		159
	Jan Dirk Harms, Cyril D'Andréa, and Nadia Fartaoui		
	22.1	The Stonefish [3, 4]	159
		22.1.1 Identification	159
		22.1.2 Habitat	160
		22.1.3 Venomous Apparatus	160
	22.2	Stings by Stonefish	160
		22.2.1 General Ideas	160
		22.2.2 Circumstances	160
		22.2.3 Wound Location	160
		22.2.4 Clinical Evidence	160
		22.2.5 Diagnosis	161
		22.2.6 Severity of the Wound Depends on Several Factors	161
		22.2.7 Medical Complications	161
		22.2.8 Treatment	162
		22.2.9 Other Used Treatments	162
	22.3	Our Experience in Réunion Island	163
	22.4	Clinical Cases	163
		22.4.1 Case 1	163
		22.4.2 Case 2	164
		22.4.3 Case 3	164
	References		164
23	**Skin Necrosis from Coma Blister**		167
	Masayuki Kashiwagi and Shin-ichi Kubo		
	23.1	Introduction	167
	23.2	Case Examination	168
		23.2.1 Immunohistochemical Examinations	168
	23.3	Features of Coma Blister	170
	23.4	Conclusion	171
	References		171

Part IV Skin Necrosis of Medical Origin

24	**Introduction of Skin Necrosis of Medical Origin**		177
	Véronique Del Marmol and Sylvie Meaume		
25	**Rheumatoid and Systemic Collagenosis Vasculitis**		179
	Masaki Fujioka		
	25.1	Introduction	179
	25.2	How Do Ulcers Develop in Patients with RA and Systemic Collagenosis Diseases?	179
		25.2.1 Vasculitis	179
		25.2.2 Neutrophilic Dermatoses	180
		25.2.3 Venous Stasis	180
		25.2.4 Arterial Disease	181
		25.2.5 Corticosteroid Therapy	181

	25.3	Ulcers in Other Connective Tissue Diseases	181
		25.3.1 Systemic Lupus Erythematosus (SLE)	181
		25.3.2 Systemic Sclerosis	182
		25.3.3 Dermatomyositis	182
		25.3.4 Sjögren's Syndrome	182
		25.3.5 Scleroderma	182
		25.3.6 Behcet's Syndrome	182
	25.4	Treatments of Ulcers in Patients with RA and Other Connective Tissue Diseases	182
		25.4.1 Systemic Approach	182
		25.4.2 Topical Wound Treatment	183
		25.4.3 Occlusive Dressings	183
		25.4.4 Approach for the Wound Infection	183
		25.4.5 Several Adjuvant Devices in the Management of Hard-to-Heal Wounds	183
	25.5	Surgical Wound Closure for Patients with RA	184
	25.6	Prevention of Recurrence	186
	References		186
26	**Giant Cell Arteritis**		**187**
	Pauline Lecerf and Sophie Golstein		
	26.1	Introduction/Physiopathology	187
	26.2	Diagnosis	187
		26.2.1 Medical Context	187
		26.2.2 Semiology	188
		26.2.3 Criteria	189
		26.2.4 Routine Evaluation	189
	26.3	Treatment	189
	26.4	Tocilizumab	190
	26.5	Methotrexate	190
	References		190
27	**Hidradenitis Suppurativa**		**193**
	Kian Zarchi, Véronique Del Marmol, and Gregor B. E. Jemec		
	27.1	Introduction	193
	27.2	Diagnosis	193
	27.3	Pathophysiology	194
	27.4	Treatment	195
	27.5	Adjuvant Therapy	196
	27.6	Conclusion	197
	References		197
28	**Martorell Hypertensive Ischemic Ulcer**		**199**
	Sylvie Meaume and Hester Colboc		
	28.1	Epidemiology	199
	28.2	Etiopathogenesis	199
	28.3	Clinical Diagnosis	199
	28.4	Histopathology	200
	28.5	Differential Diagnoses	201

		28.6	Evolution	202
		28.7	Treatment of NA	202
		28.8	Other Treatments	203
		28.9	Conclusion	203
			References	203
29	**Vasculitis**			205
	Nicolas Kluger			
		29.1	Diagnosis of Cutaneous Vasculitis Is Made on Histology	205
		29.2	Pitfalls	208
		29.3	Clinical Pathologic Correlation	208
		29.4	Clinical Manifestations	208
		29.5	Classification	210
		29.6	Approach to the Diagnosis of Cutaneous Vasculitis	210
		29.7	Management of Cutaneous Vasculitis	211
			References	212
30	**Necrobiosis Lipoidica**			215
	Miruna Negulescu			
		30.1	Introduction	215
		30.2	Epidemiology	215
		30.3	Pathogenesis and Histology	215
		30.4	Clinical Findings and Complications	215
		30.5	Treatment	216
			References	217
31	**Purpura Fulminans**			219
	Nancy Hajjar and Véronique Del Marmol			
		31.1	Introduction	219
		31.2	Epidemiology	219
		31.3	When to Suspect Purpura Fulminans	219
		31.4	Pathogenesis	219
		31.5	Clinical Presentation	220
			31.5.1 Workup	220
			31.5.2 Management	220
			31.5.3 Differential Diagnosis	220
		31.6	Long-Term Sequelae of Purpura Fulminans	220
			References	221
32	**Protein C and Protein S Deficiencies**			223
	Sébastien Humbert and Philippe Humbert			
		32.1	Physiopathology	223
		32.2	Diagnosis	223
		32.3	Treatment	224
33	**Renal Insufficiency and Necrosis**			225
	Elia Ricci			
		33.1	Comorbidity	226
		33.2	Exacerbation	227

		33.3	Direct Cause...	227
		33.4	Treatment...	228
		References..		228

34 Calciphylaxis.. 231
Mariam Kabbani, Véronique Del Marmol,
and Farida Benhadou
    34.1 Introduction... 231
    34.2 Risk Factors... 231
    34.3 Clinical Manifestation................................. 231
    34.4 Pathophysiology....................................... 232
    34.5 Diagnosis... 232
    34.6 Treatment... 232
    References.. 233

35 Livedo(id) Vasculitis.. 235
Farida Benhadou and Jean-Claude Wautrecht
    35.1 Introduction... 235
    35.2 Histology... 235
    35.3 Pathogenesis.. 235
    35.4 Clinical Presentation.................................. 235
           35.4.1 Signs and Symptoms........................ 235
           35.4.2 Location................................... 236
           35.4.3 Possible Associated Conditions............. 236
    35.5 Diagnosis... 236
    35.6 Treatment... 236
           35.6.1 General Management........................ 236
           35.6.2 Therapeutic Modalities..................... 236
           35.6.3 Perspectives............................... 237
    References.. 237

36 Pyoderma Gangrenosum.. 239
Hiroshi Yoshimoto
    36.1 Introduction... 239
    36.2 Etiopathogenesis...................................... 239
    36.3 Clinical Detailing..................................... 239
    36.4 Treatments.. 240
    References.. 241

37 Cryoglobulinemia.. 243
Alessandra Michelucci, Salvatore Panduri, Valentina Dini,
and Marco Romanelli
    37.1 Physiopathology....................................... 243
    37.2 Diagnosis... 243
    37.3 Treatment... 244
           37.3.1 Systemic Treatment........................ 244
           37.3.2 Local Treatment........................... 245
    References.. 245

38 Hand Necrosis 247
Yasser Farid, Nicolas Cuylits, Farida Benhadou, and Véronique Del Marmol
- 38.1 Introduction 247
- 38.2 Vascularization 247
- 38.3 Mechanisms 247
- 38.4 Etiologies 248
- 38.5 Clinical Presentation of Digital Ischemia 249
- 38.6 Diagnosis 249
- 38.7 Management 250
  - 38.7.1 The Localization of Necrosis 251
  - 38.7.2 The Perfusion Status and the Extent of Necrosis 251
- References 253

39 Factitious Disorders (Pathomimia) and Necrosis 255
Francoise Poot
- 39.1 Introduction 255
- 39.2 Classification 255
- 39.3 Syndromes Associated with a Denied or Hidden Pathological Behaviour 257
- 39.4 Diagnosis and Treatment 257
- 39.5 Conclusion 260
- References 260

Part V Skin Necrosis of Infectious Origin

40 Introduction to Necrosis with an Infectious Origin 263
Luc Téot

41 Necrosis and Infection 265
Farida Benhadou and Véronique Del Marmol
- 41.1 Introduction 265
- 41.2 Bacteria 265
- 41.3 Mycobacteria 266
- 41.4 Viruses 267
- 41.5 COVID-19 and Skin Necrosis 267
- 41.6 Yeast 267
- 41.7 Parasites 268
- 41.8 Pathological Mechanisms 268
- References 268

42 *Fusarium solani* 271
Raphael Masson
- References 271

43 Fournier Gangrene 273
Tristan L. Hartzell and Dennis P. Orgill
- 43.1 Introduction and History 273
- 43.2 Physiopathogenesis 274

	43.3	Diagnosis	275
	43.4	Treatment	276
	43.5	Reconstruction	278
	43.6	Conclusion	279
	References		279

44 Infection Context: Necrotizing Fasciitis 281
Sadanori Akita
- 44.1 Introduction 281
- 44.2 Epidemiology 281
- 44.3 Symptom 282
- 44.4 Clinical Course and Features of Necrotizing Fasciitis 282
- 44.5 Diagnosis and Tests 283
  - 44.5.1 Physical Diagnosis 283
  - 44.5.2 Laboratory Tests 284
- 44.6 Treatment 284
  - 44.6.1 Medical Therapy 284
  - 44.6.2 Surgical Therapy 284
- References 285

Part VI Surgical Context of Skin Necrosis

45 Introduction to Skin Necrosis in Surgical Context 289
Luc Téot

46 Skin Necrosis Over Osteosynthetic Material 293
Camille Rodaix
- 46.1 Introduction 293
- 46.2 Postoperative Skin Necrosis 293
  - 46.2.1 Debridement 293
  - 46.2.2 NPWTi 294
  - 46.2.3 Hardware Removal 294
  - 46.2.4 Soft Tissue Reconstruction 294
  - 46.2.5 Alternatives to Flap Cover 296
- 46.3 Delayed Skin Necrosis 296
- 46.4 Conclusion 296
- References 296

47 Necrotic Complications After Skin Grafts 299
Xavier Santos and Israel Iglesias
- 47.1 Introduction 299
- 47.2 Graft Survival 299
- 47.3 Graft Failure and Necrosis 300
  - 47.3.1 Recipient Site 300
  - 47.3.2 Barriers Between Bed and Graft 301
  - 47.3.3 Graft Shearing 302
  - 47.3.4 Infection 302
  - 47.3.5 Poor Systemic Conditions 303
  - 47.3.6 Technical Errors 303
- 47.4 Graft Rescue 303

48 Arterial Leg Ulcers ... 305
Josef Aschwanden, Jurg Hafner, Vincenzo Jacomella, and Severin Läuchli
- 48.1 Introduction ... 305
- 48.2 Epidemiology and Classification ... 305
- 48.3 Clinical Findings ... 306
- 48.4 Diagnosis ... 307
- 48.5 Treatment ... 308
- References ... 309

49 Prevention of Skin Necrosis in Cosmetic Medicine ... 311
Hugues Cartier, Leonie Schelke, and Peter Velthuis
- 49.1 Introduction ... 311
  - 49.1.1 Aesthetic Procedures ... 311
  - 49.1.2 Filling Products ... 311
  - 49.1.3 Lifting Effect or Collagen Stimulation by Threads ... 312
  - 49.1.4 Laser and EBD ... 312
  - 49.1.5 EBD ... 314
  - 49.1.6 Peelings ... 314
  - 49.1.7 Other Injectable Active Ingredients ... 314
- 49.2 Complications ... 314
  - 49.2.1 Inflammation and Pigmentation ... 314
  - 49.2.2 Scars ... 315
  - 49.2.3 Infectious ... 315
- 49.3 Conclusion ... 315
- References ... 315

50 Leeches in Prevention of Skin Necrosis in Flap Surgery ... 317
Luc Téot
- 50.1 Introduction ... 317
- 50.2 Mode of Action ... 317
- 50.3 Conservation and Use ... 317
- 50.4 Clinical Indications ... 318
- 50.5 Conclusion ... 318
- References ... 318

51 Revascularization Techniques to Prevent Limb Amputation Presenting Distal Necrosis ... 321
Francis Pesteil, Romain Chauvet, Lucie Chastaingt, Rami El Hage, Maxime Gourgue, Raphaël Van Damme, Loïc Prales, and Philippe Lacroix
- References ... 331

52 Skin Reconstruction Using Dermal Substitutes After Skin Necrosis ... 333
Franco Bassetto and Carlotta Scarpa
- 52.1 Introduction ... 333
- 52.2 The Different Acellular Matrices ... 334
- 52.3 Conclusion and Take-Home Messages ... 336
- References ... 336

53	**Skin Necrosis of the Diabetic Foot and Its Management** 339	
	J. Karim Ead, Miranda Goransson, and David G. Armstrong	
	53.1 Introduction 339	
	53.2 The Biochemical Consequences of Hyperglycemia 340	
	53.3 Wound Wars: The Limb Preservation Team Strikes Back! 342	
	References.. 344	
54	**Skin Necrosis of Diabetic Foot and Its Management**.......... 345	
	Joon Pio Hong	
	54.1 Introduction 345	
	54.2 Risk Factors for Diabetic Foot Skin Necrosis 345	
	54.3 Clinical Presentation 345	
	54.3.1 Detecting Early Change....................... 345	
	54.3.2 Wet Necrosis 346	
	54.3.3 Dry Necrosis 346	
	54.4 Treatment and Reconstruction 347	
	54.4.1 Debridement 347	
	54.4.2 Vascular Intervention......................... 348	
	54.4.3 Reconstruction Using Free Flaps............... 349	
	References.. 351	
55	**Exposed Necrotic Tendons** 353	
	Luc Téot	
	55.1 Introduction 353	
	55.2 Clinical Features: Staging the Living Tendinous Tissue 353	
	55.3 Mode of Treatment..................................... 355	
	55.3.1 Immobilization............................... 355	
	55.3.2 Negative Pressure Wound Therapy 356	
	55.3.3 Artificial Dermis 356	
	55.3.4 Flaps... 356	
	55.4 Causes and Specific Management 356	
	55.4.1 Burns 356	
	55.4.2 Trauma...................................... 357	
	55.4.3 Miscellaneous 357	
	References.. 357	
56	**Dissecting Haematomas in Patients Submitted to Anticoagulation**.. 359	
	Sergiu Fluieraru	
	56.1 Introduction 359	
	56.2 Clinical Signs... 359	
	56.3 Anatomical Lesions on the Skin Spreading to the Depth 359	
	56.4 Complementary Exams 360	
	56.5 Surgical Management 360	
	References.. 361	

57 Management of the Patient After Flap Failure 363
Raymund E. Horch, Justus Osterloh, Christian Taeger,
Oliver Bleiziffer, Ulrich Kneser, Andreas Arkudas,
and Justus P. Beier
  57.1 Introduction 363
  57.2 Etiology and Pathogenesis 363
  57.3 Causes of Flap Failure 364
    57.3.1 Reversible Causes Due to Outer Circumstances 364
  57.4 Reevaluation of Reconstructive Goals 366
    57.4.1 Repeat Free Flap Procedure 368
    57.4.2 Non-microsurgical Therapy 368
  References 370

Part VII Techniques Applicable to Skin Necrosis

58 Introduction to Techniques Applicable to Skin Necrosis 375
Luc Téot

59 Dressings for Necrosed Skin 377
Christine Faure-Chazelles and Sylvie Meaume
  59.1 Introduction 377
  59.2 Dressings and Autolytic Debridement 377
    59.2.1 Hydrating Dressings 377
    59.2.2 Mixed "Hydrating/Absorbent" Dressings 378
    59.2.3 Absorbent Dressings 379
  59.3 How to Use These Dressings 381
  59.4 How to Choose the Dressing 381
  References 381

60 Surgical Debridement 383
Sadanori Akita
  60.1 Introduction 383
  60.2 Pathophysiology of the Underlying Diseases and Conditions in Surgical Debridement 383
    60.2.1 Burns 383
    60.2.2 High-Energy Trauma Wound 385
    60.2.3 Pressure Injury 385
    60.2.4 Diabetic Foot Ulcer 386
    60.2.5 Leg Ulcer 388
  60.3 Choice of the Surgical Debridement 389
  References 389

61 Stabilization of Necrotic Tissue Using Cerium Nitrate Silver Sulfadiazine 391
Chloé Geri
  61.1 Introduction 391
  61.2 Burns Are the Classic Indication 391
  61.3 Contraindications and Adverse Effects 392

		61.4	Clinical Indications Outside Burns 392

- 61.4 Clinical Indications Outside Burns 392
  - 61.4.1 Arterial Leg Ulcer 392
  - 61.4.2 Heel Pressure Ulcer in the Elderly Patient. 393
  - 61.4.3 Diabetic Foot Ulcer 393
  - 61.4.4 Cutaneous Lesions of Microvascular Etiology 394
- 61.5 Other Factors of Delayed Healing 394
  - 61.5.1 Malignant Wound. 394
  - 61.5.2 Radionecrosis. 394
  - 61.5.3 Other Types of Wounds 395
- 61.6 End of Life and/or Multiple Comorbidities 395
- 61.7 Discussion and Perspectives 395
- 61.8 Conclusion. 396
- References. 396

62 Honey Debridement 399
Vijay K. Shukla and Vivek Srivastava
- 62.1 Introduction 399
- 62.2 Antibacterial Properties 399
- 62.3 Debridement. 400
- 62.4 Tissue Growth 401
- 62.5 Deodorizing 402
- 62.6 Anti-inflammatory Action 402
- 62.7 Contraindications. 402
- 62.8 Conclusion 402
- References. 403

63 Recent Technologies in Necrosis Surgical Debridement 405
Luc Téot, Christian Herlin, and Sergiu Fluieraru
- 63.1 Introduction 405
- 63.2 Description of Recently Developed Debridement Technologies 405
- 63.3 Clinical Indications 408
  - 63.3.1 Extent of Necrosis over the Wound Surface 408
  - 63.3.2 Necrotic Tissues Vary Depending on the Aetiopathogeny of the Wound. 409
- 63.4 Respective Indications of New Technologies 409
- References. 409

Part VIII Skin Necrosis in Children

64 Introduction to Skin Necrosis Treatment in Young Age 413
Luc Téot
- References. 413

65 Skin Necrosis in Children: Physical and Infectious Causes 415
Guido Ciprandi
- 65.1 Introduction 415
- 65.2 SSFTN (Skin and Subcutaneous Fat Necrosis of the Newborn: "Adiponecrosis Subcutanea Neonatorum"). 416
  - 65.2.1 General Aspects. 416
  - 65.2.2 Predisposing Factors 417

		65.2.3	Laboratory Examinations............... 417
		65.2.4	Diagnosis............................ 417
		65.2.5	Course and Outcome................... 418
	65.3	Extravasation Injuries Necrosis............. 418
		65.3.1	Introduction and Definition........... 418
		65.3.2	Actions and Injuries.................. 419
		65.3.3	Epidemiology........................ 419
		65.3.4	Distribution by Body Area and Care Setting...... 420
		65.3.5	Care................................ 420
		65.3.6	Physiology of Extravasation........... 420
		65.3.7	Factors Affecting the Pathophysiology of Extravasation...................... 420
		65.3.8	Identification of Extravasation and Risk Factors..................... 421
		65.3.9	Dangerous Substances................. 421
		65.3.10	Treatments.......................... 422
	65.4	SNSTIs (Severe Necrotizing Soft Tissue Infections)...... 424
		65.4.1	Introduction......................... 424
		65.4.2	Care................................ 425
	References.. 426

66 Neonatal Pressure Ulcer.................................. 429
Christian Herlin
  66.1 Introduction... 429
  66.2 Risk Assessment Scales............................... 430
  66.3 Principles of Treatment............................... 430
      66.3.1 Topic Treatment............................... 430
      66.3.2 Surgical Treatment............................ 430
  66.4 Main Areas Affected................................. 430
      66.4.1 The Nose..................................... 430
      66.4.2 The Foot and Leg............................. 431
      66.4.3 The Scalp and Back........................... 432
  66.5 Conclusion.. 433
  References... 433

67 Skin Necrosis in Children: Genodermatosis................ 435
Cristina Has and Agnes Schwieger-Briel
  67.1 Introduction... 435
  67.2 Genodermatoses that Manifest with Cutaneous Necrosis as a Lead Symptom......................... 435
      67.2.1 Progeroid Syndromes......................... 435
      67.2.2 Vascular Anomalies........................... 436
      67.2.3 Metabolic Disorders........................... 437
      67.2.4 Genodermatosis with Cutaneous Necrosis as a Possible Complication...................... 438
      67.2.5 Harlequin Ichthyosis.......................... 439
      67.2.6 Olmsted Syndrome........................... 439
      67.2.7 Leucocyte Adhesion Deficiency Type I......... 440
      67.2.8 Other Genetic Diseases....................... 440
  67.3 Conclusion/Take Home Messages..................... 440
  References... 441

68 Skin Necrosis in Children: Vascular Causes and Angioma..... 443
Laurence M. Boon, Valérie Dekeuleneer, and Julien Coulie
- 68.1 Ulcerated Infantile Hemangioma...................... 443
  - 68.1.1 Physiopathology 443
  - 68.1.2 Clinical Presentation 443
  - 68.1.3 Diagnosis................................. 443
  - 68.1.4 Treatment................................. 444
- 68.2 Ulcerated Congenital Hemangiomas 444
  - 68.2.1 Physiopathology 445
  - 68.2.2 Clinical Presentation 445
  - 68.2.3 Diagnosis................................. 445
  - 68.2.4 Treatment................................. 445
- 68.3 Arteriovenous Malformations 446
  - 68.3.1 Physiopathology 446
  - 68.3.2 Clinical Presentation 446
  - 68.3.3 Diagnosis................................. 447
  - 68.3.4 Treatment................................. 447
- References... 447

Part IX Skin Necrosis in the Elderly

69 Introduction: Skin Necrosis in the Elderly.................. 451
Sylvie Meaume

70 Pressure Necrosis in Geriatric Patients..................... 453
Joyce Black
- 70.1 Background 453
- 70.2 Etiology/Pathophysiology 453
- 70.3 Presentation 455
- 70.4 Differential Diagnosis 457
- 70.5 Prevention 457
- 70.6 Treatment.. 458
- References... 459

71 Deep Dissecting Haematoma: A Frequent Cause of Necrosis in Elderly Patient............................... 461
Hester Colboc and Sylvie Meaume
- 71.1 Pathophysiology................................... 461
- 71.2 Epidemiology..................................... 462
- 71.3 Clinical Signs..................................... 462
- 71.4 Differential Diagnosis 463
- 71.5 Complications 464
- 71.6 Additional Examinations 465
- 71.7 Medical and Surgical Management 466
  - 71.7.1 Medical Management 466
  - 71.7.2 Surgical Management 466
  - 71.7.3 Healing................................... 468
- 71.8 Prevention 468
- 71.9 Conclusion 469
- References... 469

Part X Education on Debridement

72 Introduction 473
Sebastian Probst
References 474

73 Education on Debridement: Non-specialized Nurses and Debridement 475
Paul Bobbink
73.1 Nurses Should Be Able to Assess a Person Living with a Chronic Wound 475
73.2 Nurses Should Have Knowledge on Basic Wound Aetiology and Wound Bed Evaluation 475
73.3 Nurses Should Be Aware of Types of Debridement 477
73.4 Nurses Should Be Able to Select the Most Suitable Type of Debridement 477
73.5 Nurses Should Have an Understanding of Moist Wound Healing to Implement an Effective After-Debridement Care Plan 478
References 479

74 How to Become an Expert in Debridement: Nurse Perspective 483
Georgina Gethin
74.1 Introduction 483
74.2 The Nurse in Advanced Practice 483
74.3 Conclusion 486
References 486

75 How to Become an Expert in Debridement? Physician Perspective 489
Kirsi Isoherranen and Virve Koljonen
75.1 Introduction 489
75.2 How to Debride 490
  75.2.1 Autolytic Debridement 490
  75.2.2 Enzymatic Debridement 490
  75.2.3 Mechanical Debridement 491
  75.2.4 Biological Debridement 491
  75.2.5 Surgical or Sharp Debridement 491
75.3 When NOT to Debride? 493
75.4 Debridement in Atypical Wounds 493
75.5 Pain Treatment During Debridement 493
  75.5.1 The Future of Debridement 493
References 494

76 Regulations for Conservative Sharp Debridement for Nurses in Europe 495
Sebastian Probst
76.1 Introduction 495
76.2 Regulations for Conservative Sharp Debridement for Nurses in Europe 495

	76.3	When to Debride?	496
	76.4	Who Can Debride?	496
	76.5	What Is the Procedure of a Sharp Debridement?	496
	76.6	Assess	496
	76.7	Pain Relief	496
	76.8	Question, What Can Be Possible Complications When Doing a Sharp Debridement	496
	76.9	Debridement Methods with Sharp Instruments	498
	76.10	Conclusions	499
		References	499
77	**Regulations for Conservative Debridement for Nurses in North America**		**501**
	Maryse Beaumier		
	77.1	Introduction	501
	77.2	The Precision of Debridement Types	501
	77.3	The Clinical Decision for Debridement's Use	502
	77.4	Regulations	503
	77.5	Conclusion	504
		References	505
78	**Distance Skin Necrosis Management**		**507**
	Chloé Geri		
	78.1	Introduction	507
	78.2	Who Is Concerned?	507
		78.2.1 The Patients	507
		78.2.2 Local or First-Line Caregivers	508
		78.2.3 The Experts	508
	78.3	Why to Choose Tele-Assistance?	508
	78.4	When? How? 'OR' What?	511
	78.5	Conclusion	512
		References	512
Index			**515**

Part I

Definitions, Physiopathology, Vascular and Imaging Investigations in Skin Necrosis

Introduction to Physiopathology, Vascular, and Imaging Investigations in Skin Necrosis

Luc Téot

Skin necrosis is a consequence of local devascularisation, induced by multiple causal factors like infection, macroangiopathy or microangiopathy, hyperpressure coming from outside or inside, or high-velocity trauma (Figs. 1.1, 1.2, 1.3, 1.4, 1.5, and 1.6). Necrosis is a consequence of cascades of events starting on the venous side and then blocking the arterioles and larger arteries.

Most of the time, the clinical context is clear enough to determine the origin of the necrosis and the potential risks of extension to the depth or over the surface. In this part, the authors resume the present knowledge on how necrotic tissue develops, which capacity of reperfusion can be expected, how to explore the extent of the necrotic process, and predominantly the vascular investigations mandatory prior to determining a debridement strategy. The capacity to properly treat ischaemic limbs as emergencies, revascularise segments of limbs (lower limbs predominantly), and prevent amputation is a real progress, allowed by early diagnosis and accurate strategies of revascularisation, using innovative performing stents and distal bypasses. In the same time, necrotic and devascularised tissues represent a potential risk for the vascular surgery itself, imposing a local debridement contemporary to the revascularisation procedure.

Keeping in mind that a freshly revascularised limb will take some days to eliminate oedema and inflammation stuck into the tissues, the risk of renecrosis remains during this period of time. Amputation itself may be the cause of hyperpressure of the suture edges, and the problem of leaving a transmetatarsal amputation open is posed, especially due to the emerging capacities of negative-pressure wound therapy (NPWT) to help local angiogenesis and improve the local granulation tissue. Imaging investigations are needed to define the limits of vascular and tissular damages, beyond which debridement is not any more possible or at risk of renecrosis issuing to an amputation.

L. Téot (✉)
Department of Plastic Surgery, Burns and Wound Healing, Montpellier University Hospital, Hôpital La Colombière, CICAT Occitanie, Montpellier, France
e-mail: l-teot@chu-montpellier.fr

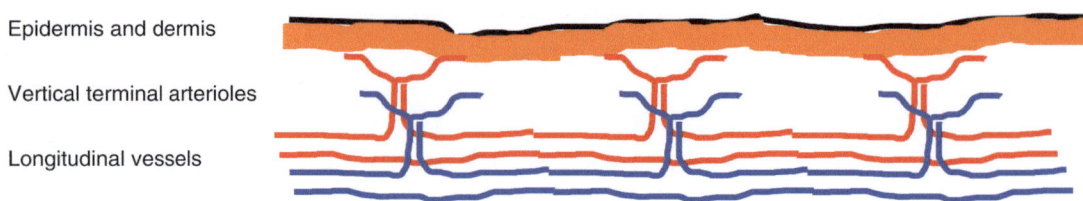

The transverse terminal arterioles form an area of vascular fragility. Any excessive mechanical force exerted on them (coming from outside like in PU of inside like in dissecting haematomas) will crush the subcutaneous fatty tissue layer, decreasing the skin perfusion.
Deeper, a blockade of longitudinal arteries or of venous return induces a complete devascularisation of the angiosome

Fig. 1.1 The vascular anatomy of the skin explains necrotic events of the skin

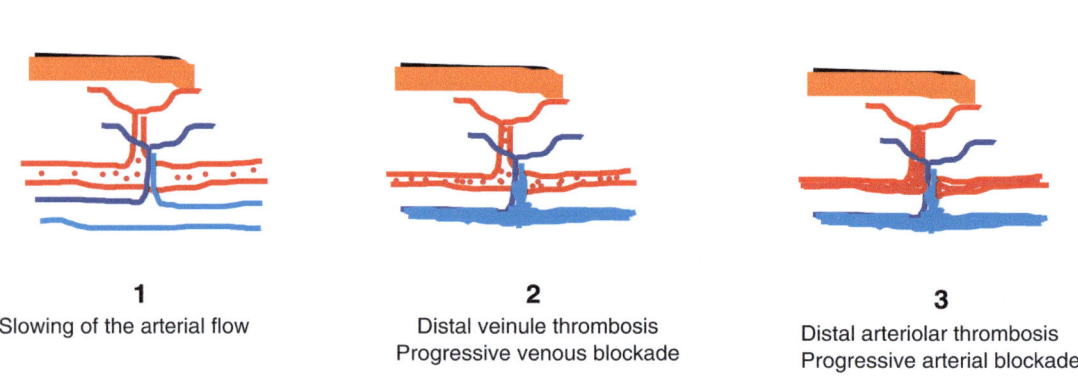

1
Slowing of the arterial flow

2
Distal veinule thrombosis
Progressive venous blockade

3
Distal arteriolar thrombosis
Progressive arterial blockade

Fig. 1.2 Sequence of skin necrosis formation

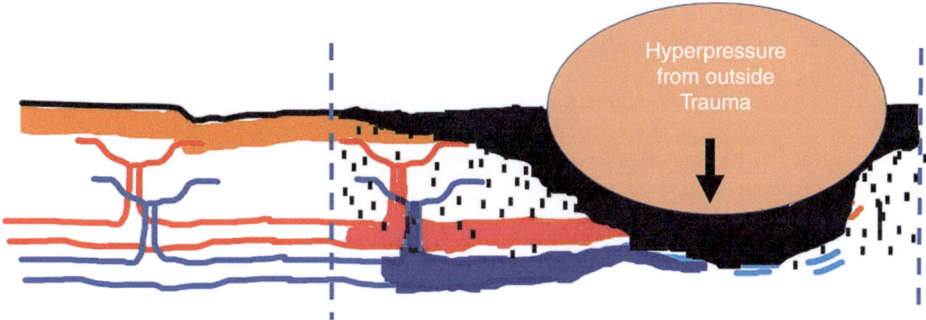

Hyperpressure induces vascular thrombosis, depending on the exerted forces:
the necrotic process remains just limited to the skin
or the underlying structures may be involved

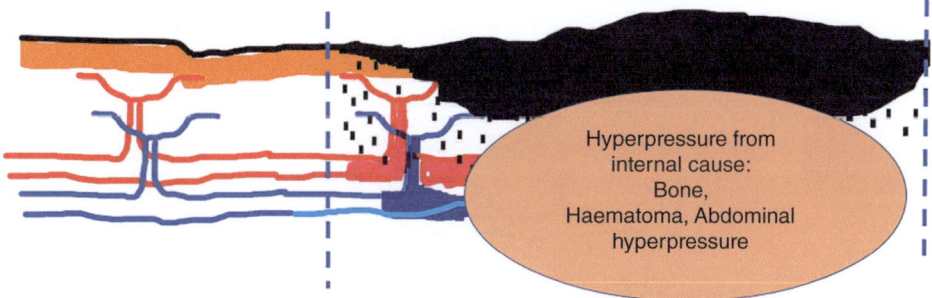

Fig. 1.3 Effect of Hyperpressure on skin tissues

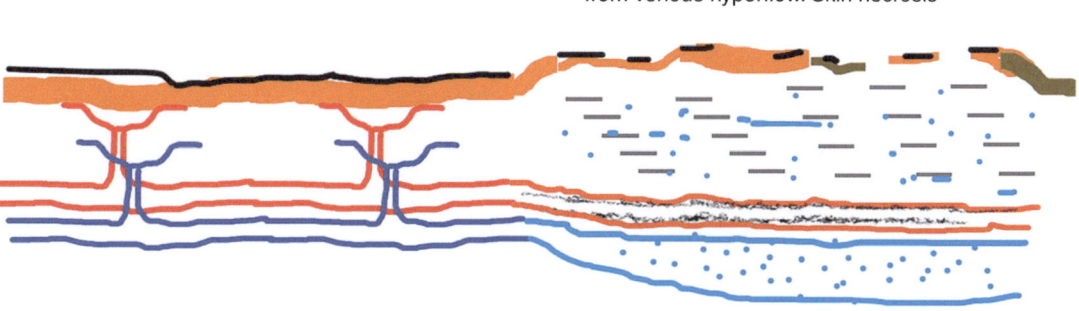

Fig. 1.4 Mixed predominantly arterial leg ulcer

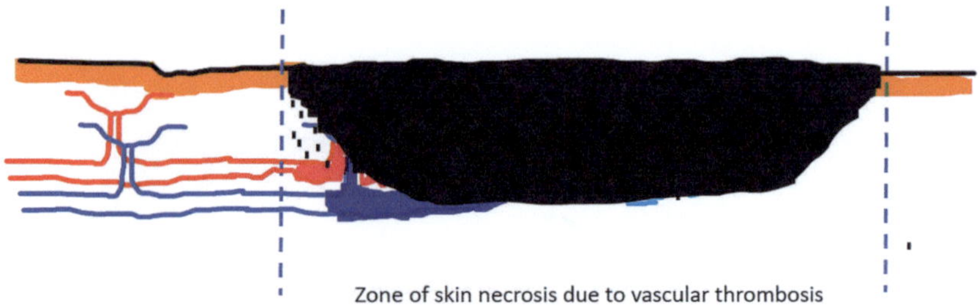

Fig. 1.5 Skin necrosis due to vascular thrombosis

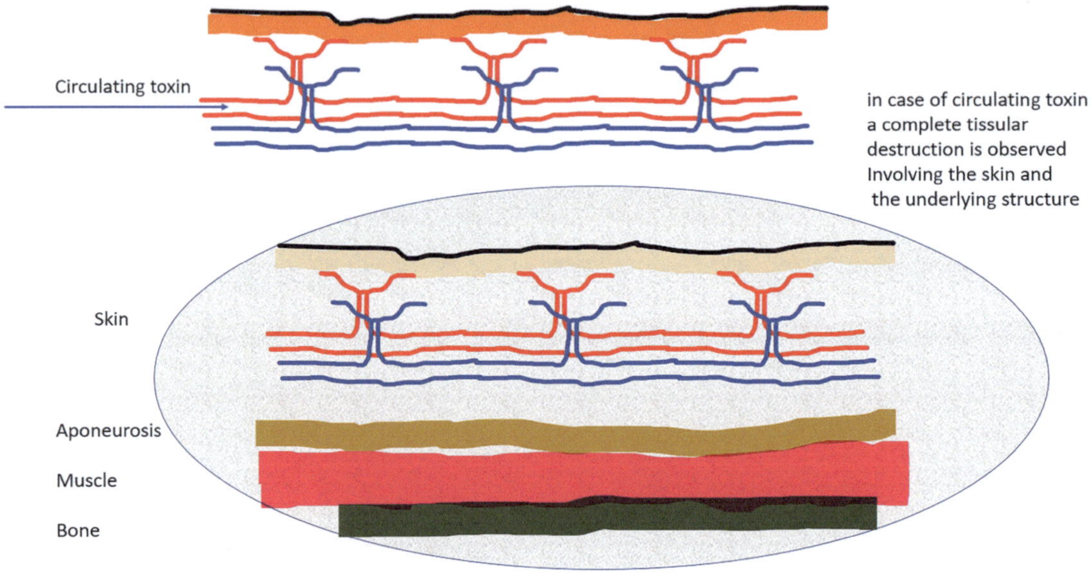

Fig. 1.6 Circulating toxin leading to tissue distruction

Open Access This chapter is licensed under the terms of the Creative Commons Attribution-NonCommercial-NoDerivatives 4.0 International License (http://creativecommons.org/licenses/by-nc-nd/4.0/), which permits any non-commercial use, sharing, distribution and reproduction in any medium or format, as long as you give appropriate credit to the original author(s) and the source, provide a link to the Creative Commons license and indicate if you modified the licensed material. You do not have permission under this license to share adapted material derived from this chapter or parts of it.

The images or other third party material in this chapter are included in the chapter's Creative Commons license, unless indicated otherwise in a credit line to the material. If material is not included in the chapter's Creative Commons license and your intended use is not permitted by statutory regulation or exceeds the permitted use, you will need to obtain permission directly from the copyright holder.

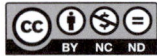

Dry Necrosis, Wet Necrosis: When to Debride, When Not to Debride

Luc Téot and Sergiu Fluieraru

2.1 Introduction

Skin necrosis is a result of several factors.

Ischaemia of a skin territory leads to venous congestion, which blocks microcirculation. The damage caused may remain reversible for a few hours, but 6 h or more of ischaemia leads to an irreversible situation and tissue loss. Several factors contribute to ischaemia. The most common is thrombosis of small arterioles, which progress, together with regional inflammatory processes, to devascularisation of a defined anatomical territory (angiosome) during the spreading of infections, necrosis is linked to the destructive effects of germs, which induce tissue damage by simple germ proliferation or induce vessel thrombosis.

The germs may also secrete toxins, which are diffused inside the arteriolar and capillary vascular systems. This leads to rapid obstruction of the vessels by chemical intimal and subintimal lesions, causing necrosis of large territories involving not only the skin but also the underlying muscles, tendons and bones.

2.2 Dry Necrosis

Subdermal necrosis may be induced by excessive pressure, leading to a mechanical crush. This is the most common factor in pressure ulcers and diabetic foot ulcers. In this situation, successive stages of skin necrosis can be observed—a situation reflected in the non-blanching stage 1 pressure ulcer following the National Pressure Ulcer Advisory Panel (NPUAP) classification, which probably corresponds to a prenecrotic stage. This is also observed in extravasation injuries [1].

Necrotic tissue and the normal skin with which it is in contact are both adherent to each other for a period of time of around 1 week. The crust that develops, including epidermis and dermis, is a mechanical obstacle to the germ penetration. After some time, a separation starts from the edges where the crust is in contact with the living tissues. The process starts with a fissure occurring between living and necrotic tissues, initiated by a difference in mechanical resistance and elasticity. This dissociation creates the "elimination fold", allowing the germs to penetrate deeply and to destroy the mechanical links between dead and living tissues. These germs proliferate in the subdermal fatty tissues. In large burns, the dissemination of germs all over the involved area is the main cause of death.

The time to complete the necrosis may vary from 6 h to 2–3 days, depending on the state of vascularisation of the limb and the exposure to air. It may be more progressive, such as observed

---

L. Téot (✉) · S. Fluieraru
Wound Healing Unit, Department of Surgery, Montpellier University Hospital, Montpellier, France
e-mail: l-teot@chu-montpellier.fr

during terminal limb ischaemia or during angiodermatitis. Microvascular impairment, autoimmune vasculitis, macroangiopathy and venous blockade are the most frequent causes, together with infection and microarterial emboli.

Other toxins and venoms may be secreted by a series of different animals (snails, mosquitoes) and may create an intense local inflammatory process leading to localised skin necrosis combined with an extensive subepidermal tissue degradation [2].

2.3 Wet Necrosis

Epidermal-dermal necrosis may rapidly appear at the skin surface. However, in some areas, such as the foot or when the depth of keratinised epidermis is thick, the necrotic tissue may resemble a subepidermal collection. This is partly because of the Tyndall effect—a light scattering observed when particles are present in colloid suspension, with blue light being much more strongly affected than red light.

When mature, this subdermal necrosis is easily confused with a deep haematoma. This situation is often observed on the heel. When the wound macerates, a wet necrosis may be observed, without any crust covering the necrosis. This situation is easily infected, with the mechanical protection of the crust being absent. Dermal necrosis may be present during a severe infection such as necrotising fasciitis, where the presence of germs secreting highly active toxins quickly involves all surrounding tissues and creates a regional progressive necrosis, a spreading infection rapidly leading to a septicaemic life-threatening shock. The proliferation of germs is facilitated inside the fatty tissue, such as in Fournier gangrene involving the perineal area and progressing very quickly in the perineum and under the abdominal skin.

In some situations, the necrotic tissue presents as wet, usually when necrosis is covered with damp dressings, allowing anaerobes to develop. This wet necrosis is often seen on the heel or other parts of the foot, the perineum, and places where maceration usually occurs. Wet skin necrosis is considered to be at high risk of local infection and should be quickly removed.

2.4 Debridement

1. Evidence-Based Medicine
   When analysing the literature from an evidence-based point of view, the Cochrane review considers that debridement has not yet demonstrated its efficacy. Nevertheless, most of the practitioners and paramedics involved in wound healing recognise the beneficial effect of debridement.
   Skin necrosis is not infected for the first few days but becomes heavily colonised when the edges are dissociated from the healthy skin. The time effect depends on a number of factors, grouped under the name of comorbidity markers. These markers may define the capacity of the patient to heal. Some of them, such as ankle brachial pressure index, albuminaemia, glycated haemoglobin and blood pressure measurement, are easily collected. Others, such as inflammatory markers or evolution with time of the wound healing process (surrogate end point), should be accurately determined.
2. Indications and Contraindications of Debridement
   Debridement in leg ulcer or heel pressure ulcer is only indicated when the limb is vascularised enough to prevent renecrosis on the edges of the wound. Lower limbs presenting an ankle brachial pressure index (ABPI) lower than 0.5 should not be debrided. When the ABPI is over 0.5, the debridement should follow an algorithm depending on multiple factors such as accessibility to surgery, availability of expertise in the use of advanced dressings such as hydrogels, hydrobalance or new debriders. Wet to dry techniques are not recommended any more.

2.4.1 Algorithm of Debridement (Fig. 2.1)

The strategic decision of debridement is multifactorial and should take into account local and systemic factors.

Depending on the first assessment, the debridement is possible or not. If the local vascularisation has not been checked, debridement is not recommended. If the patient is in a palliative situation, debridement is not recommended.

When debridement is possible, determine if a surgical debridement is needed and transfer the patient to an expert surgical team. If local availability of sharp debriding agents like scalpel or curette is poor or if expertise of the caregiver is poor, do not debride. In most of the situations, a large choice of solutions exists and can be used, depending on the local skills and the technical availabilities.

During a post-operative period after flap surgery, when the skin flap becomes necrotic, a surgical revision removing the necrotic areas is required.

2.4.2 Dissecting Haematomas

In the presence of spreading extended necrotic areas, an adapted debridement should be quickly proposed. In necrotising fasciitis, extravasation injuries, haematomas or Fournier gangrene, a large and extensive surgical debridement, including the edges of undermined cavities (decap procedure), is needed and must be considered as an emergency. The immediate post-debridement period should consider the need for repetitive debridement procedures when infection is still present. New debriders such as Versajet or NPWT Instill with VCC foam are useful in destroying local germs and preventing biofilm formation.

In the case of necrotising angiodermatitis, pain and skin necrosis may need surgical

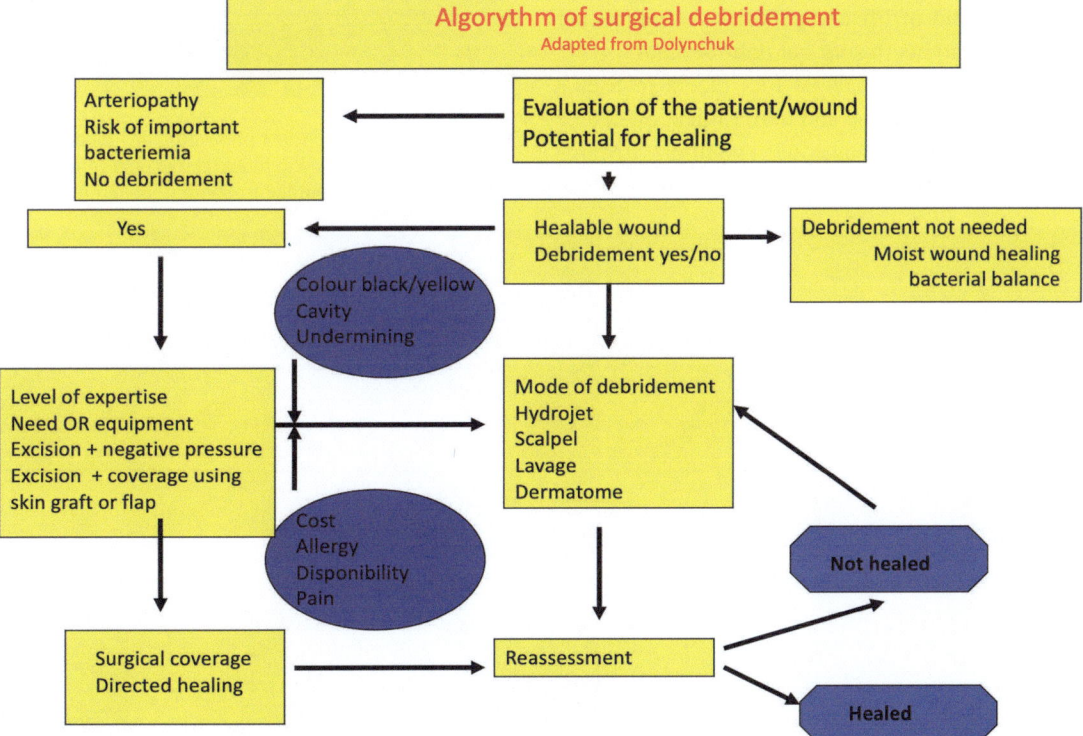

Fig. 2.1 This algorythm of surgical debridement describes the different possible strategies including or not a surgical debridement and when to redebride

debridement and rapid skin grafting using pinch grafts to stop pain.

Pressure ulcers are common causes of necrosis, particularly in the perineal area and over the heel. On the perineal area, undermining is frequently observed, as a consequence of the shearing forces exerted on the skin. The skin is more mechanically resistant than the underlying structure, with a relatively small opening covering a large undermined area being frequently observed. In this situation, all hidden cavities need to be opened to expose living edges. The granulation tissue and retraction are more rapidly obtained. Excision of the cover (decap surgery) by non-surgeon means is an option, but deep excisions along the undermined area are realised by surgeons (Figs. 2.2, 2.3, and 2.4). Concerning heel PU, a vascular assessment is mandatory (pedal pulse absence is the first sign and should indicate ABPI and Doppler ultrasound, and in case of arteriopathy, a vascular surgery consultation is needed to prevent renecrosis of the edges before any mechanical debridement). An ABPI below 0.5 is a contraindication to debride. Poor vascularisation, end-of-life and palliative situations are contraindications to surgical debridement.

Toe necrosis in diabetic foot ulcers realises a complete dry necrosis, and mummification can be recommended (spontaneous evolution towards spontaneous amputation). Below the second meta-

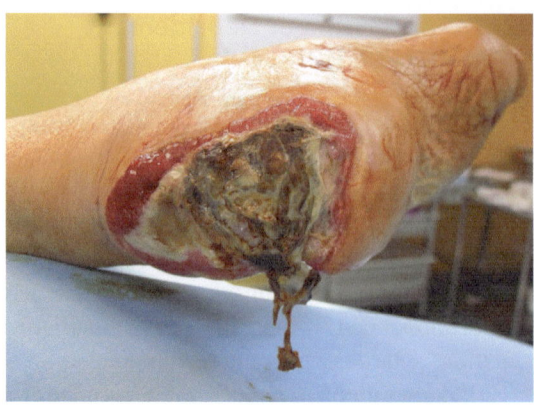

Fig. 2.2 Heel pressure ulcer: a spreading infection is observed some days after the necrotic tissue appeared

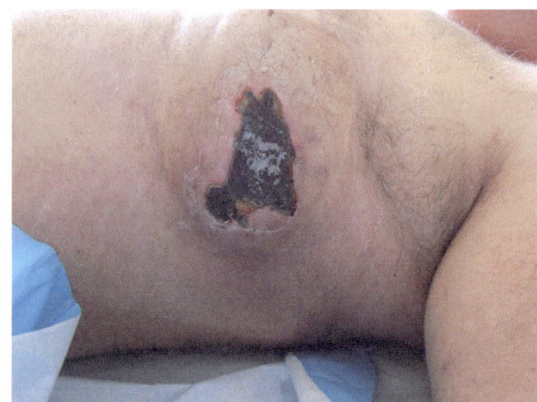

Fig. 2.3 A tigh haematoma presenting an "iceberg-like" situation. The necrotic skin hides a large undermined zone of dissecting blood, source of potential infection

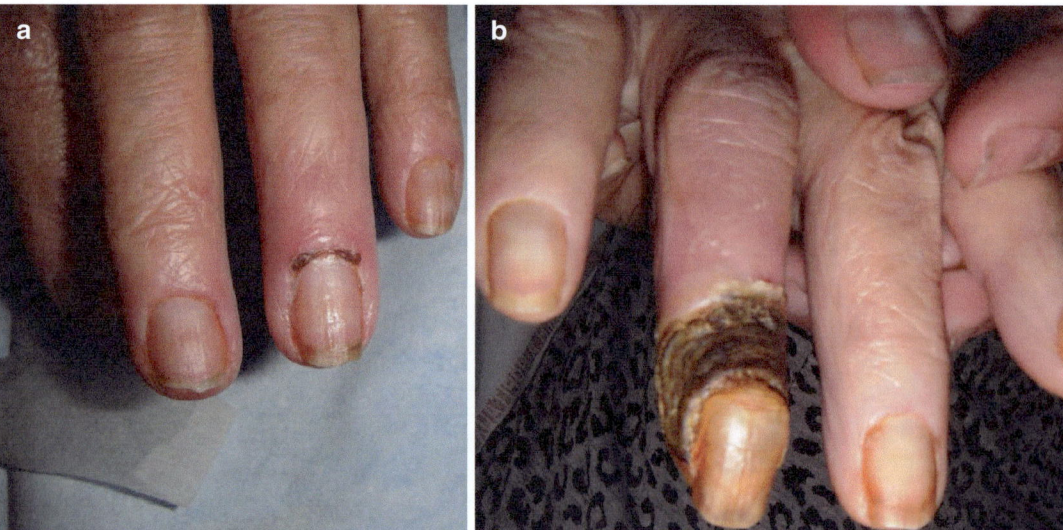

Fig. 2.4 (**a**, **b**) Progressive necrosis of the distal phalanx in a renal insufficient patient submitted to an arterial thief after arteriovenous fistula for haemodialysis

tarsal joint, plantar ulcers present as a skin necrosis reduced to a small black spot with a large cavity behind, with the foot becoming oedematous and inflammatory. Pus may leak from different zones on the foot, the dorsal aspect, the interdigital webs or from any necrotic area. Early surgical debridement may prevent amputation if carried out rapidly, in close collaboration with the vascular surgery team in order to prevent amputation.

2.5 How to Manage Skin Necrosis

1. Wet to dry is a technique used in the past to eliminate debris on the wound.
   Classically, the technique involves applying a wet gauze soaked in sterile water and waiting for its desiccation. When dry, it will be removed together with crusts, pus and debris. This painful technique will harm the granulation tissue, inducing local haemorrhage, and should not be used any more.

2. **Which techniques can be proposed?** (Fig. 2.5)
   Multiple technologies are now available for debridement. At home, grating, scalpel and syringe water projection under pressure can be easily utilised, as well as adsorbing and moisturising dressings. In advanced wound care centres, hydrojets or NPWT Instill plus VCC foam can be proposed.
   Progressive Autolytic Debridement
   Conservative solutions such as dressings providing moisture (autolytic debridement) will induce a progressive release and detachment of undesired tissues over the wound. Hydrogels are the most used dressing at home,

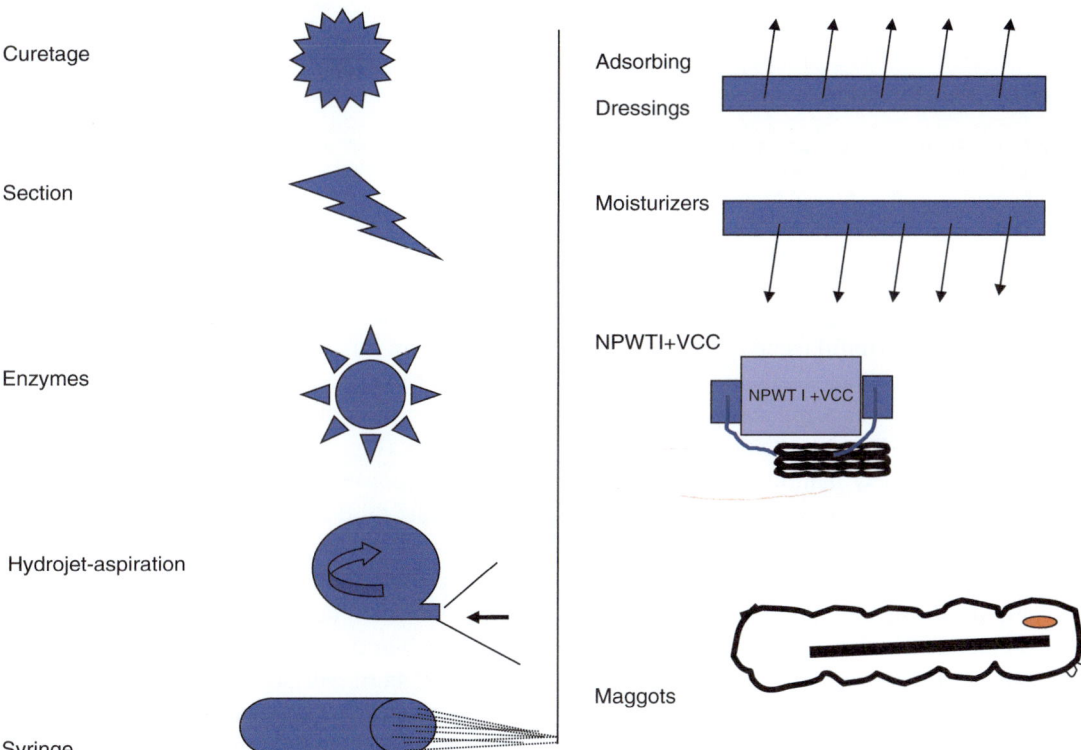

Fig. 2.5 Multiple techniques are available for debridement, depending on the availability and the skill to use them. Negative-pressure wound therapy instillation plus a specific VCC foam has recently demonstrated its capacity to debride large cavities

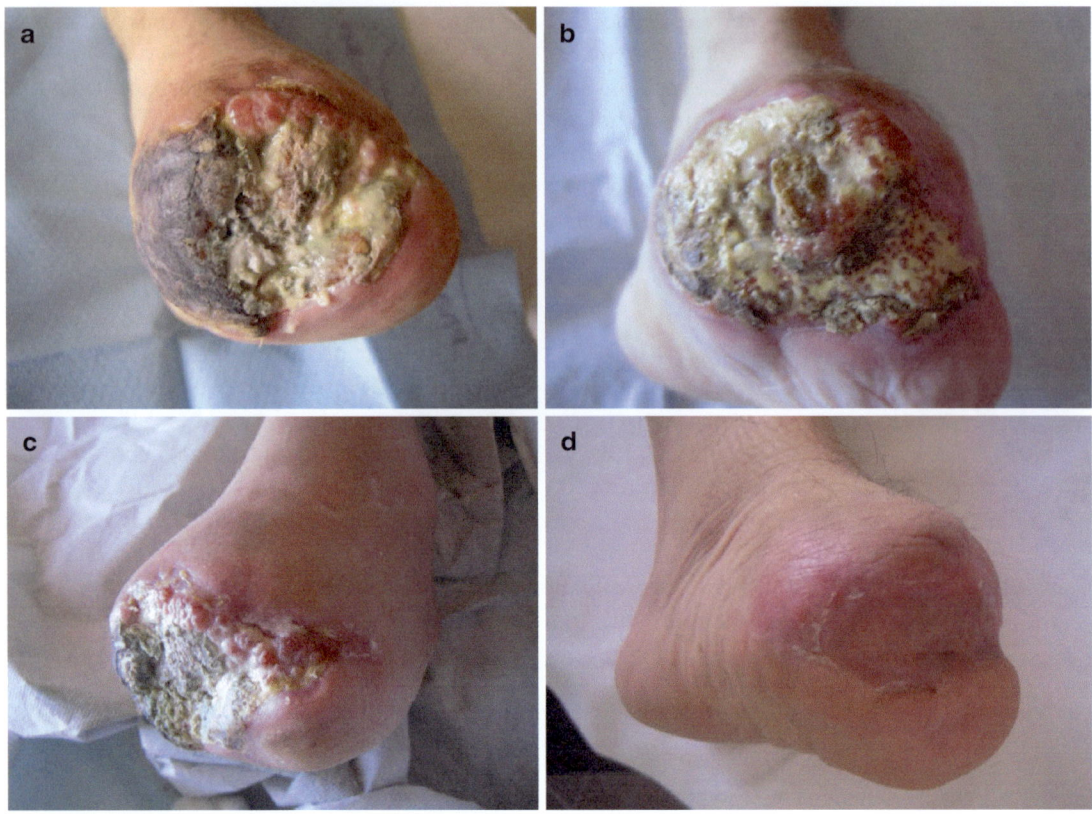

Fig. 2.6 (a–d) Midtarsal amputation after a failing flap in a young diabetes type 1 patient 42 years old; high level of comorbidities. Amputation could be prevented using local application of silver sulfadiazine plus cerium nitrate for 11 consecutive months

with the nurse moisturising the wound 1 day and gently removing the sloughy tissue the next. This less painful technique allows a better psychological management; curettage of a leg ulcer every 2 days induces pain impacting the quality of life. Mechanical debridement remains extremely painful and should be re-evaluated in the light of the new dressing performances, the capacity to remove metalloproteases from the wound surface and using local irrigating fluid. Negative-pressure wound therapy was proposed as a possible treatment for soft necrotic tissue [3].

3. Preventing Elimination Folds Around Skin Necrosis: Playing the Dry Card

Flammacerium, an antibacterial cream composed of silver sulfadiazine and 0.2% cerium nitrate, offers a solution involving stopping all possibilities for germs to penetrate the edges of necrosis and stabilising the crust in order to transform it into a protective calcified armour against infection. The dry necrotic process is stuck in its evolution and no longer becomes infected (Fig. 2.6). Flammacerium was initially proposed as a barrier to germ penetration in third-degree burns [4] and then proposed for arteriopathic necrotic wounds when revascularisation is not possible to limit or prevent amputations [5]. When applied onto extensive areas such as an 80% third-degree burn surface, methemoglobinaemia may cause life-threatening damage [6]. Blood dosage of methemoglobinaemia is required in these specific situations, but this has not yet been described for wounds presenting small surfaces [7].

2.6 Conclusion

Necrosis may present under a dry aspect, evolving spontaneously towards wet necrosis, depending on the local bacterial status. Each situation should be evaluated clinically in the context of the patient, taking care of the comorbidities, the vascularisation of the segment of limb and the availability of resources.

References

1. Doornaert M, Monstrey S, Roche N. Extravasation injuries: current medical and surgical treatment. Acta Chir Belg. 2013;113(1):1–7.
2. Kaafarani HM, King DR. Necrotizing skin and soft tissue infections. Surg Clin North Am. 2014;94(1):155–63. https://doi.org/10.1016/j.suc.2013.10.011. Epub 2013 Nov 5.
3. Teot L, Ohura N. Challenges and management in wound care. Plast Reconstr Surg. 2021;147(1S-1):9S–15S. https://doi.org/10.1097/PRS.0000000000007628.
4. Signe-Picard C, Cerdan MI, Téot L. Flammacérium in the formation and stabilisation of eschar in chronic wounds. J Wound Care. 2010;19(9):369–70, 372, 374 passim.
5. Boeckx W, Focquet M, Cornelissen M, Nuttin B. Bacteriological effect of cerium-flamazine cream in major burns. Burns Incl Therm Inj. 1985;11(5):337–42.
6. Poredos P, Gradisek P, Testen C, Derganc M. Severe methemoglobinaemia due to benzocaine-containing 'burn cream': two case reports in an adult and in a child. Burns. 2011;37(7):e63–6. https://doi.org/10.1016/j.burns.2011.05.015.
7. Barker E, Shepherd J, Asencio IO. The use of cerium compounds as antimicrobials for biomedical applications. Molecules. 2022;27(9):2678. https://doi.org/10.3390/molecules27092678.

Open Access This chapter is licensed under the terms of the Creative Commons Attribution-NonCommercial-NoDerivatives 4.0 International License (http://creativecommons.org/licenses/by-nc-nd/4.0/), which permits any non-commercial use, sharing, distribution and reproduction in any medium or format, as long as you give appropriate credit to the original author(s) and the source, provide a link to the Creative Commons license and indicate if you modified the licensed material. You do not have permission under this license to share adapted material derived from this chapter or parts of it.

The images or other third party material in this chapter are included in the chapter's Creative Commons license, unless indicated otherwise in a credit line to the material. If material is not included in the chapter's Creative Commons license and your intended use is not permitted by statutory regulation or exceeds the permitted use, you will need to obtain permission directly from the copyright holder.

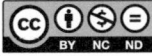

Ischemia/Reperfusion: A Potential Cause of Tissue Necrosis

Poon Apichartpiyakul, Raj Mani,
Supapong Arworn, and Kittipan Rerkasem

3.1 Introduction

Ischemia/reperfusion injury (IRI) is a sequelae following the restoration of circulatory flow to an ischemic organ. IRI can occur following different forms of acute vascular occlusion, for example acute myocardial infarction, stroke, limb ischemia, free-tissue transfer, and organ transplantation [1]. Injuries can manifest from both local and systemic effects, ranging from tissue edema, dysfunction, and necrosis to multi-organ failure. The pathophysiology of IRI includes the triggering of cellular oxidative stress and inflammatory response. Cellular oxidative stress and inflammatory response are caused by reactive oxygen species (ROS) overproduction in mitochondria. There are several preventative interventions in IRI that have shown beneficial outcomes in in vitro, in vivo, and clinical studies [2]. This chapter focuses on tissue necrosis, which is a potential local manifestation of IRI.

3.2 Pathophysiology

Tissue ischemia/reperfusion injury (IRI) manifests in either local or systemic effect. Local effect such as tissue necrosis from IRI can be found from skin to bone and muscle. Etiologies of IRI-involved muscle and skin necrosis are found in acute tissue ischemia of musculoskeletal system such as tissue free-flap transfer and acute limb ischemia, which receives immediate restoration of blood supply. Systemic effects can range from remote organ injury to multi-organ failure. IRI is a consequence of two phases of injuries. The initial ischemic phase, microcirculation to the affected tissue, has been occluded by masses of platelets in postcapillary venules [3]. Local effects, such as skeletal muscle necrosis during tissue ischemia in low collateral blood flow, were also detected in skeletal muscle model of IRI [4]. Muscle edema and systemic effects, which are observed in later phases, are not evident at this phase [5]. The reperfusion phase then follows, leading to further tissue damage. In this phase, despite successful revascularization of ischemic tissue, tissue perfusion is decreased compared to during its pre-ischemic state. This has been seen in acute myocardial infarction tissue, where up to

50% of myocardial microvasculature remained non-perfused, an event known as a "no-reflow phenomenon" [6, 7]. These findings could be caused by intravascular hemoconcentration and thrombosis, which leads to further tissue malperfusion. In the reperfusion phase, tissue necrosis, edema, and muscular contractile dysfunction are increased dramatically during reperfusion, in comparison to ischemic period [4, 8, 9]. Lactic acidosis, rhabdomyolysis, and increased pro-inflammatory cytokines were also observed in previous studies, which are affect to systemic organ during skeletal muscle IRI [5, 10, 11].

Pathology in cellular level from IRI originated from triggering oxidative stress and inflammatory response. There are studies that mimic human skeletal muscle in order to investigate subcellular and cellular pathophysiology. In vitro and in vivo studies have demonstrated that several intracellular molecules are involved in the inflammatory cascades of IRI. At a cellular level, mitochondrial dysfunction plays a crucial role in the pathogenesis of IRI [12]. Mitochondrial functions define as adenosine triphosphate (ATP) production, reactive oxygen species (ROS) generation, detoxification, metabolite synthesis, catabolism, and regulation of apoptosis. During tissue hypoxic period, ATP, a major source of energy and produced by oxidative phosphorylation, is depleted [12]. Moreover, IRI has been shown to shift mitochondrial dynamics toward mitochondrial fission, resulting in cellular apoptosis [13]. Under conditions of ischemia, xanthine dehydrogenase (D-form) is changed to xanthine oxidase (O-form), resulting in increased ROS generation [14]. These excessive ROS levels result in cellular oxidative stress, which leads to protein carboxylation, lipid peroxidation, and DNA damage. Furthermore, ATP depletion induces the translocation of Bax, Bad, and Bcl2 proteins to the mitochondrial membrane, which results in mitochondrial swelling and mitochondrial fission [15]. Additionally, an increase in intracellular calcium ions (Ca^{2+}) level during ischemia may alter mitochondrial permeability transitional pores (mPTPs) from a transient to a persistent opening state. The opening of the mPTPs allows the efflux of ROS and cytochrome c into the cellular matrix, and the influx of the Ca^{2+}, leading to mitochondrial swelling and membrane rupture, thus causing cellular apoptosis in the cells [16].

In clinical studies, there are different presentations during ischemia and reperfusion phases. In the ischemic phase, local effects in skeletal muscle tissue such as decreased intramuscular blood flow and increased cellular acidosis were observed [17]. In the case of systemic effects, oxidative stress and inflammatory markers from the peripheral blood samples were increased [18–24]. Leukocyte activation, leukocyte-adhesion molecules, and oxidative stress parameters such as glutathione and free sulfhydryl groups increased to a greater extent during the reperfusion phase than in the ischemic phase [18]. Local effects during the reperfusion phase were observed as cellular endothelial dysfunction as indicated by decreased brachial artery flow-mediated dilatation, which is observed in an healthy arm IRI model [19]. Intramuscular acidosis was decreased compared to the ischemic phase, measured by an increase in inorganic phosphate/phosphocreatine ratios, observed from ^{31}P nuclear magnetic resonance [17]. Skeletal muscle injuries including muscle edema, mortor dysfunction, and tissue necrosis were also observed after 3 h of ischemia [25]. Multi-organ failures, such as rhabdomyolysis and increased kidney, intestine, and liver injury biomarkers, were observed [21, 26]. In addition, preoperative rhabdomyolysis, positive fluid balance, poor intraoperative back bleeding, and an increase in end-organ injury markers were proposed as predictors of the occurrence of post-reperfusion compartment syndrome [20]. A summary of the proposed mechanisms in musculoskeletal tissue IRI is illustrated in Fig. 3.1.

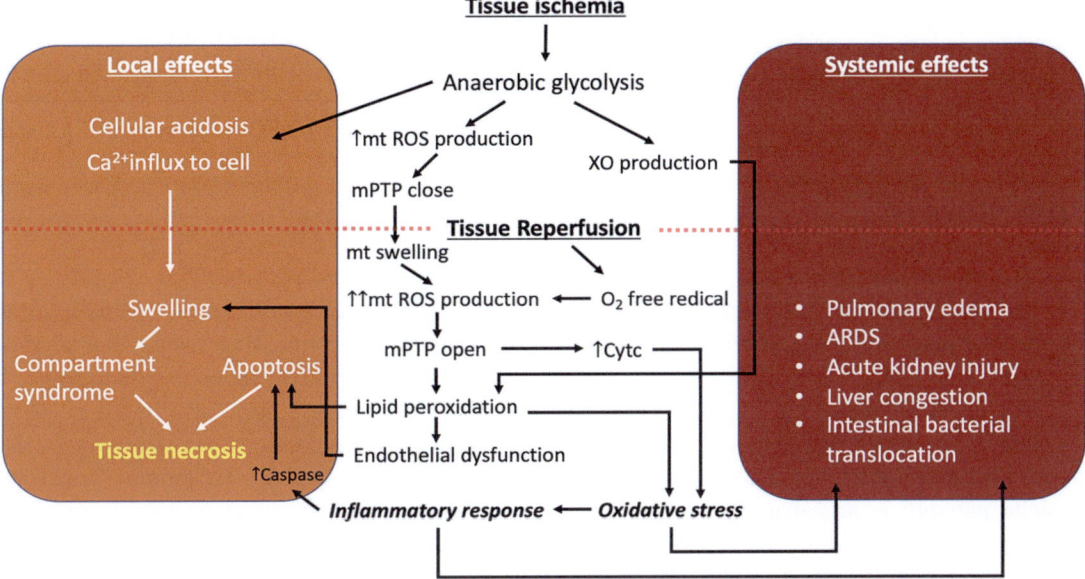

Fig. 3.1 Pathophysiology in tissue ischemia/reperfusion injury. **Abbreviations**: *ARDS* acute respiratory distress syndrome; Ca^{2+} calcium ion; *Cytc* cytochrome-C; *mt* mitochondria; *mPTP* mitochondrial permeability transition pore; O_2 oxygen; *ROS* reactive oxygen species; *XO* xanthine oxidase

3.3 Clinical Manifestations

Tissue necrosis after IRI is the end stage of injury. Tissue necrosis, including of the skin, subcutaneous fat, and skeletal muscle, as a result of IRI has been observed in acute limb ischemia and after tissue free-flap transfer surgery. Injuries begin during the ischemic phase, and more severe damage subsequently occurs in the reperfusion phase. Clinical manifestation can be well observed in the reperfusion phase. Local changes in the skin and muscle resulting from IRI are listed below.

1. *Tissue edema*

    Following reperfusion of ischemic tissue, mild tissue edema can be observed as a result of successful restoration of blood flow to the affected area. This is a result of fluid shifts from intravascular to interstitial spaces by endothelial dysfunction. However, if severe edema is observed early, venous outflow obstruction of the organ/tissue flap should be considered. Initial management of tissue edema includes elevation and adequate blood pressure raising to ensure capillary perfusion pressure of the affected tissues. IV fluid and blood transfusion should be done to keep systolic blood pressure at normal range.

2. *Acute compartment syndrome*

    Sequelae of ischemia/reperfusion injury is tissue edema in close space, such as intramuscular compartment, where the compartment pressure raises enough to compress capillary bed and compromise blood supply to tissue, are called "acute compartment syndrome." This syndrome is caused by compression of edematous tissue to venous outflow and increased venous pressure, which then results in increased fluid shifts into interstitial spaces, resulting in further tissue edema. The intramuscular pressure gradient overcomes vascular supply to skeletal muscle cell. This vicious cycle leads to acute compartment syndrome, which is defined as tissue malperfusion occurring as a result of the intra-compartment pressure overcoming the vascular bed. Lower extremity compartment syndrome manifests as massive leg edema and severe pain of the leg. Intra-compartment pressure measurement should be evaluated if clinical results are inconclusive, such as if the patient was unconscious. White side method [27] is used to evaluate absolute static intra-compartment pressure, which, when greater than 30 mmHg, indicates compartment syndrome. However, prospective studies found that dynamic pressure measurement called "delta pressure," which is diastolic blood pressure minus the intra-compartment pressure, has more value in the diagnosis of compartment syndrome than static pressure. If delta pressure is less than 30 mmHg, acute compartment syndrome could be diagnosed and therapeutic fasciotomy should be performed to release compartment pressure [28, 29] as delays in diagnosis and treatment can result in muscle dysfunction and tissue necrosis. Figure 3.2 shows the patient's necrosed skin after acute compartment syndrome. After therapeutic fasciotomy, edematous muscle was protruded out of skin.

3. *Tissue Necrosis*

End processes of local effects of IRI are tissue ischemia and necrosis. These can be the result of either process of IRI or delay in treatment of acute compartment syndrome. Preoperative factors, such as prolonged ischemia, can lead to tissue necrosis after IRI. Tissue ischemic time, which can tolerate ischemia, is different depending on the type of tissue. Summary of ischemic time is given in Table 3.1. If necrotic tissue is observed, the tissue is irreversible. Treatment should be adequate debridement of the necrotic tissue in case it will proceed to local infection and systemic bacteremia.

Table 3.1 Maximal tissue ischemia, which leads to necrosis, applied from S. Gillani et al. [30]

Type of tissues	Ischemic time (normal temperature)
Muscle	4 h
Nerve	8 h
Fat	13 h
Skin	24 h
Bone	4 days

3.4 Treatment and Prevention

Debridement of necrotic tissue is the main treatment of tissue necrosis. Adjudication of tissue viability remains primarily dependent on the clinical judgment of the healthcare team. Fixed mottling skin and noncontractile muscle are signs of irreversible tissue damage indicating tissue necrosis. Adequate tissue debridement, including amputation, until viable tissue is present is required if tissue necrosis has occurred. Unremoved necrotic tissue can lead to sepsis and drain toxic metabolites to systemic circulation. There were many investigations in therapeutic modalities to prevent tissue IRI. These have shown promised outcome in the prevention of tissue necrosis. Clinical studies in tissue and skin necrosis IRI were investigated in free-flap tissue and acute limb ischemia patients. Both pharmacological and non-pharmacological therapeutic interventions are used in studies on secondary prevention of tissue necrosis from IRI. Examples of preventive strategies, that are currently investigated in tissue necrosis after IRI, are listed in Table 3.2. Several preventive interventions have shown significant warranty but have not yet been investigated in humans [2]. Further clinical studies are needed.

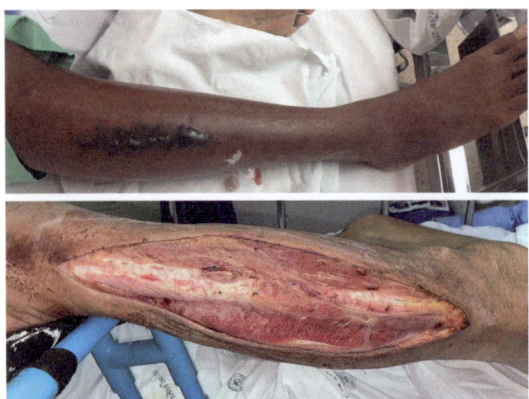

Fig. 3.2 Skin necrosis caused by acute compartment syndrome (above picture). Patient's muscle was protruded after fasciotomy (below picture)

Table 3.2 Examples of prevention in IRI-related tissue and skin necrosis—result from clinical trials

IRI models	Pharmacological treatments	Non-pharmacological treatments
Acute limb ischemia	IV mannitol [31], IV antioxidative vitamin [32]	Controlled reperfusion [33–36], RIC [37]
Free-flap	IV lidocaine [38], IV arginine [39], preconditioning with sevoflurane [40]	RIC [41, 42], NPWT [43]

Abbreviations: *IV* intravenous; *NPWT* negative-pressure wound therapy; *RIC* remote ischemic conditioning

3.5 Conclusion and Future Research

Musculoskeletal tissue IRI can result in local effects ranging from tissue edema to necrosis, leading to systemic effects such as remote organ injury to multi-organ failure. The pathogenesis of IRI is a consequence of cellular oxidative stress and inflammatory responses. To prevent IRI, investigators try to block the injuries by remediating oxidative stress and inflammation. Several interventions in the form of pharmacological and non-pharmacological treatments can prevent tissue necrosis from IRI.

References

1. Dorweiler B, Pruefer D, Andrasi TB, Maksan SM, Schmiedt W, Neufang A, et al. Ischemia-reperfusion injury: pathophysiology and clinical implications. Eur J Trauma Emerg Surg. 2007;33(6):600–12.
2. Apichartpiyakul P, Shinlapawittayatorn K, Rerkasem K, Chattipakorn SC, Chattipakorn N. Mechanisms and interventions on acute lower limb ischemia/reperfusion injury: a review and insights from cell to clinical investigations. Ann Vasc Surg. 2022;86:452–81.
3. Hammersen F, Barker JH, Gidlöf A, Menger MD, Hammersen E, Messmer K. The ultrastructure of microvessels and their contents following ischemia and reperfusion. 1989.
4. Petrasek PF, Walker PM. A clinically relevant small-animal model of skeletal muscle ischemia-reperfusion injury. J Investig Surg. 1994;7(1):27–38.
5. Kuroda Y, Togashi H, Uchida T, Haga K, Yamashita A, Sadahiro M. Oxidative stress evaluation of skeletal muscle in ischemia-reperfusion injury using enhanced magnetic resonance imaging. Sci Rep. 2020;10(1):10863.
6. Hollander MR, de Waard GA, Konijnenberg LS, Meijer-van Putten RM, van den Brom CE, Paauw N, et al. Dissecting the effects of ischemia and reperfusion on the coronary microcirculation in a rat model of acute myocardial infarction. PLoS One. 2016;11(7):e0157233.
7. Ames A 3rd, Wright RL, Kowada M, Thurston JM, Majno G, Cerebral ischemia. II. The no-reflow phenomenon. Am J Pathol. 1968;52(2):437–53.
8. Hardy SC, Homer-Vanniasinkam S, Gough MJ. The triphasic pattern of skeletal muscle blood flow in reperfusion injury: an experimental model with implications for surgery on the acutely ischaemic lower limb. Eur J Vasc Surg. 1990;4(6):587–90.
9. Forrest I, Lindsay T, Romaschin A, Walker P. The rate and distribution of muscle blood flow after prolonged ischemia. J Vasc Surg. 1989;10(1):83–8.
10. Celoria G, Zarfos K, Berman J. Effects of acute lower limb ischemia on femoral venous efflux. Angiology. 1990;41(6):439–44.
11. Hayashi M, Hirose H, Sasaki E, Senga S, Murakawa S, Mori Y, et al. Evaluation of ischemic damage in the skeletal muscle with the use of electrical properties. J Surg Res. 1998;80(2):266–71.
12. Lejay A, Meyer A, Schlagowski AI, Charles AL, Singh F, Bouitbir J, et al. Mitochondria: mitochondrial participation in ischemia-reperfusion injury in skeletal muscle. Int J Biochem Cell Biol. 2014;50:101–5.
13. Youle RJ, van der Bliek AM. Mitochondrial fission, fusion, and stress. Science. 2012;337(6098):1062–5.
14. Chambers DE, Parks DA, Patterson G, Roy R, McCord JM, Yoshida S, et al. Xanthine oxidase as a source of free radical damage in myocardial ischemia. J Mol Cell Cardiol. 1985;17(2):145–52.
15. Gao X, Bi Y, Chi K, Liu Y, Yuan T, Li X, et al. Glycine-nitronyl nitroxide conjugate protects human umbilical vein endothelial cells against hypoxia/reoxygenation injury via multiple mechanisms and ameliorates hind limb ischemia/reperfusion injury in rats. Biochem Biophys Res Commun. 2017;488(1):239–46.
16. McCully JD, Wakiyama H, Hsieh YJ, Jones M, Levitsky S. Differential contribution of necrosis and apoptosis in myocardial ischemia-reperfusion injury. Am J Physiol Heart Circ Physiol. 2004;286(5):H1923–35.
17. Brotzakis PZ, Sacco P, Jones DA, McIntyre DB, Williams R, Adiseshiah M. 31P nuclear magnetic resonance spectroscopy of acutely ischaemic limbs: the extent of changes and progress after reconstructive surgery. Cardiovasc Surg. 1995;3(3):271–6.
18. Arató E, Jancsó G, Sínay L, Kürthy M, Lantos J, Ferencz S, et al. Reperfusion injury and inflammatory responses following acute lower limb revascularization surgery. Clin Hemorheol Microcirc. 2008;39(1–4):79–85.
19. Aboo Bakkar Z, Fulford J, Gates PE, Jackman SR, Jones AM, Bond B, et al. Prolonged forearm ischemia attenuates endothelium-dependent vasodilatation and

19. plasma nitric oxide metabolites in overweight middle-aged men. Eur J Appl Physiol. 2018;118(8):1565–72.
20. Orrapin S, Orrapin S, Arwon S, Rerkasem K. Predictive factors for post-ischemic compartment syndrome in non-traumatic acute limb ischemia in a lower extremity. Ann Vasc Dis. 2017;10(4):378–85.
21. de Franciscis S, De Caridi G, Massara M, Spinelli F, Gallelli L, Buffone G, et al. Biomarkers in post-reperfusion syndrome after acute lower limb ischaemia. Int Wound J. 2016;13(5):854–9.
22. Adiseshiah M, Round JM, Jones DA. Reperfusion injury in skeletal muscle: a prospective study in patients with acute limb ischaemia and claudicants treated by revascularization. Br J Surg. 1992;79(10):1026–9.
23. Karahalil B, Polat S, Senkoylu A, Bölükbaşi S. Evaluation of DNA damage after tourniquet-induced ischaemia/reperfusion injury during lower extremity surgery. Injury. 2010;41(7):758–62.
24. Moran CG. Reperfusion injury in skeletal muscle: a prospective study in patients with acute limb ischaemia and claudicants treated by revascularization. Br J Surg. 1993;80(3):401–2.
25. Belkin M, Brown RD, Wright JG, LaMorte WW, Hobson RW 2nd. A new quantitative spectrophotometric assay of ischemia-reperfusion injury in skeletal muscle. Am J Surg. 1988;156(2):83–6.
26. Kasepalu T, Kuusik K, Lepner U, Starkopf J, Zilmer M, Eha J, et al. Remote Ischaemic preconditioning reduces kidney injury biomarkers in patients undergoing open surgical lower limb revascularisation: a randomised trial. Oxidative Med Cell Longev. 2020;2020:7098505.
27. Saikia KC, Bhattacharya TD, Agarwala V. Anterior compartment pressure measurement in closed fractures of leg. Indian J Orthop. 2008;42(2):217–21.
28. Matava MJ, Whitesides TE Jr, Seiler JG 3rd, Hewan-Lowe K, Hutton WC. Determination of the compartment pressure threshold of muscle ischemia in a canine model. J Trauma. 1994;37(1):50–8.
29. von Keudell AG, Weaver MJ, Appleton PT, Bae DS, Dyer GSM, Heng M, et al. Diagnosis and treatment of acute extremity compartment syndrome. Lancet. 2015;386(10000):1299–310.
30. Gillani S, Cao J, Suzuki T, Hak DJ. The effect of ischemia reperfusion injury on skeletal muscle. Injury. 2012;43(6):670–5.
31. Shah DM, Bock DE, Darling RC 3rd, Chang BB, Kupinski AM, Leather RP. Beneficial effects of hypertonic mannitol in acute ischemia—reperfusion injuries in humans. Cardiovasc Surg. 1996;4(1):97–100.
32. Rabl H, Khoschsorur G, Petek W. Antioxidative vitamin treatment: effect on lipid peroxidation and limb swelling after revascularization operations. World J Surg. 1995;19(5):738–44.
33. Heilmann C, Schmoor C, Siepe M, Schlensak C, Hoh A, Fraedrich G, et al. Controlled reperfusion versus conventional treatment of the acutely ischemic limb: results of a randomized, open-label, multicenter trial. Circ Cardiovasc Interv. 2013;6(4):417–27.
34. Beyersdorf F, Sarai K, Mitrev Z, Eckel L, Ihnken K, Satter P. New surgical treatment for severe limb ischemia. J Investig Surg. 1994;7(1):61–71.
35. Schmidt CA, Rancic Z, Lachat ML, Mayer DO, Veith FJ, Wilhelm MJ. Hypothermic, initially oxygen-free, controlled limb reperfusion for acute limb ischemia. Ann Vasc Surg. 2015;29(3):560–72.
36. Wilhelm MP, Schlensak C, Hoh A, Knipping L, Mangold G, Dallmeier Rojas D, et al. Controlled reperfusion using a simplified perfusion system preserves function after acute and persistent limb ischemia: a preliminary study. J Vasc Surg. 2005;42(4):690–4.
37. Bailey TG, Birk GK, Cable NT, Atkinson G, Green DJ, Jones H, et al. Remote ischemic preconditioning prevents reduction in brachial artery flow-mediated dilation after strenuous exercise. Am J Physiol Heart Circ Physiol. 2012;303(5):H533–8.
38. Del Rio M, Lopez-Cabrera P, Malagón-López P, Del Caño-Aldonza MC, Castello JR, Provencio M. Effect of intravenous lidocaine on ischemia-reperfusion injury in DIEP microsurgical breast reconstruction. A prospective double-blind randomized controlled clinical trial. J Plast Reconstr Aesthet Surg. 2021;74(4):809–18.
39. Booi DI, Debats I, Deutz NEP, van der Hulst R. Arginine improves microcirculation in the free transverse rectus abdominis myocutaneous flap after breast reconstruction: a randomized, double-blind clinical trial. Plast Reconstr Surg. 2011;127(6):2216–23.
40. Claroni C, Torregiani G, Covotta M, Sofra M, Scotto Di Uccio A, Marcelli ME, et al. Protective effect of sevoflurane preconditioning on ischemia-reperfusion injury in patients undergoing reconstructive plastic surgery with microsurgical flap, a randomized controlled trial. BMC Anesthesiol. 2016;16(1):66.
41. Min SH, Choe SH, Kim WS, Ahn SH, Cho YJ. Effects of ischemic conditioning on head and neck free flap oxygenation: a randomized controlled trial. Sci Rep. 2022;12(1):8130.
42. Kraemer R, Lorenzen J, Kabbani M, Herold C, Busche M, Vogt PM, et al. Acute effects of remote ischemic preconditioning on cutaneous microcirculation—a controlled prospective cohort study. BMC Surg. 2011;11:32.
43. Eisenhardt SU, Schmidt Y, Thiele JR, Iblher N, Penna V, Torio-Padron N, et al. Negative pressure wound therapy reduces the ischaemia/reperfusion-associated inflammatory response in free muscle flaps. J Plast Reconstr Aesthet Surg. 2012;65(5):640–9.

Open Access This chapter is licensed under the terms of the Creative Commons Attribution-NonCommercial-NoDerivatives 4.0 International License (http://creativecommons.org/licenses/by-nc-nd/4.0/), which permits any non-commercial use, sharing, distribution and reproduction in any medium or format, as long as you give appropriate credit to the original author(s) and the source, provide a link to the Creative Commons license and indicate if you modified the licensed material. You do not have permission under this license to share adapted material derived from this chapter or parts of it.

The images or other third party material in this chapter are included in the chapter's Creative Commons license, unless indicated otherwise in a credit line to the material. If material is not included in the chapter's Creative Commons license and your intended use is not permitted by statutory regulation or exceeds the permitted use, you will need to obtain permission directly from the copyright holder.

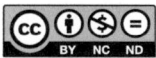

Imaging, Vascular Assessment: Extension in Depth and Vascular Anomalies

Sadanori Akita, Hideki Ishimaru, and Miho Noguchi

4.1 Introduction

Vascular anomalies are comprised of two main types: vascular tumors, which include infantile hemangioma and other rare vascular tumors in both children and adults, and vascular malformations [1]. Vascular tumors are differentiated from vascular malformations based on the clinical appearance, imaging, and pathologic characteristics [2]. Examples of vascular tumors include infantile hemangioma, congenital hemangioma (rapidly involuting congenital hemangioma (RICH), partially involuting congenital hemangioma (PICH), or non-involuting congenital hemangioma (NICH)), kaposiform hemangioendothelioma, tufted angioma, pyogenic granuloma, and hemangiopericytoma. Diagnosis of vascular malformations involves the use of various imaging methods that must be correlated with clinical findings and the purpose of imaging, whether it is for diagnosis, pre- or intra-treatment assessment, or follow-up.

The majority of infantile hemangiomas (IHs) are small and not hazardous and may recede spontaneously in three phases of proliferation, involution, and involuted phases by the age of 7 years or so. However, IH can be alarming if found in life- and function-threatening locations such as the eyelid, orbit, ear, or airway. Treatment is required for ulceration, continued infection, or hemorrhage (Fig. 4.1), which are the most common complications of IH. The incidence of ulceration in a referral population is generally reported to be about 16%. A prospective study of 1096 patients showed that the median age at ulceration was 4.0 months, which correlates with the end of the proliferative phase [3]. Risk factors for ulceration include segmental morphologic characteristics, large size, and mixed superficial and deep subtype. Early white discoloration may suggest impending ulceration [4].

Vascular malformations consist of capillary malformation (CM), venous malformation (VM), lymphatic malformation (LM), and arteriovenous malformation (AVM). Some cases involve a combination of more than one malformation and are categorized as combined vascular

---

S. Akita (✉)
Department of Plastic Surgery, Tamaki-Aozora Hospital, Tokushima, Japan

Fukushima Medical University, Fukushima, Japan
e-mail: akitas@hf.rim.or.jp

H. Ishimaru
Department of Radiological Sciences, Nagasaki University Graduate School of Biomedical Sciences, Nagasaki, Japan

M. Noguchi
Department of Plastic and Reconstructive Surgery, National Hospital Organization Nagasaki Medical Center, Ohmura, Japan

Department of Plastic and Reconstructive Surgery, Shinshu University School of Medicine, Nagano, Japan

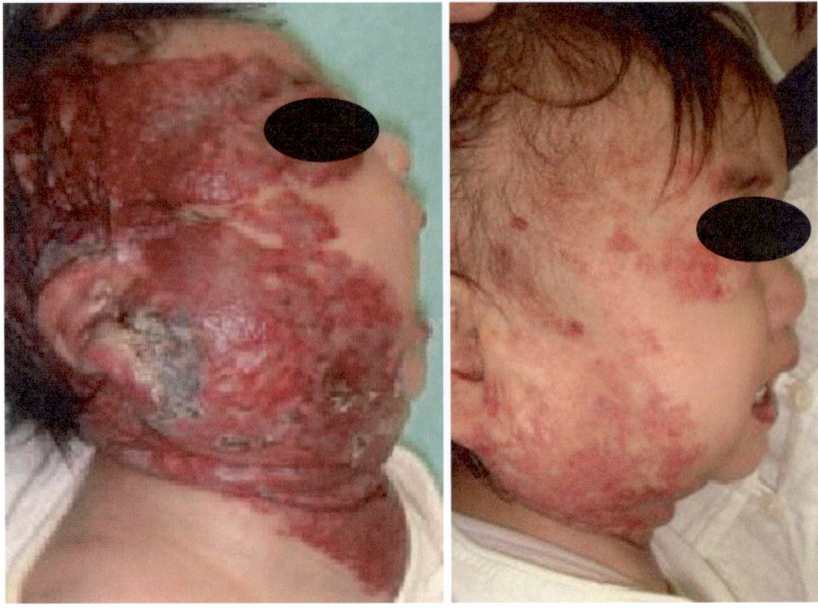

Fig. 4.1 Progression of infantile hemangioma on the right side of the face at 1 month in the first visit (*left*) and at 1.5 years (*right*). The ulcers in the preauricular, the cheek, and the submandibular areas are healed

malformations or complex syndromes such as Klippel-Trénaunay syndrome (CM + VM + LM) or Parkes Weber syndrome (AVM/or arteriovenous fistula (AVF) + skin pseudo-CM + lymphedema), which exhibit more systemic signs and symptoms. Skin necrosis is often manifested in severe AVM, LM, combined CM + LM, and minority cases of hemangiomas, such as IH.

4.2 Assessment and Imaging Tools

Many imaging tools are able to determine the diagnosis of vascular malformations.

4.2.1 Conventional X-Rays

The conventional plain X-rays outline the mass and the area of the lesions. Sometimes, they also identify the contrasted lesions. Venous malformations (VMs) may be diagnosed when phleboliths (vascular or venous stones) are visible on plain X-rays. Bone distortion is often seen in large malformations that have a soft tissue mass effect. Some diffuse and extensive VMs can cause osteolytic lesions and increase the risk of pathological fractures. AVMs affecting bones can sometimes result in osteolytic lesions due to the presence of periosteal and intraosseous nidus (nest) or large draining venous channels after the nidus.

4.2.2 Duplex Ultrasonography

This imaging is primarily used as a diagnostic and therapeutic tool [5] during the first clinical visit. It distinguishes between tumors and malformations using duplex ultrasonography. It also identifies a vascular malformation and pinpoints its type. The imaging demonstrates whether the lesion is cystic or tissular, clarifies the presence or absence of flow, and thus distinguishes between fast-flow and slow-flow malformations (Fig. 4.2). The angiostructure and vessel density can be assessed, but its reliability is not always high. Peak flow velocities and arterial output can be measured in AVMs. In head and neck or extremity AVMs, comparing the arterial output on the normal side to the abnormal contralateral side is crucial for diagnosis and prognosis, particularly regarding the possibility of cardiac failure, and therefore useful for follow-up of AVMs.

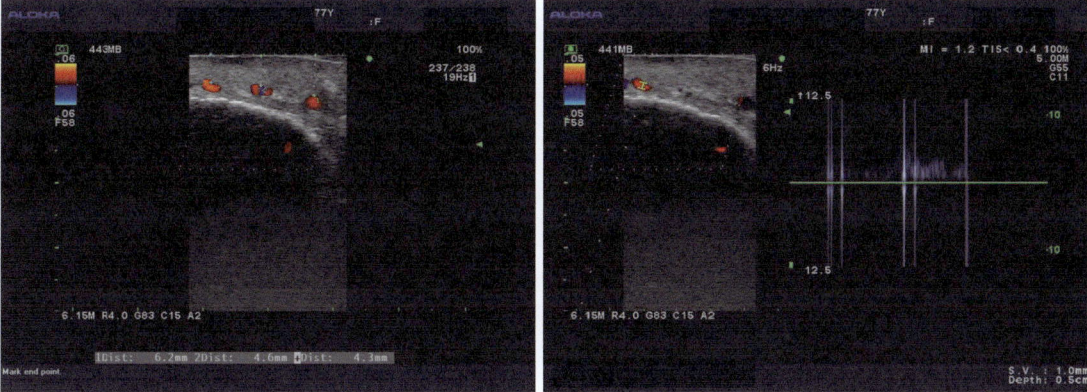

Fig. 4.2 Typical duplex ultrasonic examination. Flow patterns and localization of the lesions are depicted (*left*); flow intensity and pulse are demonstrated (*right*)

4.2.3 Computed Tomography (CT)

This method was previously considered of limited interest, even with enhanced contrast, as it only provides information on whether a lesion is highly vascularized or not. However, precise delineation and diagnosis of soft tissue lesions remain challenging, except for macrocystic LMs, where cysts are clearly depicted. The presence of phleboliths may indicate a diagnosis of venous malformation, as distinctive calcifications develop on thrombosis and debris resulting from slow flow. Bony displacement or alteration can also be seen due to long-term compression in both VMs and LMs. Pathologic fractures and absorption may be observed in bone or bone-adjacent AVMs. Currently, the less invasive 4D CT has replaced angiography and can contribute to therapeutic planning and post-therapy assessment.

4.2.4 Magnetic Resonance Imaging (MRI)

This is the best diagnostic modality for optimal analysis of soft tissue masses, as it provides proper diagnosis, distinguishes between tissular and cystic forms, and delineates fast or slow vessel flows. Venous and lymphatic malformations have their own distinct pattern. They appear as hyperintense on T2-weighted spin-echo sequences and are optimally seen in fat-suppression sequences. T1-weighted and fat-suppression sequences with contrast agents such as gadolinium demonstrate intense enhancement in infantile hemangiomas, while the enhancement is inconsistent and progressive on dynamic sequences in VMs. Gadolinium contrast allows for differential diagnosis between VMs and LMs. LMs can be distinguished from VMs as LMs show enhancement only at the margins of the cysts, whereas VMs are clearly and evenly stained.

MRI is necessary before treatment to make decisions about the extent of the lesion and its relationship to neighboring nerves, vessels, and vascular malformation. It is also necessary for the identification and diagnosis of the lesion. In fast-flow vessels, they can be identified as flow voids. MR angiography can confirm the diagnosis of fast-flow pathology, but it remains insufficient for accurately detecting AVMs' nidus and angiostructures.

4.2.5 Vascular Imaging

This procedure is primarily used for the assessment of fast-flow vascular lesions. Angiography is a powerful tool for the pretreatment evaluation of AVMs, particularly in detecting its characteristic early venous drainage. The angiostructure of an AVM can be determined by determining its location, arterial supply, draining veins, and relationship with normal neighboring arteries and veins. Angiography is also used for diagnosing quiescent AVMs, which may mimic a capillary malformation. However, with the current advancements in technology, 4D CT imaging can often replace angiography for pretreatment assessment with less invasiveness and greater accuracy.

4.3 Treatment

4.3.1 AVM

In vascular malformations, skin lesions are most commonly seen in AVMs,, which can develop ulcers during their natural clinical course or as a result of post-therapeutic side effects following embolization or sclerotherapy. A practical clinical staging system has been proposed for AVMs. This staging, as described by Schobinger, consists of four stages: (I) the lesion presents as warm, pink-blue macules; (II) it expands with pulsations, thrills, and bruits; (III) it becomes destructive with pain, hemorrhage, or ulceration; and (IV) it progresses to decompensation and congestive heart failure [6]. Treatment is ideal in stages I and II, but often the lesion goes unnoticed until stage III, when ulceration is observed as a clinically destructive sign. With a mean follow-up of 4.6 years, the cure rate for AVMs was 75% for stage I, 67% for stage II, and 48% for stage III [6]. AVMs can worsen after trauma, hormonal changes, pregnancy, or puberty. Duplex ultrasonography, as well as clinical signs and symptoms, can assist in the therapeutic decision-making process. However, a more precise and effective evaluation using contrast MRI, 4D CT, and angiography is necessary. While MRI provides information on the spatial relationship between the lesion and surrounding tissue and organs, 4D CT and angiography are most useful for abnormal vascular assessment and therapeutic evaluation during embolization, which is often required to eliminate the nidus, flow, pooling, and drainage patterns around the lesion. When the AVM lesion is localized, as is often seen in stage II, and to protect vital organs, surgical removal alone or combined with prior embolization within 24–48 h is the preferred first choice. If the defect is large, reconstruction will follow [7]. If the lesion is extensive and destructive (stage III) and the margin of the lesion is unclear, controlled reduction of the lesion should be considered. Embolization to control flow supply and drainage and subsequent percutaneous transcutaneous ultrasonic-guided sclerotherapy within 24–48 h may result in sufficient reconstruction of the wound bed (Fig. 4.3).

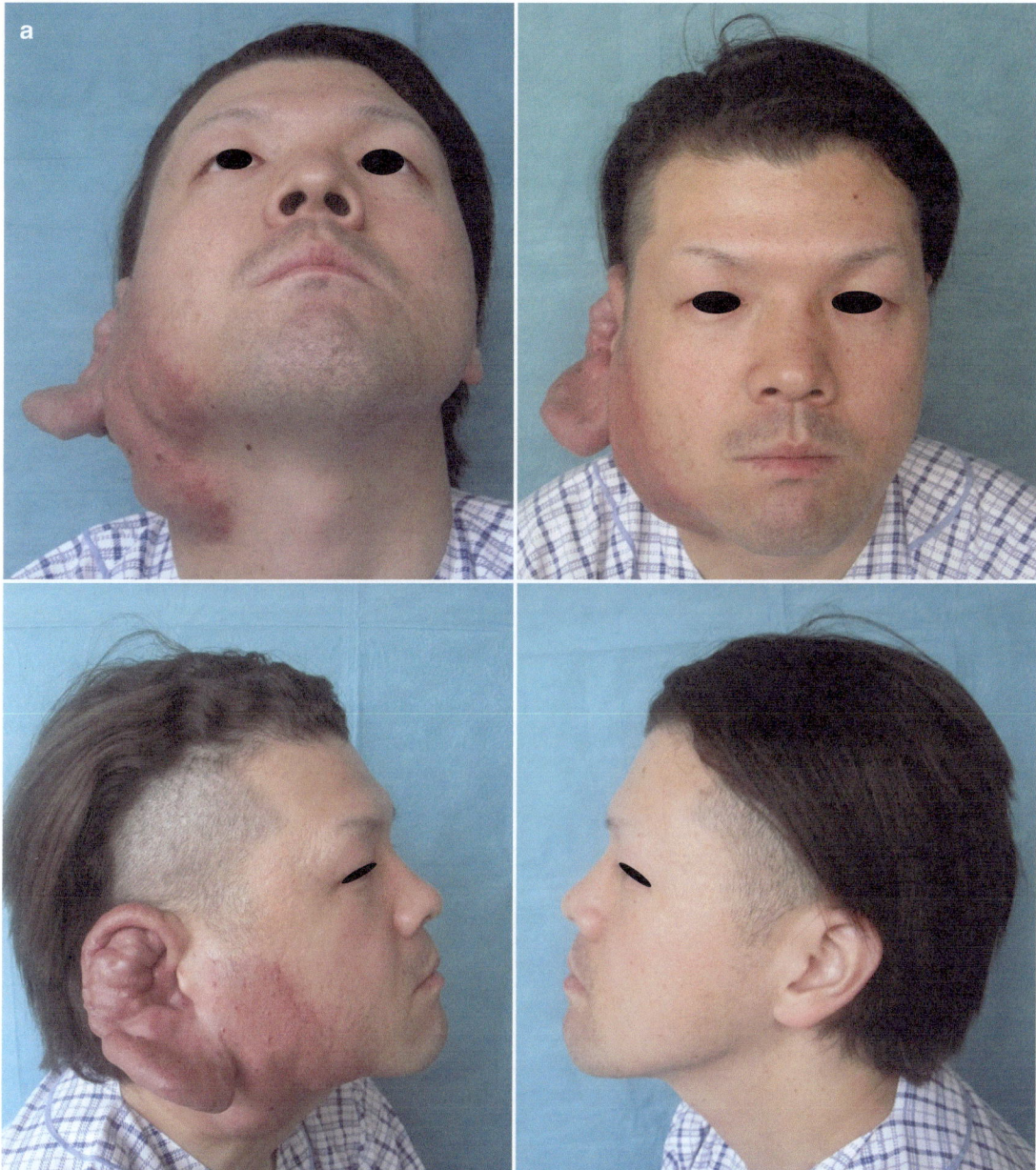

Fig. 4.3 (**a**) A 30-year-old male with capillary malformation and arteriovenous malformation (CM-AVM) in his right face including the ear. Skin discoloration and bulging in the right face due to CM-AVM are seen with minor pinhole wounds. (**b**) The imaging data of MRI, 4D CT, and ultrasonic demonstrated multiple in-flow vessels with enlarged venous pouches. (**c**) After second selective embolization, the nidus and the abnormality are controlled, but the tissue necrosis is seen. (**d**) At day 13, both necrotic tissue and exposed embolizing agents were excised, and the ear was reconstructed. (**e**) At 9 months after the final reconstruction, the angiogram and MRI imaging improved. (**f**) The patient demonstrated a satisfactory appearance, and no bruit or thrill is observed in the right face

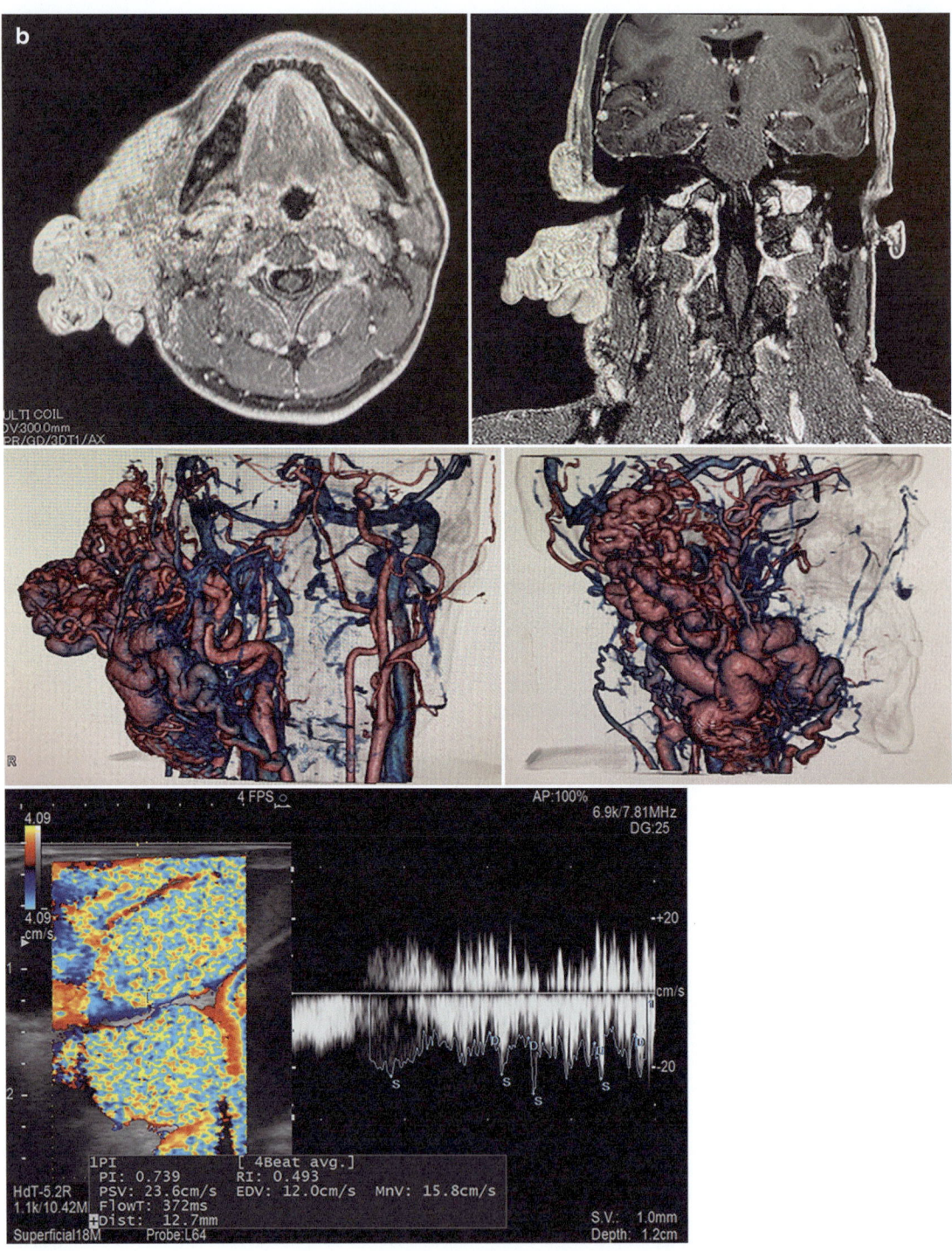

Fig. 4.3 (continued)

4 Imaging, Vascular Assessment: Extension in Depth and Vascular Anomalies

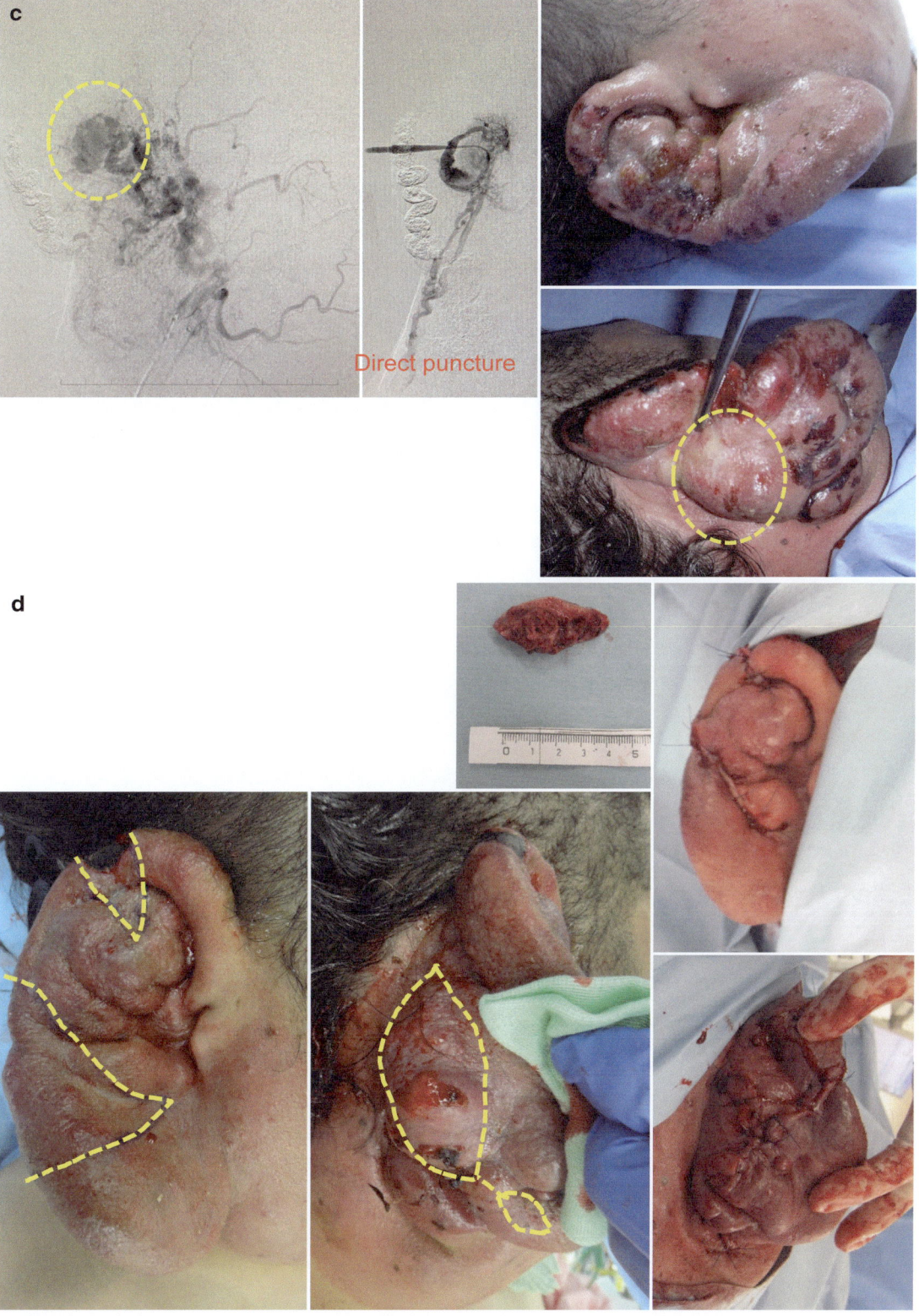

Fig. 4.3 (continued)

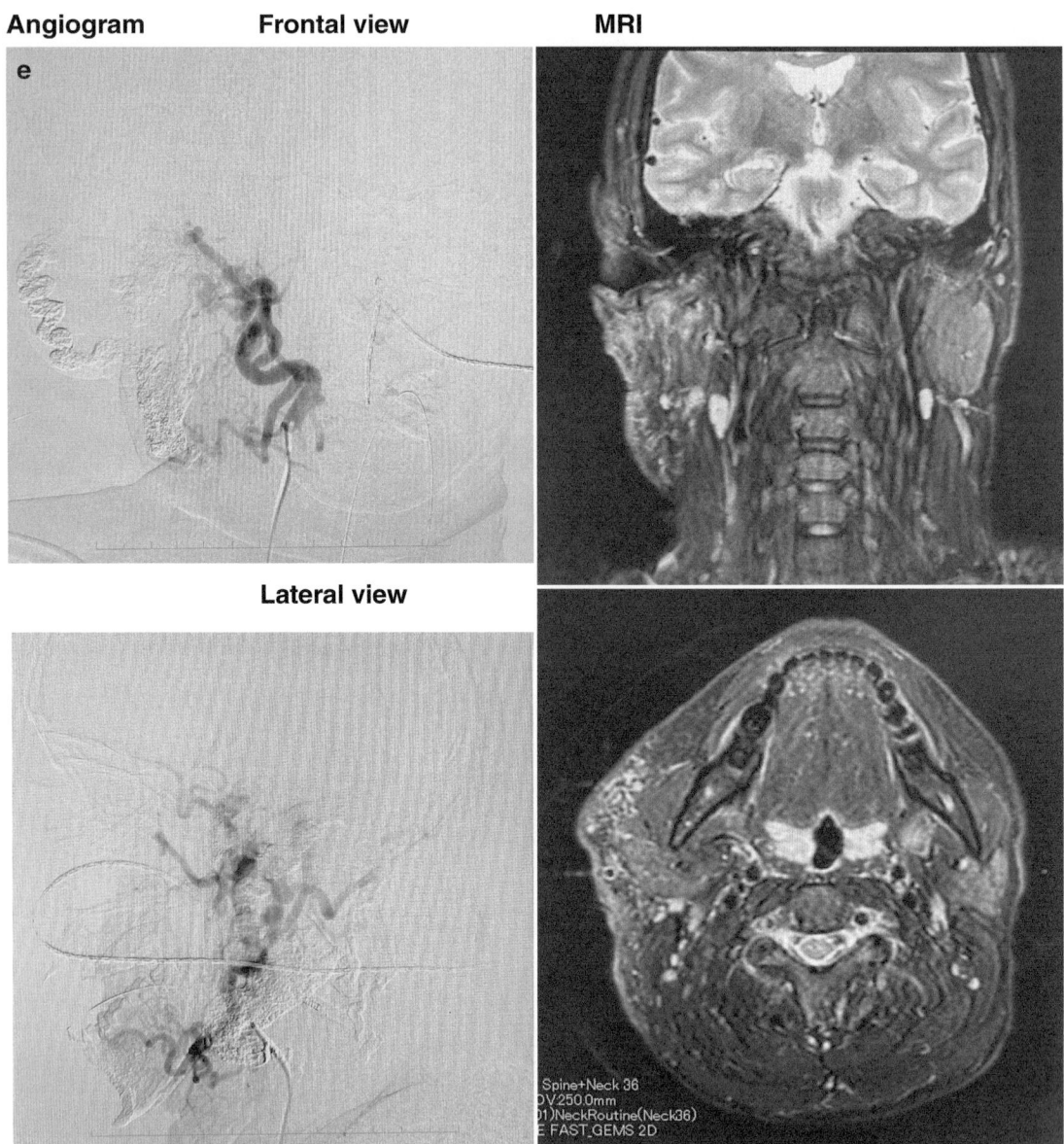

Fig. 4.3 (continued)

4 Imaging, Vascular Assessment: Extension in Depth and Vascular Anomalies

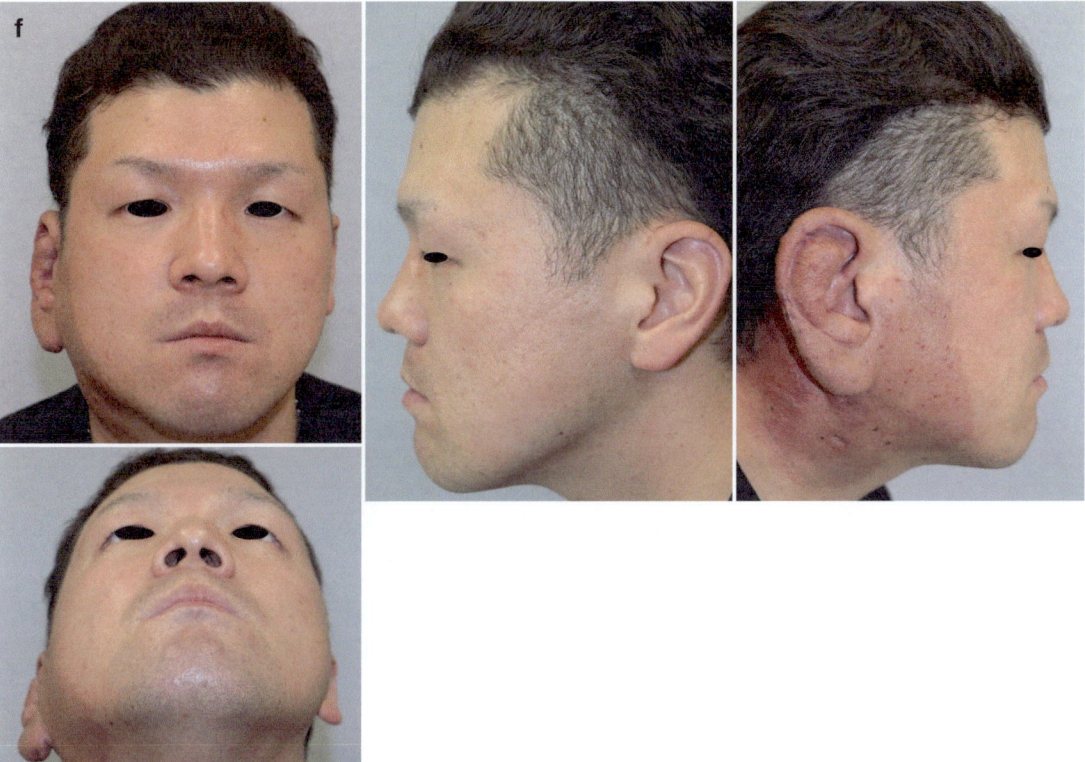

Fig. 4.3 (continued)

References

1. Enjolras O, Mulliken JB. Vascular tumors and vascular malformations. Adv Dermatol. 1997;13:375–423.
2. Wassef M, Enjolrad O. Superficial vascular malformations: classification and histopathology. Ann Pathol. 1999;19:253–64.
3. Chamlin SL, Haggstrom AN, Drolet BA, Baselga E, Frieden IJ, Garzon MC, Horii KA, Lucky AW, Metry DW, Newell B, Nopper AJ, Mancini AL. Multicenter prospective study of ulcerated hemangiomas. J Pediatr. 2007;151:684–9.
4. Maguiness SM, Hoffman WY, McCalmont TH, Frieden IJ. Early white discoloration of infantile hemangioma: a sign of impending ulceration. Arch Dermatol. 2010;146:1235–9.
5. Paltiel HJ, Burrows PE, Kozakewich HP, Zurakowski D, Mulliken JB. Soft tissue vascular anomalies: utility of US for diagnosis. Radiology. 2000;214:747–54.
6. Kohout MP, Hansen M, Pribaz JJ, Mulliken JB. Arteriovenous malformations of the head and neck: natural history and management. Plast Reconstr Surg. 1998;102:643–54.
7. Akita S, Houbara S, Hirano A. Management of vascular malformations. Plast Reconstr Surg Glob Open. 2014;2(3):e128. https://doi.org/10.1097/GOX.0000000000000079. eCollection 2014 Mar.

Open Access This chapter is licensed under the terms of the Creative Commons Attribution-NonCommercial-NoDerivatives 4.0 International License (http://creativecommons.org/licenses/by-nc-nd/4.0/), which permits any non-commercial use, sharing, distribution and reproduction in any medium or format, as long as you give appropriate credit to the original author(s) and the source, provide a link to the Creative Commons license and indicate if you modified the licensed material. You do not have permission under this license to share adapted material derived from this chapter or parts of it.

The images or other third party material in this chapter are included in the chapter's Creative Commons license, unless indicated otherwise in a credit line to the material. If material is not included in the chapter's Creative Commons license and your intended use is not permitted by statutory regulation or exceeds the permitted use, you will need to obtain permission directly from the copyright holder.

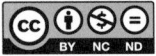

Imaging of Hypodermal Fat Necrosis

5

Ximena Wortsman

5.1 Introduction

Fat necrosis is a benign nonsuppurative inflammatory entity of the adipose tissue that results from the aseptic saponification of lipids by enzymes. The reported causes include trauma, radiotherapy, anticoagulation, inflammatory diseases, surgery, percutaneous interventions, and perinatal asphyxia, hypoxemia, or hypothermia [1]. Imaging has been growingly used for studying fat necrosis due to the often variable history and clinical findings that can simulate other conditions, which include the differential diagnosis of palpable lumps and bumps when this entity affects the hypodermis. Additionally, patients may not spontaneously refer to an inciting event such as trauma. Reports on imaging of fat necrosis started with the usage of X-rays, such as mammography, and have expanded to other imaging modalities such as ultrasound, magnetic resonance imaging (MRI), and most recently positron emission tomography-computed tomography (PET-CT). Besides the support to the clinical diagnosis, the usage of these imaging techniques may provide an anatomic perspective for evaluating the extent and characteristics of the structural changes in the tissues, as well as a support for assessing the differential diagnosis.

The aim of this chapter is to focus on the imaging characteristics of hypodermal fat necrosis with different imaging modalities and discuss some general principles, indications, advantages, and disadvantages for each method.

5.2 Imaging Methods

5.2.1 X-Ray Mammography

X-rays are the most simple and accessible form of imaging study and involve the usage of low-dose radiation for diagnostic purposes. Usually, this modality is not intended for particular study of fat necrosis; however, there are radiological signs suggestive of this condition that are frequently and incidentally found in the hypodermis, commonly during mammography screenings. The most frequent mammographic characteristic of fat necrosis is the presence of round- or oval-shaped hypodense structures, frequently showing a hyperdense calcified rim, also called "eggshell"- or "rim-like"-type calcification that corresponds to calcified lipid cysts (Fig. 5.1). This sign is almost pathognomonic of fat necrosis; therefore, the patients presenting this feature may not need additional imaging studies and should continue with the recommended screening program according to their age and history. Less frequent forms of presentation

X. Wortsman (✉)
Institute for Diagnostic Imaging and Research of the Skin and Soft Tissues, Department of Dermatology, Faculty of Medicine, Universidad de Chile, Santiago, Chile

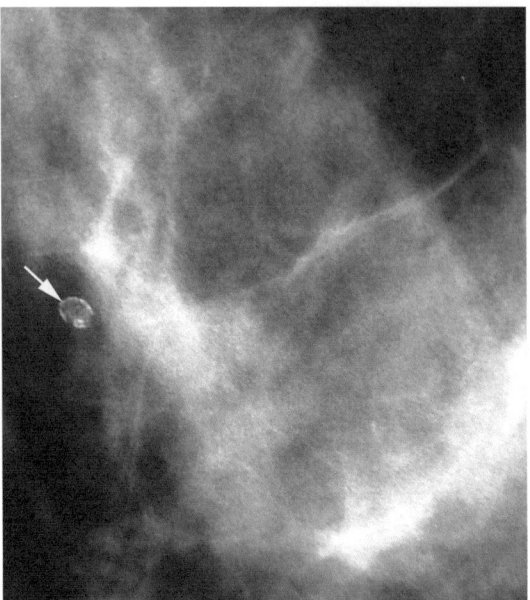

Fig. 5.1 *Fat necrosis on mammography* (lateral view) shows a "rim-like" or "eggshell" type of calcification (*arrow*) within the fatty tissue of the breast

of fat necrosis on mammography include focal asymmetries that may imply parenchymal edema. However, microcalcifications or spiculated dense masses can also be detected, with the latter being related to a major presence of fibrosis or scarring [2, 3]. Since these occasionally seen mammographic signs may mimic a breast malignancy, more imaging studies are usually needed in these particular cases.

5.2.2 Ultrasound

Also called sonography, this widely available imaging method is based on the properties of sound waves and has been increasingly used for studying fat necrosis in soft tissues due to the high-definition images of the superficial layers provided by the current machines. Besides its non-radiating nature and proved safety characteristics, there are several advantages of ultrasound such as its real-time, 2D, and 3D multiaxial and dynamic performance as well as its reasonable balance between resolution and penetration that allow us to obtain a wide range of anatomical information that can reach from the skin layers to the bony margin. Also, ultrasound can show the vascularity of the tissues through its color or power Doppler capabilities, which include the detection of the type of vessel (arterial or venous) and the velocity of blood flow (cm/s) [4, 5]. This may avoid the adverse reactions due to the use of contrast media that have been widely reported with other imaging modalities such as CT or MRI. The current limitations of ultrasound are lesions that measure <0.1 mm, with only epidermal location, and the detection of pigments such as melanin [6]. These last two limitations are not relevant for the study of fat necrosis. In fact, the hypodermis seems to be a perfect target for ultrasound use, due to its anatomically superficial location in soft tissue that makes it easily accessible with most of the linear probes that work with frequencies ≥7.5 MHz. Nevertheless, probes working with higher frequencies (≥12 MHz) are most commonly recommended for studying the hypodermis due to their higher definition at this tissue depth. On ultrasound, the most common sign of fat necrosis is the presence of well-defined round or oval-shaped anechoic pseudocystic structures, frequently with posterior acoustic enhancement, and sometimes surrounded by a hyperechoic calcified rim. These pseudocystic structures correspond to the oily cysts produced by the liquefaction of the fatty tissue. Internal echoes and a fluid–fluid level may sometimes be recognized in these pseudocysts, usually in cases with a history of trauma where the serohematic material combines with the liquefied material of the fatty lobules. Also, increased echogenicity of the hypodermis and isoechoic pseudonodules, surrounded by an anechoic or hypoechoic halo, may be detected. These latter ultrasound features indicate the degree of hypodermal inflammation. Less frequent sonographic signs are anechoic masses with a posterior acoustic shadowing artifact due to gross calcification and well- or ill-defined hypoechoic solid pseudo-masses due to prominent fibrosis and scarring. All these characteristics may appear as single or combined features in the affected region (Figs. 5.2 and 5.3). Hypo- or hypervascularity in the hypodermis may be detected according to the level of

Fig. 5.2 *Fat necrosis on ultrasound* (gray scale, transverse views) demonstrates the wide range of appearance of this condition. Symbols: *** pseudocyst; *o* pseudonodule; *x* fibrosis; *arrow* calcification; *1* and *2* fluid–fluid level. Abbreviations: *d* dermis; *h* hypodermis

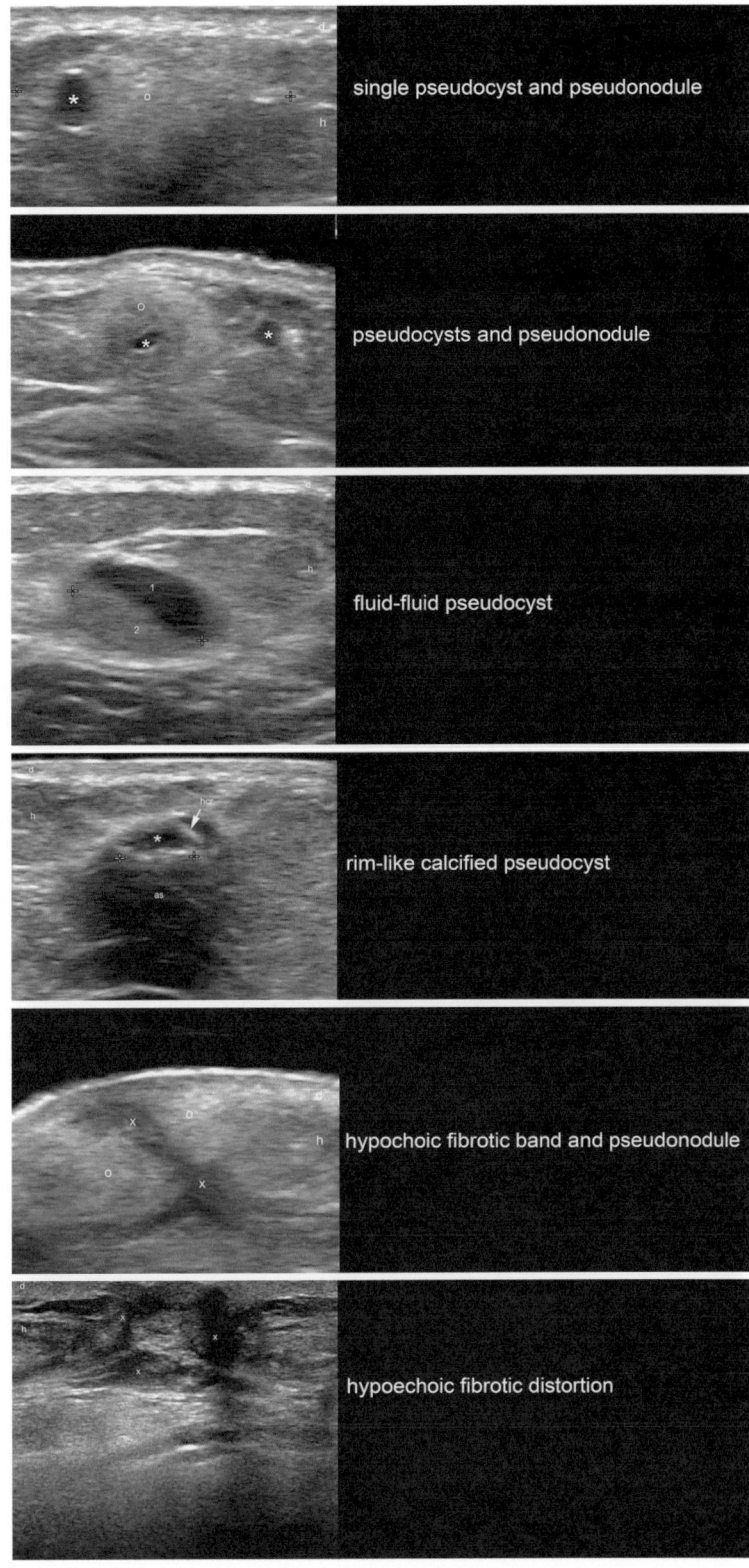

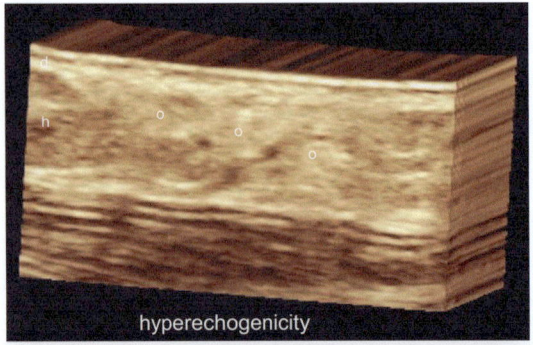
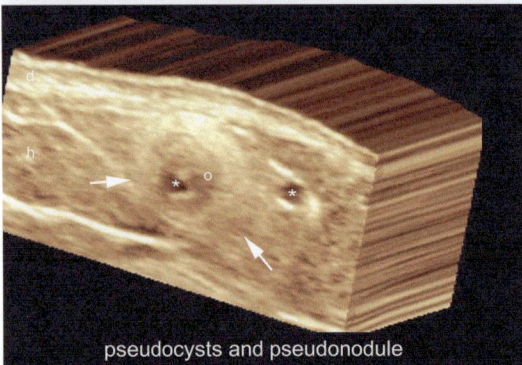
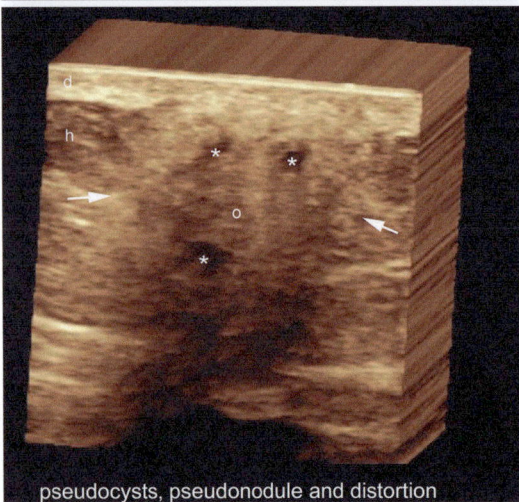

Fig. 5.3 Fat necrosis on 3D ultrasound (gray scale, 5–8-s reconstruction, transverse views) shows variable forms of presentation. Symbols: *pseudocyst; *o* hyperechogenicity (*top*) and pseudonodule (*middle* and *bottom* locations); *arrows* pointing out the lesional sites. Abbreviations: *d* dermis; *h* hypodermis

has been reported to successfully support the diagnosis [8–10]. Thus, the main indications for ultrasound in fat necrosis are to support the early diagnosis and rule out solid tumors that may be hard to differentiate on a clinical basis only.

5.2.3 Magnetic Resonance Imaging

This is an imaging method based on the response of the body's hydrogen ions in a magnetic field. This technique has been widely used in the study of soft tissues, mainly in the musculoskeletal field, due to its high-definition anatomical images. The main disadvantages of this method are its high cost and the potential adverse reactions to gadolinium, the usual contrast medium used in these examinations. Additionally, MRI has limited ability to show small calcifications, a common finding in fat necrosis which may be seen in this imaging technique as areas of signal void or may simply go undetected. On MRI, a wide spectrum of findings have been reported in fat necrosis, and some of the findings may even mimic a malignant tumor such as a breast cancer. The most typical finding on MRI is a round or oval nodule or mass with hypointense T1-weighted signal on fat-saturated images that correspond to a lipid pseudocyst. Also, fat necrosis can show as well- or ill-defined isointense or hypointense areas or pseudonodules on T1-weighted images probably due to its inflammatory and hemorrhagic characteristics. In case with strong fibrosis, architectural distortion, with or without spiculated margins, and variable degrees of intensity (low, intermediate, or high signal) on T1-weighted images are reported. Fat suppression sequences may help to differentiate fat necrosis from malignant tumors. On T2-weighted sequences, isointense, hypointense, and hyperintense appearances have been described. Pseudonodular, globular, and laminated appearances have been additionally reported (Fig. 5.4). After the injection of gadolinium contrast medium, fat necrosis can show variable appearances that can range from no enhancement to irregular or peripheral enhancement and from thin to thick rims of enhancement

inflammation present in the tissue, with hypervascularity being the most commonly found in inflamed stages [1, 3, 7]. In cases presenting subcutaneous fat necrosis of the newborn, ultrasound

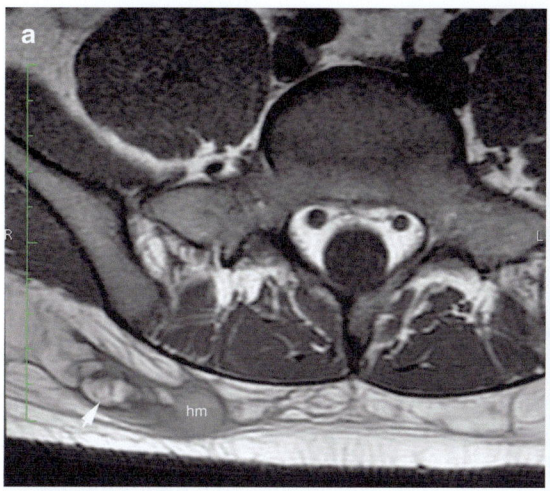 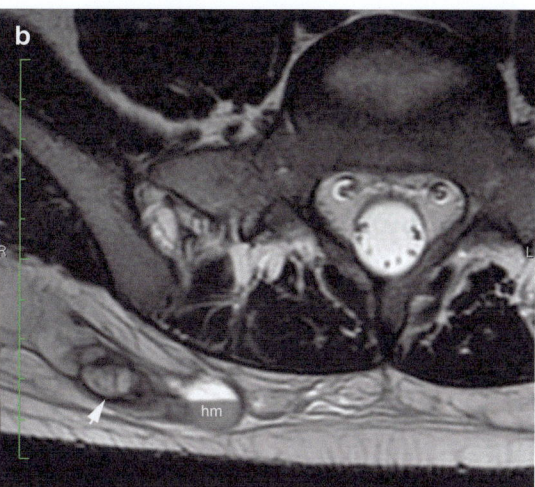

Fig. 5.4 (**a**, **b**) *Fat necrosis on MRI* (axial views). (**a**) T1-weighted sequence shows isointense pseudonodule with a hypointense rim located in the hypodermis of the right side of the lower back (*arrow*, fat necrosis area). In the vicinity, a hypointense oval-shaped hypodermal structure is detected that corresponds to a hematoma (*hm*). (**b**) T2-weighted image of the same case shows a change in the intensity of the hematoma (*hm*) with a fluid–fluid level (hyperintense/hypointense) and no change in the intensity of the pseudonodule (*arrow*, fat necrosis site) in comparison with the T1-weighted sequence. (Courtesy of Drs. Raul Valenzuela and Herly Pulgar)

[1–3, 7, 11, 12]. The most frequent indications for MRI regarding fat necrosis are to complete the imaging study in cases with mammographic abnormalities, especially the ones where a malignancy must be ruled out, and to assess the differential diagnosis in cases presenting palpable large lumps or extensive trauma.

5.2.4 Computed Tomography and Positron Emission Tomography

Computed tomography (CT) implies the cross-sectional usage of X-rays and has a broad range of applications, mainly in the neurological, cardiac, and abdominal fields. Thus, CT has been extensively used for staging malignant conditions. However, there are few reports in literature on the usage of CT for studying hypodermal fat necrosis, mostly showing isolated case reports. Advantages of CT are its wide availability and relatively short time of examination due to the new multi-slice machines that can acquire and process the images very rapidly. Disadvantages of CT are its high cost, its radiating nature, and the need for intravenous contrast media. On CT, fat necrosis has been reported as a well-defined hypodense mass with rim enhancement or a globular mass with central fat density [11].

Positron emission tomography (PET) is a nuclear imaging modality that registers the gamma rays emitted by a positron-emitting radionuclide, also called tracer. The most commonly used tracer is fluorodeoxyglucose (FDG), an analog of glucose. However, this is a radiating modality that also requires injection of an agent.

In recent years, the combination of these two modalities (PET-CT) has gained adepts due to the mix of the anatomical and biological images that have been widely used in the staging of cancerous lesions [13]. However, PET-CT has certain notable shortcomings, including the inability to perform simultaneous data acquisition and the significant radiation dose to the patient [14]. PET-CT is now used in the staging of melanoma, showing high sensitivity especially in advanced stages [15, 16]. Nevertheless, there are several reports of false positives of PET-CT due to the glycolytic activity present in inflammation that can easily mimic a malignancy in this modality [17–19]. These inflammatory features are

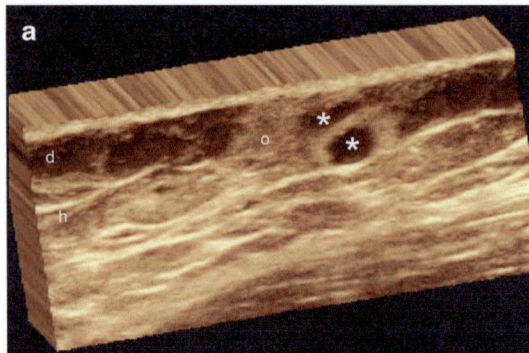

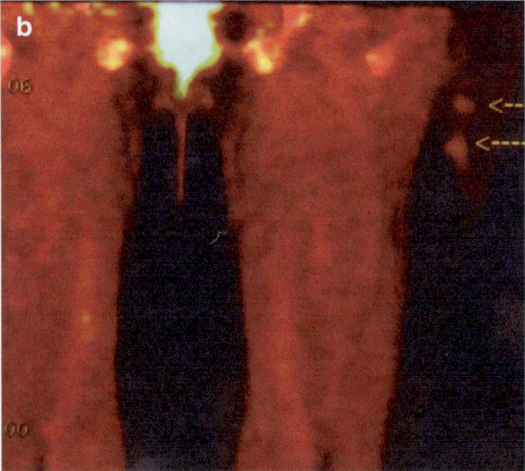

Fig. 5.5 (**a**, **b**) *Fat necrosis on 3D ultrasound and PET-CT*. Patient with a history of removed in situ melanoma in the left leg. (**a**) 3D ultrasound (gray scale, 5–8-s reconstruction, longitudinal view) shows two anechoic pseudocysts (*) surrounded by a hyperechoic pseudonodular structure (*o*) consistent with fat necrosis. (**b**) PET-CT (coronal view) demonstrates a false-positive uptake of FDG in the hypodermis of the left thigh with two hypermetabolic pseudonodules (*arrows*). Abbreviations: *d* dermis; *h* hypodermis. (PET-CT image courtesy of Dr. Vicky Roizen)

common in fat necrosis; therefore, this condition seems to be one of the most common pitfalls for PET-CT. These reports mention pseudonodular solid images with hypermetabolic activity and increased uptake of FDG (Fig. 5.5). Besides fat necrosis, other causes of false positives of PET-CT have been reported. Among them are acute and chronic inflammation or infection, physiologic lactation, and benign breast masses, including silicone granuloma, fibroadenoma, and postsurgical or radiotherapy changes. Therefore, the usage of PET-CT is not recommended as a first imaging modality in fat necrosis. Moreover, the usage of this imaging modality may cause diagnostic dilemmas in oncologic imaging [20].

5.3 Conclusion

There are several imaging methods that can reveal the anatomical characteristics of hypodermal fat necrosis. The usage of imaging in this condition is intended for the assessment of the differential diagnosis of lumps and bumps in the soft tissues and also to try to rule out malignant tumors. The advantages and disadvantages of each technique as well as the availability of these modalities in the medical institutions should be considered, when selecting the appropriate imaging modality for each case.

References

1. Atasoy MM, Oren NC, Ilica AT, Güvenç I, Günal A, Mossa-Basha M. Sonography of fat necrosis of the breast: correlation with mammography and MR imaging. J Clin Ultrasound. 2013;41(7):415–23. https://doi.org/10.1002/jcu.22061.
2. Taboada JL, Stephens TW, Krishnamurthy S, Brandt KR, Whitman GJ. The many faces of fat necrosis in the breast. AJR Am J Roentgenol. 2009;192:815–25.
3. Tan PH, Lai LM, Carrington EV, et al. Fat necrosis of the breast—a review. Breast. 2006;15:313–8.
4. Wortsman X. Common applications of dermatologic sonography. J Ultrasound Med. 2012;31:97–111.
5. Wortsman X. Ultrasound in dermatology: why, how, and when? Semin Ultrasound CT MR. 2013;34:177–95.
6. Wortsman X, Wortsman J. Clinical usefulness of variable-frequency ultrasound in localized lesions of the skin. J Am Acad Dermatol. 2010;62:247–56.
7. Walsh M, Jacobson JA, Kim SM, Lucas DR, Morag Y, Fessell DP. Sonography of fat necrosis involving the extremity and torso with magnetic resonance imaging and histologic correlation. J Ultrasound Med. 2008;27:1751–7.
8. Marszałek A, Maciejewska J, Bowszyc-Dmochowska M, Prokurat A. Subcutaneous fat necrosis of the newborn—a case report and review of literature. Pol J Pathol. 2010;61:240–4.
9. Vasireddy S, Long SD, Sacheti B, Mayforth RD. MRI and US findings of subcutaneous fat necrosis of the newborn. Pediatr Radiol. 2009;39:73–6.

10. Avayú E, Rodríguez C, Wortsman X, et al. Newborn fat necrosis: case-report. Rev Chil Pediatr. 2009;80:60–4.
11. Chan LP, Gee R, Keogh C, Munk PL. Imaging features of fat necrosis. AJR Am J Roentgenol. 2003;181:955–9.
12. Daly CP, Jaeger B, Sill DS. Variable appearances of fat necrosis on breast MRI. AJR Am J Roentgenol. 2008;191:1374–80.
13. Bockisch A, Beyer T, Antoch G, et al. Positron emission tomography/computed tomography—imaging protocols, artifacts, and pitfalls. Mol Imaging Biol. 2004;6:188–99.
14. Pichler BJ, Wehrl HF, Kolb A, Judenhofer MS. Positron emission tomography/magnetic resonance imaging: the next generation of multimodality imaging? Semin Nucl Med. 2008;38:199–208.
15. Schröer-Günther MA, Wolff RF, Westwood ME, et al. F-18-fluoro-2-deoxyglucose positron emission tomography (PET) and PET/computed tomography imaging in primary staging of patients with malignant melanoma: a systematic review. Syst Rev. 2012;1:62. https://doi.org/10.1186/2046-4053-1-62.
16. Hinz T, Voth H, Ahmadzadehfar H, et al. Role of high-resolution ultrasound and PET/CT imaging for preoperative characterization of sentinel lymph nodes in cutaneous melanoma. Ultrasound Med Biol. 2013;39:30–6.
17. Kashyap R, Lau E, George A, et al. High FDG activity in focal fat necrosis: a pitfall in interpretation of posttreatment PET/CT in patients with non-Hodgkin lymphoma. Eur J Nucl Med Mol Imaging. 2013;40(9):1330–6.
18. Akkas BE, Ucmak Vural G. Fat necrosis may mimic local recurrence of breast cancer in FDG PET/CT. Rev Esp Med Nucl Imagen Mol. 2013;32:105–6.
19. Lee SA, Chung HW, Cho KJ, et al. Encapsulated fat necrosis mimicking subcutaneous liposarcoma: radiologic findings on MR, PET-CT, and US imaging. Skeletal Radiol. 2013;42(10):1465–70.
20. Adejolu M, Huo L, Rohren E, Santiago L, Yang WT. False-positive lesions mimicking breast cancer on FDG PET and PET/CT. AJR Am J Roentgenol. 2012;198:W304–14.

Open Access This chapter is licensed under the terms of the Creative Commons Attribution-NonCommercial-NoDerivatives 4.0 International License (http://creativecommons.org/licenses/by-nc-nd/4.0/), which permits any non-commercial use, sharing, distribution and reproduction in any medium or format, as long as you give appropriate credit to the original author(s) and the source, provide a link to the Creative Commons license and indicate if you modified the licensed material. You do not have permission under this license to share adapted material derived from this chapter or parts of it.

The images or other third party material in this chapter are included in the chapter's Creative Commons license, unless indicated otherwise in a credit line to the material. If material is not included in the chapter's Creative Commons license and your intended use is not permitted by statutory regulation or exceeds the permitted use, you will need to obtain permission directly from the copyright holder.

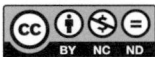

Skin Necrosis and the Need for Vascular Assessments

Saritphat Orrapin, Kittipan Rerkasem, and Rajgopal Mani

6.1 Introduction

The vascular assessment in peripheral arterial disease (PAD), which is a condition of atherosclerotic stenosis or occlusion of the peripheral arteries, plays a vital role in the diagnosis and treatment of disease. The anatomic location of the PAD involves carotid artery, vertebral artery, mesenteric artery, renal artery, upper extremity, and lower extremity artery [1, 2]. The most common location of symptomatic PAD is lower extremity. When the perfusion to the lower extremity is lower than a threshold value of resting metabolic requirement, the legs and feet turn to skin necrosis including gangrene and ischemic ulcer. The death of the cell due to ischemia is the continuing process which is associated with morbidity, amputation, and impaired quality of life. Critical limb ischemia (CLI) or chronic limb-threatening ischemia (CLTI) is the advanced stage of atherosclerotic disease due to severe impaired perfusion, which is a clinical syndrome of PAD in combination with rest pain, gangrene, or ischemic ulcer more than 2 weeks' duration [1]. There are other causes of chronic lower extremity ischemia, such as smoking arterial inflammation (thromboangiitis obliterans or Buerger's disease (TAO)), chronic arterial embolism, arterial entrapment, fungal arterial infection, Takayasu's disease, and other uncommon arteriopathies such as drug-induced arteriopathy [3–7]. The vascular assessment, which ranges from noninvasive methods such as ankle-brachial index and tissue oxygen measurement to invasive methods such as angiography, is important to differentiate the cause of disease, determine the severity of ischemia, surveil the progression of disease and prognosis, select the medication and modalities of treatment, and determine the requirement of revascularization procedure [1, 8–10].

6.2 Epidemiology of Peripheral Arterial Disease

PAD results from atherosclerotic occlusion of the blood vessels in the lower and upper limbs symptomatically expressed as pain on exercise that is

S. Orrapin
Vascular Surgery Division, Department of Surgery, Faculty of Medicine, Thammasat University, Pathum Thani, Thailand

Thammasat University – Center of Excellence for Diabetic foot care (TU-CDC), Thammasat University Hospital, Thammasat University, Pathum Thani, Thailand
e-mail: orrapins@tu.ac.th

K. Rerkasem
Research Institute for Health Sciences, Chiang Mai University, Chiang Mai, Thailand

Department of Surgery, Faculty of Medicine, Chiang Mai University, Chiang Mai, Thailand
e-mail: kittipan.r@cmu.ac.th

R. Mani (✉)
Research Institute for Health Sciences, Chiang Mai University, Chiang Mai, Thailand

relieved by transient rest: this condition is known as intermittent claudication (IC). IC worsens with reduction in blood flow and perfusion leading to CLTI. This in turn leads to cell death, ulceration, and necrosis; the pathophysiology of this condition is described in a separate section in this chapter. PAD presents a significant clinical burden. Fowkes reported that 202 million people were living with PAD worldwide: 69.7% of this population lived in low- to middle-income countries (LMICs) with a breakup of 54.8 million in Southeast Asia and 45.9 million in the Western Pacific countries [11]. Fowkes used ankle-brachial pressure index (ABI) threshold of ≤0.9 to define the presence of PAD in 34 studies from 22 high-income countries (HICs) and 12 from LMICs. Song and Fowkes [11, 12] conducted a systematic review and meta-analysis on 118 studies and, based on their modeling, estimated the global population of PAD to be 236.92 million people in 2015. Both reports found that PAD increased with age and sex: prevalence of 5.28% (95% CI 3.38–8.17%) in HIC in 45–49-year-old women and 5.41% (3.41–8.49%) in men. In the 85–89-year group, prevalence found was 18.38% (11.16–28.76%) in women and 18.83% (12.03–25%) in men. In LMIC group countries, prevalence rates were higher in women than men, especially in the younger age group, with 6.31% (4.86–8.15%) in 45–49-year group, which has implications for planning health care [11].

However, the true prevalence and incidence rate of PAD may be underestimated due to the lack of a good screening system, which makes it impossible to report the exact number of PAD patients in the group who has no symptoms or has minor symptoms [13]. According to the data registry of the Society for Vascular Surgery (SVS) and the European Society for Vascular Surgery (ESVS), 80% of PAD patients are asymptomatic, of which half of them are associated with DM and 10–30% and 20–40% are present with intermittent claudication and atypical leg pain, respectively [1, 8–10, 14–16].

The associated risk factors for PAD are the following:

- Smoking 2.72% (95 CI 2.39–3.09%) in HIC, 1.42% (1.25–1.62%) in LMIC
- Diabetes mellitus (DM) 1.86% (1.66–2.14%) in HIC, 1.47% (1.29–1.68%) in LMIC
- Hypertension 1.55% (1.42–1.71%) in HIC, 1.36% (1.24–1.50%) in LMIC
- Hypercholesterolemia 1.19% (1.07–1.33%) in HIC, 1.14% (1.03–1.25%) in LMIC

Of these risk factors, the association between DM and PAD is especially significant to this chapter. DM affects platelet aggregation and increases inflammation with raised AGE and reactive oxygen species, endothelial dysfunction, and vascular smooth muscle cell dysfunction, all of which are implicated in PAD. Pain is attenuated in people with diabetes and neuropathy. ABI could be falsely high (>1.30) owing to the presence of medial calcinosis. Estimated prevalence could be inaccurate since ABI relies on detecting two of the three vessels around the ankle, and the variation of ABI with vessel narrowing is unknown in some ethnic minorities. The narrative from these data is that the PAD is significant and an increasing burden affecting both genders: it is worse in women in the younger age range in LMIC and could be expected to affect daily life considerably: walking to work, shopping, and life in general would be affected and likely to get worse [17].

PAD is associated with morbidity and mortality due to amputation and major adverse cardiovascular events (MACEs), especially in CLTI. The major cause of death is acute coronary syndrome (ACS). Because of atherosclerotic involvement of multiple vascular beds, 50% of patients with CLTI are coronary artery disease (CAD) and cerebrovascular disease (CVD) [14, 18]. The 5-year mortality rate in patients with PAD is 10–15%. When diagnosed with CLTI, the 1-year mortality rate increases to 25%. 6.5% and 4.5% of CLTIs are fatal myocardial infarction (MI) and fatal stroke, respectively. 25% of CLTI patients undergo major amputation due to ischemic limb process or infection [19]. MACE rapidly increases during the perioperative period due to the stress from the foot infection or active comorbid disease and risk of the operation including revascularization, debridement, and amputation. Poor performance status occurs in patients with loss of ambulatory state due to amputation, limb ulceration, gangrene, rest pain, or disabling claudication, all of which are increased risk for MACE. The SVS

Objective Performance Goals (OPGs) established standardized tools to report benchmark of perioperative outcome including MACE and major adverse limb events (MALEs) after revascularization procedures in patients with CLTI [20, 21].

6.3 Pathophysiology of Peripheral Arterial Disease

Arterial obstruction can lead to skin necrosis. Atherosclerosis is the most common cause of arterial occlusion. Dyslipidemia, obesity, hypertension, DM, and smoking are the risk factors for the development of atherosclerotic lesions [22]. However, the distribution is different between the risk factors. For example, in a diabetes patient, the obstructive lesion is mainly in tibial vessel occlusion, whereas with smoking, it is in the aortoiliac segment.

The metabolic abnormality in patients with DM leads to hyperglycemia, insulin resistance, and increasing of free fatty acid [23]. Hyperglycemia increases the oxidative stress by increasing reactive oxygen species (ROS). In addition, the cellular mitogenic pathway activation through the mitochondrial generation of the superoxide anion including advanced glycation end products (AGEs), protein kinase C (PKC) activation, and nuclear factor kappa B (NF-κB) is induced by high blood glucose level. In patients with long-duration DM, insulin resistance causes endothelial dysfunction, decreasing of nitric oxide (NO) synthase, expression of adhesion molecules, and atherosclerotic lesions [23]. In addition, a thrombosis risk in DM increases through the hypercoagulation and platelet aggregation. Insulin resistance is also promoted in the atherosclerotic process due to lipid metabolism disturbance such as high triglycerides (TGs), high apolipoprotein B (ApoB), small and dense low-density lipoprotein (LDL), and low high-density lipoprotein (HDL) cholesterol [1, 16, 24]. In early atherosclerotic process, the endothelial dysfunction is associated with hypertensive patients. A reduction in NO results in a reduced vasodilatory response and thereby inflammation, thrombosis, and activate coagulation cascade [1, 16, 23–26]. The repetitive blood pressure alterations in hypertensive condition cause ongoing renin-angiotensin system activation, which impacts the atherosclerotic lesions [1, 16, 24]. Smoking causes an inflammation of vessel wall, which is related to atherosclerotic plaque formation through interleukin-6, tissue necrosis factor-α, interleukin-1-β, leukocyte, C-reactive protein (CRP), and other inflammatory markers [1, 16, 24]. The prothrombotic state of platelet activation and aggregation is created by increasing of thromboxane A2 (TXA2), von Willebrand factor (vWF), thrombin, and fibrin and decreasing of prostacyclin, antithrombotic, and fibrinolytic substances [1, 16, 24].

Detailed postmortem studies of patients of different ages show that atherosclerosis progresses from small and inconsequential fatty streaks to fibrolipid plaque and complicated lesions, which are the cause of many different clinical disorders such as skin necrosis (gangrene), myocardial infarction, or stroke. Atherosclerotic plaques begin with the subendothelial accumulation of lipid-laden foamy macrophages and T-lymphocytes (T-cells), which form non-stenotic fatty streaks. This progresses to the formation of acellular core of lipid cholesterol, bound by a fibrous cap that contains vascular smooth muscle cells (VSMCs) and inflammatory cells, especially macrophages, mast cells, and T-cells. In an advanced lesion, new blood vessels and calcium hydroxyapatite are present [1, 16, 24].

Although atherosclerosis is a systemic disease involving especially large- and medium-size arteries, atherosclerotic plaque tends to develop in certain places such as the carotid artery, the infrarenal aorta, and the arteries of the lower extremities, in particular at the sites of bifurcation, the ostia, the branchings, and the bends. This suggests that hemodynamic forces play a role in atherogenesis; many hypotheses have been proposed to explain this unique focal pattern.

6.4 Atherosclerosis and Symptomatology

There are two mechanisms by which symptoms of atherosclerotic lesions can develop. Firstly, by the time that atherosclerotic lesion has increased in size with the deposition of a necrotic core, inflammatory cells, and a fibrous cap, the lesion is so large that the downstream blood supply is not sufficient. Initially, this usually occurs because of exertion associated with increased blood flow demand such as intermittent claudication of the calf. Patients have calf pain when walking, but the symptom relieves when patients rest their leg. The muscle contraction during exercise needs much more energy (blood supply) than those with resting stage. Then in case the atherosclerotic lesion causes further obstruction, this can progress to rest pain and dry gangrene (skin necrosis). In case this dry gangrene becomes infected, this leads to wet gangrene, in which massive and rapid skin necrosis can occur (Fig. 6.1). The second mechanism begins with erosion or rupture plaque, resulting in exposure of the blood to thrombogenic lipid cores. Consequently, a rapid accumulation of platelets, deposition of fibrin, and occlusion of the vessel by thrombus or distal embolization of thrombotic material occur, which may lead to very severe problems suddenly such as acute arterial occlusion (thrombosis). This can cause massive skin necrosis in the leg (Fig. 6.2). Since these two

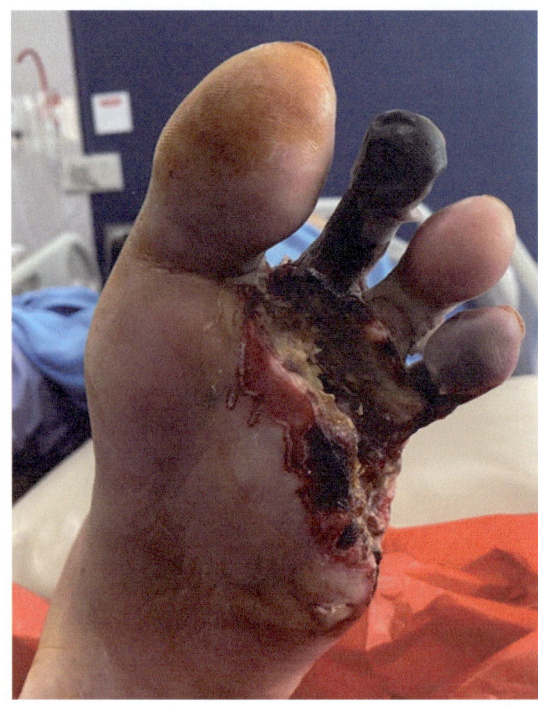

Fig. 6.1 The foot of a diabetic patient who started with gangrene in the fifth toe; then the infection resulted in massive skin necrosis of his foot in 5 days' time. This picture shows the foot after the first debridement due to wet gangrene and necrotizing fasciitis

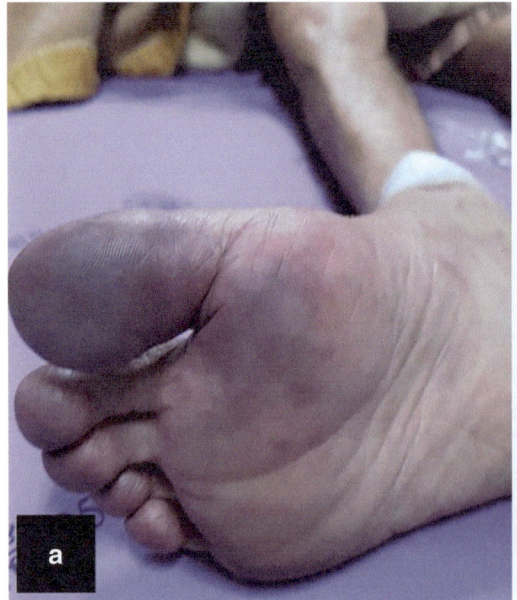
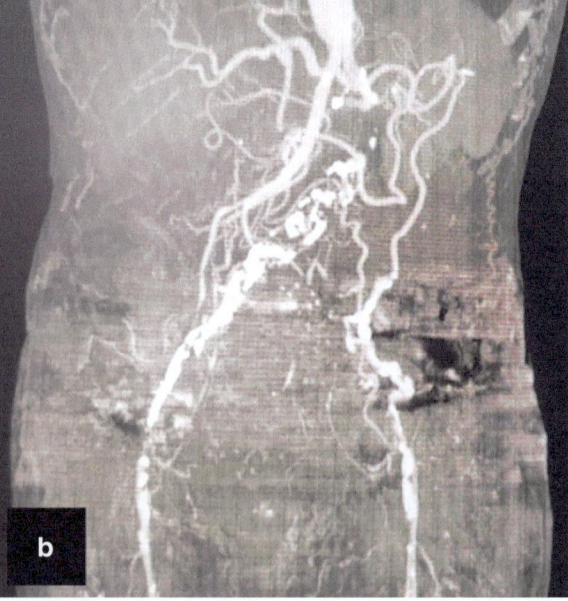

Fig. 6.2 Acute thrombosis of the aortoiliac artery shows fixed mottling skin of the foot following acute thrombosis of the aortoiliac artery (**a**), and computed tomographic arteriography demonstrated occlusion of distal aorta and bilateral common iliac artery with arterial wall calcification (**b**)

mechanisms can cause massive skin necrosis, consequently these lead to major amputation of the leg.

6.5 The Effects of Diabetes on PAD and the Diabetic Foot

DM is the major atherosclerotic risk factor that increases the risk of PAD. Chronically high blood glucose levels, increases in free fatty acids, and insulin resistance can be seen in diabetes patients. In addition, the increasing of blood glucose level activates the inflammatory response of blood vessels, leading to vasoconstriction and decreasing of thrombosis threshold [1, 16]. The diabetes patients are at risk of lower limb amputation more than normal people about 20 times. Complications from diabetes are caused by multiple factors such as hypoglycemia and high blood HbA1c level, as well as lack of knowledge of improper foot care and socioeconomic conditions of the family [1, 16, 24]. The complications of DM involve the peripheral artery that feeds the legs. Both macroangiopathy and microangiopathy cause limited blood supply to the tissue of the foot. The PAD is the part of macroangiopathy under atherosclerotic process of medium and large vessel. The incidence of PAD in patients with DM is 10–30% [9]. Most common anatomic distribution of macrovascular involvement by atherosclerosis in patients with DM is crural arteries, including tibial and peroneal arteries leading to diabetic foot ulcer (DFU) and chronic limb-threatening ischemia (CLTI) [1, 16]. In addition, the gangrene and skin necrosis can originate from microvascular involvement, which causes the capillary basement membrane thickening and decreasing of capillary blood flow and microcirculation. Another process of diabetic foot (DF) and DFU is peripheral neuropathy, which is found in 60% of DM patients and 80% of patients with DFU. Peripheral motor neuropathy causes foot deformity due to loss of muscle imbalance, causing bone and joint damage, called neuro-osteoarthropathy or Charcot foot, found in 2% of all diabetics, or causes deformed feet in other ways, such as pes cavus, claw toes, flat feet, and hallux valgus [16]. The limited ankle and feet joint mobility and their deformities cause the abnormal distribution of foot weight and repeated minor foot trauma injuries and callous formation [11, 14, 15]. A disorder of the peripheral sensory nervous system causes a decrease in the sensation of the feet [14]. The autonomic nerve involvement causes dry, cracked, and ulcerative skin to easily become ulcerative or infected in the skin layer [27]. Both vascular and neurologic involvement of DF causes chronic recurrent and high risk of infected ulcer in diabetes patients. Chronic hyperglycemias activate the inflammatory process and ongoing cell death processes (apoptosis) by oxidative stress. The neutrophil dysfunction associated with hyperglycemia causes the impairment of the immune system, which causes the infection-prone DFU or diabetic foot infection (DFI) [28, 29]. Diabetic foot infection (DFI) is caused by the invasion of microorganisms into the ulcer or tissues of the feet through the fissures of the skin in patients with diabetes. The DFI aggravates the inflammatory processes of surrounding tissue, which leads to the tissue loss and skin necrosis [29–31] (Fig. 6.3).

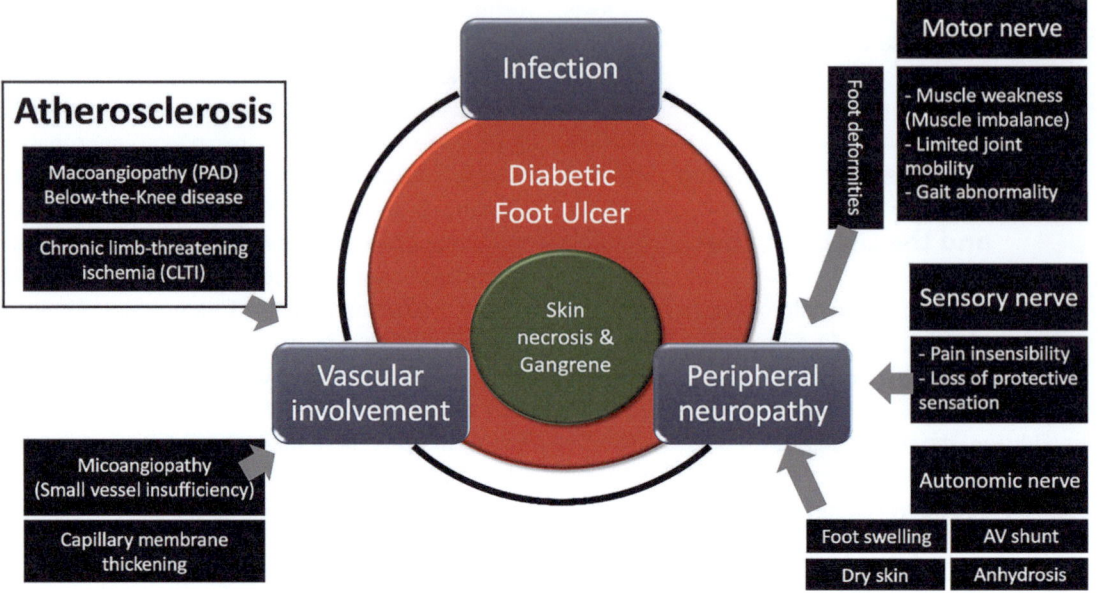

Fig. 6.3 The association between atherosclerosis, peripheral arterial disease, and diabetic foot ulcer

6.6 Macrovascular and Microvascular Assessment Tools

Vascular assessment techniques of PAD, particularly in gangrene and ischemic ulcer, are based on the severity and prognosis of disease, risk and level of amputation limit, prediction of the wound healing rate, and requirement of revascularization. Both macrovascular assessment technique such as ABI and computed tomographic angiography (CTA) and microvascular assessment technique such as skin perfusion pressure (SPP), transcutaneous oxygen tension (TcPO2), or transcutaneous oxygen measurement (TCOM) and other skin perfusion imaging are the modalities to obtain the diagnosis and anatomic distribution of PAD. When the patients indicate to lower extremity revascularization, urgently assess and treat patients, which can decrease the risk for major limb amputation [1, 16, 32, 33]. To prevent the amputation of lower extremity due to PAD, do not assume that microangiopathy, when present, is the cause of poor healing in patients with a chronic recalcitrant ulcer [34]. Although some techniques are not widely used to evaluate the perfusion of skin necrosis of the lower extremity, the appropriate use of any of the following vascular assessment modalities is useful to guide the physician to appropriate treatment modalities.

6.7 Macrovascular Assessments of Tissue Viability

The ankle-brachial index (ABI), which is the noninvasive test of chronic arterial occlusion, has been widely used for diagnosing the PAD [1, 16, 35–37]. Because of the simplicity of the measurement technique, high availability, and less expensive instrument, the ABI is recommended as the first-line screening test in patients who have high risk or are suspected of PAD [15, 36, 38]. The normal range of ABI is 1–1.3. Diagnosis of PAD is established by (1) the value of ABI less than 0.9 or (2) the value of ABI less than 0.9 after exercise or (3) the decreasing of postexercise ABI more than 20% by walking on a 3.2 km/h speed treadmill test for 5 min with the incline slope of 12° [5, 14, 35, 36, 39]. The sensitivity and specificity of ABI to diagnose PAD are 79% and 96%, respectively [40].

The ABI measurements are performed using a handheld sphygmomanometer cuff at the ankles. Doppler ultrasounds detect the signals and measure ankle systolic blood pressure at the position of the posterior tibial artery or dorsalis pedis artery and also the systolic blood pressure of the brachial artery under supine position; the ABI calculation is done using the ipsilateral highest ankle systolic blood pressure (ankle pressure) divided by the highest brachial systolic blood pressure [5, 40–42]. Lower ABI values indicate greater severity of PAD in the same patient (Table 6.1), while patients with an ABI value greater than 1.3 represent a stiffness of the arterial wall. The ABI can also determine the severity of atherosclerosis in other vascular beds and predict the risk of MACE including stroke, MI, and cardiovascular death [43]. The ankle pressure alone is less reliable due to changes in systemic blood pressure conditions such as hypertension, hypotension, shock, or heart failure that affect the ankle pressure. ABI has often been unreliable, with high false-negative rate of the test particularly for diabetes, old age, and end-stage renal disease (ESRD) patients. The false elevation of ankle pressure due to medial calcinosis causes the overestimation of ABI value and underestimation of severity of PAD (Fig. 6.4). The false elevation of ankle pressure and ABI value may present either noncompressible vessel value (ABI >1.30) or normal range of ABI (ABI 1.00–1.29) (Fig. 6.4) [1, 16, 34]. Arain's study included 17,485 consecutive patients who underwent ABI measurement to identify the incidence of noncompressible vessel. The result showed that 2781 (16%) had noncompressible vessels [44]. Randhawa's study, which is a retrospective observational study, showed that 70% of the tibial vessels that were considered to be noncompressible are actually occluded or severely stenotic by angiography [45]. So, patients who have clinical characteristics that indicate symptomatic PAD with discordant ABI result will suffer from (1) fainting, or absent pedal pulse, brittle nail, calf muscle hypotrophy, hairless leg, IC, and rest pain but will have ABI value higher than 0.90 [36], (2) ABI values greater than 1.3, (3) decreasing of the pedal pulse's intensity or systolic ankle pressure during leg lifting, and (4) monophasic or damping of Doppler waveform with a normal ABI value should evaluate the additional measurement such as toe pressure, toe-brachial index (TBI), pulse volume recorder (PVR), and Doppler waveform analysis (Fig. 6.4) [5, 38]. If TBI is less than 0.70 or toe pressure is less than 0.4, the diagnosis of PAD is established [36, 39–41, 46]. Currently, toe pressure and TBI, which are simplified, quick, and inexpensive tools for perfusion assessment, are the recommended tests of forefoot perfusion appropriately to diagnose and manage CLTI. Comparing with ABI, toe pressure assessment offers more accuracy in detecting limb ischemia in the presence of noncompressible or false elevation of ankle pressure in heavily calcified vessels. However, toe gangrene, previous toe amputation and extensive ulcer, and concomitant infection in the forefoot and toe area are limitations of toe pressure measurement [1, 47]. The vascular assessment, which included clinical history taking, physical examination and perfusion measurement of the ischemic limb, revealed that CLTI is a chronic form of limb-threatening ischemia that can result in severe limb loss due to inadequate perfusion to gangrene or ischemic ulcers. The SVS Wound, Ischemia, and foot Infection (WIfI) classification should be staging to predict a risk of amputation, likelihood of wound healing, and benefit for

Table 6.1 The severity of peripheral arterial disease related with resting and postexercise ankle-brachial index [5, 36, 39]

Disease severity	Resting ABI	Postexercise ABI
Noncompressible arteries	≥1.30	
Normal	1.00–1.29	
Borderline	0.91–0.99	
Mild PAD	0.71–0.90	0.51–0.90
Moderate PAD	0.41–0.70	0.16–0.50
Severe PAD	≤0.40	≤0.15

ABI ankle-brachial index; *PAD* peripheral arterial disease

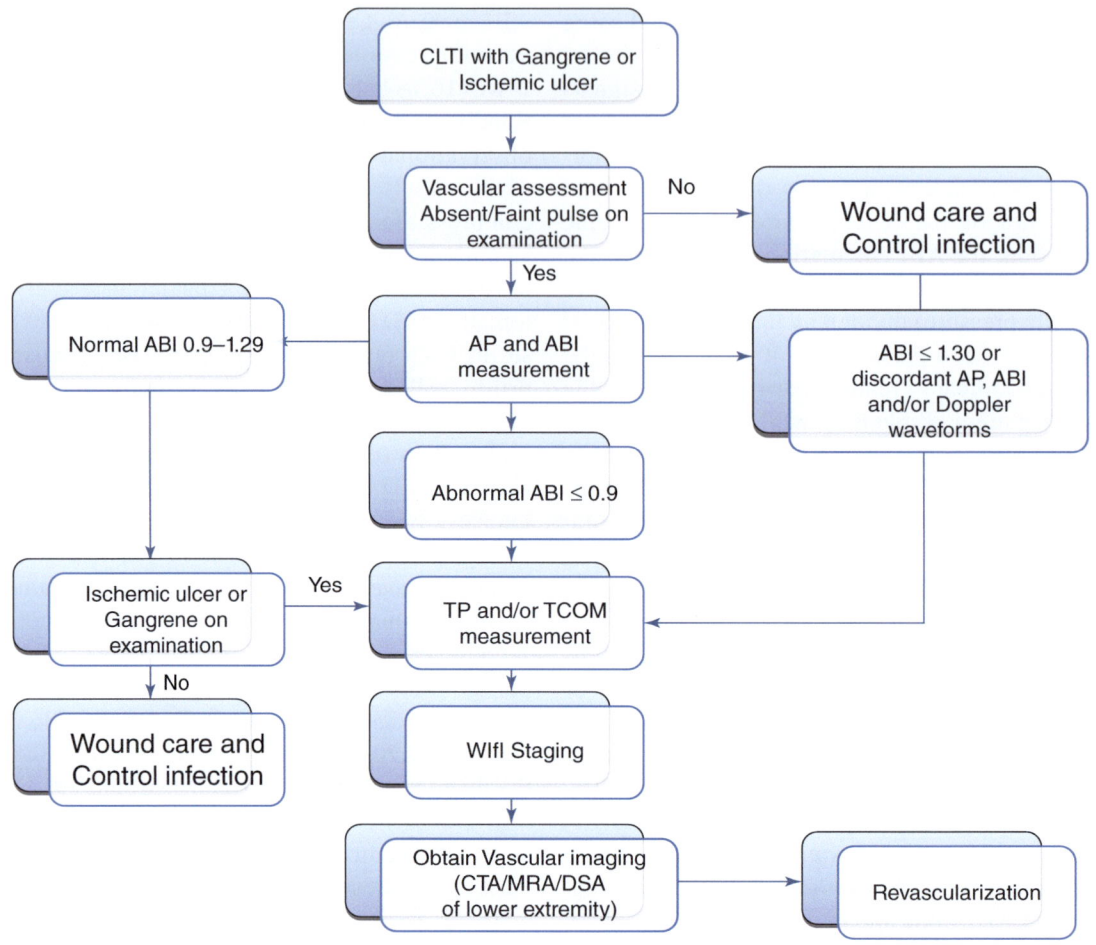

Fig. 6.4 The algorithm of decision-making for revascularization based on vascular assessment and clinical presentation of gangrene and ischemic ulcer in patients with chronic limb-threatening ischemia. *CLTI* chronic limb-threatening ischemia; *AP* ankle pressure; *ABI* ankle-brachial index; *TP* toe pressure; *TCOM* transcutaneous oxygen measurement; *CTA* computed tomographic arteriography; *MRA* magnetic resonance arteriography; *WIfI* Wound Ischemia foot Infection; *DSA* digital subtraction arteriography

revascularization. The aim of revascularization procedure is to prevent limb amputation (Fig. 6.4) [48–50].

Catheter arteriography by performing plain radiography or fluoroscopy in conjunction with the administration of contrast media intra-arterially can evaluate anatomical characteristics and dynamic blood flow of lower extremities. Because arteriography can provide a complete map of the lower limb arteries and selective catheter placement during lower extremity arteriography enhances imaging, reduces contrast material dose, and enhances sensitivity in patients with CLTI, arteriography is a gold standard diagnostic tool for PAD patients who have indicated revascularization including disabling IC and CLTI, particularly when below-the-knee to pedal artery disease is suspected (Fig. 6.5).

The arteriography shows the intraluminal anatomical characteristics of the arteries, including stenosis, occlusion, dissection, and intimal calcification. Arteriography allows intervention at the same setting such as balloon angioplasty with stenting and coil embolization (Fig. 6.5). For open vascular bypass procedure, completion arteriography immediately after an operation is recommended to identify the occult lesion to prevent restenosis of vascular bypass. Digital subtraction angiography

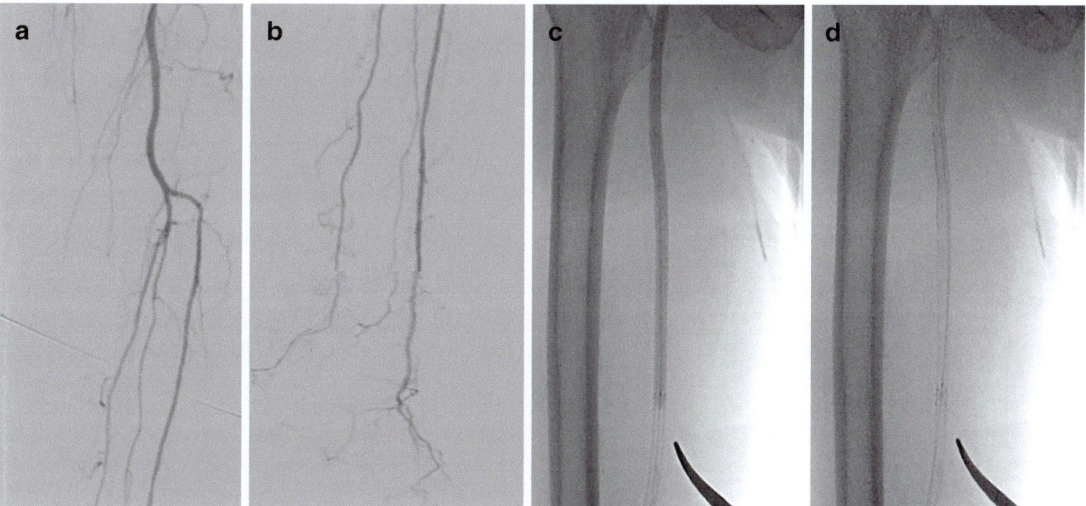

Fig. 6.5 Digital subtraction arteriography (DSA) demonstrated superficial femoral artery occlusion in chronic limb-threatening ischemia patient. (**a**) Arteriography to evaluate below-the-knee artery; (**b**) arteriography to evaluate below-the-knee and foot arteries; (**c**) balloon angioplasty of proximal superficial femoral artery; (**d**) after superficial femoral artery stenting

(DSA) is currently developed to remove the bones and opaque matter, which provides the intraluminal imaging clearly from an inflow suprainguinal aortoiliac segment to crural and foot arteries [1, 16, 47]. However, intra-arterial contrast media injection poses a higher risk of contrast-induced nephropathy (CIN) than peripheral vein injections, especially in patients who have estimated glomerular filtration rate (eGFR) less than 30 mL/min/1.73 m^2. Because of the high exposure to ionizing radiation and contrast media, the catheter angiography should be preserved in patients who are candidates for revascularization. In addition, the risk factors of catheter and wire-associated complications during arteriography include arterial dissection, thrombosis, distal embolization, and extravasation and increased risk of limb loss during the diagnostic procedure [1].

Carbon dioxide arteriography (CO_2 arteriography) by using carbon dioxide directly into the arteries can be used in patients with a chronic kidney disease to prevent CIN and allergy to contrast media. The carbon dioxide replaces the blood in artery temporarily. However, the use of CO_2 arteriography has certain limitations, including low quality of the artery image that is less clear than contrast media intra-arterially. So, CO_2 arteriography is usually used as an additional agent in conjunction with regular contrast media. CO_2 angiography is generally considered inferior to iodinated angiography but can still provide useful diagnostic images by using power injection and adjust the 30° Trendelenburg patient's position during intervention to increase carbon dioxide concentration and reduce the velocity of blood flow, respectively [51, 52].

Computed tomographic arteriography (CTA) can provide a more detailed overview of the lower limb vascular and confirm an uncertain PAD diagnosis or verify the severity and an anatomic distribution of the arterial occlusive lesion before revascularization (Fig. 6.6). In addition, the CTA composite is used for the extraluminal and intraluminal study. For extraluminal study, CTA can evaluate the source of external compression, associated organ or structural abnormalities, inflammation of the vessel wall, and surrounding structure. CTA has advanced in terms of high accuracy and acquisition times. The development of the CTA in modern era creates a multiple-plane view with high-resolution image and three-dimensional (3D) reconstructions. The sensitivity and specificity of the arterial occlusive

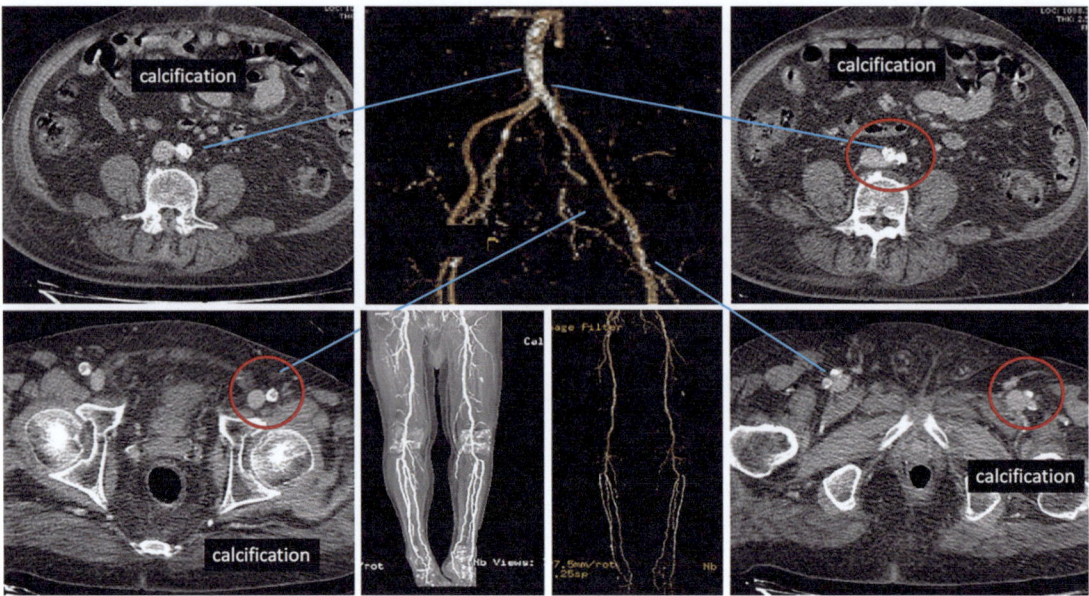

Fig. 6.6 Computed tomographic arteriography (CTA) of aortoiliac occlusive disease (AIOD) in chronic limb-threatening ischemia patient with bilateral groin calcification (right and left, Fig. 6.5, of axial view CTA) and occlusion of aortoiliac segment with heavy calcification (central, Fig. 6.5, of CTA reconstruction)

disease of CTA in the aortoiliac segment are 95% and 96%, respectively, and those of the femoropopliteal segment are 97% and 94%, respectively, and below-the-knee arteries are 95% and 91%, respectively [53, 54]. However, the limitations of the study on the CTA include the image interference on artifact, calcified artery, and limited evaluation or overestimation of below-the-knee artery lesion, especially in concomitant proximal artery occlusive disease. Because of the potentially nephrotoxic contrast agents and radiation exposure of CTA, the CTA should be performed in patients who are candidates for revascularization or who had uncertain PAD diagnosis by other modalities of investigation. Thus, the clinical value of CTA in the CLTI target population remains uncertain. Below-the-knee and below-the-ankle artery runoff vessel usually gets a complete evaluation on catheter angiography or DSA or foot magnetic resonance arteriography (MRA) due to less reliability for CTA imaging of below-the-knee artery [1].

Magnetic resonance arteriography (MRA) is a noninvasive imaging method with non-exposure to ionizing radiation, which can create the 3D images of the entire arterial map. So, the MRA is suitable for patients with CLTI who have plans for revascularization, unaffected by arterial calcification. Both sensitivity and specificity of MRA are 93–100% [40]. However, MRA interpretation depends on the availability of subspecialist vascular radiologist or expert interventionist. The overestimation with the false-positive result of the stenotic lesion is higher in MRA imaging when compared with CTA and DSA. In addition, venous contamination can obscure arteries below the knee. CLTI patients with pacemakers, defibrillators, and other metallic implantation such as cerebral clips are contraindicated to perform MRA. In addition, the metallic material can cause artifacts that mimic vessel occlusions. If MRA cannot provide the adequate below-the-knee and below-the-ankle imaging, the foot MRA or catheter arteriography is the choice of further investigation to identify the occult lesion [1, 16]. Contrast-enhanced MRA (CE-MRA) using gadolinium-based contrast agents is generally preferred because of the high contrast-to-noise ratio, better spatial resolution, more rapid acquisition, and less artifact. In addition, time-resolved techniques can improve image flow patterns and increase the accuracy to identify below-the-knee arterial occlusive disease and runoff vessel. However, CE-MRA using gadolinium-based contrast media agents has not been associated with CIN. The most severe complication of gadolinium-based contrast media agent is nephrogenic systemic fibrosis, which usually risks patients who have eGFR less than 30 mL/min/1.73 m^2 [55].

6.8 Microvascular Assessments of Tissue Viability

Tissue viability is a significant area of concern when clinicians are managing skin necrosis: depending on the cause or insult leading to necrosis, these concerns vary. Trauma, burns, pressure, underlying conditions such as ischemia, and infection require different management regimes: however, since perfusion and oxygenation are essential to growth and survival, these are also key parameters to be monitored along with others such as nutrition and pressure.

Skin blood flow was historically used to denote these parameters: skin blood is influenced by both extrinsic and intrinsic factors, which include pressure, temperature, position, humidity, sympathetic and/or autonomic control, hormonal effects, topical and/or systemic nutrition, and glycemic control. Skin blood flow was measured in mL/100 mL of tissue/min or it was a volume measurement [56, 57]. Numerous methods of skin blood flow have been described in the literature, which include isotope washout methods, volume measurements, and optical methods:

- Clearance of ^{131}iodine
- Clearance of 4-iodoantipyrine (I_{125})
- Sodium fluorescein (Na 24) clearance
- Plethysmography
- Laser Doppler flowmetry
- TV video microscopy of the capillaries
- Transcutaneous oxygen tension using skin sensors
- Optical measurement of oxygen saturation
- Laser angiography

Each method has its merits as well as limitations. Radioisotope methods yield volume flow in mL/100 ms of tissue/min, which is very important especially for research into therapeutics, but suffer the disadvantage of being difficult to repeat: in some cases, the use of 4-iodoantipyrine methods, with which there are good data to determine levels of amputation, requires a gamma camera to detect washout imposing limitations despite the inherent accuracies of the measurement.

Holstein used a photoelectric probe to measure skin reddening due to histamine release after blanching by studying the washout of ^{131}I in controls as well as $N = 24$ patients with PAD and reported excellent correlation ($r = 0.97$, $p < 0.001$) [58]. This group reported SPP of 30 mmHg, which was in overall accord with the previous work on Landis' original work on capillary pressures—clearly important observations albeit not without its limitations which were discussed in their study.

Laser Doppler flowmetry is a simple technique to use on intact skin. There is vast literature concerning its validation and many uses especially in detecting the thickness of burn wound damage [59]. Capillary microscopy and its successor, TV video-microscopy, are elegant methods even though they are limited to studying capillary blood flow, structure, and function in nail beds and the web space between thumb and first finger. This limits its applicability. Skin surface sensors to measure the partial pressure of oxygen on skin (TcPO$_2$) and optical probes to measure oxygen saturation (SO$_2$) offer reliable and accurate means to monitor tissue viability based on the use to determine amputation levels [60].

TcPO$_2$ is a noninvasive technique which relies on skin surface sensors using electrochemical means of measuring the partial pressure of oxygen in heated volume of tissue beneath skin. This skin volume may be heated between 37 and 44C, though at 43C and 44C, the reliability of the probe is not affected. Its function is dependent on the O$_2$ dissociation curve. It is reliable, reproducible, and dependent on oxygen delivered to the volume of tissue beneath the probe as well as the oxygen consumed locally and the resistance to diffusion in tissue beneath [61]. So, edema and infection will affect readings. It helps to assess tissue viability around wound sites [62]. On a cautionary note, TcPO$_2$ sensors must be moved from a test site after 2 h to prevent burns. A systematic review and meta-analysis of data from four studies including 901 patients ($n = 911$ wounds) showed that prediction of healing was accurate and reliable using cutoff values <30 or <20 mmHg, with $TcPO_2$ odds ratio being 3.21 (95% CI 1.07–9.69) with $I^2 = 77\%$. Note that most studies used a value of 20 mmHg to predict nonhealing [63].

SO_2 probes rely on detecting reflected light from a volume of tissue beneath to measure oxygen saturation; it is based on the Beer's law of exponential decay of light through tissues. The ratio of the intensity of reflected (or transmitted) light to that of the incident beam is a measure of the optical impedance/transmittance of the medium: the amount of transmission/reflection of light is a function of the wavelength light as well as the tissues. At 805 nm, the amount reflected is affected by the volume of tissues: at 633 nm, it is affected maximally by the color as well as the volume of tissues. Since oxygenated hemoglobin and deoxygenated hemoglobin are cherry red and dark blue in color, respectively, measurements at both wavelengths permit the level of oxygen saturation to be computed using Beer's law. In practice, the transmittance/reflectance of small samples of blood contained in cuvettes are measured over a range of wavelengths to calibrate the detection of oxygen saturation in tissues. Early oximeters were worn on the earlobe which, in healthy, is richly perfused. These devices do not heat tissues, which is a great advantage. In current practice, oximeters are more like clips to fit on to a forefinger and widely used in emergency medicine departments. Such probes can be used on toes to measure SO_2 on toes or on the proximal edge of a nonhealing wound. Castronuovo studied the use of SO_2 probes to measure SPP in a cohort with critical limb ischemia, ulcers, and gangrene and reported that SPP <30 mmHg was 85% sensitive and 73% specific with an overall accuracy of 79.3% ($p < 0.002$) [60]. This principle is used with a laser source for angiography [64].

Apelqvist and Lepantalo, in a bid to determine the most useful device to detect tissue viability, studied SO_2 and $TcPO_2$ probes against ankle-brachial index (ABI) measurements and concluded that both SO_2 and $TcPO_2$ techniques are in the 25–40 mmHg range: 30 mmHg is a safe threshold for tissue viability [65]. ABI, a measure at ankle level, was less sensitive to tissue viability. SO_2 and $TcPO_2$ are recommended to be used on the proximal edge of lesions [37].

Laser angiography is a skin perfusion imaging by tissue infusion visualization technique. Indocyanine green (ICG), which is a water-soluble contrast, nonradioactive, nonionizing, and nontoxic contrast agent that is approved by the US Food and Drug Administration (FDA) for administering intravascularly, is used to determine the real-time tissue perfusion under the near-infrared laser light spectrum (650–900 nm) via a camera system. Laser angiography is an invasive technique of skin perfusion imaging due to requiring of intravascular ICG administration. ICG is infused to tissue by the binding to plasma proteins [32, 66]. For PAD and CLTI, the ICG fluorescence angiography is used for patients with PAD. Zimmermann's study demonstrated the value of ICG angiography in the determination of tissue perfusion in patients with PAD, which showed significant difference in the perfusion index indicating the severity of PAD. A receiver-operating characteristic (ROC) curve demonstrated a positive likelihood ratio and negative likelihood ratio of 6.00 and 0.00, respectively, with an area under the curve (AUC) of 0.949 to discriminate the CLI and non-CLI patients [67]. The ICG angiography is used to evaluate the success of revascularization immediately after the procedure and intraoperative assessment [33, 68]. Colvard studied the measurement of plantar perfusion by laser-assisted fluorescence angiography (LAFA), which also showed a significant increase in the fluorescence intensity and peak perfusion on the plantar surface during LAFA, from 7.1 to 12.4 units/s ($P < 0.001$) and 97.1 to 143.9 units ($P < 0.001$), respectively. The result of the study also showed a strong correlation of different LAFA parameters with an overall change in ABI [66]. The ICG fluorescence angiography can be used to evaluate superficial tissue perfusion of the foot and leg because of the tissue penetration in the range of 3–7 mm [66,

67, 69]. However, ICG fluorescence angiography may have limited efficacy in patients with asymptomatic and early PAD and who need more penetration depth. ICG is prohibited in patients with a history of sulfa allergy. In addition, the recent systematic review demonstrated the multiple unclear and high risk of bias with low quality of six included cohort studies on tissue perfusion by laser angiography [33].

Indigo carmine is another agent for skin perfusion imaging, which is used in evaluating limb perfusion, microcirculation, and angiosomal revascularization immediately after the procedure [47]. The organic salt property, which is commonly used as a food-coloring agent, guarantees the safety of indigo carmine administration intra-arterially. DIESEL study demonstrated that if revascularization is a success and the wound is adequately perfused, the indigo carmine stains the wound and demarcation of the arterial perfusion distribution is visualized [70]. However, the data on the use of indigo carmine in patients with PAD are limited and need further studies to determine the possibility of wound healing.

A lot of studies have demonstrated the correlation between measurements of the ABI, TcPO2, and perfusion parameters from LAFA [66, 71, 72]. The 85 and 100% of sensitivity and specificity correlated to ABI are reported, respectively [73]. They are useful for evaluating amputation limits and predicting the further wound healing process. However, a recent cohort study reported the paradoxical decrease in perfusion following successful angioplasty, possibly due to microemboli, vasospasm, or microvascular disease. The result reported no significant correlation between the ABI and perfusion parameters. Inflow perfusion rate correlated significantly with Rutherford stage (Spearman rho 0.398, $P = 0.036$). Thirty-nine percent had a decrease in inflow rate, and 57% had a decreased total inflow after successful angioplasty. So, real-time perfusion imaging is not correlated with angiographic outcome and may not predict the possibility of wound healing [47]. Because of LAFA measurements affected by temperature and vasoactive medication, the limitation of LAFA is a severe ischemic ulcer or extensive gangrene and concomitant foot infection [66, 71, 72].

Two-dimensional perfusion angiography (2D PA) is the skin perfusion imaging method, which is used for standard DSA runs without extra ionizing radiation or contrast agents. 2D PA provides a functional status of foot perfusion. The advantages of 2D PA are providing a quantitative data for the diagnosis of PAD and success of revascularization procedures. However, DSA acquisition protocols are heterogeneous. The motion artifacts are seen in up to 10% of the patients. Ikeoka's study demonstrated the increase of mean ABI significantly from 0.87 ± 0.14 to $1.030.17$ ($p < 0.001$). Mean systolic ankle pressure increased significantly from 120 ± 24 mmHg to 137 ± 24 mmHg ($p = 0.025$) [74]. However, majority of studies have not demonstrated the correlation analysis between 2D PA parameters and ABI. Kim's study reports no significant correlation between the degree of change in 2D parameters (arrival time (AT), time to peak (TTP), AUC, peak, wash in rate, width, mean transit time (MTT), and degree of change in the ABI) [75]. Other noninvasive skin perfusion imaging methods include laser speckle contrast imaging (LSCI), micro-lightguide spectrophotometry (O_2C), near-infrared spectroscopy (NIRS), and plantar thermography (PT). Invasive techniques include contrast-enhanced ultrasound (CEUS) and computed tomography (CT) perfusion imaging. However, none of these techniques is currently widely used peri-procedurally because of lack of strong evidence-based data, high cost, and expensive imaging system [32, 33, 47].

6.9 Treatment Strategy for Limb Salvage

After all patients undergo limb staging by a classification system, such as WifI which correlates with the risk of amputation, likelihood of wound healing, and benefit for revascularization, the wound infection must be controlled, before considering the need for revascularization by surgical procedure to remove all infected tissues; then, revascularization is carried out as indicated. The diagnostic tools to complete anatomic imaging of lower extremity arterial tree should be performed [48–50]. Although catheter arteriography or DSA is the gold standard imaging technique, the CTA and MRA are preferred to investigate before revascularization in some institutions to decide the choice of revascularization and the strategic planning such as endovascular treatment or open vascular bypass procedure. DSA is typically used only when MRA or CTA is not available or imaging fails to identify the arterial anatomy, or for those patients expected to proceed to endovascular treatment at the same setting especially in below-the-knee arterial occlusive disease. Finally, physicians should not assume microangiopathic cause of unhealed ulcer or gangrene and should always consider additional high-resolution vascular imaging and revascularization in a patient with a gangrene or ischemic ulcer and PAD, irrespective of the results of initial diagnostic tests such as ABI or TBI, when the wound is not healing within 4–6 weeks despite optimal management. Without complete angiography of lower extremity artery to the foot, the physician should not deny the revascularization procedure in candidate patients [34].

6.10 Revascularization Procedure

The CLTI patients require urgent revascularization if the patient's status and arterial lesion are feasible for bypass surgery or endovascular therapy. Limb salvage rates have been reported as high as 80% for ischemic ulcers and gangrene undergoing urgent revascularization [1, 76]. The revascularization modality of choice for lower limb revascularization is multifactorial, which is determined by the patient and disease characteristics. The comorbidities, anatomic distribution and severity of disease, clinical presentation, degree of tissue loss, availability of venous conduit, as well as physician's preference and experience determine the revascularization strategy. In the new era, the "endovascular-first strategy" or "endovascular-first approach" for revascularization in patients with CLTI is generated to decrease the morbidity and mortality of the open vascular bypass procedure [77]. There are a lot of publications reporting the endovascular treatment in CLTI patients. Complex, severe, atherosclerotic occlusive disease can be treated by revascularization through endovascular-first approach, which is associated with the improvement of amputation-free survival but relative increased risk of reintervention [78]. Although the study of CLTI in the Vascular Quality Initiative (VQI) reports that the endovascular treatment procedures are more offered to older patients and who are with more comorbidities, the patients who underwent endovascular treatment still demonstrated lower perioperative mortality when compared with open vascular bypass [79]. However, long-term patency and freedom from reintervention rate of open vascular bypass procedures are better than endovascular treatment. The selection of CLTI patients for open vascular bypass or endovascular treatment should be done carefully. Finally, the endovascular-first strategy is the preferred approach for the CLTI patients. The open vascular bypass procedures are more likely to be performed for reintervention procedures, young patients, and those with few comorbidities [79]. The patient-based individual approach and risk-benefit consideration including the risk of perioperative MACE, limb amputation, reintervention, quality of life, morbidity, and mortality of each procedure are very important [80, 81].

6.11 Wound Care and Biological Therapy

Not only the revascularization procedure is mandatory in CLTI to limb salvage, but also proper wound care is promoting wound healing until the complete closure of the wound [1, 76]. In addition, the risk of revascularization should be weighed against the patient's life-threatening comorbidities. During the preoperative and postoperative periods of revascularized patients, wound care acts as an adjuvant therapy and improves the healing of ischemic ulcer. Revascularization that restores the blood flow to the foot is perfused only with the macrocirculation but does not involve microcirculation that feeds oxygen and nutrients to the ulcer directly. An ischemic process of tissue may persist in the microcirculation system, which prohibits healing process. Although wound care cannot replace surgical and endovascular revascularization, when they are used in combination, the outcome of wound healing can be significantly improved. Currently, there are a lot of advance wound therapies such as oxygen, biophysical, and biological therapies. Growth factor, platelet-rich plasma (PRP), cellular and acellular tissue-based treatment, stem cell therapies, and other bioactive wound dressing products are categorized in the biological therapy, which are the most recent advances in wound care technology. All of them are the additional modalities which are available if the ischemic wounds do not adequately heal with standard treatment after revascularization [10, 37].

6.12 Nonoperative Treatment

Nonoperative treatment in patients with CLTI is very important to stop the process of atherosclerosis [40, 52, 82]. Lifestyle modifications such as exercise with diet control and control of atherosclerotic risk factor, including blood glucose, HbA1C, LDL level, systemic blood pressure, and smoking cessation with administration of statin therapy and antiplatelet (aspirin or clopidogrel) in symptomatic PAD and CLTI, can decrease both MACE and adverse limb events such as limb amputation and reintervention rate [15, 37]. The medical treatment is related to the improvement of the clinical outcome in patients with PAD including antithrombotic therapy, lipid-lowering therapy, and antihypertensive therapy. The single antiplatelet such as aspirin or clopidogrel as well as the combination of low-dose aspirin and rivaroxaban, 2.5 mg twice, are recommended to prevent MACE in patients with CLTI. The Critical Leg Ischaemia Prevention Study (CLIPS) group which demonstrated the benefit of 100 mg of aspirin per day in patients with symptomatic PAD reported a 64% risk reduction in vascular events compared with a 24% reduction in the placebo group [83]. The Vascular Outcomes Study of Acetylsalicylic Acid Along With Rivaroxaban in Endovascular or Surgical Limb Revascularization for PAD (VOYAGER PAD) trial reported that the MACE and adverse limb event rates at 3 years of low-dose aspirin and rivaroxaban, 2.5 mg twice, and low-dose aspirin alone are 17.3% and 19.9%, respectively (hazard ratio, 0.85, 95% confidence interval [CI], 0.76–0.96; $P = 0.009$) [84]. HMG-CoA reductase inhibitors or statin therapy is associated with the inhibition of plaque rupture process. In addition, moderate- to high-intensity statin therapy may reduce cardiovascular death and MACE in patients with CLTI. Angiotensin-converting enzyme inhibitor (ACEI), angiotensin receptor blocker (ARB), calcium channel blocker, and diuretic drugs are recommended for antihypertensive therapy in PAD patients [36, 37, 52]. Phosphodiesterase III inhibitor, which is a smooth muscle cell proliferation inhibition, can increase a maximal walking distance (MWD) in IC patients and increase the patency outcome after revascularization especially in femoropopliteal arterial occlusive disease [1, 84, 85].

The Sufficient Treatment of Peripheral Intervention by Cilostazol (STOP-IC) study found that the angiographic restenosis rate at 12 months is 20% in the cilostazol group versus 49% in the noncilostazol group ($P = 0.0001$) [85]. Other medications which have showed beneficial outcome in patients with CLTI for MWD or pain-free walking distance include methylxanthine derivative (pentoxifylline), serotonin antagonist (naftidrofuryl), and prostanoid (prostaglandin E1) [1].

6.13 Conclusion

Appropriate use of vascular assessment modalities in patients with PAD and CLTI is guiding the patients to proper treatment. The delayed diagnosis of PAD and CLTI causes limb loss and increasing of the perioperative and long-term MACE. The initial diagnostic tools for macrocirculation assessment are ABI and TBI. In patients who indicate revascularization, the completion of anatomic imaging, including CTA, MRA, and DSA of lower extremity artery, is necessary for planning of the revascularization strategy. The catheter arteriography or DSA is the gold standard imaging technique, which is typically used when there is uncertain diagnosis by other imaging modalities or endovascular treatment is expected to be performed at the same setting, especially in below-the-knee segment. The microcirculation assessment plays a vital role in evaluating tissue viability, which is a significant area of concern when clinicians are managing skin necrosis. The TcPO2, SPP, SO_2, skin perfusion imaging, and other microcirculation assessment tools are advance technologies to evaluate the perfusion of the foot, which aim to evaluate the response of revascularization procedure and evaluate the possibility of wound healing. Both microcirculation and macrocirculation are used to determine the outcome after revascularization and requirement of biotherapy and other adjunctive treatments.

Acknowledgements This study was supported by the research group in surgery, Faculty of Medicine, Thammasat University.

References

1. Conte MS, Bradbury AW, Kolh P, White JV, Dick F, Fitridge R, et al. Global vascular guidelines on the management of chronic limb-threatening ischemia. Eur J Vasc Endovasc Surg. 2019;58:S1–S109.e133.
2. Orrapin S, Rerkasem K. Carotid endarterectomy for symptomatic carotid stenosis. Cochrane Database Syst Rev. 2017;6:CD001081.
3. Orrapin S, Reanpang T, Orrapin S, Arwon S, Kattipathanapong T, Lekwanavijit S, et al. Case series of HIV infection-associated arteriopathy: diagnosis, management, and outcome over a 5-year period at Maharaj Nakorn Chiang Mai Hospital, Chiang Mai University. Int J Low Extrem Wounds. 2015;14:251–61.
4. Dosluoglu HH. Chapter 108: Lower extremity arterial disease: general considerations. 8th ed. Cronenwett JL, Johnston KW, editors. Philadelphia: Elsevier; 2014.
5. Kullo IJ, Rooke TW. Clinical practice. Peripheral artery disease. N Engl J Med. 2016;374:861–71.
6. Brunicardi FC. Schwartz's principle of surgery. 10th ed. The McGraw-Hill Companies, Inc.; 2015.
7. Reanpang T, Orrapin S, Orrapin S, Arworn S, Kattipatanapong T, Srisuwan T, et al. Vascular Pythiosis of the lower extremity in northern Thailand: ten years' experience. Int J Low Extrem Wounds. 2015;14:245–50.
8. Orrapin S, Kosachunhanun N, Sony K, Inpankaew N, Sritara P, Phrommintikul A, et al. Predictive factors to determine good atherosclerotic risk factor control for diabetes patients with peripheral arterial disease [abstract]. Ann Vasc Dis. 2016;53:A05–8.
9. Orrapin S, Kosachunhanun N, Sony K, Inpankaew N, Sritara P, Phrommintikul A, et al. Undertreatment for peripheral arterial disease in diabetic patients [abstract]. Ann Vasc Dis. 2015:A09–A06.
10. Orrapin S, Rekasem K. Role of topical biological therapies and dressings in healing ischemic wounds. Int J Low Extrem Wounds. 2018;17:236–46.
11. Fowkes FGR, Rudan D, Rudan I, Aboyan V, O'Dennenerg J, McDermott MM, et al. Comparison of global estimates of prevalence and risk factors for peripheral artery disease in 2002 and 2010: a systematic review and meta-analysis. Lancet. 2013;382:1329–40.
12. Song P, Rudan D, Zhu Y, Fowkes FGI, Rahimi K, Fowkes FGR, et al. Global, regional and national prevalence and risk factors for peripheral artery disease in 2015. An updated systematic review and meta-analysis. Lancet Glob Health. 2019, 7: e1020–30.
13. Sritara P, Sritara C, Woodward M, Wangsuphachart S, Barzi F, Hengprasith B, et al. Prevalence and risk factors of peripheral arterial disease in a selected Thai population. Angiology. 2007;58:572–8.
14. Norgren L, Hiatt WR, Dormandy JA, Nehler MR, Harris KA, Fowkes FG. Inter-society consensus for the management of peripheral arterial disease (TASC II). J Vasc Surg. 2007;45 Suppl S:S5–67.
15. Olin JW, White CJ, Armstrong EJ, Kadian-Dodov D, Hiatt WR. Peripheral artery disease: evolving role of exercise, medical therapy, and endovascular options. J Am Coll Cardiol. 2016;67:1338–57.
16. Aboyans V, Ricco J-B, Bartelink M-LEL, Björck M, Brodmann M, Cohnert T, et al. Editor's choice; 2017 ESC guidelines on the diagnosis and treatment of peripheral arterial diseases, in collaboration with the European Society for Vascular Surgery (ESVS). Eur J Vasc Endovasc Surg. 2018;55:305–68.
17. Soyoye DO, Abiodun OO, Ikem RT, Kolawole BA, Akintomide O. Diabetes and peripheral artery disease. World J Diabetes. 2021;12:827–38.
18. Carmo GA, Calderaro D, Gualandro DM, Pastana AF, Yu PC, Marques AC, et al. The ankle-brachial index is associated with cardiovascular complications after noncardiac surgery. Angiology. 2016;67:187–92.
19. Alberts MJ, Bhatt DL, Mas JL, Ohman EM, Hirsch AT, Rother J, et al. Three-year follow-up and event rates in the international REduction of

Atherothrombosis for continued health registry. Eur Heart J. 2009;30:2318–26.
20. Conte MS, Geraghty PJ, Bradbury AW, Hevelone ND, Lipsitz SR, Moneta GL, et al. Suggested objective performance goals and clinical trial design for evaluating catheter-based treatment of critical limb ischemia. J Vasc Surg. 2009;50:1462–73.
21. Saraidaridis JT, Patel VI, Lancaster RT, Cambria RP, Conrad MF. Applicability of the Society for Vascular Surgery's objective performance goals for critical limb ischemia to current practice of lower-extremity bypass. Ann Vasc Surg. 2016;30:59–65.
22. Castelli WP. Epidemiology of coronary heart disease: the Framingham study. Am J Med. 1984;76:4–12.
23. Ross R. The pathogenesis of atherosclerosis: a perspective for the 1990s. Nature. 1993;362:801–9.
24. Creager MA, Belkin M, Bluth EI, Casey DE Jr, Chaturvedi S, Dake MD, et al. 2012 ACCF/AHA/ACR/SCAI/SIR/STS/SVM/SVN/SVS key data elements and definitions for peripheral atherosclerotic vascular disease: a report of the American College of Cardiology Foundation/American Heart Association task force on clinical data standards (writing committee to develop clinical data standards for peripheral atherosclerotic vascular disease). J Am Coll Cardiol. 2012;59:294–357.
25. Pearson TA, Mensah GA, Alexander RW, Anderson JL, Cannon RO, Criqui M, et al. Markers of inflammation and cardiovascular disease. Circulation. 2003;107:499.
26. Gerhard-Herman MD, Gornik HL, Barrett C, Barshes NR, Corriere MA, Drachman DE, et al. 2016 AHA/ACC guideline on the Management of Patients with Lower Extremity Peripheral Artery Disease: executive summary: a report of the American College of Cardiology/American Heart Association task force on clinical practice guidelines. Circulation. 2017;135:e686–725.
27. Kosachunhanun N, Tongprasert S, Rerkasem K. Diabetic foot problems in tertiary care diabetic clinic in Thailand. Int J Low Extrem Wound. 2012;11:124–7.
28. Lipsky BA, Aragón-Sánchez J, Diggle M, Embil J, Kono S, Lavery L, et al. IWGDF guidance on the diagnosis and management of foot infections in persons with diabetes. Diabetes Metab Res Rev. 2016;32:45–74.
29. Kayssi A, Rogers LC, Neville RF. Chapter 113: General considerations of diabetic foot ulcers. In: Sidawy AN, Perler BA, editors. Rutherford's vascular surgery and endovascular therapy. 9th ed. Philadelphia: Elsevier; 2019. p. 5001–38.
30. IWGDF Editorial Board. IWGDF definitions and criteria. 2019. https://iwgdfguidelines.org/definitions-criteria/. Accessed 23 Apr 2019.
31. IWGDF Editorial Board. IWGDF Guideline on the diagnosis and treatment of foot infection in persons with diabetes. 2019. https://iwgdfguidelines.org/infection-guideline/. Accessed 23 Apr 2019.
32. Rother U, Lang W. Noninvasive measurements of tissue perfusion in critical limb ischemia. Gefässchirurgie. 2018;23:8–12.
33. Wermelink B, Ma KF, Haalboom M, El Moumni M, de Vries J-PPM, Geelkerken RH. A systematic review and critical appraisal of peri-procedural tissue perfusion techniques and their clinical value in patients with peripheral arterial disease. Eur J Vasc Endovasc Surg. 2021;62:896–908.
34. Hinchliffe RJ, Forsythe RO, Apelqvist J, Boyko EJ, Fitridge R, Hong JP, et al. Guidelines on diagnosis, prognosis, and management of peripheral artery disease in patients with foot ulcers and diabetes (IWGDF 2019 update). Diabetes Metab Res Rev. 2020;36:e3276.
35. Skelly CL, Cifu AS. Screening, evaluation, and treatment of peripheral arterial disease. JAMA. 2016;316:1486–7.
36. Gerhard-Herman MD, Gornik HL, Barrett C, Barshes NR, Corriere MA, Drachman DE, et al. 2016 AHA/ACC guideline on the management of patients with lower extremity peripheral artery disease: executive summary. Vasc Med. 2017;22:NP1–NP43.
37. Mani R, Margolis DJ, Shukla V, Akita S, Lazarides M, Piaggesi A, et al. Optimizing technology use for chronic lower-extremity wound healing: a consensus document. Int J Low Extrem Wounds. 2016;15:102–19.
38. Rooke TW, Hirsch AT, Misra S, Sidawy AN, Beckman JA, Findeiss LK, et al. 2011 ACCF/AHA focused update of the guideline for the Management of Patients with Peripheral Artery Disease (updating the 2005 guideline): a report of the American College of Cardiology Foundation/American Heart Association task force on practice guidelines. J Am Coll Cardiol. 2011;58:2020–45.
39. Aboyans V, Criqui MH, Abraham P, Allison MA, Creager MA, Diehm C, et al. Measurement and interpretation of the ankle-brachial index: a scientific statement from the American Heart Association. Circulation. 2012;126:2890–909.
40. Tendera M, Aboyans V, Bartelink ML, Baumgartner I, Clement D, Collet JP, et al. ESC guidelines on the diagnosis and treatment of peripheral artery diseases: document covering atherosclerotic disease of extracranial carotid and vertebral, mesenteric, renal, upper and lower extremity arteries: the task force on the diagnosis and treatment of peripheral artery diseases of the European Society of Cardiology (ESC). Eur Heart J. 2011;32:2851–906.
41. Crawford F, Welch K, Andras A, Chappell FM. Ankle brachial index for the diagnosis of lower limb peripheral arterial disease. Cochrane Database Syst Rev. 2016;2016(9):Cd010680.
42. Alahdab F, Wang AT, Elraiyah TA, Malgor RD, Rizvi AZ, Lane MA, et al. A systematic review for the screening for peripheral arterial disease in asymptomatic patients. J Vasc Surg. 2015;61:42S–53S.
43. Hyun S, Forbang NI, Allison MA, Denenberg JO, Criqui MH, Ix JH. Ankle-brachial index, toe-

brachial index, and cardiovascular mortality in persons with and without diabetes mellitus. J Vasc Surg. 2014;60:390–5.
44. Arain FA, Ye Z, Bailey KR, Chen Q, Liu G, Leibson CL, et al. Survival in patients with poorly compressible leg arteries. J Am Coll Cardiol. 2012;59:400–7.
45. Randhawa MS, Reed GW, Grafmiller K, Gornik HL, Shishehbor MH. Prevalence of Tibial artery and pedal arch patency by angiography in patients with critical limb ischemia and noncompressible ankle brachial index. Circ Cardiovasc Interv. 2017;10:e004605.
46. Aboyans V, Ho E, Denenberg JO, Ho LA, Natarajan L, Criqui MH. The association between elevated ankle systolic pressures and peripheral occlusive arterial disease in diabetic and nondiabetic subjects. J Vasc Surg. 2008;48:1197–203.
47. Misra S, Shishehbor MH, Takahashi EA, Aronow HD, Brewster LP, Bunte MC, et al. Perfusion assessment in critical limb ischemia: principles for understanding and the development of evidence and evaluation of devices: a scientific statement from the American Heart Association. Circulation. 2019;140:e657–72.
48. Cerqueira LO, Duarte EG, Barros ALS, Cerqueira JR, de Araújo WJB. WIfI classification: the Society for Vascular Surgery lower extremity threatened limb classification system, a literature review. J Vasc Bras. 2020;19:e2019.
49. Darling JD, McCallum JC, Soden PA, Meng Y, Wyers MC, Hamdan AD, et al. Predictive ability of the Society for Vascular Surgery Wound, ischemia, and foot infection (WIfI) classification system following infrapopliteal endovascular interventions for critical limb ischemia. J Vasc Surg. 2016;64:616–22.
50. Mills JL Sr, Conte MS, Armstrong DG, Pomposelli FB, Schanzer A, Sidawy AN, et al. The Society for Vascular Surgery Lower Extremity Threatened Limb Classification System: risk stratification based on wound, ischemia, and foot infection (WIfI). J Vasc Surg. 2014;59:220–34.e221–222.
51. Stegemann E, Tegtmeier C, Bimpong-Buta NY, Sansone R, Uhlenbruch M, Richter A, et al. Carbondioxide-aided angiography decreases contrast volume and preserves kidney function in peripheral vascular interventions. Angiology. 2016;67:875–81.
52. Cronenwett JL, Johnston KW. Rutherford's vascular surgery. Philadelphia: Elsevier; 2014.
53. Edwards AJ, Wells IP, Roobottom CA. Multidetector row CT angiography of the lower limb arteries: a prospective comparison of volume-rendered techniques and intra-arterial digital subtraction angiography. Clin Radiol. 2005;60:85–95.
54. Ota H, Takase K, Igarashi K, Chiba Y, Haga K, Saito H, et al. MDCT compared with digital subtraction angiography for assessment of lower extremity arterial occlusive disease: importance of reviewing cross-sectional images. Am J Roentgenol. 2004;182:201–9.
55. Thomsen HS. Nephrogenic systemic fibrosis: a serious adverse reaction to gadolinium–1997–2006–2016. Part 2. Acta Radiol. 2016;57:643–8.
56. Petrovsky JS. Control of skin blood flow. Aging Skin. 2018.
57. Swain ID, Grant LJ. Methods of measuring skin blood flow. Phys Med Biol. 1989;124:34–45.
58. Holstein P, Nilsson PE, Lund P, Gyntelberg F, et al. Skin perfusion pressures in the legs measured as external pressure required for skin reddening after blanching: a photo-electric technique compared to isotope washout. Scand J Clin Lab Invest. 1980;40:535–43.
59. McKinnell T, Pape S. Measurements in burns. In: Mani R, Romanelli M, Shukla VK, editors. Measurements in wound. Healing: Springer; 2012.
60. Castronuovo JJ Jr, Adera HM, Smiell JM, Price RM. Skin perfusion pressure is valuable in the diagnosis of critical limb ischemia. J Vasc Surg. 1997;26:629–37.
61. Mani R. Transcutaneous measurements of oxygen tension in venous ulcer disease. Vasc Med Rev. 1995;6:121–31.
62. Kolari PJ, Pekenmaki K, Pohjola RT. Transcutaneous oxygen tension in patients with post-thrombotic leg ulcers: treat with intermittent pneumatic compression. Cadiovasc Res. 1988;22:138–41.
63. Arsenault KA, McDonald J, Devereaux PJ, Thorlund K, Titley JG, Whitlock PR. The use of transcutaneous oximetry to predict complications of chronic wound healing: a systematic review and meta-analysis. Wound Repair Regen. 2011;19:657–63.
64. Gurtner GC, Jones GE, Neligan PC, Newman MI, Phillips BT, Sacks JM, et al. Intraoperative laser angiography using the SPY system: a review of the literature and recommendations for use. Annals of Surg Innovations and Research. Ann Surg Innov Res. 2013;7:1.
65. Apelqvist JAP, Lepantalo MJA. The ulcerated leg when to vascularise. Diabetes Metab Res Rev. 2012;28:30–5.
66. Colvard B, Itoga NK, Hitchner E, Sun Q, Long B, Lee G, et al. SPY technology as an adjunctive measure for lower extremity perfusion. J Vasc Surg. 2016;64:95–201.
67. Zimmermann A, Roenneberg C, Reeps C, Wendorff H, Holzbach T, Eckstein HH. The determination of tissue perfusion and collateralization in peripheral arterial disease with indocyanine green fluorescence angiography. Clin Hemorheol Microcirc. 2012;50: 157–66.
68. Unno N, Suzuki M, Yamamoto N, Inuzuka K, Sagara D, Nishiyama M, et al. Indocyanine green fluorescence angiography for intraoperative assessment of blood flow: a feasibility study. Eur J Vasc Endovasc Surg. 2008;35:205–7.
69. Rother U, Lang W, Horch RE, Ludolph I, Meyer A, Gefeller O, et al. Pilot assessment of the angiosome concept by intra-operative fluorescence angiography after Tibial bypass surgery. Eur J Vasc Endovasc Surg. 2018;55:215–21.
70. Higashimori AA-OX, Takahara M, Utsunomiya M, Fukunaga M, Kawasaki D, Mori SA-OX, et al. Utility of indigo carmine angiography in patients with criti-

cal limb ischemia: prospective multi-center intervention study (DIESEL-study). Catheter Cardiovasc Interv. 2019;93:108–12.
71. Rother U, Lang W, Horch RE, Ludolph I, Meyer A, Regus S. Microcirculation evaluated by intraoperative fluorescence angiography after Tibial bypass surgery. Ann Vasc Surg. 2017;40:190–7.
72. Braun JD, Trinidad-Hernandez M, Perry D, Armstrong DG, Mills JL Sr. Early quantitative evaluation of indocyanine green angiography in patients with critical limb ischemia. J Vasc Surg. 2013;57:1213–8.
73. Igari K, Kudo T, Uchiyama H, Toyofuku T, Inoue Y. Intraarterial injection of Indocyanine green for evaluation of peripheral blood circulation in patients with peripheral arterial disease. Ann Vasc Surg. 2014;28:1280–5.
74. Ikeoka K, Hoshida S, Watanabe T, Shinoda Y, Minamisaka T, Fukuoka H, et al. Pathophysiological significance of velocity-based microvascular resistance at maximal hyperemia in peripheral artery disease. J Atheroscler Thromb. 2018;25:1128–36.
75. Kim AH, Shevitz AJ, Morrow KL, Kendrick DE, Harth K, Baele H, et al. Characterizing tissue perfusion after lower extremity intervention using two-dimensional color-coded digital subtraction angiography. J Vasc Surg. 2017;66:1464–72.
76. Frykberg RG, Banks J. Challenges in the treatment of chronic wounds. Adv Wound Care (New Rochelle). 2015;4:560–82.
77. Lin JH, Brunson A, Romano PS, Mell MW, Humphries MD. Endovascular-first treatment is associated with improved amputation-free survival in patients with critical limb ischemia. Circ Cardiovasc Qual Outcomes. 2019;12:e005273.
78. Wiseman JT, Fernandes-Taylor S, Saha S, Havlena J, Rathouz PJ, Smith MA, et al. Endovascular versus open revascularization for peripheral arterial disease. Ann Surg. 2017;265:424–30.
79. Abu Dabrh AM, Steffen MW, Asi N, Undavalli C, Wang Z, Elamin MB, et al. Bypass surgery versus endovascular interventions in severe or critical limb ischemia. J Vasc Surg. 2016;63:244–53.
80. Kaweewan R, Orrapin S, Kosachunhanun N, Sony K, Inpankaew N, Rerkasem K. Chronic leg ulcer is a strong predictor to determine the major cardiovascular events in diabetic patients with peripheral arterial disease in Thailand. Int J Diabetes Dev Ctries. 2018;38:461–70.
81. Patel MR, Conte MS, Cutlip DE, Dib N, Geraghty P, Gray W, et al. Evaluation and treatment of patients with lower extremity peripheral artery disease: consensus definitions from peripheral academic research consortium (PARC). J Am Coll Cardiol. 2015;65:931–41.
82. Antoniou GA, Hajibandeh S, Hajibandeh S, Vallabhaneni SR, Brennan JA, Torella F. Meta-analysis of the effects of statins on perioperative outcomes in vascular and endovascular surgery. J Vasc Surg. 2015;61:519–32. e511.
83. Catalano M, Born G, Peto R. Prevention of serious vascular events by aspirin amongst patients with peripheral arterial disease: randomized, double-blind trial. J Intern Med. 2007;261:276–84.
84. Bonaca MP, Bauersachs RM, Anand SS, Debus ES, Nehler MR, Patel MR, et al. Rivaroxaban in peripheral artery disease after revascularization. N Engl J Med. 2020;382:1994–2004.
85. Iida O, Yokoi H, Soga Y, Inoue N, Suzuki K, Yokoi Y, et al. Cilostazol reduces angiographic restenosis after endovascular therapy for femoropopliteal lesions in the sufficient treatment of peripheral intervention by cilostazol study. Circulation. 2013;127:2307–15.

Open Access This chapter is licensed under the terms of the Creative Commons Attribution-NonCommercial-NoDerivatives 4.0 International License (http://creativecommons.org/licenses/by-nc-nd/4.0/), which permits any non-commercial use, sharing, distribution and reproduction in any medium or format, as long as you give appropriate credit to the original author(s) and the source, provide a link to the Creative Commons license and indicate if you modified the licensed material. You do not have permission under this license to share adapted material derived from this chapter or parts of it.

The images or other third party material in this chapter are included in the chapter's Creative Commons license, unless indicated otherwise in a credit line to the material. If material is not included in the chapter's Creative Commons license and your intended use is not permitted by statutory regulation or exceeds the permitted use, you will need to obtain permission directly from the copyright holder.

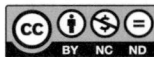

Arterial and Mixed Leg Ulcer

Monira Nou Howaldt

7.1 Introduction

Leg ulcers are chronic wounds which are unable to heal spontaneously after 4–6 weeks. The incidence of leg ulcers in the general population is around 1–2% of industrialized countries, with up to 5% of the over-80s affected. 80–90% of leg ulcers are of vascular origin, with venous involvement predominating. Arterial etiology accounts for 10–15% of leg ulcers, while mixed etiology (i.e., involving both arterial and venous involvement) accounts for 15–20% [1]. Arterial insufficiency is linked to the presence of peripheral arterial disease (PAD). Atherothrombosis is the most frequent cause of PAD. The management of arterial and mixed ulcers requires a vascular assessment involving vascular explorations and specific vascular imaging. The prognosis for healing depends on the severity of arterial ischemia: in the case of arterial ulcers, revascularization is the reference treatment, whereas in the case of mixed ulcers, the choice of revascularization will depend on the severity of arterial insufficiency and must be weighed against venous insufficiency [1].

M. Nou Howaldt (✉)
Vascular Medicine, University Hospital Center of Montpellier, Montpellier, France
e-mail: m-nou@chu-montpellier.fr

7.2 Metabolic Origin

Atherothrombosis is by far the most frequent cause of arterial ulceration. Other causes of PAD include thromboembolic causes, inflammatory vascular diseases (Horton, Takayasu, Behcet diseases), Buerger's disease, iatrogenic causes (corticosteroids, chemotherapy, etc.), and degenerative causes (fibromuscular dysplasia) [1].

Mixed ulcer combines PAD and chronic venous insufficiency, which is secondary to venous hyperpressure. The main causes of venous insufficiency are varicose veins, post-thrombotic syndrome, and functional causes [1].

7.3 Pathophysiology

- **PAD Related to Atherothrombosis**
  Artery is made up of three tunics. The innermost is the intima, made up of endothelial cells; the media is the intermediate layer, made up of smooth muscle cells; and the adventitia is the outermost layer, acting as an envelope. Atherothrombosis develops slowly over several decades, starting early but progressing very slowly as it alters the function of the intimal endothelial cells. Gradually, a thickening will appear, giving way to a plaque which may become complicated (rupture, bleeding, ulceration, etc.). Atherothrombotic plaque forms as follows: LDL cholesterol penetrates the intima and oxidizes. This leads

to endothelial cell activation, migration, and leukocyte adhesion. The accumulation of oxidized LDL leads to the agglomeration of foam cells between intima and media and the proliferation and migration of smooth muscle cells. Gradually, a lipid core forms, creating a plaque that is covered by a fibrous cap of muscle cells. In the event of plaque rupture or bleeding, arterial thrombosis may occur, obstructing the vessel lumen (Fig. 7.1). Arterial obstruction generates ischemia and tissue hypoxia, leading to skin necrosis [2–4].
- **Mixed ulcers are associated with venous insufficiency**
Ninety percent of venous return is provided by the deep veins and 10% by the superficial veins (saphenous veins and their tributaries). The two networks communicate via perforating veins (Dodd, Hunter, Boyd, and Cockett), saphenous junctions, and Giacomini's vein, which provides an anastomosis between the saphenous veins. The veins are equipped with valves that prevent the blood from flowing back downwards in an orthostatic position. Pressure in the veins is determined by two components: hydrostatic pressure (weight of the blood column) and hemodynamics resulting from muscle contraction. In a static position, venous pressure is around 90 mmHg at the ankles. On initiation of walking, this pressure gradually decreases to an average of 30 mmHg, thanks to the contraction of the calf muscles (muscular pump) and the crushing of the plantar sole, which

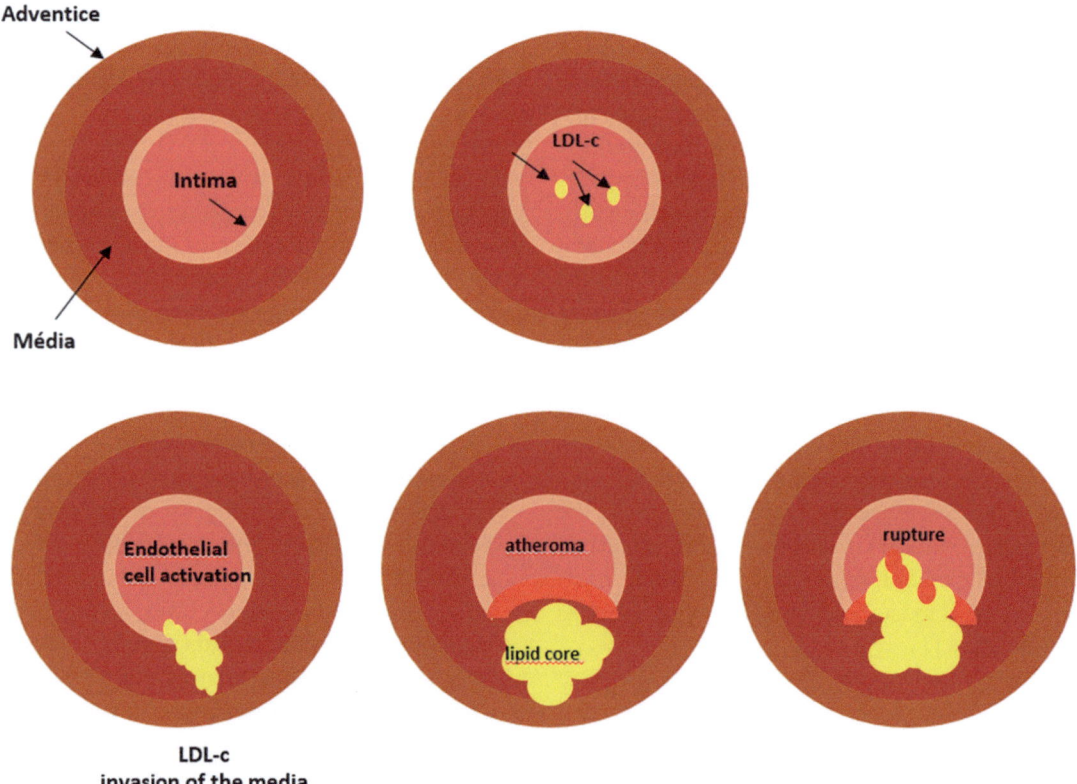

Fig. 7.1 From top to bottom: Atherothrombotic plaque formation in an artery

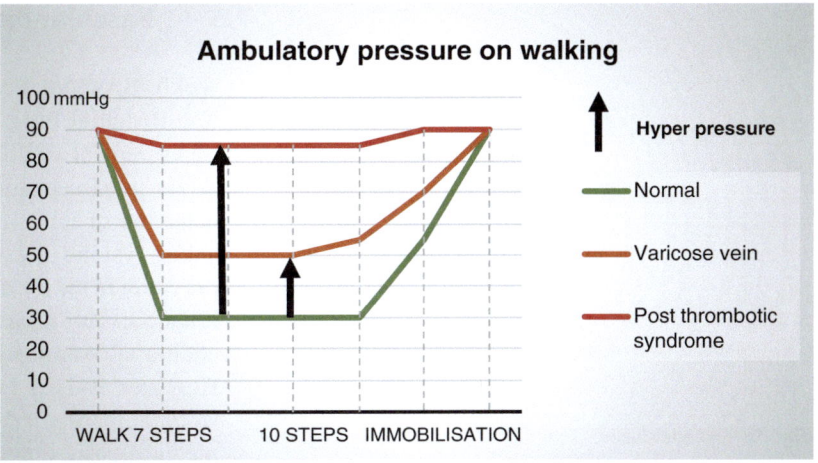

Fig. 7.2 Evolution of venous pressure in the lower limbs when walking. Hyperpressure in subjects with varicose veins or post-thrombotic syndrome

behaves like a veritable blood-filled sponge (Fig. 7.2). The valvular system ensures segment-by-segment return of the blood column, and the abdominodiaphragmatic system acts on hydrostatic pressure [5, 6].

Chronic venous insufficiency is linked to poor venous return, which generates venous and veno-capillary hyperpressure. The result is capillary and venous dilatation, increased endothelial cell permeability, and leukocyte infiltration, leading to toxin accumulation and cellular hypoxia, which in turn leads to the production of inflammatory mediators. Ultimately, this leads to skin remodeling, culminating in the appearance of skin ulceration [5, 6].

7.4 Clinical Diagnosis

- **Arterial ulcer**
  Arterial ulcers are painful trophic disorders. Most often of recent onset (a few days to a few weeks), it is located on both the leg and the foot. The patient has cardiovascular risk factors (hypertension, diabetes, smoking, dyslipidemia, etc.). The characteristics of arterial ulcers are as follows: rounded, clean edges, possible exposure of underlying structures (tendon, bone), low exudation, and presence of necrosis (Fig. 7.3) [1].
  Skin involvement is accompanied by signs of arterial insufficiency: intermittent claudication of the lower limbs (i.e., pain in the lower limbs when walking), pain at rest, coldness, paleness of the limb with declivity erythrocyanosis, coldness of the foot, disorders of the *Phanera* (thin skin; thick, brittle nails; depilation; dry skin, etc.), and sometimes amyotrophy when the PAD has been evolving for a long time [3].

- **Mixed ulcer**
  Mixed ulcers combine signs of arterial ulceration with signs of chronic venous insufficiency. Signs of venous stasis include edema, phlebalgia (pain along the veins), and corona radiata phlebectatica. Skin changes such as ochre dermatitis (brown pigmentation of the leg due to hemosiderin deposition), lipodermatosclerosis, inflammatory hypodermatitis, and Milian's white atrophy may also be present [1]. The mixed ulcer is exudative and can be painful, and the peri-ulcer skin is pathological (erythema, maceration, hyperkeratosis,

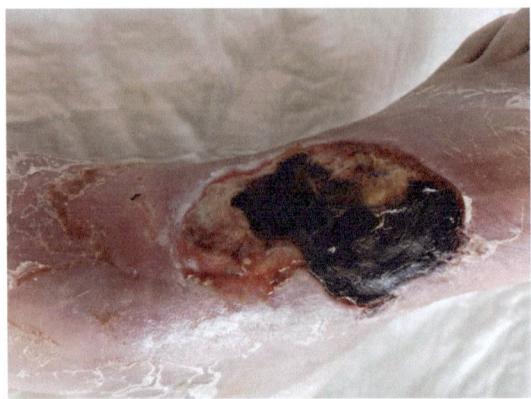

Fig. 7.3 Arterial ulcer

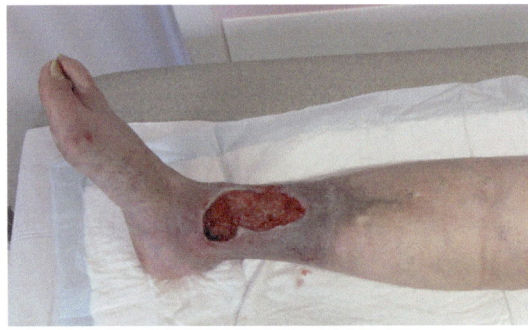

Fig. 7.4 Mixed ulcer predominantly venous

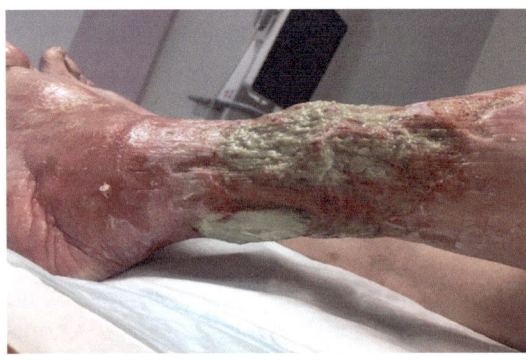

Fig. 7.5 Mixed ulcer predominantly arterial with exposed tendon

eczema). The difficulty lies in assessing the predominant vascular component, as this will determine the choice of treatment (Figs. 7.4 and 7.5).

7.5 Vascular Explorations

- **Ankle-Brachial Pressure Index (ABI) and Toe-Brachial Index (TBI)**
  Measurement of ABI is recommended, as it offers good sensitivity and specificity in the detection of PAD (Fig. 7.6). It is the ratio of ankle systolic pressure to humeral systolic pressure. In the event of a result <0.91 or >1.4, it is necessary to search for PAD by means of additional examinations [2–4, 7].
  However, PAD is less accurate in the case of wounds, particularly if there is Mönckeberg mediacalcosis (calcium deposits in the arterial wall responsible for parietal stiffness). The guidelines recommend measuring toe systolic pressure and calculating the TBI, which is the ratio of toe systolic pressure to humeral systolic pressure, in patients with diabetes and kidney failure and the very elderly (Fig. 7.7). The pathological threshold is a ratio <0.7 [2, 3, 7].

- **Arterial Doppler Ultrasound of the Lower Limbs**
  Arterial Doppler ultrasound is a noninvasive, first-line examination for leg ulcers. It is thus possible to visualize hemodynamically significant arterial lesions (stenoses or occlusions) that may explain the ischemic picture [7].
  In the case of mixed ulcers, arterial assessment must be complemented by an analysis of the venous network, in order to identify the cause of superficial venous insufficiency (varicose veins) or deep venous insufficiency (post-thrombotic syndrome). In the case of varicose veins, there is venous reflux, and in the case of post-thrombotic syndrome, there may be obstructive sequelae or valvular incompetence [8].

- **Venous Doppler Ultrasound of the Lower Limbs**
  This exploration is indicated in case of venous insufficiency signs in order to detect varicosis or to research a post-thrombotic syndrome. This test can be used to detect venous reflux.

Figs. 7.6 and 7.7 Measurement of ankle-brachial pressure index (ABI) and toe-brachial index (TBI)

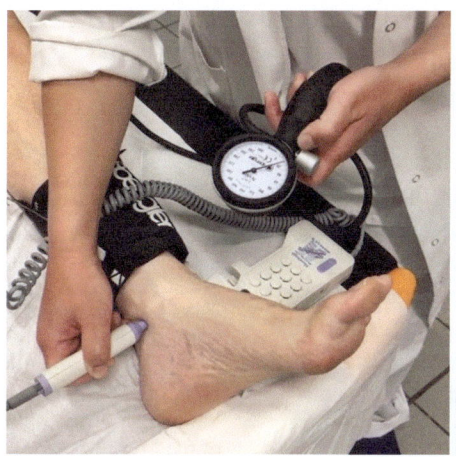
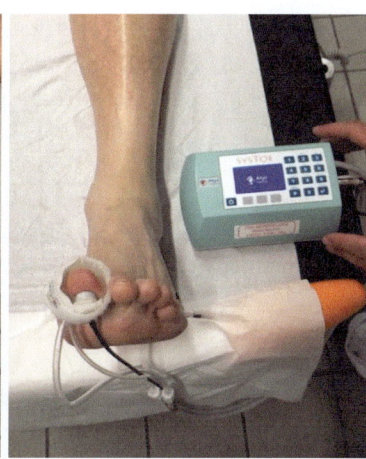

- **TcPO$_2$**
  This is a subcutaneous oxygen pressure measurement. Using polarographic sensors (Clark electrodes) positioned close to the trophic disorder, an automaton will record an 02 pressure value expressed in mmHg. The cutoff value for healing is 30 mmHg. Below this value, the prognosis for healing is very poor, and impossible if <10 mmHg [7].

- **Vascular Imaging**
  Vascular imaging (CT angiography, MRI angiography, or arteriography of the lower limbs) is essential if revascularization is to be performed. These examinations enable a more detailed analysis of the lesions detected by echo-Doppler. Arteriography is used in cases where the sub-popliteal arterial axes of the leg are affected, as it is more effective than MRI or CT angiography in exploring the leg axes, especially if there is mediacalcosis.

7.6 Treatment

Arterial ulcer treatment aims to correct arterial ischemia. Revascularization may be proposed either by surgery or by transluminal angioplasty. Medical treatment of PAD combining lipid-lowering therapy, antiplatelet therapy, and a converting enzyme inhibitor is systematically associated with the control of cardiovascular risk factors and a healthy lifestyle including daily walking [2–4, 7].

There are no recommendations to guide the therapeutic management of mixed ulcers, and the role of compression therapy for patients with ABI <0.8 is controversial as there is thought to be a greater risk of iatrogenic skin damage with the use of compression therapy in the presence of arterial disease. However, it has been demonstrated that modified compression therapy, using short stretch or inelastic material with a pressure <40 mmHg, is very effective in obtaining healing of a mixed ulcer, provided that the absolute value of the ankle pressure is >60 mmHg, the toe pressure >30 mmHg, and the ABI >0.6 [8–11]. In addition, curative treatment of superficial venous insufficiency would be effective in treating mixed ulcers [8–10]. In case of post-thrombotic syndrome, for patients with iliac vein outflow obstruction and severe symptoms/signs, endovascular treatment should be considered [8].

Revascularization may nevertheless be necessary if compression is no longer tolerated and the wound no longer progresses, or if it worsens under compression.

7.7 Conclusion

Since 80–90% of leg ulcers have a vascular cause, a vascular assessment using ABI, TBI, and arterial and/or venous Doppler ultrasound should be carried out systematically in the case of chronic leg or foot wounds. Arterial ulceration is a serious pathology resulting from arterial insufficiency and responsible for ischemia. The appearance of necrosis is often a clinical element that guides the diagnosis, and revascularization is the only curative treatment. In the case of mixed ulcer, management will depend on the degree of severity of the PAD, which can be quantified and assessed using the various vascular function tests. Venous insufficiency must not be neglected, as this may delay healing. Appropriate venous compression is often necessary in the case of mixed ulcers and warrants monitoring of treatment tolerance and efficacy.

References

1. Nou Howaldt M, et al. Vascular assessment for chronic wounds of the lower limbs. La Lettre du Médecin Vascul. 2022.
2. Franck U, et al. Guideline on peripheral arterial disease. Vasa. 2019;48(Suppl 102). https://doi.org/10.1026/a000002.
3. Task Force Members. 2017 ESC guideline on the diagnosis and treatment of peripheral arterial diseases, in collaboration with the European Society for Vascular Surgery (ESVS). Eur Heart J. 2018;39:763–816. https://doi.org/10.1093/eurheartj/ehx095.
4. Criqui MH, et al. Lower extremity peripheral artery disease: contemporary epidemiology, management gaps and future directions: a scientific statement from the American Heart Association. Circulation. 2021;144:e171–91.
5. Nou Howaldt M, Quéré I, Godin SM, Henneton P, Tapon M, Laroche JP. Venous chronic insufficiency. In: Guillevin L, Mouthon L, Lêvesque H, editors. Traîté de médecine. 5th ed. Paris: Tdm Edition; 2018. p. 1–8.
6. Youn YJ, Lee J. Chronic venous insufficiency and varicose veins of the lower extremities. Kor J Intern Med. 2019;34:269–83.
7. Mahé G, et al. Disparities between international guidelines (AHA/ESC/ESVS/ESVM/SVS) concerning lower extremity peripheral arterial disease. Consensus of the French Society of Vascular Medicine (SFMV) and the French Society for Vascular and Endovascular Surgery (SCVE). Ann Vasc Surg. 2020;72:1–56.
8. De Maeseneer MG, et al. European Society for Vascular Surgery (ESVS) 2022 clinical practice guidelines on the management of chronic venous disease of the lower limbs. Eur J Vasc Endovasc Surg. 2022;63:184–267. https://doi.org/10.1016/j.ejvs.2021.12.024.
9. Mosti G, et al. Compression therapy in mixed ulcers increases venous output and arterial perfusion. J Vasc Surg. 2012;55:122–8.
10. Mosti G, et al. Recalcitrant venous leg ulcers may heal by outpatient treatment of venous disease even in the presence of concomitant arterial occlusive disease. Eur J Vasc Endovasc Surg. 2016;52:385–91.
11. Lim SLX, et al. Modified compression therapy in mixed arterial–venous leg ulcers: an integrative review. Int Wound J. 2021;18:822–42.

Open Access This chapter is licensed under the terms of the Creative Commons Attribution-NonCommercial-NoDerivatives 4.0 International License (http://creativecommons.org/licenses/by-nc-nd/4.0/), which permits any non-commercial use, sharing, distribution and reproduction in any medium or format, as long as you give appropriate credit to the original author(s) and the source, provide a link to the Creative Commons license and indicate if you modified the licensed material. You do not have permission under this license to share adapted material derived from this chapter or parts of it.

The images or other third party material in this chapter are included in the chapter's Creative Commons license, unless indicated otherwise in a credit line to the material. If material is not included in the chapter's Creative Commons license and your intended use is not permitted by statutory regulation or exceeds the permitted use, you will need to obtain permission directly from the copyright holder.

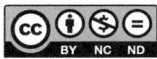

Part II

Different Clinical Context of Skin Necrosis Physical Injuries

Introduction to Physical Injuries in Skin Necrosis

Sebastian Probst

Skin necrosis, a distressing condition characterized by the death of skin cells and tissues, is a medical concern with a range of underlying causes [1]. Physical injuries leading to skin necrosis are one of the most common triggers for this condition, posing serious challenges to patients and healthcare professionals alike. Whether the result of trauma, extremes of temperature, radiation exposure, or electric shock, skin necrosis can have devastating consequences, impacting the affected individuals' quality of life and often requiring complex medical interventions. This chapter aims to explore the various forms of physical injuries that can lead to skin necrosis, their underlying mechanisms, and the potential treatment strategies employed to manage and alleviate the distressing effects of this condition. Understanding the complexities of skin necrosis due to physical injuries is crucial for early detection, prompt intervention, and, ultimately, improvement of patient outcomes. Through enhanced awareness and comprehensive research, health care professionals can strive to prevent and mitigate the burden of skin necrosis in those vulnerable to its development.

Reference

1. Hakkarainen TW, Kopari NM, Pham TN, Evans HL. Necrotizing soft tissue infections: review and current concepts in treatment, systems of care, and outcomes. Curr Probl Surg. 2014;51(8):344–62. https://doi.org/10.1067/j.cpsurg.2014.06.001.

S. Probst (✉)
HES-SO University of Applied Sciences and Arts Western Switzerland, Geneva, Switzerland
e-mail: sebastian.probst@hesge.ch

Open Access This chapter is licensed under the terms of the Creative Commons Attribution-NonCommercial-NoDerivatives 4.0 International License (http://creativecommons.org/licenses/by-nc-nd/4.0/), which permits any non-commercial use, sharing, distribution and reproduction in any medium or format, as long as you give appropriate credit to the original author(s) and the source, provide a link to the Creative Commons license and indicate if you modified the licensed material. You do not have permission under this license to share adapted material derived from this chapter or parts of it.

The images or other third party material in this chapter are included in the chapter's Creative Commons license, unless indicated otherwise in a credit line to the material. If material is not included in the chapter's Creative Commons license and your intended use is not permitted by statutory regulation or exceeds the permitted use, you will need to obtain permission directly from the copyright holder.

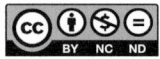

9

Skin Mechanobiology: From Basic Science to Clinical Applications

Aleksei Orlov and Amit Gefen

9.1 Introduction

The skin forms the physical interface between the human body and the environment, and its mechanical properties are therefore important in both health and disease. Among other functions, this largest organ of the human body constantly counteracts external and internal mechanical forces during all daily activities. For tolerating these forces, the human skin has evolved to have remarkable biomechanical properties that are uniquely suited to its function, both locally and overall. While it is relevant to know how skin tissue deforms and fails from a basic science aspect, it is even more important, from an applied medical-clinical perspective, to understand how mechanical forces act on skin tissue to maintain normal tissue physiology and to regulate inherent biological processes such as wound healing. In addition to its protective mechanical function and ability to conform to the changing body structure, the skin maintains water equilibrium in the body, reduces heat and water loss, and contains nerve fibers for sensation and immune-responsive cells [1, 2].

The external layer of the skin, called the epidermis, varies in thickness depending on its anatomical location and function. This layer consists of a stratified squamous epithelium of keratinocytes, delimited by the basal membrane and containing melanocytes, Langerhans cells, and Merkel cells [3, 4]. The internal skin layer, termed the dermis, is a connective tissue that represents most of the skin substance and structure. The dermis is composed of fibroblasts and extracellular matrix (ECM) enriched in collagen and elastin fibers and can be divided into two sublayers: the upper papillary and the thicker lower reticular dermis. The skin mechanical properties at a certain anatomical site, such as the stiffness and strength, are mostly due to the local composition, organization, and directional preference of the ECM microarchitecture in the dermis [5]. Lastly, beneath the dermis is the hypodermis which is composed primarily of adipocyte cells that store lipids and triglycerides; this is often not regarded as an integral part of the skin organ.

Healthy skin tissue is normally "pre-stretched" over the body surfaces, that is, has inherent residual tension internally (known as residual tension stresses), but upon even a small incisional wound, the skin relaxes as cell-cell and cell-matrix forces

A. Orlov
Department of Biomedical Engineering, Faculty of Engineering, Tel Aviv University, Tel Aviv, Israel
e-mail: alexeyorlov@mail.tau.ac.il

A. Gefen (✉)
Department of Biomedical Engineering, Faculty of Engineering, Tel Aviv University, Tel Aviv, Israel

Skin Integrity Research Group (SKINT), University Centre for Nursing and Midwifery, Department of Public Health and Primary Care, Ghent University, Ghent, Belgium

Department of Mathematics and Statistics, Faculty of Sciences, Hasselt University, Hasselt, Belgium
e-mail: gefen@tauex.tau.ac.il

are disrupted at the wound margins, and the wound may thereby extend with respect to its original shape. Skin damage can be the result of an extrinsic trauma such as a mechanical, thermal, or chemical insult. Alternatively, skin cell and tissue damage may develop over time due to a chronic disease or condition that increases the fragility of the skin itself or disables the protective discomfort and pain sensation, which originates in the skin, or compromises the supportive vascular and lymphatic structures leading to, for example, skin tears, frictional blisters, diabetic foot ulcers, venous leg ulcers, and pressure ulcers/injuries; all of these wounds may deteriorate to involve infection or even cause sepsis and osteomyelitis [6].

9.2 Skin Biomechanics on a Tissue Scale

For those patients who suffer from loss of mobility, the skin viability and integrity are constantly challenged by external factors, particularly frictional forces at the skin surface that typically intensify due to moisture and wetness, and are further affected by the characteristics of the clothing and bedsheet materials, the body habitus, the posture, and any relative motion between the skin and contacting objects (Fig. 9.1) [7, 8]. Frictional forces may strip the stratum corneum, which triggers inflammation and opens a portal for infections. A combination of pressures and shear stresses, which is always present in real-world conditions, may, above a critical level, further cause the dermal blood vessels to be distorted and angulated in a manner that compromises perfusion and, thereby, normal skin metabolism [9]. Specifically, moisture on the skin is known to increase the coefficient of friction (COF) between the skin and any contacting object (Fig. 9.1), which in turn elevates the frictional forces and shear stresses on and within the skin, as the frictional force is proportional to the COF [7, 8, 10]. Moisture or wetness also weakens the dermal-epidermal anchoring complex and dissolves collagen, which eventually manifests macroscopically as skin maceration [11, 12]. The tolerance of skin to the intensity and duration of frictional forces and shear stresses depends on numerous factors such as the age, chronic conditions affecting the skin structure, function, vascular status, and inflammatory status such as diabetes, obesity, and central nervous system injuries, as well as the anatomical site, the individual orientation of the Langer lines, and the level of dryness of the skin [9, 13]. In particular, it was shown that shear stresses in the superficial skin (stratum corneum) increase with the depth of age wrinkles or development of nonage-related wrinkles [7, 8, 14]. It was further demonstrated that a rise in the local skin temperature, or in the ambient temperature or in the relative humidity, as well as a decreased permeability of the support surface materials in contact with the skin or in close proximity to the skin, all raise the risk for pressure ulcers/injuries [10]. Related to that, repositioning an elderly bed-bound patient with their aged, stiffer and wrinkled skin, under moist or wet conditions, increases the risk of superficial pressure ulcers/injuries forming during the repositioning (Fig. 9.1) [15]. Accordingly, in individuals confined to wheelchairs or beds, wetness of the skin in weight-bearing body regions should be avoided.

An effective biomechanical means to mitigate pressure and friction damage to skin in the context of pressure ulcer/injury prevention is through the use of multilayer silicone-foam prophylactic dressings. Schwartz and colleagues [16] investigated relationships between design features and biomechanical efficacy of sacral prophylactic dressings. Using computer modeling, they simulated a commercial anisotropic multilayer dressing and another hypothetical dressing with different mechanical properties, under dry and three levels of moist/wet conditions. They developed 16 finite element model variants representing the buttocks with applied dressings. Their model variants utilized slices of a weight-bearing female buttocks for segmentation of the pelvic

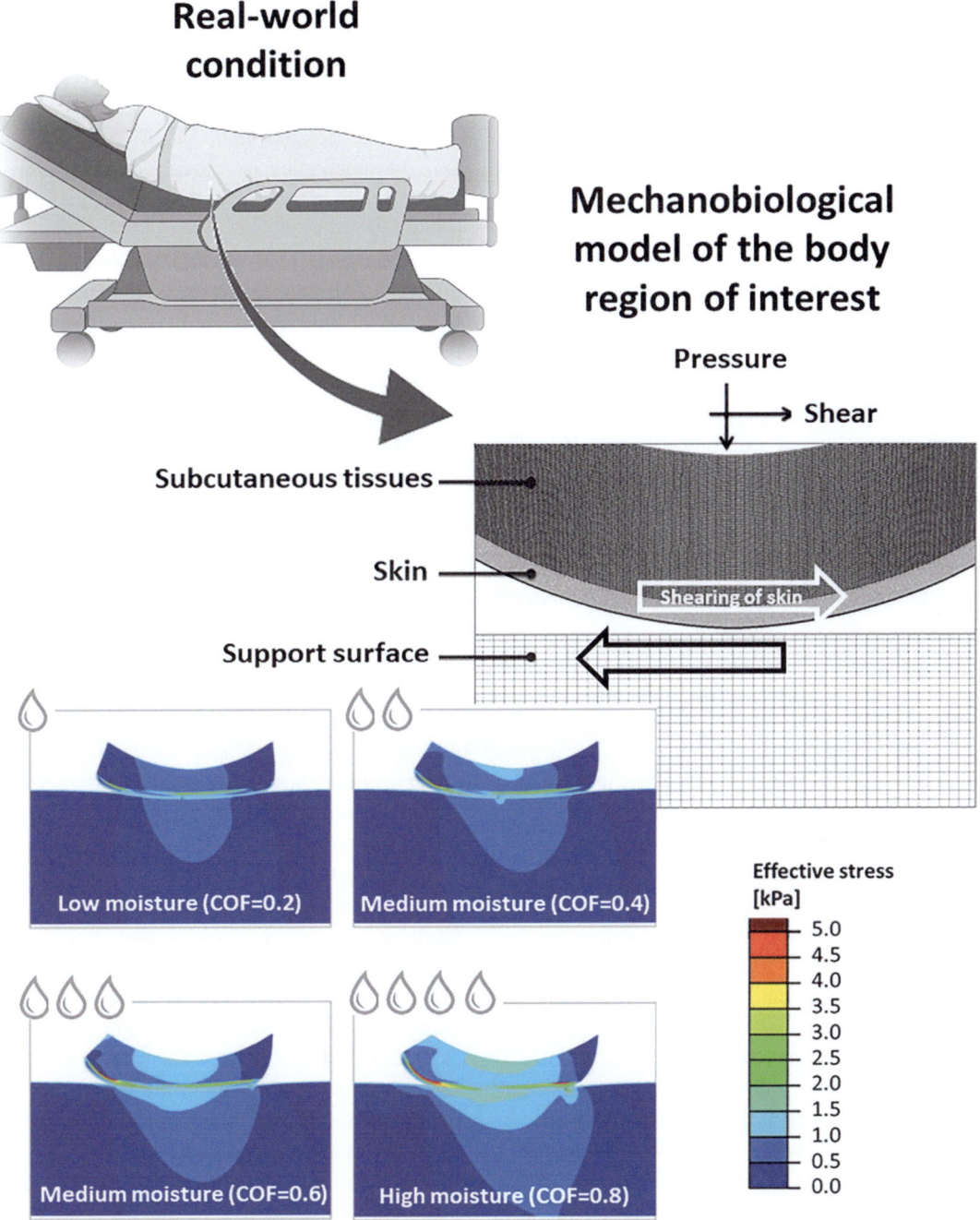

Fig. 9.1 Biomechanical computational modeling of a skin region under a bony prominence in a person lying supine in a hospital bed (top frame). As gravity pulls the patient's body towards the foot of the bed, skin is sheared between the support surface and the underlying tissues (middle frame). With the level of moisture that exists in the microenvironment, the coefficient of friction (COF) increases, e.g., due to perspiration or incontinence, which intensifies the level of shear stress and the overall stress magnitudes that the skin experiences (bottom frame). The detailed study results are reported in [17]

bones and soft tissues [16]. Effective stresses and maximal shear stresses in a volume of interest of soft tissues surrounding the sacrum were calculated from the simulations, and a protective endurance index was further calculated for the different dressing cases [16]. Resistance to tissue deformations along the direction of the spine in the presence of wetness was determined by rating simulation outcomes (i.e., the volumetric exposures to effective stress) for the different dressing conditions. Based on this analysis, the studied commercial anisotropic multilayer prophylactic dressing exhibited superior protective endurance (80%), which was approximately four times that of the hypothetical dressing (22%) [16]. The above Schwartz et al.'s study provided important insights regarding the optimal design of prophylactic dressings for effective skin protection in individuals who are at a risk of developing pressure ulcers/injuries, especially when exposed to moisture [16].

Bioengineering studies of how the skin interacts with prophylactic dressings are not only limited to protecting the sacral area. For example, prone positioning is used for surgical access and also, more recently, was used widely while treating COVID patients who are ventilated prone. To reduce the risk for a facial pressure ulcer/injury, prophylactic dressings can be used on the head. Peko and colleagues [17] evaluated facial soft tissue exposures to sustained mechanical loads in a prone position, with versus without multilayer silicone foam dressings applied as tissue protectors at the forehead and chin. They used an anatomically realistic validated computer (finite element) model of an adult male head to determine the contribution of the dressings to the alleviation of the sustained tissue loads. They found that the application of the dressings considerably relieved the tissue exposures to loading [17]. Specifically, with respect to the forehead, the application of a prophylactic dressing of the studied type on the facial skin resulted in 52 and 71% reductions in soft tissue exposures to effective stresses and strain energy densities, respectively. Likewise, a chin dressing of the type under investigation lowered the soft tissue exposures to stresses and strain energy densities by 78% and 92%, respectively.

Another related field where knowledge on skin biomechanics is critical for effective skin protection is in the prevention of medical device-related pressure ulcers/injuries [18]. Peko-Cohen and colleagues [19] studied the biomechanical efficacy of prophylactic dressings in protection from facial injuries caused by noninvasive ventilation masks, which are commonly used for respiratory support where intubation (or a surgical procedure) can be avoided, including in COVID patients who suffer a respiratory distress syndrome. However, prolonged use of respiratory masks involves risk to facial skin, which is subjected to sustained deformations caused by tightening of the mask and humid microclimate conditions. The risk of developing such medical device-related pressure ulcers/injuries can be reduced substantially by providing additional cushioning at the mask-face interface. Accordingly, the Peko-Cohen study [19] determined differences in facial tissue stresses while using a respiratory mask with versus without using foam dressing cuts. First, they developed a force measurement system that was used to experimentally determine the local forces applied to skin at the bridge of the nose, cheeks, and chin while using a mask. They further demonstrated facial temperature distributions after use of the mask using infrared thermography [19]. Next, using the finite element method, Peko-Cohen et al. [19] delivered the measured compressive forces per site of the face in the model and compared maximal facial effective stresses with versus without the dressing cuts. The dressings have shown substantial biomechanical effectiveness in protecting facial skin from device-related pressure ulcers/injuries by providing localized cushioning to skin sites at risk. Taken together, the above studies clearly demonstrate the importance of understanding skin tissue biomechanics for the development and evaluation of clinical methods for skin protection.

9.3 The Mechanobiology of Skin at a Cell Scale: Focus on Fibroblasts

Dermal fibroblasts are the main cell type present in the dermis. These fibroblasts interact with epidermal cells and immune cells and play an essential role during cutaneous wound healing. Fibroblasts are known to be highly mechanoresponsive; namely, if a wound forms, the mechanical properties and deformations of the wound and peri-wound skin influence the proliferation and collective migration of fibroblasts into the wound site [20], which are essential for epithelization of the wound bed, granulation, revascularization, and, eventually, tissue repair and scar formation [21]. The adhesive interactions, likelihood of apoptosis, and velocity and directionality of the collective cell migration are also affected by the wound environment, and specifically by its mechanical environment such as the tissue stiffness characteristics and the level and regime of deformations that apply within and in the vicinity of the wound (Fig. 9.2) [22].

The above understanding led to the development of the biological theory for the mode of action of negative-pressure wound therapy at the cell niche, which is supported by robust experimental evidence from cell culture assays (Fig. 9.2). Specifically, during the proliferative phase of the normal wound healing cascade, dermal fibroblasts proliferate and migrate into the wound bed to fill the gap, synthesize growth factors, and, ultimately, produce new ECM. This collective fibroblast migration followed by collagen synthesis by the arriving cells results in the scarring of wounded skin [23]. As such, dermal fibroblast migration into wounds is vital for wound healing, and therefore, in vitro "wound healing" assays typically focus on the kinematics of migration of these cells, e.g., through transwell assays, stopper-based assays, and scratch assays [24, 25]. The cell migration behavior observed in monolayer fibroblast culture models in vitro was found to be informative and useful with respect to understanding the in vivo cell migration process, specifically with regard to factors that accelerate or inhibit collective fibroblast migration, including mechanobiological factors such as the substrate stiffness and pre-stretch levels (Fig. 9.2) [26–28]. With regard to the latter factor, it has been shown that the mechanical stretching of cells and their environment (within a certain optimal domain) triggers intracellular biochemical signaling, which increases the expression of various proteins (e.g., fibronectin), alters gene expression, and activates molecular pathways of proliferation, differentiation, or angiogenesis [23]. Mechanobiology work in fibroblast cultures revealed that these cells are irresponsive to low strains below 0.5%; however, fibroblasts may accelerate their collective migration towards a damaged site in response to strains above 3%. Given that it was demonstrated that the plasma membranes of cells may be damaged above strains of ~12%, there must be a strain sweet spot within the 0.5–12% range for optimally stimulating fibroblasts to migrate in response to mechanical perturbations [23, 29, 30]. This new mechanobiological knowledge, implemented in the design of advanced negative-pressure wound therapy system hardware and treatment protocols, will improve both clinical outcomes and cost-benefit measures in skin and wound care.

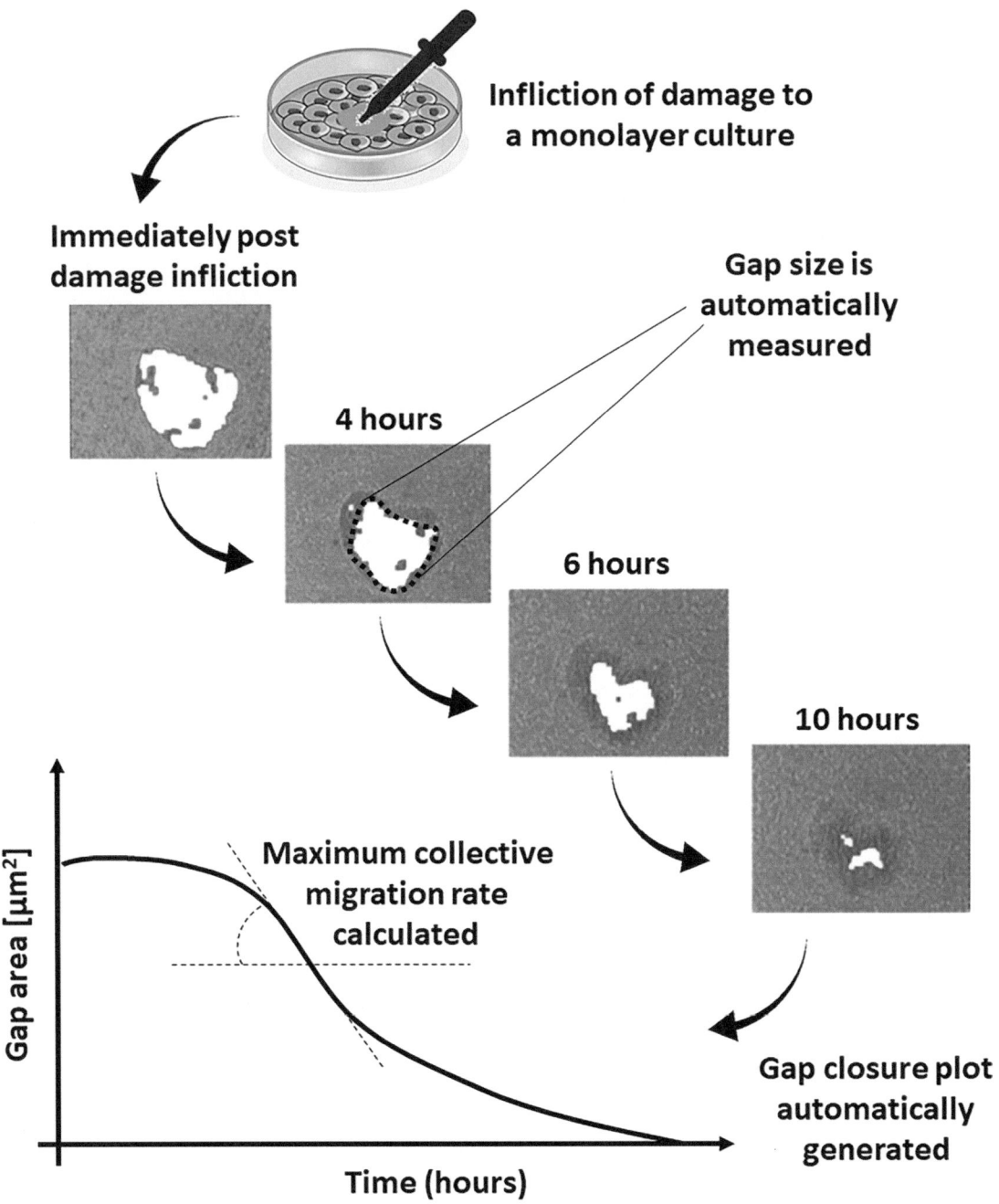

Fig. 9.2 Fibroblasts are skin-repairing cells which are stimulated by an immune response to migrate into sites of cell and tissue damage for synthesis of collagen in order to form scar tissue. Automated migration assays developed at Professor Gefen's research group ([21] and articles cited therein), which are illustrated here, allow objective, quantitative, standardized, and cost-effective tracking of the collective cell migration for studies of environmental factors such as the mechanobiological conditions (e.g., the level of stretch or the stiffness of the substrate) or the biochemical conditions (e.g., the pH level or certain medium supplements) and how they may affect damage accumulation and repair. The size of the gap in fibroblast cultures over time and the dynamics of the repair process automatically captured by digital optical microscopy allow to determine characteristic closure times and speeds, per specific experimental conditions, using custom-made image processing software developed for these studies, as reported in [21] and the previous Gefen group articles cited there

9.4 Conclusion

Understanding the mechanobiology of human skin at both the macroscopic and microscopic scales not only has a basic science objective; it is also essential for protecting the skin integrity and viability. This was demonstrated in this chapter in the context of bioengineering studies to achieve more effective pressure ulcer/injury prevention using prophylactic dressings, and as related to repairing damaged skin by promoting dermal fibroblast migration into a wound site using contemporary negative-pressure wound therapy systems.

The bioengineering work conducted at the senior author's (AG) research group for the last two decades utilizes an integrated approach including studies of skin physiology and microclimate conditions, e.g., by means of infrared thermography, subepidermal moisture measurements, analysis of skin inflammatory markers, anatomically realistic computer (finite element) modeling and simulations (Fig. 9.1), cell culture studies including microscopy and image processing methods (Fig. 9.2), and, importantly, a combination of all of these together, to form a hierarchical description of the mechanobiology of human skin, from the cell to the organ level. As the above research methods continue to improve and reveal the mechanobiology of skin in health and disease, bioengineers can now create better skin and wound care technologies, including enhanced dressings for prophylaxis and treatment of wounds, non-dressing-based skin protection methods, novel negative-pressure wound therapy systems for superior wound closure, etc.

Acknowledgements This work has received funding from the European Union's Horizon 2020 research and innovation programme under the Marie Skłodowska-Curie Grant Agreement No. 811965, project STINTS (Skin Tissue Integrity under Shear). This work was also partially supported by the Israeli Ministry of Science and Technology (Medical Devices Program Grant no. 3-17421, awarded to Professor Amit Gefen in 2020).

References

1. Groves RB. Quantifying the mechanical properties of skin in vivo and ex vivo to optimise microneedle device design. Cardiff University; 2016.
2. Groves RB, Coulman SA, Birchall JC, Evans SL. Quantifying the mechanical properties of human skin to optimise future microneedle device design. Comput Methods Biomech Biomed Engin. 2012;15:73–82. https://doi.org/10.1080/10255842.2011.596481.
3. Kamel RA, Ong JF, Eriksson E, Junker JPE, Caterson EJ. Tissue engineering of skin. J Am Coll Surg. 2013;217:533–55. https://doi.org/10.1016/J.JAMCOLLSURG.2013.03.027.
4. Gantwerker EA, Hom DB. Skin: histology and physiology of wound healing. Clin Plast Surg. 2012;39:85–97. https://doi.org/10.1016/J.CPS.2011.09.005.
5. Oxlund H, Manschot J, Viidik A. The role of elastin in the mechanical properties of skin. J Biomech. 1988;21:213–8. https://doi.org/10.1016/0021-9290(88)90172-8.
6. Lawton S. Maintaining skin health in older people. Nurs Older People. 2018;30:42–8. https://doi.org/10.7748/NOP.2018.E1082.
7. Gerhardt LC, Mattle N, Schrade GU, Spencer ND, Derler S. Study of skin-fabric interactions of relevance to decubitus: friction and contact-pressure measurements. Skin Res Technol. 2008;14:77–88. https://doi.org/10.1111/J.1600-0846.2007.00264.X.
8. Gerhardt LC, Strässle V, Lenz A, Spencer ND, Derler S. Influence of epidermal hydration on the friction of human skin against textiles. J R Soc Interface. 2008;5:1317–28. https://doi.org/10.1098/RSIF.2008.0034.
9. Garcia AD, Thomas DR. Assessment and management of chronic pressure ulcers in the elderly. Med Clin North Am. 2006;90:925–44. https://doi.org/10.1016/J.MCNA.2006.05.018.
10. Gefen A. How do microclimate factors affect the risk for superficial pressure ulcers: a mathematical modeling study. J Tissue Viability. 2011;20:81–8. https://doi.org/10.1016/J.JTV.2010.10.002.
11. Agam L, Gefen A. Pressure ulcers and deep tissue injury: a bioengineering perspective. J Wound Care. 2013;16:336–42. https://doi.org/10.12968/JOWC.2007.16.8.27854.
12. Schwartz D, Gefen A. The biomechanical protective effects of a treatment dressing on the soft tissues surrounding a non-offloaded sacral pressure ulcer. Int Wound J. 2019;16:684–95. https://doi.org/10.1111/IWJ.13082.
13. Flynn C, McCormack BAO. Simulating the wrinkling and aging of skin with a multi-layer finite ele-

ment model. J Biomech. 2010;43:442–8. https://doi.org/10.1016/J.JBIOMECH.2009.10.007.
14. Sopher R, Gefen A. Effects of skin wrinkles, age and wetness on mechanical loads in the stratum corneum as related to skin lesions. Med Biol Eng Comput. 2011;49:97–105. https://doi.org/10.1007/S11517-010-0673-3.
15. Shaked E, Gefen A. Modeling the effects of moisture-related skin-support friction on the risk for superficial pressure ulcers during patient repositioning in bed. Front Bioeng Biotechnol. 2013;1:1. https://doi.org/10.3389/FBIOE.2013.00009.
16. Schwartz D, Levy A, Gefen A. A computer modeling study to assess the durability of prophylactic dressings subjected to moisture in biomechanical pressure injury prevention. Ostomy Wound Manage. 2018;64:18–26.
17. Peko L, Barakat-Johnson M, Gefen A. Protecting prone positioned patients from facial pressure ulcers using prophylactic dressings: a timely biomechanical analysis in the context of the COVID-19 pandemic. Int Wound J. 2020;17:1595–606. https://doi.org/10.1111/IWJ.13435.
18. Gefen A, Alves P, Ciprandi G, Coyer F, Milne CT, Ousey K, et al. Device-related pressure ulcers: SECURE prevention. Second edition. J Wound Care. 2022;31:S1–72. https://doi.org/10.12968/JOWC.2022.31.SUP3A.S1.
19. Peko Cohen L, Ovadia-Blechman Z, Hoffer O, Gefen A. Dressings cut to shape alleviate facial tissue loads while using an oxygen mask. Int Wound J. 2019;16:813–26. https://doi.org/10.1111/IWJ.13101.
20. Lee KN, Ben-Nakhi M, Park EJ, Hong JP. Cyclic negative pressure wound therapy: an alternative mode to intermittent system. Int Wound J. 2015;12:686–92. https://doi.org/10.1111/IWJ.12201.
21. Singer AJ, Clark RAF. Cutaneous wound healing. N Engl J Med. 1999;341:738–46. https://doi.org/10.1056/NEJM199909023411006.
22. Van Helvert S, Storm C, Friedl P. Mechanoreciprocity in cell migration. Nat Cell Biol. 2017;20:8–20. https://doi.org/10.1038/s41556-017-0012-0.
23. Katzengold R, Orlov A, Gefen A. A novel system for dynamic stretching of cell cultures reveals the mechanobiology for delivering better negative pressure wound therapy. Biomech Model Mechanobiol. 2020;20:193. https://doi.org/10.1007/s10237-020-01377-6.
24. Rodriguez-Menocal L, Salgado M, Ford D, Van Badiavas E. Stimulation of skin and wound fibroblast migration by mesenchymal stem cells derived from normal donors and chronic wound patients. Stem Cells Transl Med. 2012;1:221–9. https://doi.org/10.5966/SCTM.2011-0029.
25. Lin JY, Lo KY, Sun YS. Effects of substrate-coating materials on the wound-healing process. Mater (Basel, Switzerland). 2019;12(17):2775. https://doi.org/10.3390/MA12172775.
26. Pinto BI, Cruz ND, Lujan OR, Propper CR, Kellar RS. In vitro scratch assay to demonstrate effects of arsenic on skin cell migration. J Vis Exp. 2019. https://doi.org/10.3791/58838.
27. Pijuan J, Barceló C, Moreno DF, Maiques O, Sisó P, Marti RM, et al. In vitro cell migration, invasion, and adhesion assays: from cell imaging to data analysis. Front Cell Dev Biol. 2019;7:107. https://doi.org/10.3389/FCELL.2019.00107.
28. Monsuur HN, Boink MA, Weijers EM, Roffel S, Breetveld M, Gefen A, et al. Methods to study differences in cell mobility during skin wound healing in vitro. J Biomech. 2016;49:1381–7. https://doi.org/10.1016/J.JBIOMECH.2016.01.040.
29. Toume S, Gefen A, Weihs D. Low-level stretching accelerates cell migration into a gap. Int Wound J. 2017;14:698–703. https://doi.org/10.1111/iwj.12679.
30. Slomka N, Gefen A. Relationship between strain levels and permeability of the plasma membrane in statically stretched myoblasts. Ann Biomed Eng. 2012;40:606–18. https://doi.org/10.1007/S10439-011-0423-1.

Open Access This chapter is licensed under the terms of the Creative Commons Attribution-NonCommercial-NoDerivatives 4.0 International License (http://creativecommons.org/licenses/by-nc-nd/4.0/), which permits any non-commercial use, sharing, distribution and reproduction in any medium or format, as long as you give appropriate credit to the original author(s) and the source, provide a link to the Creative Commons license and indicate if you modified the licensed material. You do not have permission under this license to share adapted material derived from this chapter or parts of it.

The images or other third party material in this chapter are included in the chapter's Creative Commons license, unless indicated otherwise in a credit line to the material. If material is not included in the chapter's Creative Commons license and your intended use is not permitted by statutory regulation or exceeds the permitted use, you will need to obtain permission directly from the copyright holder.

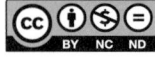

Necrosis in Burns

10

Christoph Hirche, Holger Engel, Thomas Kremer, and Ulrich Kneser

10.1 Pathophysiology of Burns with Respect to Necrosis

Burn wound progression refers to the phenomenon of continued tissue necrosis in the zone of stasis after termination of the initial thermal or toxic exposition. It includes partial- or full-thickness dermal burns.

The basis of necrosis in burns has been introduced in 1953, when Jackson described the three concentric zones of a burn wound as the basis of research on burn wound necrosis and progression: the central zone of coagulation, the intermediate zone of stasis, and the outer zone of hyperemia [1]. The zone of coagulation received the greatest damage due to direct thermal or toxic exposition and has been characterized by irreversible necrosis with complete destruction of the subdermal capillary network. In 1969, the zone of stasis was observed to have the ability to recover with bleeding from a small number of arterioles [2]. Subsequently, investigations focused on the questions regarding what factors may contribute to or even ameliorate the progression of tissue destruction in the zone of stasis [3]. The answer to this question was expected to lead to interventional measures with high clinical significance. It was expected that improved perfusion in the zone of stasis may influence the depth and total body surface area determining both mortality and morbidity, rates of delayed wound healing, hypertrophic scarring, dyspigmentation, contractures, infection, and shock [3–5].

A cascade of various endogenous factors triggers the local pathophysiologic process of burn wound progression [3]. The continuous release of cytotoxic mediators and free radicals maintains inflammation. In addition, an increase in secretion of neutrophils has been demonstrated which leads to clotting of obliterated dermal venules. The decrease of venous drainage leads to increased vascular permeability and interstitial hydrostatic pressure. Capillary leakage contributes to augmented interstitial fluid retention and hydrostatic pressure and thus leads to edema with potential ischemia. In accordance, hypercoagulability and venous thrombosis impair blood flow, and hypoxia-induced mediators lead to endothelial cell damage with compromised arteriole and capillary circulation. Singh et al. reviewed all peer-reviewed, original, and review articles published in English-language literature relevant to the topic of burn wound conversion and furthermore described infection, tissue desiccation, circumferential eschar, metabolic derangements,

---

C. Hirche · H. Engel · T. Kremer · U. Kneser (✉)
Department of Hand, Plastic and Reconstructive Surgery, Burn Centre, BG Trauma Centre Ludwigshafen, Ludwigshafen, Germany

Department of Plastic and Hand Surgery, University of Heidelberg, Heidelberg, Germany
e-mail: ulrich.kneser@bgu-ludwigshafen.de

advanced age, and poor general health as further factors with influence on necrosis [6].

Various authors have approached the mechanisms of burn wound progression and necrosis in order to investigate strategies and agents which aim to reduce inflammation, capillary leakage, edema, hypercoagulability, and venous thrombosis in acute burns [7–10].

Nevertheless, the clinical benefit and applicability of the results still raise controversial discussions. Further research is necessary to improve the understanding of all interrelated mechanisms and the convergence of burn wound progression in order to limit cell apoptosis as the basis of burn necrosis (Fig. 10.1) [3].

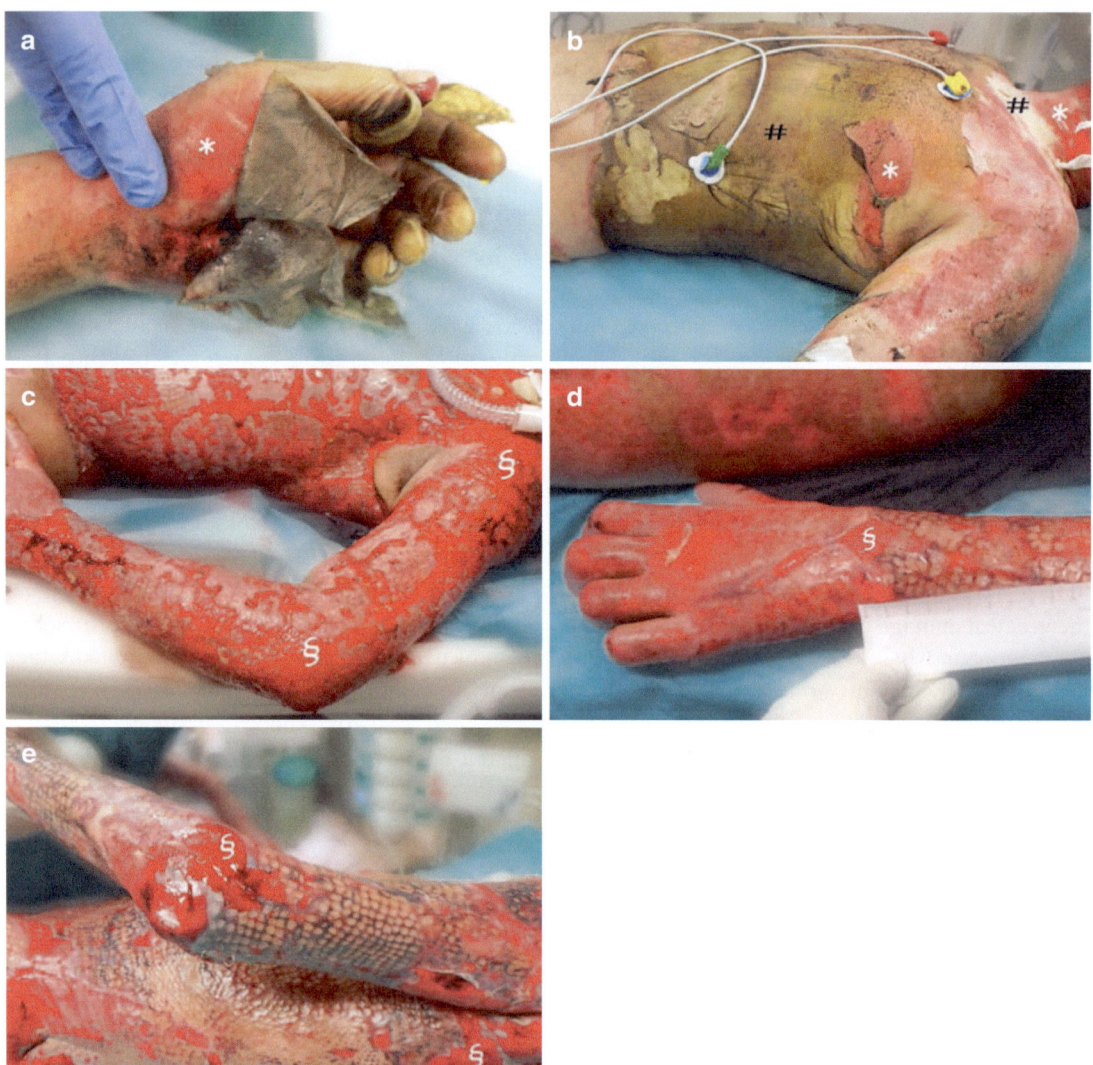

Fig. 10.1 Origination of burn necrosis. The acute trauma induced by heat or chemical toxin exposition leads to partial (*) dermal primary necrosis with necrotic epidermis layer (a). In case of partial necrosis (*), reduction of inflammation can limit full-thickness necrosis (#) (b). If inflammation continues, secondary necrosis with necessity of split- or full-thickness skin transplantation occurs. In case of tertiary necrosis of burns, transplant loss may lead to secondary healing (§) or requires retransplantation (c–e)

10.2 Apoptosis and Oncosis in Burn Wounds

Apoptotic dermal cells are found in normal, unburned skin, in superficial partial-thickness and in full-thickness burns. Nevertheless, a higher rate is found in deep partial-thickness burns than in normal skin, superficial partial-thickness burns, and full-thickness burns [9, 11]. These results suggest that apoptosis has an impact on burn wound progression of deep partial-thickness wounds. Apoptosis has been shown to continue for at least 23 days after the initial burn injury, which represents the window for pharmacologic intervention [12]. Apoptotic rates are mainly influenced by the local conditions in the zone of stasis.

Further investigation by Singer et al. showed that both apoptosis and oncosis to cell death in the zone of stasis play a role in burn wound necrosis and progression [13]. In order to approach apoptosis in the zone of stasis, Giles et al. developed a pharmaceutical agent to block the mechanism of apoptosis before irreversible loss of cell viability [14]. Giles et al. investigated inhibition of c-Jun, a transcription factor involved in multiple cell processes, including inflammation, proliferation, and apoptosis in an animal model. They found that direct application of the c-Jun inhibitor to full-thickness burn wounds in mice resulted in improved reepithelialization and a reduction in apoptotic cells at 24 h after burn injury [14].

10.3 Inflammation as a Key Step in Burns

Inflammation has an important key role in promoting local wound healing. Nevertheless, depending on the extent, it may constrain the healing process. Positive effects of local inflammation include local clearance of cellular fragments and local immunoactivity against microbial agents [15]. In contrast, prolonged inflammation mediated by neutrophil and macrophage release may increase secretion of proinflammatory cytokines. This secretory imbalance may trigger collagen degradation and keratinocyte cell apoptosis, adherence of neutrophils to the venular endothelium, production of oxygen-derived free radicals with disruption of plasma membranes, DNA cross-links and strand breaks, and peptide fragmentation [3, 16]. Further regulatory steps which keep up an imbalanced inflammation are delayed neutrophil apoptosis, local neutrophil aggregation, venule occlusion, and cytokine production. Wound infection has a major impact on inflammation due to endotoxin production and protease release that destroy tissue but also perpetuate the prolonged inflammatory response [3, 16, 17].

Deep partial-thickness burns are subject to these pathophysiological changes surrounding the primary zone of thermally induced coagulation, with potential expansion within 48 h postburn. From the clinical point of view, intervention by pharmacological interaction aims at reducing the need for surgical debridement and the area requiring skin grafting by keeping a balanced inflammation level, but potential systemic reactions have to be taken into consideration with limitation of application.

10.4 How to Prevent Necrotic Burns

In this chapter, primary necrosis is defined as resulting initially after the thermal or chemical exposition and is irreversible, while secondary necrosis results from conversion of the zone of stasis due to insufficient perfusion. Tertiary necrosis is defined as necrosis after transplantation with need for revision or secondary healing.

10.4.1 Primary Necrosis

The emergency preclinical and clinical therapy may have an early influence on burn wound progression and necrosis. With reference to the national and international guidelines, the early steps include stopping the burn, cooling the wound with care, appropriate dressings, and goal-directed, individual burn wound care [18].

At the site of the accident, the burning process has to be stopped or rather extinguished. All burnt clothing and any jewelry should be removed unless it is merged with the patient (e.g., polyvinyl chloride, polyester). There are controversial discussions about cooling of burns, especially regarding the correct time, temperature, timeframe, and medium. Many patients are mistakenly cooled down and arrive with mild to severe hypothermia. Cooling has a high analgesic potency and can reduce area of the zone of stasis where capillary perfusion is reduced when applied correctly. If the burnt body surface area is small (<10%), cooling of the burn should be performed [19]. Medium-tempered running tap water (approximately 15–20 °C) with a maximum cooling time of 15 min is recommended, while specially manufactured burn dressings (Water–Gel®, Burn–Pack®) have raised concerns regarding hypothermia following application due to handling errors. Dressings are important for pain management and to prevent the burnt area from contamination as a potential source of infection and inflammation. Dressings also play a role in thermal balance. Customary metal films (e.g., Metalline®) can reduce the risk of undercooling as a further external measure with impact on burn progression [20, 21].

Goal-directed, individual burn wound care includes specialist treatments, regular antiseptic dressing with appropriate wound climate, balanced fluid supply to prevent unnecessary edema, and analgesia in order to reduce pain-associated vasoactive mediator release.

10.4.2 Secondary Necrosis

Although research is going on, current milestones of treatment include adequate fluid resuscitation, nutritional support, and local wound care, with focus on topical antimicrobial agents and dressings. With potential therapeutic application, resolvins, a class of endogenous mediators derived from omega-3 polyunsaturated fatty acids, have been shown to regulate the resolution of inflammation in an animal model. By preserving the microvascular network, the agent was shown to enhance neutrophil access to the dermis, but prevented neutrophil-mediated damage [8].

Ipaktchi et al. hypothesized that topical attenuation of burn wound inflammatory signaling will control the dermal inflammatory source, attenuate SIRS, and reduce acute lung injury. They applied a topical p38 mitogen-activated protein kinase (MAPK) inhibitor to wounds. Topical p38 MAPK inhibition resulted in significantly less pulmonary inflammatory response by reducing pulmonary neutrophil sequestration, pulmonary cytokine expression, and a significant reduction in pulmonary microvascular injury and edema formation. They concluded that there is a strong interaction between dermal inflammation and systemic inflammatory response; thus, attenuating local inflammatory signaling appears effective in reducing SIRS and subsequent systemic complications after burn injury [22].

10.4.3 Tertiary Necrosis

In order to prevent tertiary necrosis, adequate necrectomy remains the key factor in the preparation of high-rate transplant take. In addition, a balanced specialist and multidisciplinary therapy includes adequate fluid supply, nutritional support, and local wound care. Vasoactive mediators may lead to capillary occlusion impairing transplant take. If epithelial islands are surrounded by tertiary necrosis, secondary wound healing vs. retransplantation have to be evaluated on the basis of affected burned area, localization, and expected healing period. Hypertrophic scarring, dyspigmentation, and potential contractures can result from tertiary necrosis.

Key Messages for Necrosis in Burns
Primary necrosis:
Inflammation, capillary leakage, edema, hypercoagulability, venous thrombosis, and arteriole and capillary stasis lead to burn progression and involve a number of factors which are linked.
Establish early diagnosis of primary necrosis and debridement and adequate initial care.
Secondary necrosis:
Try to prevent or limit inflammation.
Conversion zones may lead to secondary necrosis.

Tertiary necrosis:

Sufficient necrectomy enables high rate of transplant take.

Loss of transplant may lead to tertiary necrosis.

Tertiary necrosis necessitates secondary healing or retransplantation.

References

1. Jackson DM. [The diagnosis of the depth of burning]. Br J Surg. 1953;40:588–96.
2. Jackson DM. Second thoughts on the burn wound. J Trauma. 1969;9:839–62.
3. Shupp JW, Nasabzadeh TJ, Rosenthal DS, et al. A review of the local pathophysiologic bases of burn wound progression. J Burn Care Res. 2010;31:849–73.
4. Gravante G, Filingeri V, Delogu D, et al. Apoptotic cell death in deep partial thickness burns by coexpression analysis of TUNEL and Fas. Surgery. 2006;139:854–5.
5. Shakespeare P. Burn wound healing and skin substitutes. Burns. 2001;27:517–22.
6. Singh V, Devgan L, Bhat S, Milner SM. The pathogenesis of burn wound conversion. Ann Plast Surg. 2007;59:109–15.
7. Kremer T, Harenberg P, Hernekamp F, et al. High-dose vitamin C treatment reduces capillary leakage after burn plasma transfer in rats. J Burn Care Res. 2010;31:470–9.
8. Bohr S, Patel SJ, Sarin D, et al. Resolvin D2 prevents secondary thrombosis and necrosis in a mouse burn wound model. Wound Repair Regen. 2012;21(1):35–43.
9. Gravante G, Palmieri MB, Esposito G, et al. Apoptotic cells are present in ischemic zones of deep partial-thickness burns. J Burn Care Res. 2006;27:688–93.
10. Gravante G, Palmieri MB, Delogu D, Montone A. Apoptotic cells in cutaneous adnexa of burned patients. Burns. 2007;33:129–30.
11. Gravante G, Palmieri MB, Esposito G, et al. Apoptotic death in deep partial thickness burns vs. normal skin of burned patients. J Surg Res. 2007;141:141–5.
12. Gravante G, Delogu D, Palmieri MB, et al. Inverse relationship between the apoptotic rate and the time elapsed from thermal injuries in deep partial thickness burns. Burns. 2008;34:228–33.
13. Singer AJ, McClain SA, Taira BR, et al. Apoptosis and necrosis in the ischemic zone adjacent to third degree burns. Acad Emerg Med. 2008;15:549–54.
14. Giles N, Rea S, Beer T, et al. A peptide inhibitor of c-Jun promotes wound healing in a mouse full-thickness burn model. Wound Repair Regen. 2008;16:58–64.
15. Chitnis D, Dickerson C, Munster AM, Winchurch RA. Inhibition of apoptosis in polymorphonuclear neutrophils from burn patients. J Leukoc Biol. 1996;59:835–9.
16. Parihar A, Parihar MS, Milner S, Bhat S. Oxidative stress and anti-oxidative mobilization in burn injury. Burns. 2008;34:6–17.
17. Ogura H, Hashiguchi N, Tanaka H, et al. Long-term enhanced expression of heat shock proteins and decelerated apoptosis in polymorphonuclear leukocytes from major burn patients. J Burn Care Rehabil. 2002;23:103–9.
18. Hirche C, Hrabowski M, Kolios L, et al. Emergency prehospital care of burn injuries: thermal, electrical and chemical burns. J Paramed Prat. 2011;3:10–8.
19. Krämer PF, Grützner PA, Wölfl CG. Care of burn victims. Preclinical management. Notfall Rettungsmed. 2010;13:23–30.
20. Allison K, Porter K. Consensus on the pre-hospital approach to burns patient management. J R Army Med Corps. 2004;150:10–3.
21. Lonnecker S, Schoder V. [Hypothermia in patients with burn injuries: influence of prehospital treatment]. Chirurg. 2001;72:164–7.
22. Ipaktchi K, Mattar A, Niederbichler AD, et al. Attenuating burn wound inflammatory signaling reduces systemic inflammation and acute lung injury. J Immunol. 2006;177:8065–71.

Open Access This chapter is licensed under the terms of the Creative Commons Attribution-NonCommercial-NoDerivatives 4.0 International License (http://creativecommons.org/licenses/by-nc-nd/4.0/), which permits any non-commercial use, sharing, distribution and reproduction in any medium or format, as long as you give appropriate credit to the original author(s) and the source, provide a link to the Creative Commons license and indicate if you modified the licensed material. You do not have permission under this license to share adapted material derived from this chapter or parts of it.

The images or other third party material in this chapter are included in the chapter's Creative Commons license, unless indicated otherwise in a credit line to the material. If material is not included in the chapter's Creative Commons license and your intended use is not permitted by statutory regulation or exceeds the permitted use, you will need to obtain permission directly from the copyright holder.

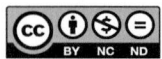

Electrical Burns

Christian Herlin

11.1 Introduction

Electrical burns are rare but can be particularly severe or injuring and sometimes fatal. They represent approximately 5% of burns [1]. In addition, it is estimated that 4000 people every year undergo an electrocution in France.

This type of burn affects mainly *two categories of patients:*

- The young child exploring his environment.
- The adult in his workplace.

They are of *two types:*

- Damage by direct contact with the electric current. The lesions spreading from an entry point to an exit point of the current (our focus of interest in this chapter).
- Injury by electric arcs in accidents at very high voltage. That is mainly thermal burns but at a very high temperature (>2000 °C).

They can be divided into *two groups:*

- Low-voltage injuries (<1000 V) occurring mainly at home.
- High-voltage injuries (>1000 V) occurring more often in the workplace.

In a recent review of the literature [2] 44% of patients presented low-voltage injuries (LVIs) and 38.3% high-voltage injuries (HVIs), and some studies did not characterise outcomes according to LVIs vs. HVIs. Psychological outcomes such as post-traumatic stress disorder were poorly documented. Mortality rates from electrical injuries are 2.6% in LVI, 5.2% in HVI, and 3.7% in not otherwise specified situations with a ratio of 2.4:1 for deaths caused by LVI compared with HVI. HVIs lead to greater morbidity and mortality than LVIs. However, the results may suggest that immediate mortality from LVI may be underestimated.

They mainly concern *two locations:*

- The upper limb.
- The face.

Mechanisms of tissular injury appear to be of *three different types:*

- The Joule effect: generating heat depending on tissue resistance—"$J = R\,I^2\,T$." The amount of the heat intensity generated (J) depends indeed on voltage U because $U = RI$. T is the

C. Herlin (✉)
Wound Healing Unit, Department of Surgery, Montpellier University, Montpellier, France
e-mail: c-herlin@chu-montpellier.fr

duration in seconds of the contact, R is the resistance in ohms, and I is the intensity in amperes.
- The higher the resistance, the greater the heat generated will be and the more serious the injuries are, but less current will travel through.
- Actually, two parameters influence tissue resistance:
- Its category (with decreasing resistance): Bone > fat > skin > muscle > mucosa > vessel > nerve.
- Its diameter: the smaller the diameter (wrist, elbow, and ankle), the higher the resistance, and thus the damage related to the Joule effect is significant [2].
- Cell membrane destruction by electric shock (electroporation) [3] increasing tissue damage and promoting the release of myoglobin.
- Massive depolarisation, which will result in the damage of muscle and cardiac and nervous cells. The "shock" causes the phenomenon of tetanisation, which increases the contact time of the victim with the electric current source (cable grasps, feeling of being "stuck" to the source). Furthermore, tetanisation allows the joint's jump of current by hyperflexion of the joints [4].

11.2 Tissue Injury

11.2.1 Entry and Exit Skin Points

These points are most often located at the extremities. The entry point is centred by a sore indicating carbonisation. This area is surrounded by a burn of decreasing depth ("cockade aspect"). On the way to the exit point, an area of deep burn should be suspected, following theoretically the path of sensory and motor nerves (the superficial veins also).

However, the current path remains unpredictable. Meanwhile, the exit point more often represents a whitish area. During the impact, it links the body to the ground or other external elements connected to it (Fig. 11.1).

11.2.2 Muscle Injury

It is always more severe than suggested by skin lesions and is due to the action of depolarisation and Joule effect. It represents the most important vital and functional prognosis factor in this type of burn. Muscles submitted to high voltage will undergo a very significant oedema, which can

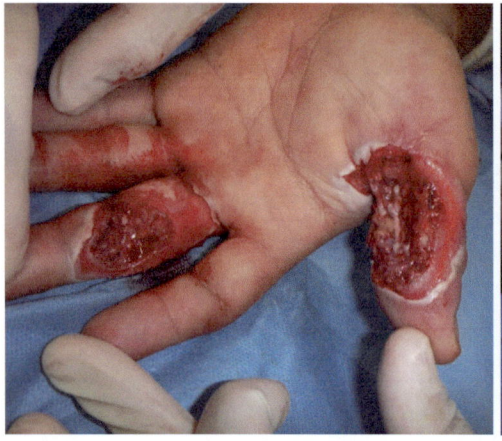 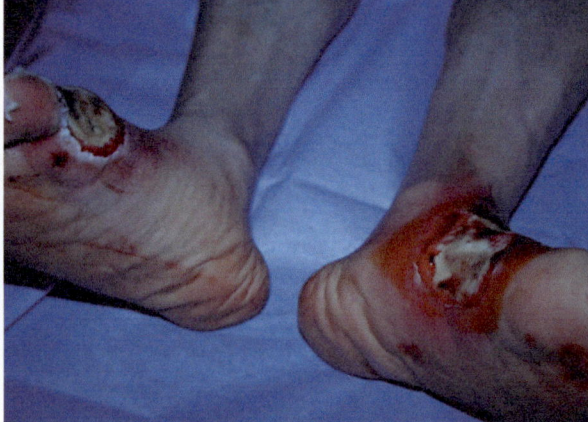

Fig. 11.1 Example of multiple points of entry and exits in the same patient

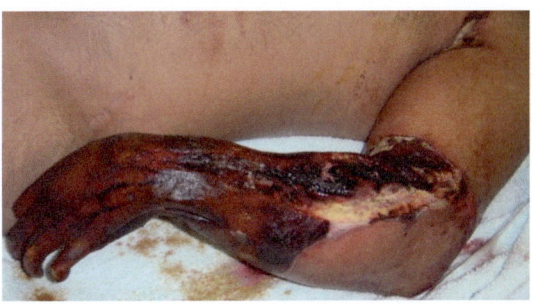

Fig. 11.2 Carbonisation of upper limb responsible for major and composite tissue lesions

lead quickly to a compartment syndrome (>30 mmHg). This syndrome, if not managed by a fasciotomy, will significantly increase muscle, nerve, and vascular damage, by direct compression, thrombosis [5], and necrosis, leading to local acidosis. This vicious cycle is to be broken as soon as possible (Fig. 11.2).

11.2.3 Myocardial Damage

Except the acute cardiac fibrillation, approximately 10% of patients admitted for electrical burn present electrocardiographic abnormality. This is most often represented by bundle branch block, supraventricular tachycardia, or non-specific repolarisation disorder. To these mechanisms is added necrosis by coronary thrombosis according to the same mechanisms mentioned above.

11.2.4 Buccal Mucosa Damage

It is typical of young children biting electric cables. The lesions are most often at the commissures, gums, and tongue. Full necrosis occurs most often before the end of the second week. Spontaneous wound healing is often adequate, but sometimes secondary interventions are required [6]. Their objective is in fact to reconstruct the anatomical subunits. The establishment of a shaper must be compulsory if there is a risk of microstomia.

11.2.5 Nerve Damage

It is most often a direct injury of axons by the current, causing paralysis or sensory disturbances more or less permanent. Indirect injury, often persistent, is caused by thrombosis or compression.

11.2.6 Deep Damage (Except Viscera)

They are the consequences of the Joule effect. With the bone and fascia being poor conductors, the heat effect is very significant, causing periosteal bone necrosis. In addition to that, fractures and serious sprains (typical posterior glenohumeral dislocation) are not uncommon due to tonic muscle tetanisation.

11.2.7 Other Damages

- Renal: damage by renal parenchymal necrosis, thrombosis, or *disseminated intravascular coagulation* (DIC) and acute tubular necrosis by accumulation of myoglobin.
- Visceral damage represented by gastrointestinal perforation, paralytic ileus, hepatorenal syndrome, liver injury, or acute pancreatitis. Liver enzymes as well as amylase/lipase are to be obtained.

11.3 Medical Management

11.3.1 Monitoring

The intensive care management (cardiovascular monitoring, rehydration, coagulation, CPK, K^+, etc.) must be rigorous and precautionary [7]. Compartment syndrome is to be ruled out (increased pressure of the compartments, hypoaesthesia, impaired distal perfusion, etc.).

11.3.2 Assessment of the Lesions

If entry and exit skin points are usually obvious, the path and the internal damages are sometimes more difficult to assess. Scintigraphy (99mTc; 133X) and MRI can provide important information on the condition about the deep integuments [8].

11.4 Surgical Management

11.4.1 First Surgery

It must be determined by the existence of a compartment syndrome, which must be managed within 6 h of the injury [9]. Deep exploration is to be done while carrying out escharotomies and fasciotomies. Necrotic tissue should be removed; the damaged muscles and nerves have to be preserved if we consider a possible recovery especially after fasciotomy (Fig. 11.3).

Immediate flap coverage is recommended by many authors to limit devascularisation, but in emergency cases, we think that it must be reserved for vital organ coverage [10]. Besides these situations, we believe that we must avoid performing locoregional or free flaps before 3 weeks to allow time for oedema to decrease and promote drainage of all local toxins (free radicals, lactate) leached after the trauma. Immediate amputation is limited to extreme cases with anuria or shock; it will aim to keep a length always compatible with future equipment.

11.4.2 Second Look

It is carried out 2–3 days later. We have to spare the maximum of tissue (tendon, nerve, etc.) even if they fall in a grey zone. Skin coverage remains our priority; the damaged nerves will be repaired in a second time. Even if not widely practised, these interventions bring some interest as they will allow being less aggressive in the first surgery and opening a window for a new debridement of secondary necrotic tissue after the removal of the ischemia-reperfusion syndrome

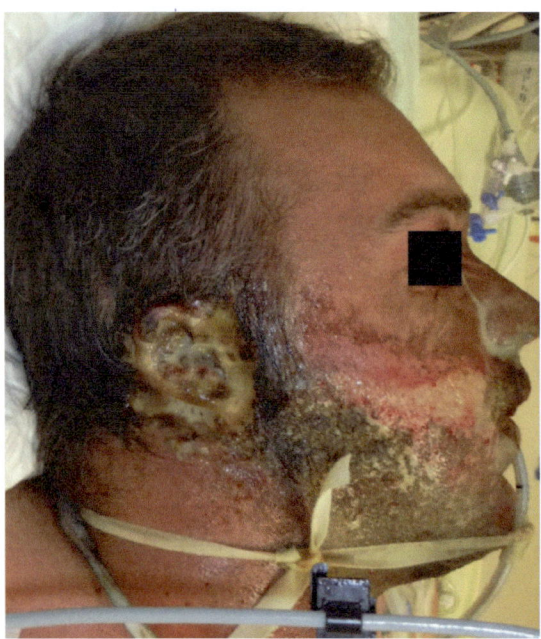 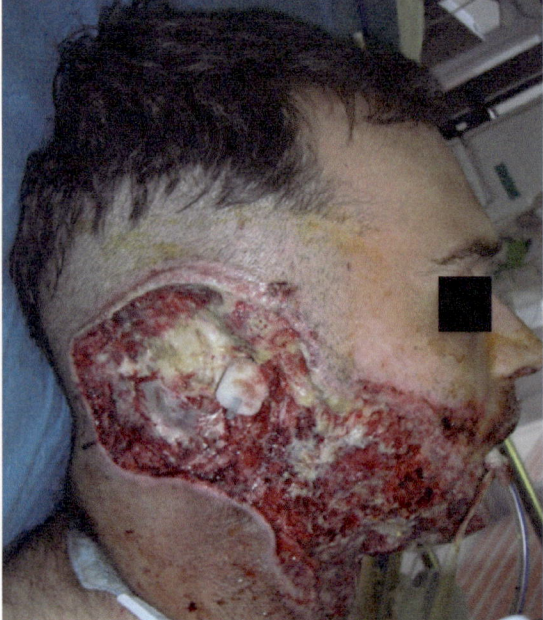

Fig. 11.3 Deep burn of the lateral side of the face due to a very-high-voltage electric arc

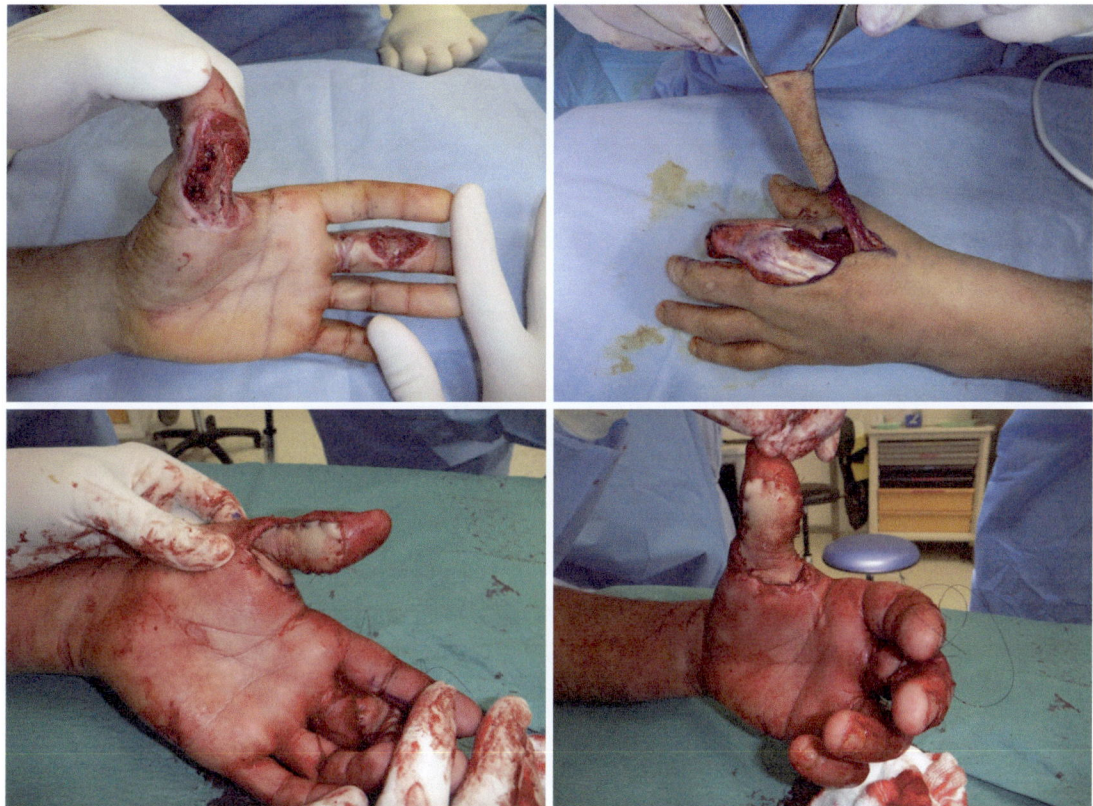

Fig. 11.4 Realisation of an island flap for the reconstruction of the proximal defect. Skin graft was used for the middle finger

(when fasciotomy is performed). Ultimately, a third or a fourth revision is sometimes necessary to achieve complete debridement of large areas (Fig. 11.4).

Furthermore, a polymicrobial infection of necrotic tissue can occur with plurimicrobiens processes often including anaerobes or *Pseudomonas aeruginosa*. Bacteriological samples are systematically taken, and antibiotics are given as needed.

11.5 Global Management

This type of patients requires hospitalisation in specialised burn unit with experienced teams. Supervision by physiotherapists to limit retractions is necessary, but also the psychological side should not be neglected.

It is indeed known that electrocution can have a psychological impact and even cause psychiatric diseases.

The final healing is often long and delayed. Thus, 3–4 weeks may be required to obtain granulation tissue after debridement and 2–3 months to hope for healing of the entry and exit skin points.

11.6 Prevention

In developed countries, electrical burns occurring in working conditions as well as paediatric burns have decreased, and most of the patients are admitted with low-voltage burns, whereas in developing countries, patients are more frequently admitted with high-voltage burns, with an extensive need for acute and reconstructive surgical interventions. Voltage of the burn injury is a determinant factor in the severity of the necrotic lesions. A reduction in paediatric high-voltage injuries was observed over the past two decades, likely due to the enhancement of electrical safety [11, 12].

11.7 Conclusion

The electrical burns are rare but often severe. The initial management is dominated by the detection of deep lesions and the prevention of organ failure. Management of muscle injury is important for vital and functional outcomes; however, it remains very difficult to assess in the early days. Surgery is often delayed and should usually aim, after a second look, to restore the original anatomy and function. Cosmetic and functional sequelae will be supported later, usually at 18–24 months.

References

1. Koumbourlis AC. Electrical injuries. Crit Care Med. 2002;30(11 Suppl):S424–30. PubMed PMID: 12528784
2. Shih JG, Shahrokhi S, Jeschke MG. Review of adult electrical burn injury outcomes worldwide: an analysis of low-voltage vs high-voltage electrical injury. J Burn Care Res. 2017;38(1):e293–8.
3. Hunt JL. Electrical injuries of the upper extremity. Major Probl Clin Surg. 1976;19:72–83. PubMed PMID: 1256066
4. Lee RC, Gaylor DC, Bhatt D, Israel DA. Role of cell membrane rupture in the pathogenesis of electrical trauma. J Surg Res. 1988;44(6):709–19. PubMed PMID: 3379948
5. Skoog T. Electrical injuries. J Trauma. 1970;10(10):816–30. PubMed PMID: 5506363
6. Holliman CJ, Saffle JR, Kravitz M, Warden GD. Early surgical decompression in the management of electrical injuries. Am J Surg. 1982;144(6):733–9. PubMed PMID: 7149133
7. Garson S. Les levres brulees [Burned lips]. Ann Chir Plast Esthet. 2002;47(5):547–55. PubMed PMID: 12449878
8. Purdue GF, Hunt JL. Electrocardiographic monitoring after electrical injury: necessity or luxury. J Trauma. 1986;26(2):166–7. PubMed PMID: 3944840
9. Ligen L, Hongming Y, Feng L, Huinan Y, Quan H, Guang F. Magnetic resonance imaging features of soft tissue and vascular injuries after high-voltage electrical burns and their clinical application. Injury. 2012;43(9):1445–50. PubMed PMID: 21764053
10. Teot L, Griffe O, Brabet M, Gavroy JP, Thaury M. Severe electric injuries of the hand and forearm. Ann Hand Upper Limb Surg. 1992;11(3):207–16. PubMed PMID: 1382511
11. Zhu ZX, Xu XG, Li WP, Wang DX, Zhang LY, Chen LY, et al. Experience of 14 years of emergency reconstruction of electrical injuries. Burns. 2003;29(1):65–72. PubMed PMID: 12543048
12. Depamphilis MA, Cauley RP, Sadeq F, Lydon M, Sheridan RL, Driscoll DN, Winograd JM. Surgical management and epidemiological trends of pediatric electrical burns. Burns. 2020;46(7):1693–9. https://doi.org/10.1016/j.burns.2020.03.005. Epub 2020 Mar 31.PMID: 32245570

Open Access This chapter is licensed under the terms of the Creative Commons Attribution-NonCommercial-NoDerivatives 4.0 International License (http://creativecommons.org/licenses/by-nc-nd/4.0/), which permits any non-commercial use, sharing, distribution and reproduction in any medium or format, as long as you give appropriate credit to the original author(s) and the source, provide a link to the Creative Commons license and indicate if you modified the licensed material. You do not have permission under this license to share adapted material derived from this chapter or parts of it.

The images or other third party material in this chapter are included in the chapter's Creative Commons license, unless indicated otherwise in a credit line to the material. If material is not included in the chapter's Creative Commons license and your intended use is not permitted by statutory regulation or exceeds the permitted use, you will need to obtain permission directly from the copyright holder.

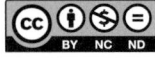

12 Gunshot Wounds

Supaporn Opasanon
and Apirag Chuangsuwanich

12.1 Introduction

Gunshot wounds (GSWs) are one of the most fatal traumatic injuries. Bullets not only cause direct vital organ damage, but also further problems from undermanagement of the wounds [1–3]. Soft tissue damage, foreign bodies, and bacterial contamination at GSW sites and along the wound tract are the factors that may cause infection and delay wound healing [4, 5]. After the Advanced Trauma Life Support (ATLS®) protocol [2] for life-threatening condition, GSWs should be managed thoroughly. In this chapter, we describe the updated knowledge and principle of GSW management.

12.2 Etiopathogeny

Gunshot causes tissue damages by disrupting the tissue, through bleeding, and by permitting entrance of infection [1–3, 6]. The mechanism of tissue injuries is mixed, blunt, and penetrating trauma injuries. For penetrating trauma, destruction of flesh tissue is due to passing of the bullet through it and the large amount of kinetic energy transferred to the tissue. Some blunt trauma is due to displacement of tissue adjacent to the track of the penetrating bullet. The bullet's shock wave may damage the adjacent structure. Severity of a bullet wound may be expressed by the formula $KE = \frac{1}{2} MV^2$. This formula expresses the amount of the energy transfer to the body by a bullet. Contusion and hemorrhage will occur. Increasing the velocity of the bullet will have more tissue destruction than increasing its mass. A bullet is not sterilized and may carry viable bacteria and clothing into a wound [4, 5].

12.3 Clinical Detailing

12.3.1 Characteristics of GSWs

Tissue destruction relies on the kinetic energy of the bullet. A high-velocity bullet causes more tissue damage than a low-velocity bullet. The anatomy of the wounds is also an important factor of severity:

S. Opasanon
Faculty of Medicine, Division of Trauma Surgery, Department of Surgery, Siriraj Hospital, Mahidol University, Bangkok, Thailand

A. Chuangsuwanich (✉)
Faculty of Medicine, Division of Plastic Surgery, Department of Surgery, Siriraj Hospital, Mahidol University, Bangkok, Thailand

12.3.1.1 Cavity

Kinetic energy dissipates forward and laterally away from the bullet and pushes the surrounding tissue aside causing a cavity (Figs. 12.1 and 12.2). Entrance wound is round with abrasion ring and shows soot deposition or blackening of the skin edge (Fig. 12.3). Stellate-shaped entrance wound may be found in near-contact shooting due to tearing of the skin from expanding gas (Fig. 12.4). Exit wound is typically larger and more irregular than the entry. If the path of the bullet is long, entrance and exit wounds may be small. Negative pressure may suck debris into the wound track.

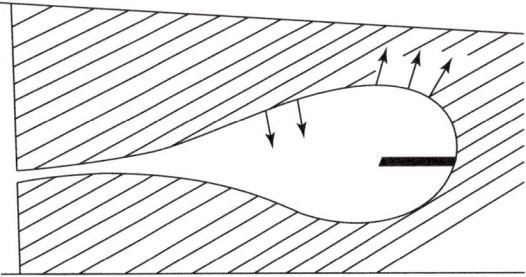

Fig. 12.1 Kinetic energy of the bullet dissipates in the wound track and another way, which causes damage outside the track

12.3.1.2 Abrasion Ring (Marginal Abrasion, Contusion Ring)

Bullet indents the skin and abrades the margin of entrance wound.

12.3.1.3 Crush and Laceration

Direct laceration and disruption of the tissues occur along the track with any penetrating object and effects of gases.

12.3.1.4 Secondary Shock Wave

Tissue damage may occur in the remote tissue caused by the kinetic energy of a high-velocity bullet, which produces a shock wave.

12.3.1.5 Skin Burn

The bullet's kinetic energy is converted to heat. Heat is transmitted to the surrounding tissues.

12.3.1.6 Bullet Wipe

Lubricant and debris on bullet surface wiped off onto the wound edge.

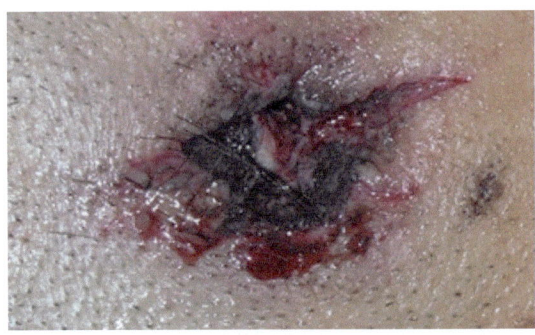

Fig. 12.4 Stellate-shaped entrance wound with soot

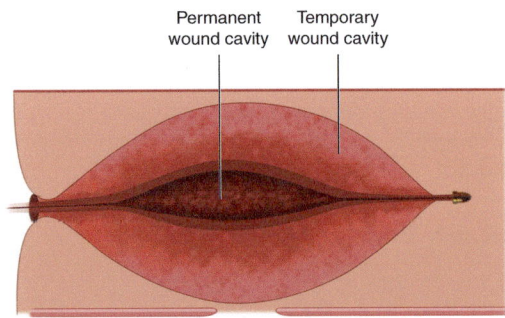

Fig. 12.2 The energy and heat expand explosively, causing a cavity in the tissue

Fig. 12.3 Round entrance gunshot wound showing dark soot deposition with marginal abrasion

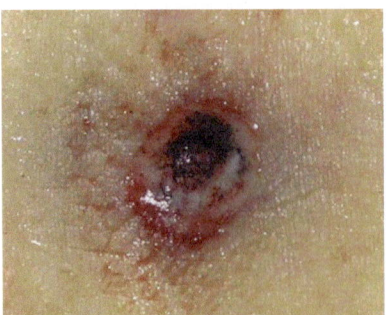

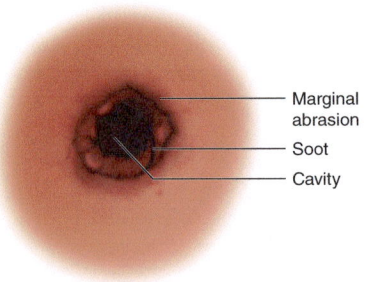

12.3.1.7 Smudging

Soot from partially burnt gases.

12.3.1.8 Tattooing

Burning propulsive grains embedded in the skin.

12.3.1.9 Retained Foreign Materials

GSWs penetrate the soiled clothing and introduce foreign bodies such as lubricant, debris, and bacteria into the wound track. They are the source of wound contamination. Retained wadding and bone fragment should be removed.

12.4 General Principles of GSW Management

12.4.1 Save Life

- For initial management, ATLS protocol should be performed.

12.4.2 Local Wound Care to Prevent Infection

- Control bleeding: Wound hematomas (Fig. 12.5) lead to infection [4].
- Cleansing.

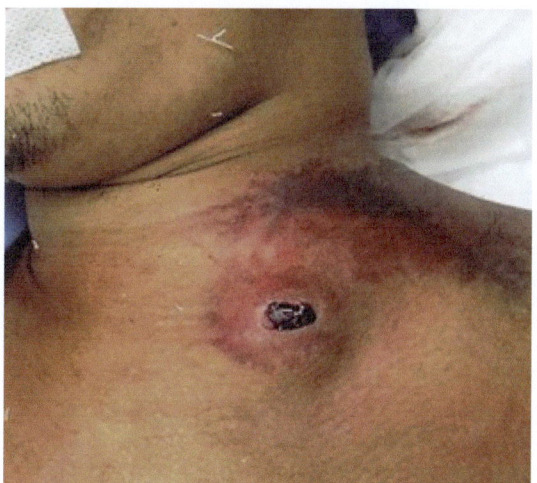

Fig. 12.5 Gunshot wound with hematoma

- Adequate debridement [4]: Debridement of all grossly nonviable tissues should be undertaken.
- Remove foreign materials: soot, clothing, lubricant, and bone fragment.
- Antibiotics [4]: Bullets are not sterile. Puncture wound is a risk factor for serious infection. Antibiotic prophylaxis is recommended in GSWs.
- Tetanus immunization [4]: GSWs are at risk for tetanus, and the patient should receive tetanus prophylaxis.

12.5 Gunshot Wound Management

12.5.1 Initial Dressing

Bleeding should be controlled with direct pressure. As always, GSWs should be treated as soon as possible in a hospital.

12.5.2 Wound Surgery

"Treat the wound, not the weapon" is the key of GSW management [7].

12.5.3 Irrigation and Debridement

Gunshot wounds are contaminated wounds and are at high risk of infection. Wound must be cleaned as much as possible. Wound irrigation with copious volumes of saline can reduce the number of bacteria in the wound. Soot and lubricant are removed. *High-pressure irrigation* may be as effective in removing contamination [4, 8].

Adequate debridement is very important. Skin necrosis and damaged subcutaneous fat are removed by sharp debridement. *High-pressure hydrosurgery* [4] is one of the new debridement techniques. It is very effective to cut and debride the abrasion ring and laceration and clean bullet wipe. In addition, hydrosurgery is an easy method to clean the cavity wounds.

12.5.4 Dressing and Closure

Wound should be left open [4, 8]. Closing a contaminated wound can trap bacteria inside and lead to infection. Wide excision may be required to clear foreign materials. Moist saline gauze is inserted directly into the wound to allow drainage twice a day for the first few days or until there is no more fluid draining from it. Reinspection at 72–96 h should be considered. After reevaluation, if there is no remaining fluid or other contaminants with no excessive loss of skin, delayed primary closure is accepted [4]. If the patient has deep cavity or large skin and soft tissue defect, flap reconstruction should be considered. The principle of wound management is to keep the wound environment moist [9]. *Hydrogel* supports autolytic debridement and provides a moist wound bed. It is a good choice for relatively desiccated wounds. Fluid in cavity wound can cause infection. Absorbent dressing is needed. *Calcium alginate* [9] and *hydrofiber* dressings are appropriate to control exudates. Alginates are available in rope form, which is very easy to apply in the cavity wound. An ionic-silver dressing is also a good choice for GSWs.

12.5.5 Instructions for Special Areas

12.5.5.1 A Bullet Wound to the Head

Bone fragment should be removed. It is easy to miss these in hairy parts of the body such as the scalp, axilla, and perineum, so careful examination is very important.

12.5.5.2 A Bullet Wound to the Face

A good examination with attention to possible nerve damage and parotid gland and Stensen's duct injuries should be performed. The skin at the face is highly vascular and tends to heal better than other areas of the body. It can be sutured after good wound cleansing. In case of *through-and-through GSWs*, connecting between the skin and mucosa, such as the cheek and mouth, primary closure of mucosal wound must be done and thorough wound irrigation is recommended. Delayed primary closure of the skin may be considered.

12.5.5.3 A Bullet Wound to the Arm or Leg [8, 10]

Evaluation of injury to the neurovascular structures, muscle, and bone should be done. Massive debridement is required to clear the dead tissue, foreign material, and bone fragment. Close monitoring of compartment syndrome is mandatory. Hyperbaric oxygen therapy (HBO) [11] may help to reduce swelling and inflammation in pending case or be used as adjunctive treatment. However, complete fasciotomy is the primary treatment for compartment syndrome. Retained foreign material and inadequate debridement may lead to late infection.

12.6 Conclusion

GSWs can cause immediate life-threatening conditions that should be treated first followed by associated injuries. The severity of tissue damage depends on the bullet's kinetic energy and location of the wounds. Thorough wound evaluation, effective wound debridement, and prevention of infection are the principles of GSW management. Hydrosurgery with high pressure and hydrogel may be the tools for debridement with good outcome.

References

1. Alexandropoulou CA, Panagiotopoulos E. Wound ballistics: analysis of blunt and penetrating trauma mechanisms. Health Sci J. 2010;4(4):225–36.
2. American College of Surgeons Committee on Trauma. Advanced trauma life support student course manual. 9th ed. Chicago, IL: ACS; 2012.
3. Denton JS, Segovia A, Filkins JA. Practical pathology of gunshot wounds. Arch Pathol Lab Med. 2006;130:1283–9.
4. Adams CA, Heffernan DS, Cioffi WG. Wound, bites, and stings. In: Mattox KL, Moore EE, Feliciano DV, editors. Trauma. 7th ed. New York, NY: McGraw-Hill Books; 2013. p. 896–921.
5. Yildiz O, Alp E, Simsek S, Selcuklu A, Doganay M. Gunshot wounds and late infection. Turk J Med Sci. 2005;35:269–72.
6. PathologyOutlines.com, Inc. Forensics: types of injuries-Gunshot wounds [Internet]. [cited 2014 Jan 6]. http://www.pathologyoutlines.com/topic/forensicsgunshotwounds.html

7. Lindsey D. The idolatry of velocity, or lies, damn lies, and ballistics. J Trauma. 1980;20(12):1068–9.
8. Bowyer GW, Ryan JM, Kaufmann CR, Ochsner MG. General principles of wound management. In: Ryan JM, Rich NM, Dale RF, Morgans BT, Cooper CJ, editors. Ballistic trauma. London: Edward Arnold; 1997.
9. Opasanon S, Muangman P, Namviriyachote N. Clinical effectiveness of alginate silver dressing in outpatient management of partial-thickness burns. Int Wound J. 2010;7(6):467–71.
10. Bowyer GW, Rossiter ND. Management of gunshot wounds of the limbs. J Bone Joint Surg Br. 1997;79(6):1031–6.
11. Gesell LB, editor. Hyperbaric oxygen therapy indications. The hyperbaric oxygen therapy committee report. 12th ed. Durham: Undersea and Hyperbaric Medical Society; 2008.

Open Access This chapter is licensed under the terms of the Creative Commons Attribution-NonCommercial-NoDerivatives 4.0 International License (http://creativecommons.org/licenses/by-nc-nd/4.0/), which permits any non-commercial use, sharing, distribution and reproduction in any medium or format, as long as you give appropriate credit to the original author(s) and the source, provide a link to the Creative Commons license and indicate if you modified the licensed material. You do not have permission under this license to share adapted material derived from this chapter or parts of it.

The images or other third party material in this chapter are included in the chapter's Creative Commons license, unless indicated otherwise in a credit line to the material. If material is not included in the chapter's Creative Commons license and your intended use is not permitted by statutory regulation or exceeds the permitted use, you will need to obtain permission directly from the copyright holder.

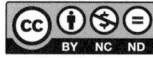

Frostbite 13

Marc-James Hallam, Steven J. Lo, and Christopher Imray

Frostbite is defined as the injury sustained by tissues subjected to temperatures below their physiological freezing point (−0.55 °C). The severity of a frostbite injury is related to the temperature, wind chill and duration of exposure to that temperature, as well as the volume of tissue subjected to cooling. As a result, a description of a frostbite injury is somewhat of an umbrella term used to describe wounds ranging from those with minimal tissue damage over small areas to substantial necrosis of entire limbs, necessitating amputation. Advances in frostbite management have improved the potential outcome in frozen injuries, and thus, it is important that front-line medical staff can recognise and treat frostbite effectively [1].

13.1 Aetiology

Frostbite typically affects the extremities with 90% of injuries affecting the fingers and toes although the nose, ears and external genitalia are also commonly affected [2]. Although historically it was most frequently observed in military personnel, there has been a shift over the last few decades with increasing numbers of civilians being affected. Modern epidemiological evidence suggests that high-risk groups still include those in military organisations but also the homeless, extreme sports enthusiasts, those in poor health, and individuals intoxicated through drink or drug use and genetic susceptibility, e.g. people from warm climates (see Table 13.1) [1, 2].

13.2 Classification of Frostbite

There are a number of ways one can classify frostbite injuries, and the most commonly utilised classification is simply one of mild or severe injury, but the first predictive outcome classification was suggested by Cauchy et al. (2001) [3]. Cauchy's classification is based on the anatomical location, radiotracer uptake on technetium scanning and skin blistering. This was based on a retrospective study of 70 frostbite patients presenting to the Department of Mountain Medicine in Chamonix, France (Table 13.2).

M.-J. Hallam (✉)
Aberdeen Royal Infirmary, Aberdeen, UK

S. J. Lo
Canniesburn Plastic Surgery Unit, Glasgow, UK

C. Imray
UHCW NHS Trust, Division of Translational and Systems Medicine, Warwick Medical School, Aberdeen, UK

Table 13.1 Aetiological factors predisposing to frostbite injury

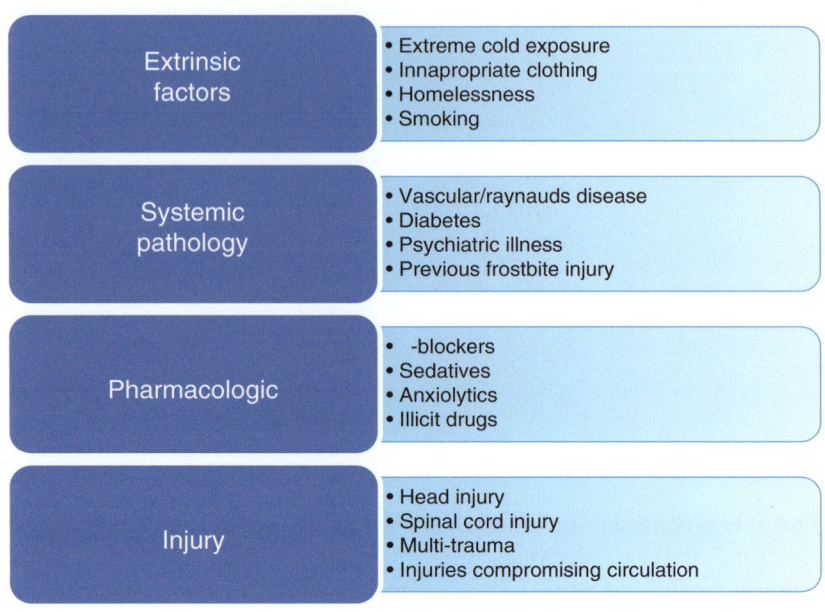

Table 13.2 Predictive classification of frostbite injuries affecting the limb extremities

Severity grade	Lesion location (day 0)	Radioactive tracer uptake on bone scan (day 2)	Character of blistering (day 2)	Likely outcome
1.	Not visible	N/A	None	No tissue loss or long-term sequelae
2.	Distal phalanx	Hypo-fixation	Clear	Soft tissue loss with nail changes
3.	Mid-phalanx	Absence of uptake at phalanx	Haemorrhagic	Amputation of digit. Functional sequelae
4.	Carpus/tarsus	Absence of uptake at carpus/tarsus	Haemorrhagic	Extensive amputation with likely sepsis or thrombosis. Functional sequelae

(Reproduced and adapted with permission from Grieve et al. [2], © BMJ, All Rights Reserved)

13.3 Pathology

A frostbite injury results from both direct and indirect effects of freezing and pathologically is characterised by a continuum of overlapping pathological phases that ultimately cumulate in cellular ischaemia and necrosis of the affected tissues. These phases can be broadly divided into the following:

- Pre-freeze phase.
- Freeze-thaw phase.
- Vascular stasis phase.
- Late ischaemic phase.

13.3.1 Intracellular Effects

The direct effects of freezing are principally due to the formation of ice crystals within the tissues themselves. These crystals increase the oncotic pressure within the extracellular space, dehydrating cells via the osmotic movement of water out of the cellular membranes and disturbing the intracellular homeostasis. With the rewarming of tissues, the crystals melt producing interstitial tissue oedema. Indirectly, the freezing injury stimulates the release of a variety of pro-inflammatory cytokines.

13.3.2 Extracellular Effects: The Freeze-Thaw-Refreeze Injury

Initial exposure to cold temperatures results in an immediate, localised vasoconstriction. This may sometimes be followed by a transient vasodilatory reflex known as the "hunting response" or cold-induced vasodilatation. This physiological reflex results in a redistribution of flow from the core and is thought to be a primitive reflex to protect the extremities from freezing. Ultimately, this results in a drop in core body temperature and furthermore is ineffective in protecting the peripheries against extreme cold stress. The reduced blood flow secondary to vasoconstriction in turn further exacerbates localised cooling producing a vicious cycle of ever-increasing vasoconstriction and tissue cooling. An oedematous state results through a combination of increased plasma viscosity, microvascular damage and fluid migration. The microvascular (endothelial) damage produces a pro-thrombotic environment through activation of the clotting cascade in which microthrombi form, occluding the capillaries, resulting in ischaemia. When such a time as tissue rewarming occurs, further microvascular clot occlusion occurs due to the promotion of a pro-thrombotic state through the lysis of frozen cells. Local mast cells degranulate in response to the lytic cell membranes, releasing histamine which further increases vascular permeability and oedema. The end point of all of these processes is potentially devastating local tissue ischaemia, and as first noted by Baron Larrey, Surgeon General to Napoleon, the most significant ischaemia, and therefore tissue necrosis, is seen in injuries that freeze and thaw and are then frozen again.

13.3.3 Long-Term Sequelae

It should also be appreciated that aside from these immediate-type effects seen following a freezing injury, there is also long-term pathological damage sustained by tissues, which may result in chronic dysfunction or impact upon the patient many years post-injury. Although rare, one of the most serious observed syndromes is probably related to chronic vasomotor dysfunction, manifesting clinically as chronic pain affecting the previously frostbitten area that is often unresponsive to conventional analgesia and requires anaesthetic or pain specialist input. Those that develop these complex regionalised pain syndromes frequently also suffer with associated problems such as paraesthesia and cold intolerance. It should also be noted that all patients who have experienced frostbite are at increased risk of further future episodes (presumably again secondary to vasomotor dysfunction), and all patients must be warned of this and given appropriate preventive advice. More serious long-term sequelae of frostbite that have been reported include the malignant transformation of frostbitten tissues and bone and joint pathologies including osteoporosis and arthritic changes [1].

13.4 Clinical Evaluation of Frostbitten Patients

13.4.1 History

Critical details of the patient history include the likely temperature, duration and timing of exposure, as this will help predict the severity of injury and may affect subsequent management. It is also important to obtain information relating to the patient's premorbid state such as peripheral vascular disease and pertinent risk factors such as smoking or use of β-blockers.

13.4.2 Examination

In rare cases, frostbite injuries may present as a purely uniform frozen injury, but more frequently, there is a mixed clinical picture with overlapping areas between deeper frozen tissues and more superficial nonfrozen tissues. Even in the case of a purely frozen injury, there is much variation in severity from the lesser affected forms (frostnip) to large areas of frozen tissues or indeed whole limbs.

It can be seen that frostbite presents in variable fashions and the injury evolves with time, and thus one is often unable to determine the full or likely extent of injury for some time after the injurious cooling from clinical examination alone, illustrating the importance of a thorough history. Nonfreezing injuries may be managed locally without the need for specialist intervention, and they typically follow a short exposure to (relatively) warmer temperatures and involve the feet most commonly with patients complaining initially of localised numbness and/or paraesthesia. As the tissues rewarm, severe pain is experienced with the rapid onset of a reactive hyperaemia and tissue oedema. The pain is usually transient but may become chronic with patients suffering long after tissues have recovered. Actual tissue loss is uncommon in these cases with most injuries only exhibiting mild discolouration, and very occasionally small areas of watery blisters may develop.

Any potentially serious frostbite injury however must be discussed with a suitably experienced unit for consideration of patient transfer, especially if the patient has presented less than 24 h post-injury as they may be a candidate for thrombolytic therapy.

13.4.3 Radiological Investigations in Frostbite

Due to some of the difficulties outlined in accurately assessing the initial severity of tissue devitalisation in frostbite injuries (hence avoiding early surgical debridement), a variety of radiological investigations have been suggested as clinical assessment adages. It is important to appreciate however that no radiological investigation is currently predictive in isolation and these studies are designed only to augment clinical opinion in cases that may be unclear.

Many investigations have been suggested over the years to image frostbite injuries, but the most clinically useful appear to be technetium 99 (Tc-99) triple-phase scanning and magnetic resonance angiography. There is convincing evidence from a large retrospective review of 92 patients with severe frostbite injuries that Tc-99 scanning in the first few days can predict the subsequent level of amputation in up to 84% of cases [4]. However, further large-scale studies are required in this area, and currently, there is little role for complex imaging in routine and less severe frostbite cases. Possible exceptions to this include severe injury with early presentation and no associated traumatic injuries, those rare cases where early surgery is being undertaken, or if thrombolytic therapy is being considered.

13.5 Acute Frostbite Management

13.5.1 Prioritisation of Life-Threatening Injuries and Specialist Referral

It is vital to appreciate that patients presenting with frostbite frequently present with coexisting severe and life-threatening emergent conditions such as hypothermia or significant traumatic injury. In line with the management of any emergency situation, such coexisting morbidities must be treated and stabilised before commencing treatment or transferring a patient to an expert centre for localised frostbitten tissue(s). Hypothermia should be corrected, and core temperature should be raised to 34 °C [2]. In any case, frostbite injuries often occur in remote regions where transfer or access to expert centres is not immediately possible and immediate management must be commenced locally. In today's technologically advanced age, those treating frostbitten patients can seek expert advice through the use of satellite phones and the Internet; indeed, many remote facilities rely on such technology.

13.5.2 Prevention of Refreezing and Differential Approach to Rewarming

It is also imperative that rewarming of the locally frostbitten tissues must only be commenced once there is absolutely no risk of refreezing as this will result in further tissue damage; similarly, it is advised that frostbitten tissues should not be rubbed or massaged for similar reasons. Once a patient with a frozen injury has been secured in a safe environment and any emergent conditions are stabilised, directed therapy can be commenced. In such injuries (be they minor areas of freezing or more extensive), the principal goal of treatment is to rapidly rewarm the affected area in a water bath with an antiseptic agent such as chlorhexidine in an attempt to preserve the dermal circulation. State of Alaska guidelines suggest a warming bath of 37–39 °C, whilst others suggest 40–41 °C [1, 5]; in practice, especially if in the field, it is nearly impossible to maintain exact water temperatures, and the critical factor is that the water should be warm, not hot, as the tissue will be neuropathic and one must avoid scalding. The rewarming should continue for a minimum of 30 min or as long as necessary for all affected tissues to be defrosted, thoroughly rewarmed and pliable exhibiting a deep-red or purple colour, carefully monitoring the water temperature throughout. This 30-min regime of rewarming should be repeated at twice-daily intervals until such a time that there is either evidence of tissue regeneration or clear demarcation of necrotic tissues, and the tissues should be kept warm and dry during in-between periods. There are a variety of commercial whirlpool or foot spa devices suitable for this purpose. It should be noted that a differential approach to rewarming is used in true frozen injuries in comparison to milder, nonfrozen cases. Milder cases should be warmed more slowly at normal room temperature, as rapid rewarming may exacerbate injury.

13.5.3 Pharmacological Support During Rewarming

Patients with frostbite require pharmacological support with respect to analgesia, vasodilatation and antibiosis, but certain caveats apply to the drugs that should be used and those that should be avoided. The rewarming of frozen tissues is frequently accompanied with severe pain, and all patients must therefore be provided with judicious amounts of analgesia. Analgesia should always, where possible, include ibuprofen due to its selective anti-prostaglandin activity, which may improve tissue perfusion in addition to providing analgesia. Some authors have recommended avoiding aspirin-based analgesia as it irreversibly blocks prostaglandin function and some vasodilatory prostacyclins, which may be beneficial in the healing wound [6]. Regarding vasodilators, surgical sympathectomy used to be used routinely but has now been superseded by vasodilatory drugs such as iloprost. Iloprost should be infused over a 5-day period in an appropriate high-care facility that is capable of performing regular (at least every 30 min) patient observations. Most units have locally approved infusion protocols for iloprost, but a suggested regime is to commence a 10 mL/h infusion of 100 mcg iloprost in 500 mL 0.9% saline. The dose can then be titrated up incrementally to a maximum of 50 mL/h or until there are observed side effects and should be run over a period of 6 h in any 1 day. Necrotic or devitalised tissues are at risk of infection, which may secondarily worsen tissue damage, and prophylactic broad-spectrum antibiotics, such as co-amoxiclav, should be administered together with tetanus vaccination where appropriate.

Thrombolytic therapy (see Table 13.3) with tissue plasminogen activator (t-PA) aims to lyse the multiple small intravascular thromboses that occur during the vascular stasis phase of frostbite and restore perfusion to the affected area, improving tissue survival. The use of t-PA reduced amputation rates from 41% to 10% in a study when administered within the first 24 h of injury [7]. Treatment with thrombolytic agents is not without risk (severe haemorrhage), and thrombolysis should only be reserved for patients presenting with severe frostbite within 24 h of injury and without any contraindications to treatment such as concurrent traumatic injuries. This form of treatment should only be considered in facilities that are equipped with high-dependency care facilities and are familiar with caring for patients undergoing thrombolytic therapy. Aside from the risk of associated major haemorrhage, the restoration of perfusion following thrombolysis to a

Table 13.3 Treatment algorithm for t-PA infusion

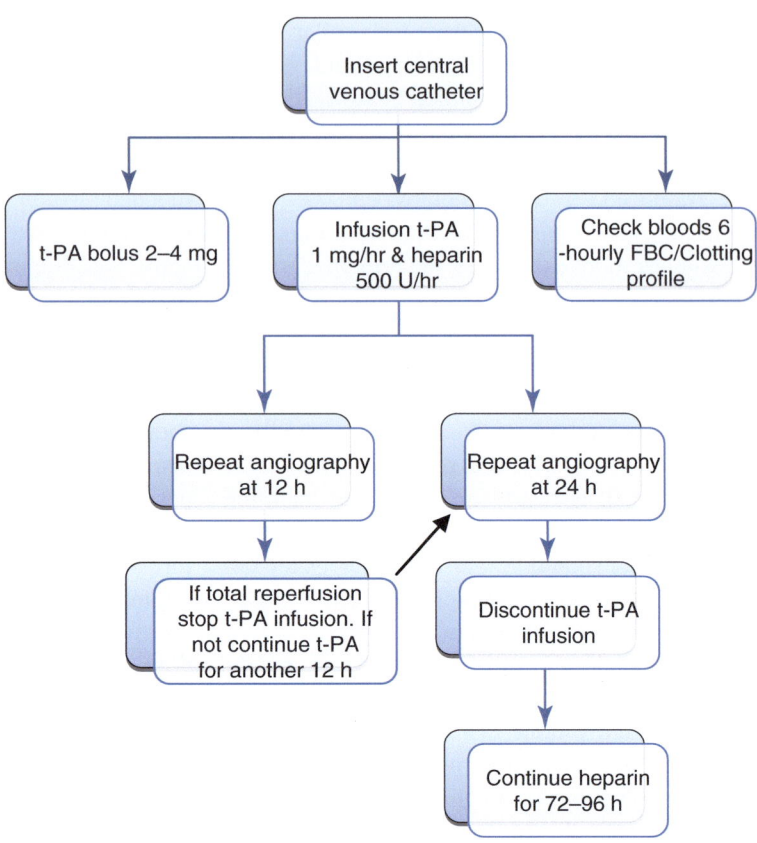

limb may cause a compartment syndrome (secondary to oedema from damaged capillaries), and the requirement for prophylactic fasciotomies must always be considered. The vasodilatory agent iloprost has been shown to be a suitable alternative to t-PA in a randomised controlled trial [8]. Cauchy et al. randomised 47 patients with frostbitten digits to receive either buflomedil, iloprost or iloprost + t-PA treatments following rewarming and antiplatelet therapy. Results showed that the risk of amputation was significantly lower in the iloprost and the iloprost + t-PA groups compared with the group that received buflomedil alone. No evidence was gained to suggest superiority of either treatment, and the study recommends that prostacyclin (iloprost) be used in patients with severe (grade 3) frostbite and the addition of t-PA be reserved for severe (grade 4) frostbite [8].
Adapted from Bruen et al. [7]

13.6 Post-thaw Frostbite Care

13.6.1 Management of Blisters

Areas subject to a freezing insult will frequently exhibit blistering, and a clinical decision must be taken as to the management of such areas. Generally speaking, small blistered areas that are not tense with clear fluid should be left intact as de-roofing these blisters may increase susceptibility to opportunistic infection. Blisters are sterile until they burst, and immunoglobulins have been shown to be present in blister fluid [9]. However, in most circumstances, more extensive areas of tense blistering or haemorrhagic blisters should be carefully de-roofed in aseptic conditions by a specialist. In rare cases where the patient is at particular risk of opportunistic infection, such as in dirty wounds, or if the patient is known to be colonised with a resistant organism, then it may be appropriate to leave all blistered areas intact to reduce the risk of a potentially devastating tissue infection, and all such cases must be discussed with a specialised unit. Topical aloe vera is a commonly suggested therapy in minor frostbite cases due to its anti-prostaglandin actions, and whilst there is little evidence to recommend its use, it may be considered in minor cases [1, 2].

13.6.2 Physiotherapy Protocols

Regardless of the clinical appearance, the affected area needs to be elevated in order to reduce venous stasis and tissue oedema. Similarly, all affected tissues will be fragile and easily disrupted through even gentle mechanical stresses; thus, all lower limb injuries must be placed on a strictly non-weight-bearing status to protect against ischaemia. These measures are designed to prevent extension of injury through progressive tissue oedema, thrombosis and ischaemia, and frequently areas that initially appeared non-salvageable will recover.

13.6.3 Surgery

Early surgical debridement of frostbite injuries is nearly always contraindicated, as the reversibility and progression of the frostbite injury cannot be quantified in the early stages. Debridement is best delayed until definitive demarcation of devitalised tissues at approximately 6–8 weeks post-injury. With appropriate management, surgery is frequently not required, despite the initial appearance of the injury. Similarly, it may be appropriate to leave demarked areas to auto-amputate if expert surgical input is not available or if the patient has substantial comorbidities making anaesthesia unsafe. Exceptions to this conservative approach to surgery include injuries with uncontrolled severe infection, concurrent severe limb trauma and compartment syndrome, all of which may require urgent limb surgery. Fortunately, these are infrequent and are more commonly seen in freeze-thaw-refreeze injuries (Table 13.4).

Adapted from Hallam et al. [1]

Table 13.4 Treatment algorithm for frostbite (Reproduced and adapted with permission from Hallam et al. [1], © BMJ, All Rights Reserved)

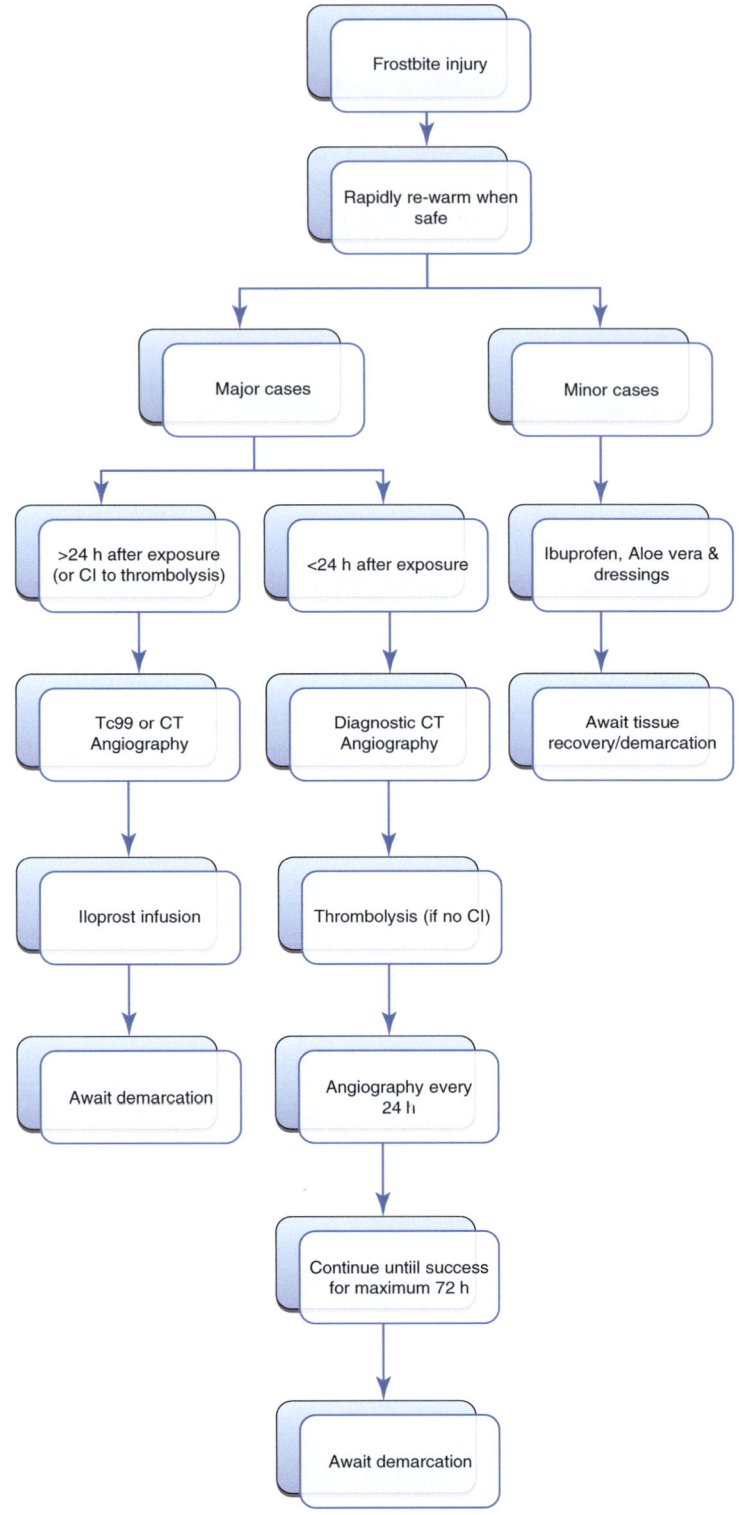

13.7 Summary Points

- Prevention is paramount.
- Treat any serious or life-threatening conditions as a priority.
- Do not rewarm frozen tissues until there is no risk of refreezing occurring.
- Rewarm nonfreezing cold injuries slowly in air.
- Rewarm freezing cold injuries at 37–39 °C or 40–41 °C in a whirlpool device or foot spa for a minimum 30 min with a mild antiseptic, and continue treatment twice daily until improvement is seen.
- Any patient with actual tissue loss should be given empirical broad-spectrum antibiotics.
- Discuss all significant cases with a specialised unit.
- Consider treatment adjuncts such as thrombolysis following discussion with a specialised unit.
- Avoid early surgical debridement.

References

1. Hallam M-J, Cubison T, Dheansa B, Imray C. Managing frostbite. BMJ. 2010;341:c5864. http://www.ncbi.nlm.nih.gov/pubmed/21097571
2. Grieve AW, Davis P, Dhillon S, Richards P, Hillebrandt D, Imray CHE. A clinical review of the management of frostbite. J R Army Med Corps. 2011;157(1):73–8. http://www.ncbi.nlm.nih.gov/pubmed/21465915
3. Cauchy E, Chetaille E, Marchand V, Marsigny B. Retrospective study of 70 cases of severe frostbite lesions: a proposed new classification scheme. Wild Environ Med. 2001;12(4):248–55. http://www.ncbi.nlm.nih.gov/pubmed/11769921
4. Cauchy E, Marsigny B, Allamel G, Verhellen R, Chetaille E. The value of technetium 99 scintigraphy in the prognosis of amputation in severe frostbite injuries of the extremities: a retrospective study of 92 severe frostbite injuries. J Hand Surg. 2000;25(5):969–78. http://www.ncbi.nlm.nih.gov/pubmed/11040315
5. State of Alaska Cold-Injury Guidelines. 2003:1–60. www.chems.alaska.gov
6. Imray C, Grieve A, Dhillon S. Cold damage to the extremities: frostbite and non-freezing cold injuries. Postgrad Med J. 2009;85(1007):481–8. http://www.ncbi.nlm.nih.gov/pubmed/19734516
7. Bruen KJ, Ballard JR, Morris SE, Cochran A, Edelman LS, Saffle JR. Reduction of the incidence of amputation in frostbite injury with thrombolytic therapy. Arch Surg (Chicago, Ill: 1960). 2007;142(6):546–51; discussion 551–3. http://www.ncbi.nlm.nih.gov/pubmed/17576891
8. Cauchy E, Cheguillaume B, Chetaille E. A controlled trial of a prostacyclin and rt-PA in the treatment of severe frostbite. N Engl J Med. 2011;364(2):189–90. http://www.ncbi.nlm.nih.gov/pubmed/21226604
9. Robson MC, Heggers JP. Evaluation of hand frostbite blister fluid as a clue to pathogenesis. J Hand Surg. 1981;6(1):43–7. http://www.ncbi.nlm.nih.gov/pubmed/7204918

Open Access This chapter is licensed under the terms of the Creative Commons Attribution-NonCommercial-NoDerivatives 4.0 International License (http://creativecommons.org/licenses/by-nc-nd/4.0/), which permits any non-commercial use, sharing, distribution and reproduction in any medium or format, as long as you give appropriate credit to the original author(s) and the source, provide a link to the Creative Commons license and indicate if you modified the licensed material. You do not have permission under this license to share adapted material derived from this chapter or parts of it.

The images or other third party material in this chapter are included in the chapter's Creative Commons license, unless indicated otherwise in a credit line to the material. If material is not included in the chapter's Creative Commons license and your intended use is not permitted by statutory regulation or exceeds the permitted use, you will need to obtain permission directly from the copyright holder.

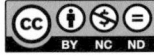

How to Manage Radiation Injuries

Chikako Senju, Masaki Fujioka, Katsumi Tanaka, and Sadanori Akita

14.1 Introduction

Complex chronic ulcers due to irradiation are sometimes seen in patients who have undergone radiation therapy for malignancies or X-ray fluoroscopic procedures for ischemic heart disease or radiation accidents. Radiation-induced ulcers are difficult to treat because of the poor state of the wound bed. Radiation of tissues results in insufficient vascularity and tissue damage, leading to erythema and dermal atrophy with resultant tissue necrosis, infection, and later fibrosis, all of which are characteristics of chronic radiation injury syndrome [1]. More specifically, 95% of cancer patients receiving radiation therapy will develop some form of radiodermatitis, including erythema, dry desquamation, and moist desquamation [2]. These undesirable complications cause continuous distress for patients and impair their quality of life.

14.2 Ionizing Radiation

Exposure to ionizing radiation generates a burst of free radicals, causing damage to deoxyribonucleic acid (DNA) and altering proteins, lipids, carbohydrates, and complex molecules [3]. The most sensitive cells are those that divide rapidly, such as the cells of the skin, bone marrow, and gastrointestinal tract. The severity of radiation-induced morbidity depends on the dose received, the time over which the dose is received, the volume of tissue irradiated, and the quality or type of radiation [4]. There are individual differences in the appearance of radiation-induced symptoms. Symptoms of acute radiation injury such as redness, blisters, sores, and skin ulcers occur within a few weeks after treatment. In contrast, late complications such as skin ulceration, tissue necrosis, and osteomyelitis may take months or years to develop and are often permanent.

The technique of radiation therapy for malignant tumors is improving, and the number of patients who develop radiation ulcers is thus decreasing. The technique of cardiac catheterization has advanced in recent years, and the procedure has become complicated. As a consequence, the irradiation time has become longer, and the number of people who develop radiation ulcers is

C. Senju (✉)
Department of Plastic and Reconstructive Surgery, Specified Medical Corporation Yuhakukai Senju Hospital, Nagasaki, Japan

M. Fujioka
Department of Plastic and Reconstructive Surgery, National Hospital Organization Nagasaki Medical Center, Nagasaki, Japan

K. Tanaka
Department of Plastic and Reconstructive Surgery, Nagasaki University Hospital, Nagasaki, Japan

S. Akita
Department of Plastic and Reconstructive Surgery, Medical Corporation Meiwakai Tamaki-Aozora Hospital, Tokushima, Japan

Fukushima Medical University, Fukushima, Japan

increasing. Therefore, despite these advancements, patients still experience the clinical consequences of radiation ulcers.

14.3 Radiation Ulcers

Radiation causes endothelial damage and fibrosis, leading to impairment of vascular and lymphatic flow. This impairment produces hypoxic, hypocellular, and hypovascular tissue that is unable to maintain normal tissue turnover, resulting in tissue necrosis, infection, and ulceration [5]. The naturally progressive wound-healing stage, which includes the hemostasis, inflammatory, proliferative, and remodeling phases, is impaired by collagen deposition and excessive extracellular matrix and fibrogenesis [6]. If wound healing is unsuccessful, a serious radiation ulcer will occur.

14.4 Management of Radiation Ulcers

Conservative treatments are not effective in most patients when a wound does not heal naturally. In such cases, surgical procedures are often required.

14.4.1 Debridement

Radiation ulcers are intractable and difficult to heal naturally because of the progression of necrosis. The underlying ischemia sets in motion a cycle of infection and necrosis, leading to the development of additional ulcers in the surrounding tissue and finally to gangrene. The principle of treatment is to perform sufficient excision including the surrounding red and pigmented tissue affected by radiation. However, there is no established index for the excision range, and it is often difficult to determine how much debridement should be performed. When the damage extends deep into the muscles and bones, extensive wound resection should extend to the area that has soft and sufficient blood flow. Although magnetic resonance imaging can help to diagnose infected bone presenting as osteomyelitis [7], it is generally difficult to determine the extent of bone resection required. Checking for bleeding from the bone marrow during surgery will allow the surgeon to determine the extent of resection required. If important tissues such as large blood vessels or nerves are damaged, as much tissue as possible should be excised without leaving any serious dysfunction. In case of calcification, resection including the calcified tissue will be required [8]. In addition, refractory radiation ulcers may require histological examination because they may include radiation-induced squamous cell carcinoma, skin cancer such as sarcoma, or recurrence of the original tumor [9, 10].

14.4.2 Methods of Wound Closure

After debridement, proper treatment that aids wound closure by surgery or stem cell transplantation is required.

14.4.2.1 Surgical Treatment
Local cutaneous flaps located within the radiation field are unreliable; they result in partial necrosis and rarely provide stable wound closure because of the poor blood flow of the surrounding skin [11]. Because skin grafts lack blood flow, adequate blood flow in the wound bed is required for skin engraftment. Thus, one of the two conditions is necessary: either thorough debridement to expose muscle with adequate blood flow or formation of good granulation tissue for successful skin engraftment [11, 12]. The most widely recommended method to heal these complex wounds is placement of musculocutaneous flaps harvested from nonirradiated areas; such flaps provide good blood circulation for effective results. This technique is also useful when

important organs such as the carotid artery, nerves, or bronchi are exposed [9]. Additionally, free flaps are useful for covering wounds. However, if the blood vessel on the recipient side is within the irradiation range, the condition of the vascular endothelial cells may be poor, and the blood vessel may be clogged. Therefore, to the greatest extent possible, it is necessary to perform anastomosis with a well-conditioned blood vessel outside the irradiation range on the recipient side [13].

14.4.2.2 Stem Cell Therapy

Many studies have confirmed that stem cells can improve tissue damage and dysfunction and that they may have clinical applications. Adipose-derived stem cells can differentiate into fibroblasts, keratinocytes, and endothelial cells. They can also secrete some cytokines that may promote their proliferation and migration. This increases angiogenesis and granulation, which promote wound healing [14]. Autologous adipose-derived regenerative cells (ADRCs) comprise several types of stem and regenerative cells, including adipose-derived stem cells. ADRCs can be collected via minimally invasive surgery by liposuction through a small incision [15]. When artificial dermis is used in combination with adipose stem cells, the artificial dermis becomes a scaffold for wounds, and the stem cells enter the artificial dermis to perform wound healing. By this process, intractable ulcers such as radiation ulcers can be healed [16].

14.5 Case Reports

14.5.1 Case 1

A 77-year-old man underwent cardiac catheterization. Nine months after irradiation, pigmentation, redness, and dermal atrophy were observed at the irradiation site (Fig. 14.1a). Twelve months after irradiation, the skin inflammation had progressed, resulting in the development of dry necrosis (Fig. 14.1b). Seventeen months after irradiation, an inadequate wound bed was observed after the necrotic tissue was removed (Fig. 14.1c). Debridement was performed, including adipose tissue and muscle that had been exposed to radiation, because healing had not occurred with conservative treatment (Fig. 14.1d). Nevertheless, the adipose tissue and muscle necrosis progressed (Fig. 14.1e). Because the wound did not heal properly, the patient was referred for plastic surgery. Extensive, deep debridement of the skin, adipose tissue, and muscles was performed, including the normal tissue around the irradiated area, and the wound was covered with a latissimus dorsi musculocutaneous flap (Fig. 14.1f). One year after surgery, the patient showed favorable wound resurfacing and no recurrence of the skin ulcers (Fig. 14.1g).

14.5.2 Case 2

A 66-year-old woman underwent radiation therapy 40 years previously for the treatment of breast cancer after ablation of the tumor. Redness of the skin was seen in the precordium, and a pus-draining fistula reached the sternum (Fig. 14.2a). Intraoperative examination revealed necrosis of the sternum and ribs, which were ablated with the parietal pleura (Fig. 14.2b). The thorax and pleura were restored using artificial substances (Fig. 14.2c). The wound was covered with a vertical rectus abdominis musculocutaneous flap. Nine months after surgery, the patient showed favorable wound resurfacing and no recurrence of skin ulcers (Fig. 14.2d).

14.5.3 Case 3

A 77-year-old woman underwent radiation treatment for breast cancer after ablation of the tumor. Examination revealed chronic chest ulcers that formed fistulae penetrating to the rib (Fig. 14.3a). Intraoperative examination showed necrosis of

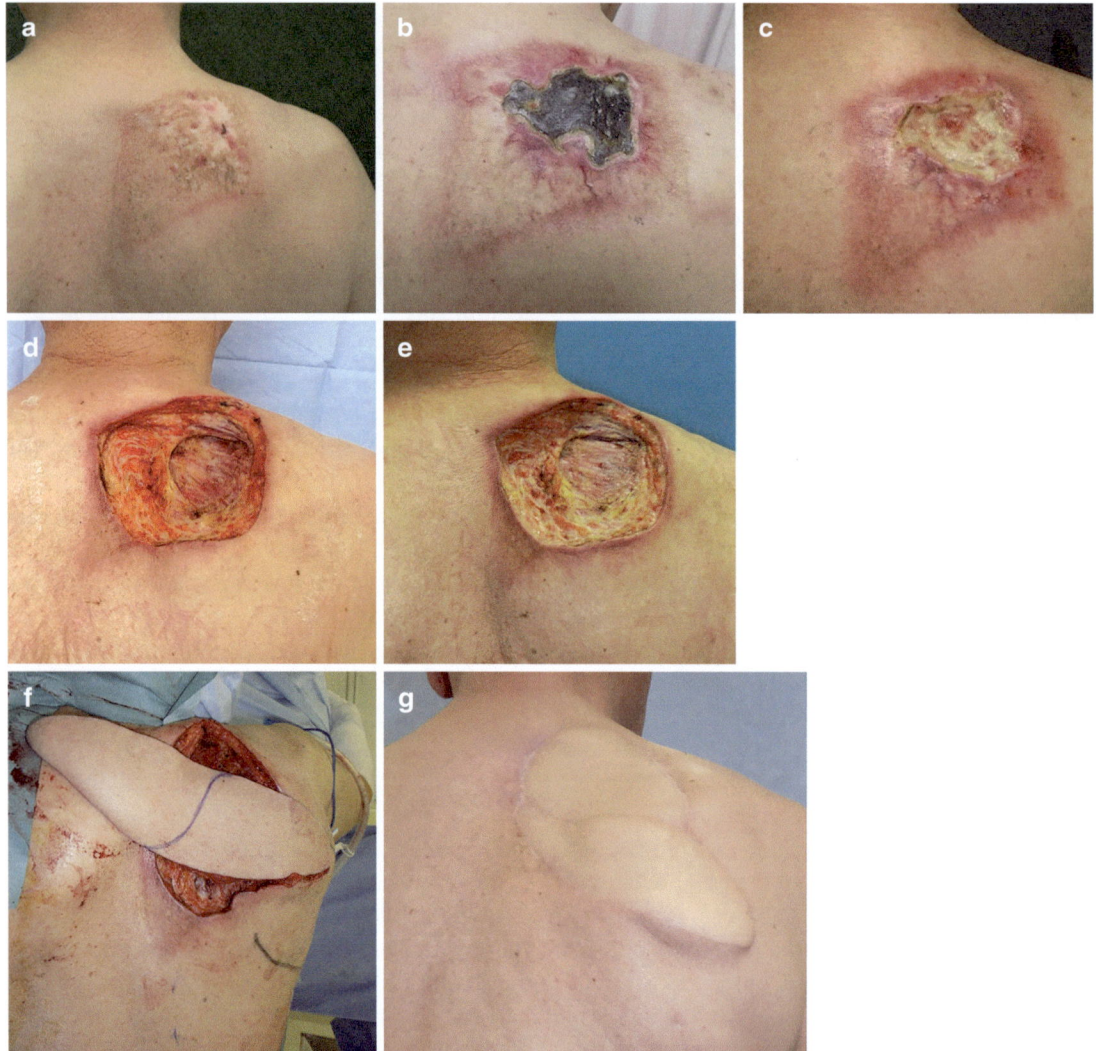

Fig. 14.1 (**a**) A 77-year-old man who underwent cardiac catheterization had developed irradiation, pigmentation, and redness after 9 months. (**b**) Twelve months after irradiation, the skin inflammation had progressed, leading to dry necrosis. (**c**) Seventeen months after irradiation, the necrotic tissue was removed. (**d**) Debridement was performed. (**e**) Five days after debridement, progression of adipose tissue and muscle necrosis was observed. (**f**) The debridement excision was enlarged, and a latissimus dorsi musculocutaneous flap was constructed. (**g**) One year after the surgery, the wound was resurfaced

the ribs, which were ablated with the parietal pleura. The pleura was restored using artificial material (Fig. 14.3b). The wound was covered by transfer of a latissimus dorsi musculocutaneous flap from the back (Fig. 14.3c). Six months after surgery, the radiation ulcer was reconstructed without disruption of shoulder movement (Fig. 14.3d).

14.5.4 Case 4

A 52-year-old woman developed intractable chronic radiation wounds. The thyroid cartilage was exposed, and the carotid artery was adjacent to the exposed cartilage (Fig. 14.4a). After surgical debridement, the size of the defect was 25 × 17 mm and reached partially to the left thy-

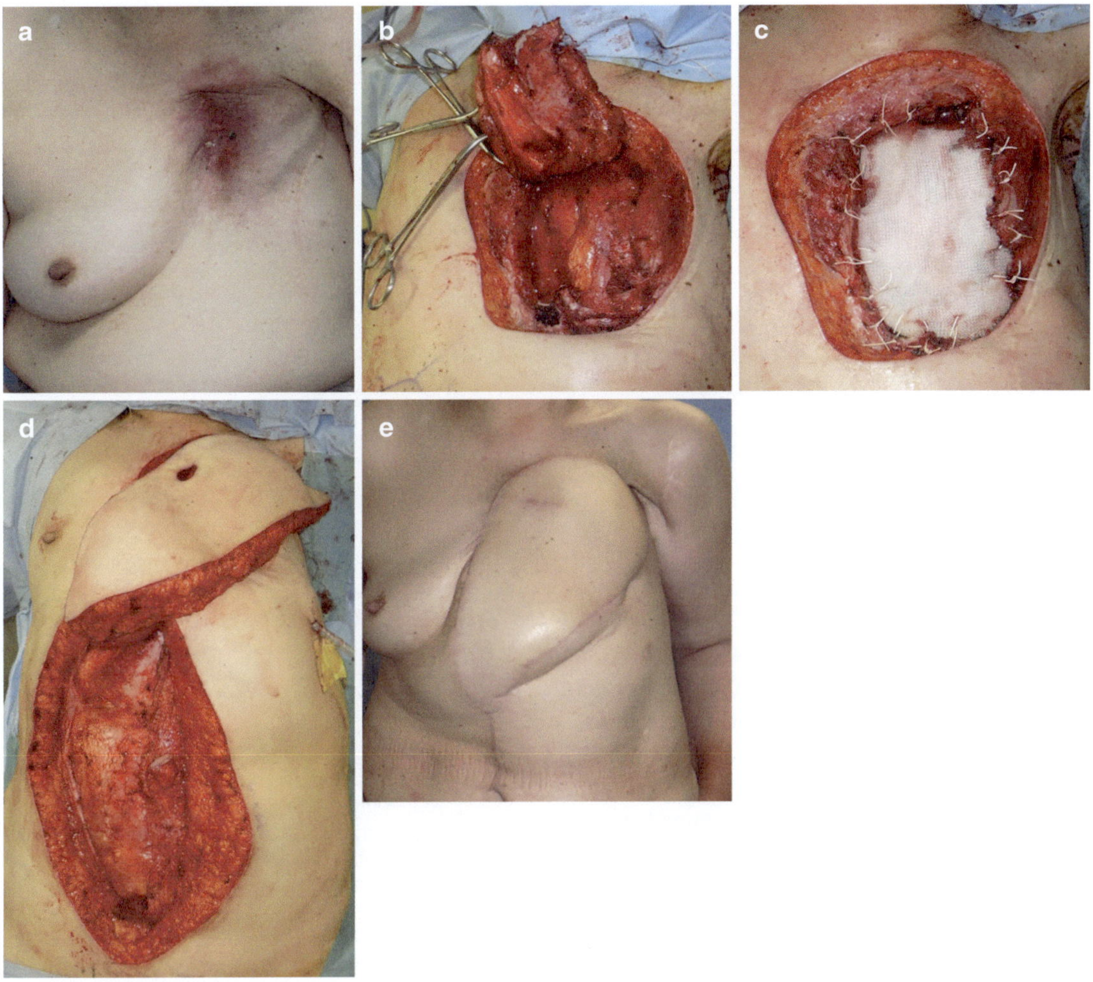

Fig. 14.2 (**a**) A 66-year-old woman underwent radiation therapy 40 years previously for the treatment of breast cancer after ablation of the tumor. The necrotic sternum was exposed. (**b**) Intraoperative examination showed necrosis of the sternum and ribs. (**c**) After debridement, the thorax and pleura were restored using artificial substances. (**d**) The radiation ulcer was reconstructed using a vertical rectus abdominis musculocutaneous flap. (**e**) Nine months after the surgery, the wound was resurfaced

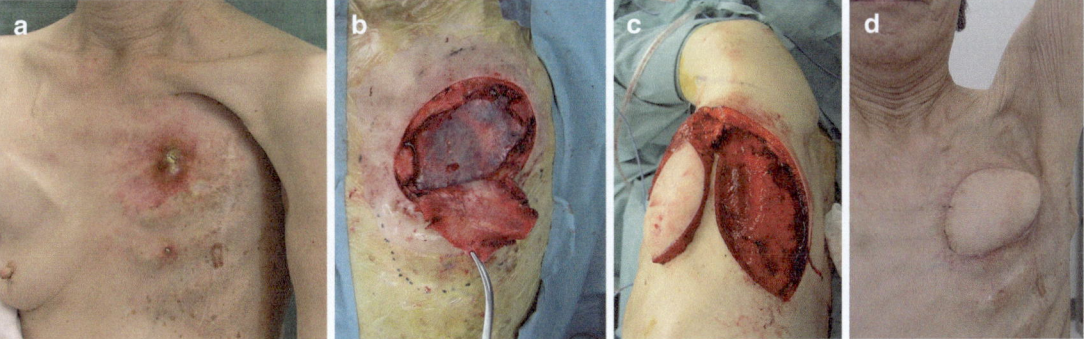

Fig. 14.3 (**a**) A 77-year-old woman underwent radiation treatment of breast cancer after ablation of the tumor. The necrotic rib was exposed. (**b**) After debridement, the pleura was restored using artificial substances. (**c**) A latissimus dorsi musculocutaneous flap was transferred from the back. (**d**) Six months after the surgery, the wound was resurfaced

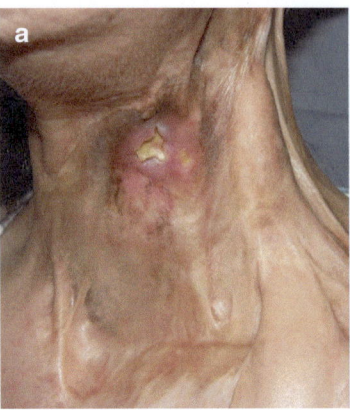 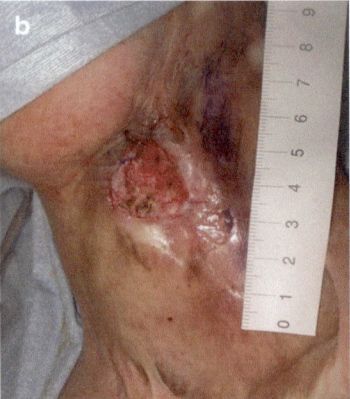 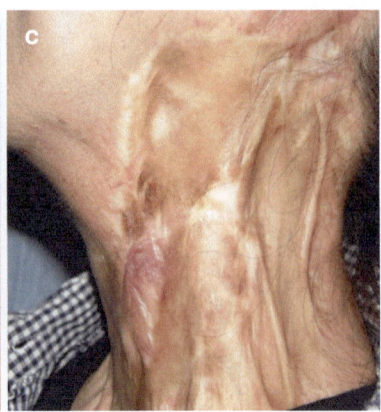

Fig. 14.4 (a) The thyroid cartilage was exposed because of a neck radiation-induced injury. (b) After debridement, the wound defect measured 25 × 17 mm. ADRCs were injected around the wound and into the artificial dermis. (c) Six months after the surgery, the wound was resurfaced

roid cartilage. Approximately 335 mL of adipose tissue containing 4.1×10^7 ADRCs was harvested by liposuction. Artificial dermis was used, and ADRCs were injected into the debrided wound margin, wound base, and artificial dermis (Fig. 14.4b). The wound had healed completely by 75 days after surgery. Six months later, the injected subcutaneous lesion maintained its soft texture and exhibited thick and vascularized soft tissue (Fig. 14.4c).

14.6 Conclusion

Radiation ulcers impair blood circulation in the irradiation field. The resulting wound becomes intractable because the natural healing process is unsuccessful. Radiation ulcers require treatment with adequately deep and wide debridement of the necrotic skin, adipose tissue, muscle, and sometimes bone. After debridement, healing must be promoted by covering the wound with well-circulated tissue or using adipose stem cells.

References

1. Olascoaga A, Vilar-Compte D, Poitevin-Chacón A, Contreras-Ruiz J. Wound healing in radiated skin: pathophysiology and treatment options. Int Wound J. 2008;5(2):246–57.
2. Singh M, Alavi A, Wong R, Akita S. Radiodermatitis: a review of our current understanding. Am J Clin Dermatol. 2016;17(3):277–92.
3. Denham JW, Hauer-Jensen M. The radiotherapeutic injury—a complex 'wound'. Radiother Oncol. 2002;63(2):129–45.
4. Gieringer M, Gosepath J, Naim R. Radiotherapy and wound healing: principles, management and prospects (review). Oncol Rep. 2011;26(2):299–307.
5. Wei KC, Yang KC, Mar GY, Chen LW, Wu CS, Lai CC, et al. STROBE—radiation ulcer: an overlooked complication of fluoroscopic intervention: a cross-sectional study. Medicine (Baltimore). 2015;94(48):e2178.
6. Bentzen SM. Preventing or reducing late side effects of radiation therapy: radiobiology meets molecular pathology. Nat Rev Cancer. 2006;6(9):702–13.
7. Pineda C, Espinosa R, Pena A. Radiographic imaging in osteomyelitis: the role of plain radiography, computed tomography, ultrasonography, magnetic resonance imaging, and scintigraphy. Semin Plast Surg. 2009;23(2):80–9.
8. Nakanishi T, Kuwahara M, Sasaki C, Ando J, Harada M, Takeuchi M. A radiation ulcer that required partial lung resection and recurred in a small residual area of ectopic calcification. Int J Surg Case Rep. 2021;85:106201.
9. Fujioka M. Surgical reconstruction of radiation injuries. Adv Wound Care (New Rochelle). 2014;3(1):25–37.
10. Kuwahara M, Yurugi S, Ando J, Takeuchi M, Miyata R, Harada M, et al. Squamous cell carcinoma developed in a chronic radiation-induced chest wall ulcer that is difficult to undergo thorough preoperative histological examination. Int J Surg Case Rep. 2020;72:467–70.
11. Wei KC, Yang KC, Chen LW, Liu WC, Chen WC, Chiou WY, et al. Management of fluoroscopy-induced

radiation ulcer: one-stage radical excision and immediate reconstruction. Sci Rep. 2016;6:35875.
12. Winaikosol K, Punyavong P, Jenwitheesuk K, Surakunprapha P, Mahakkanukrauh A. Radiation ulcer treatment with hyperbaric oxygen therapy and haemoglobin spray: case report and literature review. J Wound Care. 2020;29(8):452–6.
13. Ma X, Jin Z, Li G, Yang W. Classification of chronic radiation-induced ulcers in the chest wall after surgery in breast cancers. Radiat Oncol. 2017;12(1):135.
14. Huang SP, Huang CH, Shyu JF, Lee HS, Chen SG, Chan JY, et al. Promotion of wound healing using adipose-derived stem cells in radiation ulcer of a rat model. J Biomed Sci. 2013;20(1):51.
15. Akita S. Treatment of radiation injury. Adv Wound Care (New Rochelle). 2014;3(1):1–11.
16. Akita S, Yoshimoto H, Ohtsuru A, Hirano A, Yamashita S. Autologous adipose-derived regenerative cells are effective for chronic intractable radiation injuries. Radiat Prot Dosim. 2012;151(4):656–60.

Open Access This chapter is licensed under the terms of the Creative Commons Attribution-NonCommercial-NoDerivatives 4.0 International License (http://creativecommons.org/licenses/by-nc-nd/4.0/), which permits any non-commercial use, sharing, distribution and reproduction in any medium or format, as long as you give appropriate credit to the original author(s) and the source, provide a link to the Creative Commons license and indicate if you modified the licensed material. You do not have permission under this license to share adapted material derived from this chapter or parts of it.

The images or other third party material in this chapter are included in the chapter's Creative Commons license, unless indicated otherwise in a credit line to the material. If material is not included in the chapter's Creative Commons license and your intended use is not permitted by statutory regulation or exceeds the permitted use, you will need to obtain permission directly from the copyright holder.

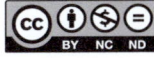

Excessive Internal Pressure (Dissecting Hematoma, Abdominal Hyperpressure, Abscesses, etc.) Leading to Skin Necrosis

Luc Téot

15.1 Introduction

Hyperpressure coming from inside is encountered in different clinical situations potentially leading to skin necrosis. Abdominal hyperpressure, dissecting hematoma, excessive edema, and infected collection are the most encountered causes of a progressive skin devascularization, leading to an occlusion of the dermal arteriolar system, causing necrosis of the skin.

15.2 Gastroschisis

Early management of large open abdomen occurring in gastroschisis during the neonatal period is mostly realized using mesh prosthesis. This very specialized surgical procedure should take care about the potential pulmonary hyperpressure together with an abdominal hyperpressure if an excessive tension is exerted over the abdominal fascial edges. The use of foreign implant material (Teflon, polytetrafluoroethylene patch) was reported to enhance the risk of mechanical hyperpressure and infection. This technique also imposes some degree of skin undermining, with potential complications, from a transient ischemia to a complete necrosis, leading in some cases to an infected prosthesis varying from 3% to 10% [1, 2]. Surgical procedures like myocutaneous flaps are needed in case of large skin necrosis [3].

15.3 Dissecting Hematoma

Hyperpressure induced by a progressing collection between the muscular fascia and the skin may be devastating for the skin. Blood impregnation of the fatty subcutaneous tissues transforms the mechanical properties of the skin, limiting the skin elasticity and creating a bumpy surface over a nonmobile area.

Elderly women are more affected than men, and the leg is the affected part; a predisposing factor is the dermatoporotic skin encountered in the elderly. Systemic corticosteroids and anticoagulation are also frequently observed.

Skin necrosis appears after a period of edema, confounding the clinical aspect with erysipelas, and an antibiotherapy was often started. Dissecting hematomas are rarely seen by an expert before 2–3 weeks. The diagnosis is confirmed by echography or RMI. Deep incision, clot evacuation, and debridement are the key elements to prevent local infection and allow wound healing [4].

L. Téot (✉)
Department of Plastic Surgery, Burns and Wound Healing, Montpellier University Hospital, Hôpital La Colombière, CICAT Occitanie, Montpellier Cedex 5, France
e-mail: l-teot@chu-montpellier.fr

15.4 Foreign Bodies and Paraosteoarthropathy

Pressure ulcers occurring in neurologically deficient patients presenting paraosteoarthropathy can be found in the literature [5]. The mechanisms generating a PU are comparable to pressure ulcers, with an extended risk linked to the heterotopic bone formation located superficially in the deep part of the skin. These heterotopic formations are usually located under the subcutaneous tissues, forming a nonelastic sheet with anarchic surface. In paraplegic patients, the position inside a rolling chair may induce an excessive pressure over the heterotopic subcutaneous bone formation in regard to the hip. Large hematomas may be observed, with the risk of heterotopic bone infection leading to the difficulty to heal and adding a risk of hip septic arthritis. Large debridement including all foreign bodies followed by NPWT Instill preparing flap surgery may be considered as the standard of care.

Heterotopic ossifications may be observed in leg ulcers [6] and in the extremities of amputated limbs, both in BK and AK amputations.

Calciphylaxis is observed in patients presenting a chronic renal insufficiency under frequent hemodialysis. Calcification of subdermal fat may induce rigid calcified blocks capable of skin perforation leading to severe infection (Fig. 15.1).

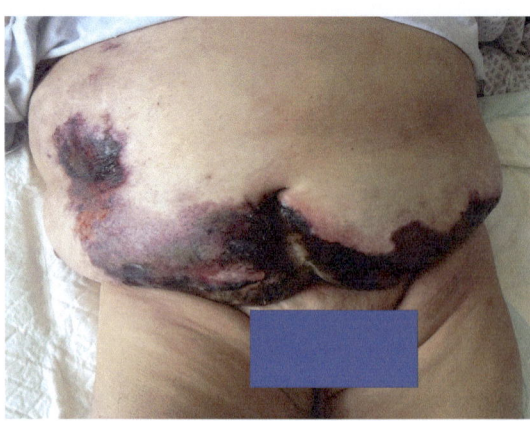

Fig. 15.1 Large abdominal calciphylaxis in a patient presenting a chronic renal insufficiency under hemodialysis

15.5 Diabetic Foot Abscesses

Wagner stage 4 cases involving large cavities in a diabetic foot should be considered as a surgical emergency and admitted rapidly in a specialized center [7, 8]. However, when this organization of care cannot be realized, some emergency protocols may save tissue.

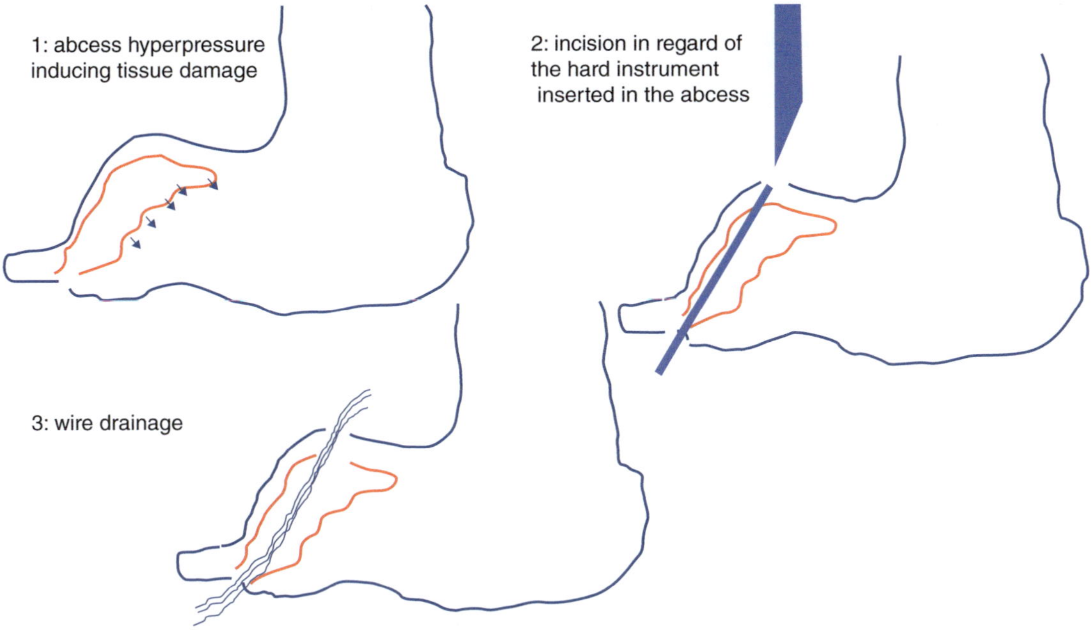

15 Excessive Internal Pressure (Dissecting Hematoma, Abdominal Hyperpressure, Abscesses, etc....

Fig. 15.2 Schematic emergency procedure to drain a hyperpressure linked to a diabetic foot abscess

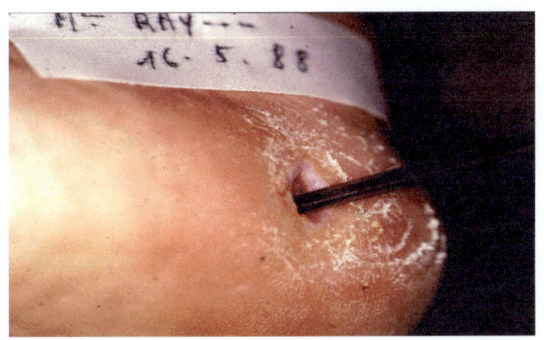

Fig. 15.3 Drainage of an infected DFU

In large abscesses with an infected tense, inflammatory foot showing a single minimal skin perforation in an interdigital web space, wound exploration of the depth of the cavity using a forceps measuring the length of undermining is crucial. Usually directed toward the dorsal aspect of the foot, the forceps can raise the skin at the extremity. A small incision using a scalpel will allow a drainage using polyethylene wires, rapidly reducing the tissue damage induced by the abscess hypertension (Figs. 15.2 and 15.3).

References

1. Debeugny P, Canarelli JP, Bonnevalle M, Besson R, Ricard J, Herlin P, Ducloux B. Laparoschisis. Indications for a teflon patch in wall repair. Chir Pediatr. 1990;31(1):18–25.
2. Trupka AW, Schweiberer L, Hallfeldt K, Waldner H. Management of large abdominal wall hernias with foreign implant materials (Gore-Tex patch). Zentralbl Chir. 1997;122(10):879–84.
3. Balén EM, Díez-Caballero A, Hernández-Lizoáin JL, Pardo F, Torramadé JR, Regueira FM, Cienfuegos JA. Repair of ventral hernias with expanded polytetrafluoroethylene patch. Br J Surg. 1998;85(10):1415–8. https://doi.org/10.1046/j.1365-2168.1998.00849.x.
4. Vanzi V, Toma E. Deep dissecting haematoma in patients with dermatoporosis: implications for home nursing. Br J Community Nurs. 2021;26(Sup3):S6–S13. https://doi.org/10.12968/bjcn.2021.26.Sup3.S6.
5. Yang K, Graf A, Sanger J. Pressure ulcer reconstruction in patients with heterotopic ossification after spinal cord injury: a case series and review of literature. J Plast Reconstr Aesthet Surg. 2017;70(4):518–28. https://doi.org/10.1016/j.bjps.2016.11.026. Epub 2016 Dec 21
6. Cafasso DE, Bowen DK, Kinkennon SA, Stanbro MD, Kellicut DC. Heterotopic ossificans in chronic venous insufficiency: a new consideration for clinical, aetiology, anatomy and pathophysiology stag-

ing. Phlebology. 2013;28(7):361–5. https://doi.org/10.1258/phleb.2012.012050. Epub 2013 May 6
7. Hingorani A, LaMuraglia GM, Henke P, Meissner MH, Loretz L, Zinszer KM, Driver VR, Frykberg R, Carman TL, Marston W, Mills JL Sr, Murad MH. The management of diabetic foot: a clinical practice guideline by the Society for Vascular Surgery in collaboration with the American Podiatric Medical Association and the Society for Vascular Medicine. J Vasc Surg. 2016;63(2 Suppl):3S–21S. https://doi.org/10.1016/j.jvs.2015.10.003. PMID: 26804367
8. Duane TM, Huston JM, Collom M, Beyer A, Parli S, Buckman S, Shapiro M, McDonald A, Diaz J, Tessier JM, Sanders J. Surgical infection society 2020 updated guidelines on the management of complicated skin and soft tissue infections. Surg Infect. 2021;22(4):383–99. https://doi.org/10.1089/sur.2020.436. Epub 2021 Feb 26

Open Access This chapter is licensed under the terms of the Creative Commons Attribution-NonCommercial-NoDerivatives 4.0 International License (http://creativecommons.org/licenses/by-nc-nd/4.0/), which permits any non-commercial use, sharing, distribution and reproduction in any medium or format, as long as you give appropriate credit to the original author(s) and the source, provide a link to the Creative Commons license and indicate if you modified the licensed material. You do not have permission under this license to share adapted material derived from this chapter or parts of it.

The images or other third party material in this chapter are included in the chapter's Creative Commons license, unless indicated otherwise in a credit line to the material. If material is not included in the chapter's Creative Commons license and your intended use is not permitted by statutory regulation or exceeds the permitted use, you will need to obtain permission directly from the copyright holder.

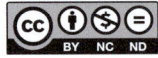

Telemedicine and Skin Necrosis

16

Anne Dompmartin and Véronique Hyppolite

16.1 Introduction

Tissue death or skin necrosis can occur from an injury, trauma, radiation treatment, chemical exposure, or inflammatory disease. DNA structure damage appears within the cells, preventing mitosis which is an essential process of healthy and normal cell duplication. Removing all the tissue necrosis is mandatory to heal the wound and prevent infection [1]. The level of tissue necrosis depends on the etiology of the lesion. Withdrawal of these tissues can be performed by surgery, but it may be difficult as necrosis has to be circumscribed. Therefore, nurse care needs to be performed to accelerate the process. Communication technology devices currently available can adequately support the need of tele-assistance for this specific wound care.

16.2 Diagnosis of Skin Necrosis

There are two main types of necrotic tissue present in wounds. One is a dry, thick, leathery tissue, usually tan, brown, or black in color. The other is often yellow, slough, tan, green, or brown and might be moist, loose, and stringy in appearance. Necrotic tissue will eventually become black, hard, and leathery. Before any wound care, the knowledge of the etiology of the skin necrosis is mandatory. It will guide wound care and global follow-up of the patient. Management of a necrotic ulcerated skin tumor (Fig. 16.1) is different from a calciphylaxis (Fig. 16.2).

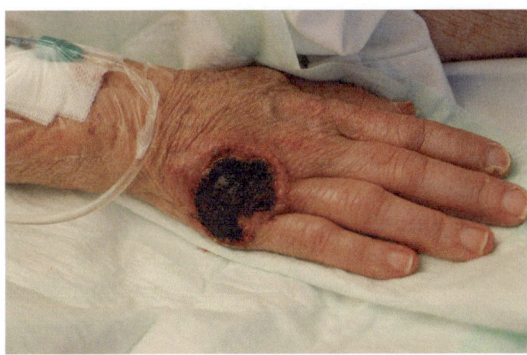

Fig. 16.1 Necrotic ulceration of a carcinoma on the dorsum of the hand

A. Dompmartin (✉) · V. Hyppolite
Dermatology Department, CHU Caen, Caen, France
e-mail: dompmartin-a@chu-caen.fr;
hyppolite-v@chu-caen.fr

© The Author(s) 2024
L. Téot et al. (eds.), *Skin Necrosis*, https://doi.org/10.1007/978-3-031-60954-1_16

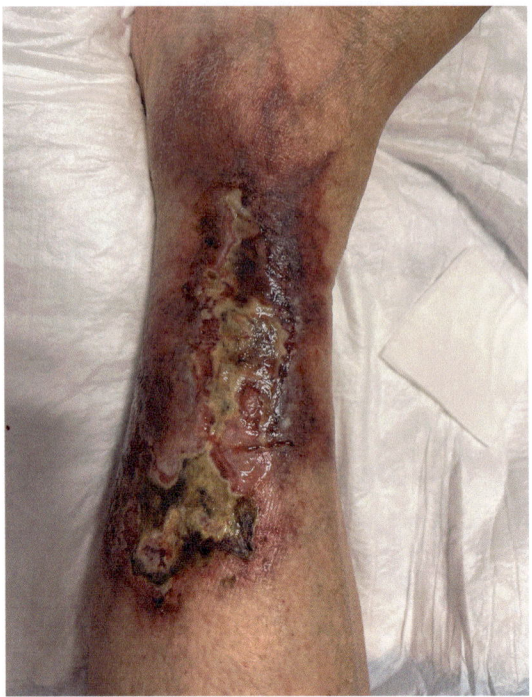

Fig. 16.2 Calciphylaxis of the leg in a patient with renal insufficiency

16.3 Tele-Assistance

Telemedicine can be performed with two modalities: live interactive and store and forward. The live interactive systems operate in real time and include a video monitor and high-resolution camera [2–5]. The store and forward technology can be described as e-mail pictures; the clinical history collected is accompanied by radiologic and/or photographic images to support the clinical history. Tele-consultation and tele-assistance need synchronous communication via video conferencing or telephone calls to allow real-time interaction between the home nurse and the physician or the expert nurse during the wound care. The store and forward technology is used for tele-expertise: dermatoses, interpretation of biologic examinations, etc. There is a need for a common clear regulation for practicing telemedicine, encompassing privacy issues and data management, and these rules have been established in most countries.

16.4 Technology

Technology is adapted according to the different countries. Initially only for medical care, it has been widened to other healthcare professionals to decrease professional isolation through mutual aid. It uses a wireless technology, which is an audiovisual communication system that has the capacity for synchronous electronic voice and image transfer. The bedside nurse has a mobile phone or a computer tablet, and an expert nurse observes the wound on her computer screen. All data are transmitted via a secure connection.

The expert nurses are enterostomal therapy nurses or nurses with strong knowledge (diploma in wound care) and clinical experience in complex wound care. They need to write reports of virtual clinical sessions, which are inserted in the medical file of the patient and sent to all the healthcare professionals of the patient. Expert and resource nurses need familiarization with the service and the related technologies but have also to be convinced of the importance of secure transmission of medical data [6].

16.5 Telemedicine and Skin Necrosis

Prior to the removal of the death tissue, the first step is clinical assessment of the necrosis in order to decide if the necrosis needs to be softened or hardened before removal. Swelling, edema, and inflammation need to be detected as the main problems are the underlying tissues, which will be the bed of wound healing. This first step is usually decided in specialized centers before remote follow-up and wound care analgesia are prescribed. Acral lesions are usually mummified so that hard necrosis is circumscribed and comes off easily (Fig. 16.3a, b). Wound care is simple with dressing that absorbs exudates. Necrosis can also be softened with hydrogel and removed progressively with a scalpel, on the face, limbs, or trunk (Fig. 16.4). Therefore, the type of wound care has to be clearly explained to the resource nurses before the patient comes back home.

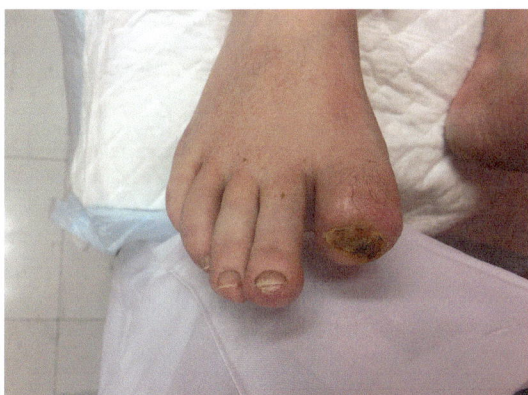

Fig. 16.3 Acral necrosis of a patient in intensive care unit; mummification of the lesions. The aim is to dry and circumscribe the necrosis. Wound care allowed to cut the distal necrosis of the finger

Tele-assistance is proposed as a remote follow-up to remove necrosis. Removal of skin necrosis is often difficult at home for bedside nurses who feel isolated and need clinical support. It is an interventional care that needs a team to reassure the bedside nurse. It is also an opportunity for the resource nurses to widen their knowledge and feel more comfortable for wound debridement. This knowledge transfer is also closely linked to the rise of professional autonomy and reduces professional isolation. Another important benefit of tele-assistance is to reduce the travel of patients to hospitals, which promotes time and cost savings [7, 8].

16.6 Conclusion

Tele-assistance helps to support resource nurses and improves nurse practice and quality of care. The resource nurse needs to trust the experience and the knowledge of the expert nurse or the medical doctor who assists them remotely. Contrary to tele-consultation, tele-assistance is not integrated in most healthcare systems although the benefit is widely recognized. Removal of skin necrosis that needs specific care is a good illustration of the interest of remote wound care assistance.

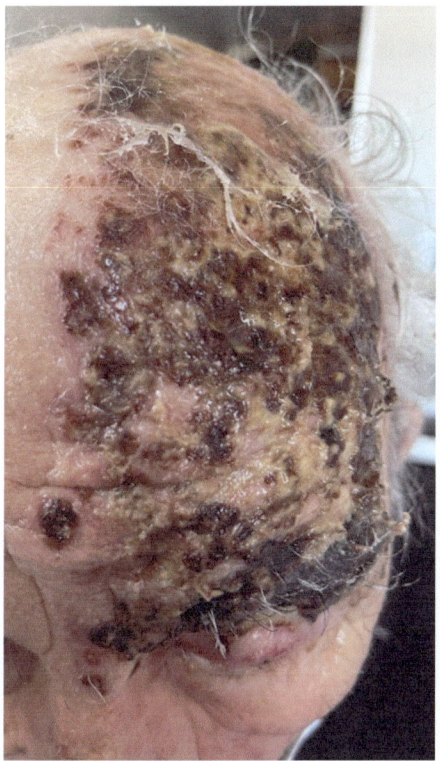

Fig. 16.4 Necrotic herpes zoster of the face: necrosis has to be softened and removed with a scalpel

References

1. Mosti G. Wound care in venous ulcers. Phlebology. 2013;28(Suppl 1):79–85.
2. Singh G, Pal US, Mishra M, Gaur A, Pathak D, Singh YB. Teleassistance and teleconsultation using smartphone and its contribution in clinical progress of oral and maxillofacial surgery. Natl J Maxillofac Surg. 2020;11(1):10–3.
3. De Cola MC, Maresca G, D'Aleo G, Carnazza L, Giliberto S, Maggio MG, Bramanti A, Calabrò RS. Teleassistance for frail elderly people: a usability and customer satisfaction study. Geriatr Nurs. 2020;41(4):463–7.

4. Loh CH, Chong Tam SY, Oh CC. Teledermatology in the COVID-19 pandemic: a systematic review. JAAD Int. 2021;5:54–64.
5. Ekeland AG, Bowes A, Flottorp S. Effectiveness of telemedicine: a systematic review of reviews. Int J Med Inform. 2010;79(11):736–71.
6. Chaet D, Clearfield R, Sabin JE, Skimming K, Council on Ethical and Judicial Affairs American Medical Association. Ethical practice in telehealth and telemedicine. J Gen Intern Med. 2017;32(10):1136–40.
7. Corriveau G, Couturier Y, Camden C. Developing competencies of nurses in wound care: the impact of a new service delivery model including teleassistance. J Contin Educ Nurs. 2020;51(12):547–55.
8. Gagnon MP, Breton E, Courcy F, Quirion S, Côté J, Paré G. The influence of a wound care teleassistance service on nursing practice: a case trial in Quebec. Telemed J E Health. 2014;20(6):593–600.

Open Access This chapter is licensed under the terms of the Creative Commons Attribution-NonCommercial-NoDerivatives 4.0 International License (http://creativecommons.org/licenses/by-nc-nd/4.0/), which permits any non-commercial use, sharing, distribution and reproduction in any medium or format, as long as you give appropriate credit to the original author(s) and the source, provide a link to the Creative Commons license and indicate if you modified the licensed material. You do not have permission under this license to share adapted material derived from this chapter or parts of it.

The images or other third party material in this chapter are included in the chapter's Creative Commons license, unless indicated otherwise in a credit line to the material. If material is not included in the chapter's Creative Commons license and your intended use is not permitted by statutory regulation or exceeds the permitted use, you will need to obtain permission directly from the copyright holder.

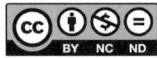

Part III

Skin Necrosis of Toxic Origin

Introduction to Skin Necrosis of Toxic Origin

Sadanori Akita

Medical toxic agents and animal or insect bites can cause skin necrosis. In addition, there are clinical and forensic signs of opioid abuse. Coma-induced blisters are a rare condition associated with prolonged impairment of consciousness levels, which is relatively well known in adults following an overdose of barbiturates. This chapter covers skin ulcers and necrosis due to medications, snakebites, jellyfish and stonefish, spider *Loxosceles reclusa*, scorpions, and "drugs" such as *Cannabis sativa*, cocaine, and heroin. It also discusses the systemic conditions of the toxic syndrome and how to resuscitate foot necrosis. Each theme can bring about a better understanding of how it develops and how to treat it properly.

S. Akita (✉)
Department of Plastic Surgery, Tamaki-Aozora Hospital, Tokushima, Japan

Fukushima Medical University, Fukushima, Japan
e-mail: akitas@hf.rim.or.jp

Open Access This chapter is licensed under the terms of the Creative Commons Attribution-NonCommercial-NoDerivatives 4.0 International License (http://creativecommons.org/licenses/by-nc-nd/4.0/), which permits any noncommercial use, sharing, distribution and reproduction in any medium or format, as long as you give appropriate credit to the original author(s) and the source, provide a link to the Creative Commons license and indicate if you modified the licensed material. You do not have permission under this license to share adapted material derived from this chapter or parts of it.

The images or other third party material in this chapter are included in the chapter's Creative Commons license, unless indicated otherwise in a credit line to the material. If material is not included in the chapter's Creative Commons license and your intended use is not permitted by statutory regulation or exceeds the permitted use, you will need to obtain permission directly from the copyright holder.

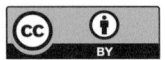

Resuscitation Foot Necrosis: A New Entity for a Complex Management?

Franck Duteille

18.1 Introduction

As in every medical discipline, resuscitation techniques are regularly progressing, allowing more and more patients to survive. In these departments, acute skin problems are observed, particularly those linked to the use of vasopressive drugs prescribed to maintain a stable patient haemodynamics.

Once the acute phase is solved and the patients are stabilised, the consequence of the use of these vasopressive drugs may appear and become the main difficult problem. The context is variable, but most of these patients have presented or still present with prolonged haemodynamic shocks (septic shock, purpura fulminans, etc.) [1].

Since the last decade, we have been confronted with a series of patients presenting with skin and tissular distal extremity necrosis following intensive care. Problems were essentially involving the hands and feet. This new capacity of resuscitating desperate life-threatening situations in patients who already died creates a series of new challenging tissular reconstruction. The management of these patients is delicate in terms of the therapeutic decisions (amputation or limb salvage) but also of the OR planning and modalities. We hereby propose action to be taken and the elements of management, which have shown to be important in view of our clinical experience.

18.2 Clinical Presentation

This dry necrosis has probably evolved from the superficial to the deep structures. The whole skin and subcutaneous tissues may be affected (skin, subcutaneous cellular tissue, muscles). The damage is essentially located at the level of the toes but also involves the plantar vault leaving intact the calcaneal area, a sign of pejorative evolution.

Lesions appearing on the dorsal aspect of the foot are usually less extended than on the plantar aspect and appear secondarily. The pathophysiology is linked to vasoconstriction (linked to amines) potentialised by the existence of a haemodynamic failure already present in these patients. This drop in blood flow linked to vasoconstriction may lead to small-diameter vessel thrombosis explaining the clinical situation: necrosis from superficial to deep toe necrosis with thrombosis of the collateral arteries.

18.3 The Therapeutic Decision

18.3.1 Evolution

The choices made during the surgical debridement procedure should be carefully balanced

F. Duteille (✉)
Department of Plastic, Reconstructive and Aesthetic Surgery, Burn Centre, Hotel Dieu, Nantes Cedex 01, France

because of their impact on the whole success. This decision must be made in careful consultation with the critical care team. The evolution of this necrosis is different to that found in arterial patients. In fact, intensive care patients are often young and do not present with preliminary vascular lesions or permanent heart failure. The vascular injury observed in resuscitation is therefore an epiphenomenon, and the improvement of the haemodynamic status associated with the limitation of vasopressive drug administration will sometimes allow the partial recovery of tissue which initially appeared as destroyed. Also in Fig. 18.1, this patient presents with an extremely disturbing situation of the foot arch and for which we observed a complete or partial tissue recovery (with the disappearance of the shock associated with the suppression of amines). The necrosis was limited to the superficial part of the cutaneous tissue; the toes could not be saved. There is therefore a real danger in planning a surgical procedure before the patient is in a completely stable status. In our experience, the surgical procedure started 15 days at the earliest after the stabilisation of the clinical status and the suppression of amines. An earlier debridement can conduce to excise tissue with uncertain evolution. This is equally true of a certain number of intensive care specialists who 'push' to debridement partly because the fever presented by the patients may be linked to necrotic tissue (Fig. 18.2).

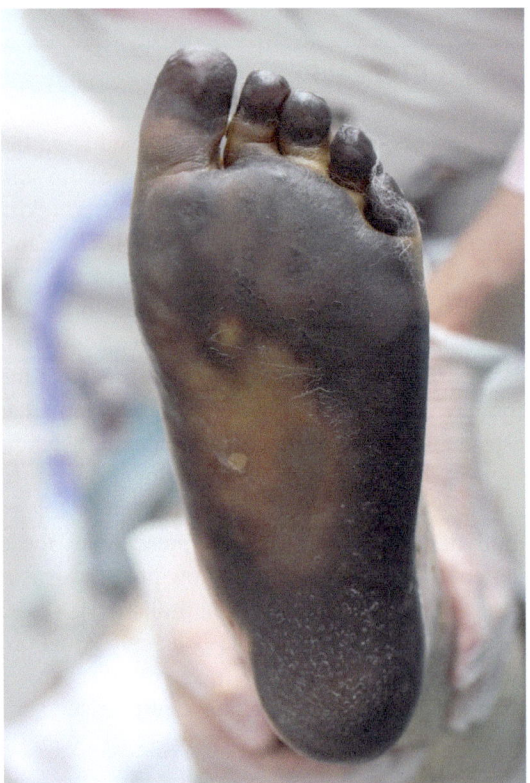

Fig. 18.1 Initial state of a patient still taking vasopressive drugs

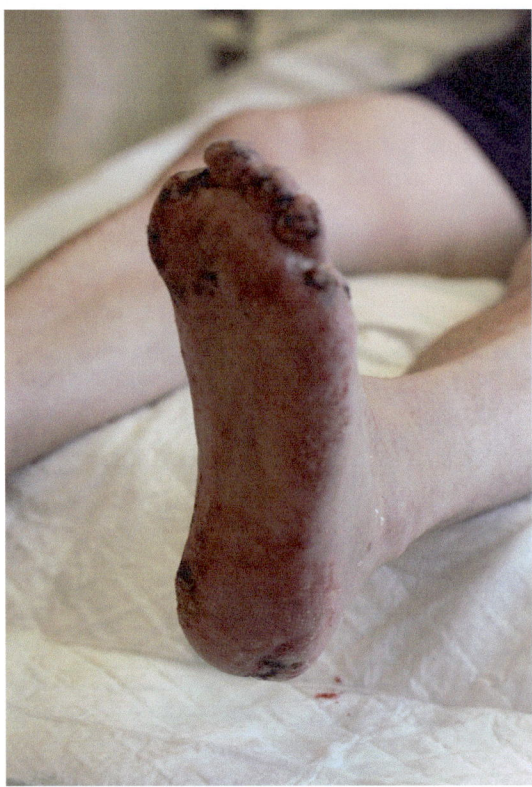

Fig. 18.2 Evolution 3 weeks after and the stopping of vasoactive drugs and amputation of the toes

18.3.2 The Strategy Concerning the Therapeutic Attitude

The therapeutic decision is complex and does not comply with the established decision tree. It mainly depends on the experience of the practitioner, but the final decision often comes from the patient himself.

We exclude the situations relying on classical techniques of healing (skin graft, treatment by negative pressure, etc.). We have limited ourselves to the most serious situations where the only solution is to perform a free flap to avoid the amputation of the leg [2].

Some authors describe the interest of hyperbaric oxygen. But it was only one case report and in a child [3]. And the study did not describe the importance of tissue necrosis; thus, it is difficult to evaluate the real interest of this treatment. Situations exist where all attempts at salvage are excluded due to the clinical situation: necrosis affecting the entire foot (plantar side, dorsal side, and heel cup) and especially when the necrosis reaches the proximal aspect of the ankle (Fig. 18.3), the contraindications to microsurgery

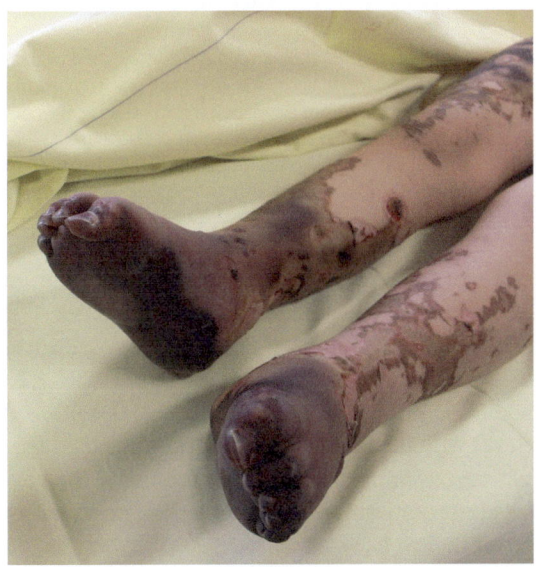

Fig. 18.3 A young boy 6 years of age presenting with necrosis of 2 ft. going up to the ankle. Surgical exploration having confirmed this extensive necrosis with notable necrosis in the two ankle bones; no solution has unfortunately been envisioned

(arterial patient, heart failure, renal failure, etc.), and a patient who has no donor site (latissimus dorsi muscle). When a solution seems conceivable, the patient must be seen awake and the therapeutic stake must be clearly explained, as well as the risks of amputation, in case of failure. These patients should be in complete physiological and mental recovery, and this decision does not need to be taken urgently. It is also necessary to see the patient several times to be sure that the situation and the potential complications are completely understood. Of course, all the elements will be taken into account in the therapeutic option (age, professional activity, uni- or bilateral injury, etc.). As in many of these difficult decision-making moments, care must be taken to avoid increasing the number of people involved as this makes the decision process more complicated for the patient. Nevertheless, we ask a rehabilitation doctor specialised in limb prostheses to visit the patient, so that the patient has a complete picture of the problems. The options can be simplified to salvage or amputation of one or more limbs or parts of the limbs. The objective is saving the foot, but toes were usually not saved. The aim is therefore to anticipate a back-to-normal walking. However, running will definitively be compromised.

The salvage requires a microsurgical muscle transfer. Usually, the latissimus dorsi muscle is used (isolated or associated with the dental muscle) to cover this large loss of substance. The choice of muscle (versus cutaneous flap) is fundamental. This choice remains controversial [4], but for us, it will be the only way to fill the dead space volume after debridement, it is the only way to be sufficiently thick to ensure a secondary support and avoid the soaping phenomenon, and it is the best way to reduce the risk of infection. In addition, we think that the blood reserve that represents the muscle allows debridement to be limited because certain undefined tissue limits may benefit the vascular supply brought locally by the revascularised muscle. The only negative in this strategy is the sacrifice of the latissimus dorsi muscle, which may be detrimental if the intervention fails, and the use of crutches proves to be necessary.

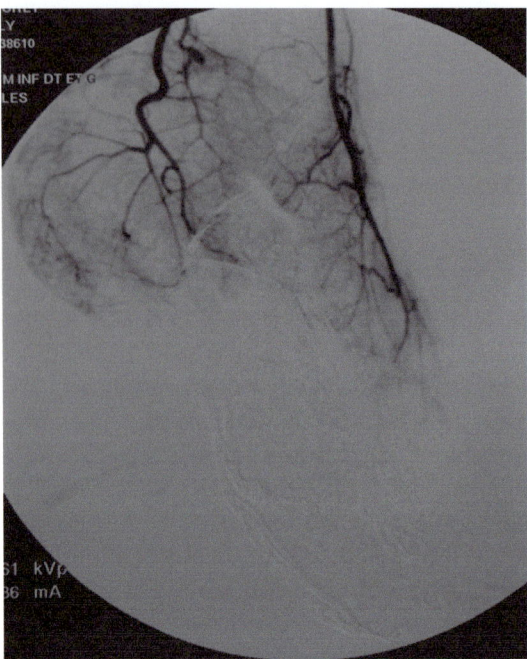

Fig. 18.4 Arteriogram of a 42-year-old patient presenting with a 'resuscitation foot' with a clear interruption of the flow and a desert afterwards

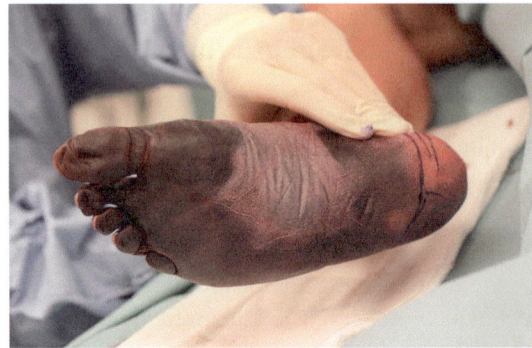

Fig. 18.5 A 42-year-old patient presenting with necrosis of almost all of the insteps following a visit in rehabilitation for septic shock and the use of vasoconstrictive drugs

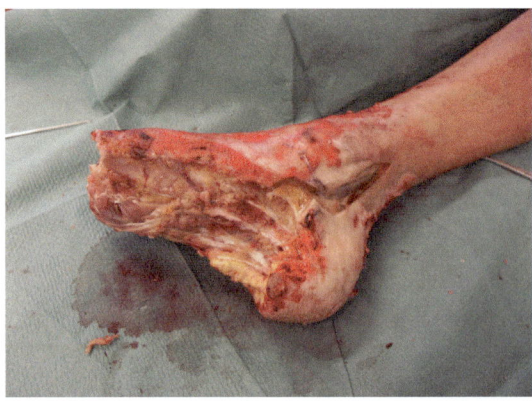

Fig. 18.6 The foot of the same patient after the surgical debridement (we may note that the heel cup is partially preserved, which is often the case), the debridement is not exhaustive, and certain tissues have uncertain vitality but are left in place because we hope for a certain part of 'revascularisation' contributed from the free flap

If the decision is taken, a vascular assessment is performed in order to explore the arteries of the lower limbs. The choice of an arteriogram or an echo/Doppler with a flux calculation may be performed. The arteriogram usually shows a clear interruption of the arteries with a healthy network before and a vascular desert after (Fig. 18.4).

18.3.3 Surgical Intervention

Debridement and free flap will be performed during the same operation. Debridement must remove all the necrotic tissue but must try to leave in place the tissue which is in doubt or especially limit the bone structures for the reasons explained earlier. The flap specimen will only be started (by a second team if possible) once the debridement has been performed and the salvage indication has been confirmed (Figs. 18.5 and 18.6). The vessels must be addressed in a healthy zone. On the strategic plan, it is necessary to expect an option for covering pedicle anastomoses of the free flap because complete debridement does not offer any option of covering the remaining tissue on the foot. For these, the Z incisions (allowing a V/Y closure) are made opposite to the recipient vessels. In addition, the entire latissimus dorsi is removed (level with the tendinous insertion). The high part of the muscle may also be redriven over the vessels after anastomosis completion in order to cover them.

The recipient vessels have always been of good quality, in our experience (Fig. 18.7), because it concerns a young patient with no mechanical avulsion and trauma. The limit between the healthy and pathological zone is

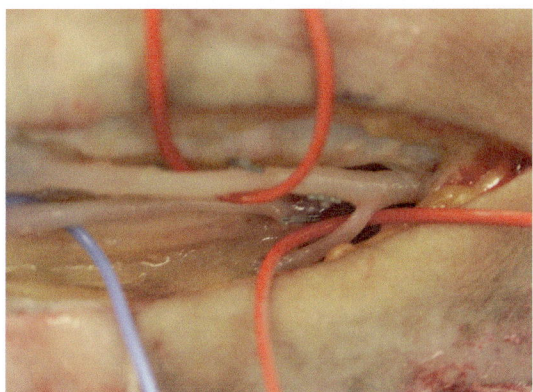

Fig. 18.7 Expose the vessels of the patient; these appear healthy during the surgical exploration

actually extremely clean. Technically, this microsurgical act does not at all differ from the standard free flap. During the follow-up period, we apply the normal protocols: fasting during 12 h in case it is necessary to perform further surgery, bed rest for 5 days, and regular monitoring of the flap. The dermo-epidermal skin graft on the muscle is performed between the fifth and eighth days associated with the restructuring of the flap.

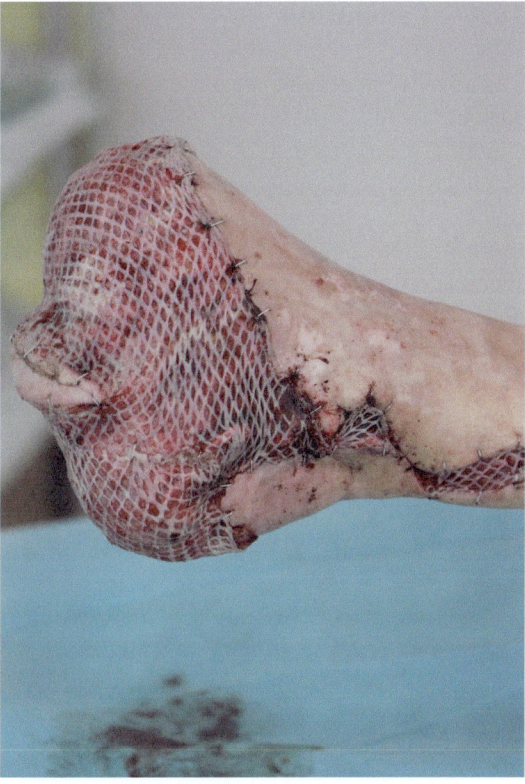

Fig. 18.8 The flap is put in place and grafted 15 days after the intervention. Its bulky appearance is only temporary

18.3.4 Follow-Up

When complete healing of the flap has been achieved, it is necessary to be sure of its very bulky aspect and especially its temporary characteristics (Fig. 18.8). Volume reduction will take place progressively and may require between 2 and 6 months (Fig. 18.9). Compression stockings are applied 21 days after the surgical intervention as well as when leaving the rehabilitation centre where walking will be gradually recommenced.

Patients are seen every 3 months and then every 6 months; often, there are inflammation episodes which translate into an inflamed pressure, most often on a fragment of necrotic bone. Surgical action must be done sparingly. Usually, walking limitation by a 10-day course of antibiotics allows the problem to be resolved. Sometimes, the radiographic assessment highlights a bony fragment potentially in relation with the clinical signs. A surgical excision may then be suggested, preferably conducted by the

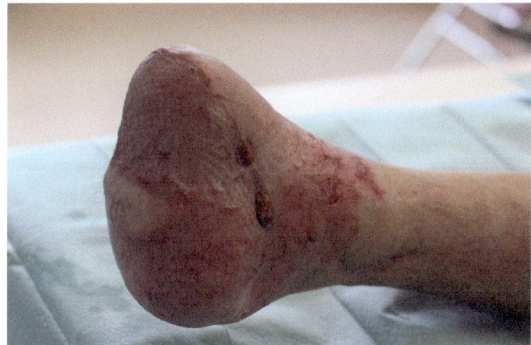

Fig. 18.9 The result at 4 months with slight decrease in the size of the flap allowing a normal walking for the foot supported by adapted shoe inserts

same physician who performed the free flap. We would not cover all aspects of rehabilitation here (learning to walk again, shoes and adapted shoe inserts, etc.), which remain a fundamental part of the patient learning to walk normally again.

18.4 Conclusion

The advancement in resuscitation has led to the appearance of a new type of pathology that we commonly call 'pied de réanimation'. It refers to a necrosis of all or part of the foot (and sometimes other extremities) by a phenomenon resulting from a combination of haemodynamic shock and the use of vasopressive drugs in high doses.

These necroses are often a major challenge for the plastic surgeon to envisage the possibilities of 'limb salvage'. This is done via the execution of a large-sized muscular free flap (still the latissimus dorsi) in our experience. This surgery presents an increased failure rate than the usual rate of failure, but a 77% success rate is still acceptable.

The follow-up of patients nevertheless shows a large majority who are able to walk, enjoy leisure activities, and live a normal life, and this pushes us to continue this method of treatment (Figs. 18.7 and 18.8).

Bibliography

1. Korenberg RJ, Landau-Price D, Penney S. Vasopressin-induced bullous diseases and cutaneous necrosis. J Am Acad Dermatol. 1986;57:393–8.
2. Duteille F, Thibault F, Perrot P, Renard B, Pannier M. Salvaging limbs in case of severe purpura fulminans: advantages of free flap. Plast Reconstr Surg. 2006;118:681–5.
3. Takak I, Kvolik S, Divkovic K, Kalajdžić-Čandrlić J, Pulsejic S, Izakovic S. Conservative surgical management of necrotic tissues following meningococcal sepsis: case report of a child treated with hyperbaric oxygen. Undersea Hyperb Med. 2010;37(2):95–9.
4. Chan JK, Harry L, William G, Nanchahol J. Soft tissue reconstruction of open fracture of the lower limb: muscle versus fasciocutaneous flap. Plast Reconstr Surg. 2012;130:284–95.

Open Access This chapter is licensed under the terms of the Creative Commons Attribution-NonCommercial-NoDerivatives 4.0 International License (http://creativecommons.org/licenses/by-nc-nd/4.0/), which permits any non-commercial use, sharing, distribution and reproduction in any medium or format, as long as you give appropriate credit to the original author(s) and the source, provide a link to the Creative Commons license and indicate if you modified the licensed material. You do not have permission under this license to share adapted material derived from this chapter or parts of it.

The images or other third party material in this chapter are included in the chapter's Creative Commons license, unless indicated otherwise in a credit line to the material. If material is not included in the chapter's Creative Commons license and your intended use is not permitted by statutory regulation or exceeds the permitted use, you will need to obtain permission directly from the copyright holder.

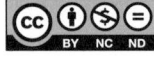

Skin Necrosis and Ulcers Induced by Medications

Joachim Dissemond

19.1 Introduction

In recent decades, it has been reported for numerous medications that their systemic administration can lead to the development of skin necrosis and subsequently to ulcerations. Allergic as well as nonallergic etiologic mechanisms have been described. Most of the relevant pathological reactions induced by these medications are a type of vasculitis or vasculopathy. Although these reactions often manifest as rashes or other skin diseases, some medications can also cause skin necrosis and ulcers [1]. Therefore, in this chapter, an exemplary number of medications are presented, which had been discussed to be responsible for the development of skin or mucosal necrosis and ulcers (Table 19.1).

19.2 Medications

19.2.1 Hydroxyurea

Hydroxyurea, synonym referred to as hydroxycarbamide, is a hydroxylated urea derivative which inhibits as an S-phase-specific inhibitor of ribonucleotide reductase during the DNA synthesis. It is clinically used for example for the treatment of patients with chronic myelogenous leukemia, essential thrombocythemia, and polycythemia vera.

In a retrospective study, 41 patients were presented in which a leg ulcer was caused by hydroxyurea. In these patients with a mean age of 67 years, ulcers occurred after an average treatment period of 5 years with hydroxyurea. Clinically, in most patients, multiple ulcerations in the area of the malleoli could be found. In total, 80% of patients with ulcers healed after dis-

Table 19.1 Overview of the systemically given medications associated with the development of skin necroses and ulcerations

Amezinium methylsulfate [2]
Anagrelide [3, 4]
Barbituric acid [5]
Coumarins [6–10]
Diltiazem [11]
Erythropoietin [12]
Estrogen combinations [13]
Furosemide [14]
Heparin [15, 16]
Hydralazine [17]
Hydroxyurea [18–20]
Leflunomide [21–23]
Levamisole [24–26]
Methotrexate [27, 28]
Nicorandil [29–32]
Nifedipine [33]
Pentazocine [34–37]
Pentamidine [38]
Propylthiouracil [39, 40]
Tyrosine kinase inhibitors [41–45]

J. Dissemond (✉)
Department for Dermatology, Venerology and Allergology, University of Essen, Essen, Germany
e-mail: joachim.dissemond@uk-essen.de

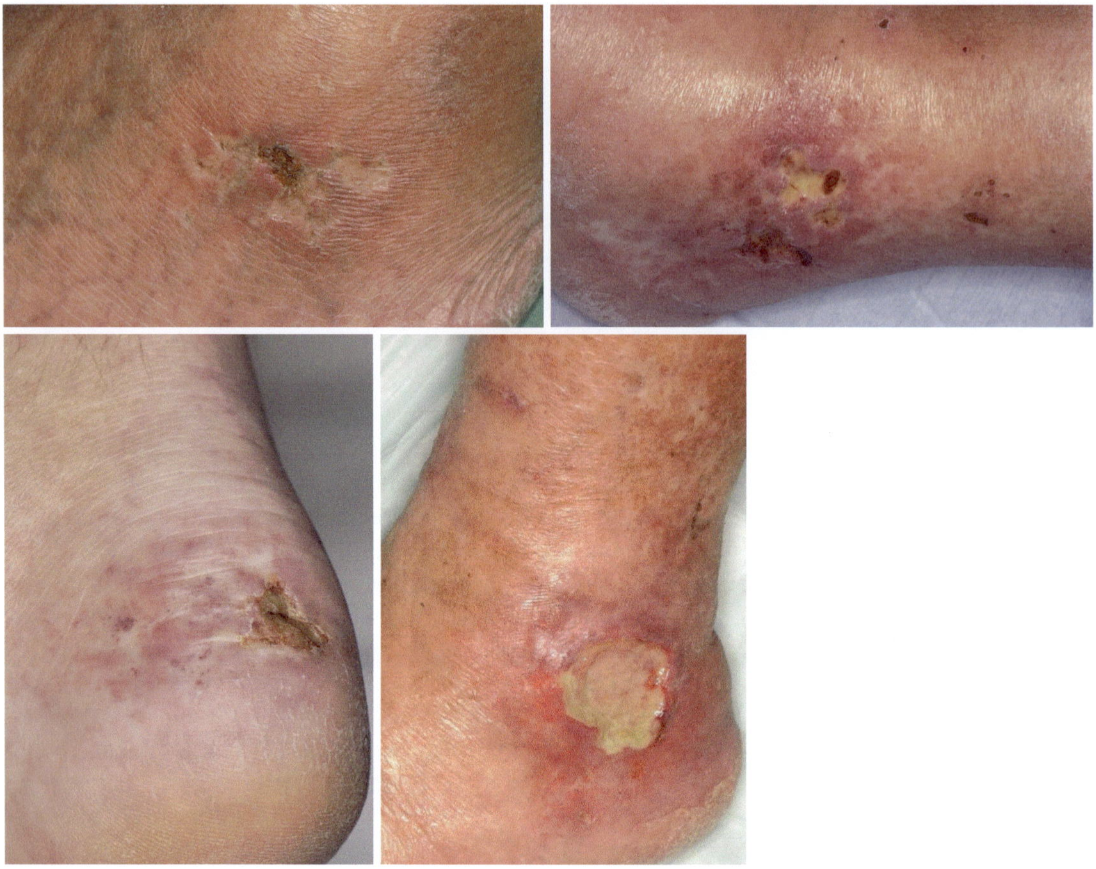

Fig. 19.1 Extremely painful ulcerations of the lower legs in different patients after long-term intake of hydroxyurea

continuation of the medication [20]. Comparable data have been presented by Best et al. in a study of 14 patients [18].

Hydroxyurea is the most widely publicized medication that is associated with the development of leg ulcers. It has been described that the first appearance of this extremely painful ulcerations is usually 1–10 years after starting therapy with hydroxyurea [19, 46, 47]. Hydroxyurea-induced ulcers are manifested in particular symmetrically in the area of the malleoli, dorsum of the foot, or heel (Fig. 19.1). In rare cases, genital wounds also occurred [48].

The underlying pathogenesis is so far not fully understood. It is discussed that a graft-versus-host-like reaction with degeneration of the basal keratinocytes and an epidermodermal gap formation could be directly related to cytostatic effects of hydroxyurea on the basal keratinocytes. In addition, a disturbance of microcirculation by

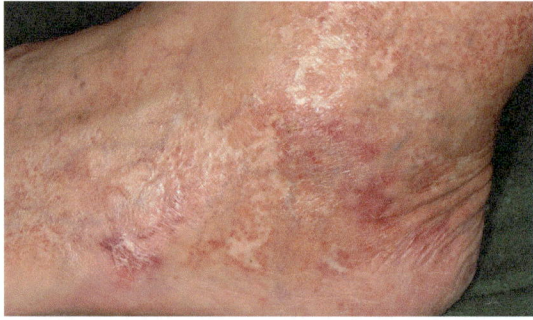

Fig. 19.2 Livid erythema with clinically typical but not specific atrophie blanche in a patient after many years of taking hydroxyurea

effects on erythrocytes with decrease in their number, increase of their mean volume, and thus reduced deformability has been described [20, 49]. The typical but not specific atrophie blanche was discussed as a clinical indicator for an underlying impaired microcirculation (Fig. 19.2).

Since some of these lesions are not reversible, it is also observed that despite discontinuation of therapy, in some patients, the wounds persist for long periods of time or recur [50].

19.2.2 Anagrelide

Anagrelide is an imidazoquinazoline derivative, which is used for the treatment of patients with myeloproliferative diseases such as essential thrombocythemia. The inhibitory effect of anagrelide on human platelets is mediated by the formation of a delay of maturation of megakaryocytes by inhibiting cyclic AMP phosphodiesterase III.

In a case report, our group reported a 38-year-old patient with extremely painful ulcers with atrophie blanche on both outer ankles, which occurred 6 weeks after starting treatment with anagrelide (Fig. 19.3). Despite an intensified advanced wound therapy, the wounds were refractory. A complete healing of the ulcer was achieved after stopping of the medication. An underlying disturbed microcirculation comparable to hydroxyurea effects was discussed [3]. Another case report was of a 77-year-old woman who developed a very painful ulcer on the dorsum of the foot and outer ankle with marked atrophie blanche in the surrounding skin. The drug had been taken for 1 year at the time of the first symptoms [4].

19.2.3 Coumarins

Coumarins derived from 4-hydroxycoumarin compounds are well known as drugs with an inhibitory effect on coagulation. Coumarins have a structure similar to vitamin K. They are used clinically as for the treatment and prophylaxis of thrombosis and embolism. The effect as anticoagulants is based on the inhibition of plasmatic coagulation. Coumarins bind instead of vitamin K to the enzyme vitamin K epoxide reductase, block it, and thus inhibit competitively the formation of active clotting factors. The two most commonly used in medicine are phenprocoumon coumarins and warfarin.

In a case series report, three patients were described in which it came within 5 days after initiation of therapy with warfarin to painful, sharply defined erythema, which ulcerated secondarily. All patients were obese. The authors discussed the fact that the coexistence of may be other individual factors is important for the devel-

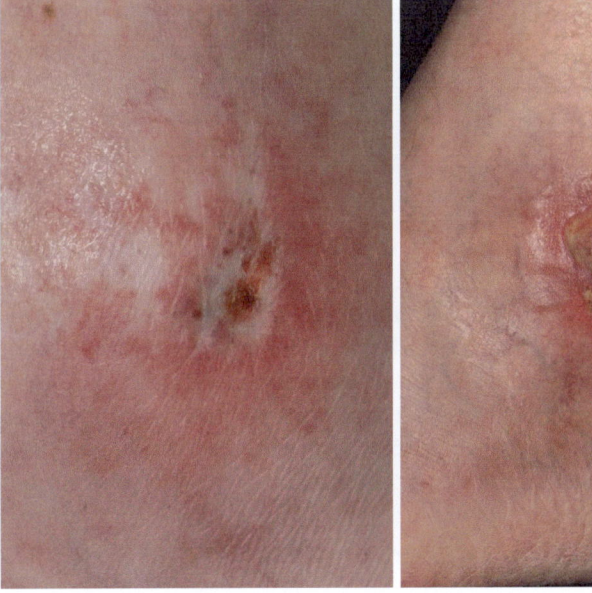

Fig. 19.3 Patient who developed an atrophie blanche 6 weeks after he started taking anagrelide and shortly later very painful ulcerations in the area of both lateral ankles

opment of coumarin necrosis [7]. Another case report described a 67-year-old patient with the occurrence of a cutaneous leukocytoclastic vasculitis of the lower limb 4 weeks after he started coumarin therapy [51]. Skin necrosis occurred at 0.01–0.1% of all patients after started taking coumarins. This necrosis can be observed more frequently in patients with congenital protein C deficiency or rarely described association with a deficiency of protein S [9]. In addition, the affected patients may be more common in obese women. A systematic search of the literature found 90 case reports involving 111 patients with warfarin-induced skin necrosis. The mean age of these patients was 52.5 years. A total of 20.7% of patients died from associated complications [10].

Skin necroses usually appear symmetrically on the chest, abdomen, or buttocks. Besides severe pain, often petechiae, erythema, and ecchymoses are the first clinical signs. As the condition progresses, crusts, hemorrhagic bullae, necrosis, or ulcer can be observed. As the underlying pathophysiology at the beginning of therapy with coumarins, hypercoagulative statuses by the imbalance of the various anticoagulant mechanisms have been discussed. The resulting microvascular thrombotic occlusions typically cause necroses. The first clinical symptoms start within 1–10 days, usually on days 3–6 [6]. Only in rare cases can it also occur even after several years of the onset of necrosis [8]. The median age of onset is 54 years; about 75% are women, and about 60% of the necroses are localized at the legs, breasts, or buttocks [6].

19.2.4 Heparin

Heparin is a mucopolysaccharide polysulfate, which binds to among others antithrombin III, causing the inactivation of many coagulation factors. Thereby, its anticoagulant effects are enhanced. Heparin preparations are used for the prophylaxis and treatment of thromboembolic disorders. The occurrence of purpura with necrosis in the injection areas and in other parts of the body has been reported. As a potential pathogenic mechanism, a leukocytoclastic vasculitis is described.

Another pathological reaction is the heparin-induced thrombocytopenia type II (HIT II), which may lead to arterial and venous thrombosis with necrosis. HIT is caused by the formation of autoantibodies against the heparin platelet factor 4 (PF4) complexes and occurs in 0.1–2% of all patients treated with heparin. After the beginning of heparin treatment, HIT II usually occurs within 10–14 days. If a heparin treatment has been done in the previous 100 days, the disease can manifest itself much more rapidly [15].

In a 66-year-old woman with diabetes and hemodialysis who received intravenous heparin during hemodialysis, the occurrences of ulcers of the lower legs were described [16]. Our group already described a 38-year-old patient in whom HIT II led to multiple necroses and ulcers on the mucous membrane and integument. The painful, sharply defined necroses with inflammatory surroundings were not localized at the injection sites [15].

19.2.5 Methotrexate

Methotrexate (MTX) is an analog of folic acid and competitively inhibits dihydrofolate reductase. As an antimetabolite, it inhibits DNA and RNA synthesis. The drug is dosed higher in oncologic patients as part of chemotherapy. Lower doses are widely used in the treatment of patients with rheumatoid arthritis or psoriasis vulgaris.

In the literature, a 39-year-old woman with non-Hodgkin's lymphoma was described. Two months after starting a therapy with 15 mg MTX once weekly, painless ulcerations on the malleoli appeared. One year ago, similar ulcerations occurred after a combination therapy with 7.5 mg MTX, and indomethacin was initiated. After discontinuation of the therapy within 2 months, the ulcers healed completely [28]. The occurrence of generalized erosions and ulcerations of psoriatic plaques was described in a case series report on 47 patients. As a risk factor, the co-medication with NSAIDs has been described [52]. In a systematic literature search, 114 patients experienced cutaneous ulcerations under methotrexate. Of these, men accounted for 57.9% with a mean age of 61 years. Erosions on psoriatic plaques were found most frequently with 33.3% of the case reports. Because these are often toxic effects of the drug, the authors specifically point out the frequent lack of folic acid supplementation, which can prevent the occurrence of this side effect [27].

19.2.6 Leflunomide

Leflunomide is a drug from the group of immunosuppressants, which is used as a therapy for patients with rheumatoid arthritis and psoriasis. The active metabolite of leflunomide, A771726, inhibits the enzyme dihydroorotate dehydrogenase, a key enzyme for de novo biosynthesis of pyrimidine [53].

Our group described a 68-year-old woman with rheumatoid arthritis who developed ulcers during treatment with leflunomide. Three months after starting treatment with leflunomide, the patient described the appearance of a purpura, which ulcerated in the following days. As the result of a vasculitis, an extremely painful, sharply demarcated ulceration with livid edges above the right malleolus occurred [21, 23]. Another case report described a 78-year-old woman with rheumatoid arthritis and ulcers, which appeared 6 months after starting treatment with leflunomide. It was discussed that a direct toxic effect of leflunomide on epidermal cells could be relevant, since leflunomide blocked in vitro, for example, epidermal growth factors [54]. In another case report, a 63-year-old patient who had suffered for 14 years from rheumatoid arthritis developed spontaneous ulcerations on both lower legs 10 months after initiation of leflunomide treatment. Neither serological nor histological signs for an underlying vasculitis could be found. After discontinuation of leflunomide therapy, the ulcers healed after 8 months [22].

19.2.7 Hydralazine

Hydralazine is a derivative of phthalazine. In some countries, it is used therapeutically as hydralazine hydrochloride in combination, for example, with atenolol or metoprolol and hydrochlorothiazide or for the treatment of essential hypertension.

In a 50-year-old man, very painful ulcers on the Achilles' tendon were described after the intake of hydralazine for 3 years. The histology showed newly occurred autoantibodies comparable to the first manifestation of systemic lupus erythematosus. The authors discussed the occurrence of the ulcer as a manifestation of a drug-induced lupus erythematosus. After discontinuation of hydralazine, the ulcer healed quickly and completely [17].

19.2.8 Amezinium Methylsulfate

Amezinium methylsulfate is an indirect α-sympathomimetic, which is used therapeutically in patients with essential and symptomatic hypotension. Amezinium methylsulfate inhibits the intra-dimensional monoamine oxidase, thus causing decreased norepinephrine degradation. Furthermore, it inhibits norepinephrine reuptake in the sympathetic neuron. Through these mechanisms, the noradrenalin amount increases in the peripheral receptors. This leads to vasoconstriction, and the blood pressure rises.

A case report described a 52-year-old patient, who suffered for 22 years from a chronic glomerulonephritis, had hemodialysis, and had already developed a generalized vascular calcification. One year after starting treatment with amezinium methylsulfate, he developed painful leg ulcers which were refractory to different treatments for over 7 months. After discontinuation of the drug, the ulcers healed within a few weeks. The authors discussed that the vasoconstrictive effects of the drug can be an important cause for the ulceration [2].

19.2.9 Diltiazem

Diltiazem belongs to the group of calcium antagonists. The drug is used as diltiazem hydrochloride in patients with coronary heart disease or angina pectoris. As an antiarrhythmic drug for the treatment of cardiac arrhythmias, diltiazem can be used preventively against paroxysmal supraventricular tachycardia and in patients without Wolff-Parkinson-White (WPW) syndrome in slowing the heart rate in atrial fibrillation and atrial flutter. Another application of diltiazem is the treatment of arterial hypertension.

In a 59-year-old man with leg edema, livid erythema and ulceration of both lower legs as a result of a cutaneous vasculitis arose 2 months after starting a therapy with diltiazem. After discontinuation of the drug, the ulcerations healed completely after 3 months of therapy [11].

19.2.10 Propylthiouracil

The thiouracils are thioureylenes that belong to the family of thioamides. Propylthiouracil inhibits the intrathyroidal peroxidase system. Therefore, it is used as a thyroid drug in patients with hyperthyroidism.

The intake of propylthiouracil over a period of 13 years for the treatment of Graves' disease was described in a 26-year-old woman. After increasing the dose to 50 mg/day, she developed livid erythema and painful ulcers on both lower legs 2 months later. Five months after discontinuation of propylthiouracil, the wounds healed. After retaking the medication, it came after a period of only 5 days to a relapse [40]. In another case report, a 27-year-old man with Graves' disease was described. Two years after beginning a therapy with propylthiouracil, it came to the occurrence of very painful ulcers on both lower legs. These ulcers developed from erythematous plaques with pustules, were sharply demarcated, and showed bizarre configured wound edges. A pyoderma gangrenosum was diagnosed, and a causal relationship with the medication was discussed. After discontinuation of propylthiouracil therapy and initiation of treatment with prednisolone and cyclosporin A, the ulcerations healed after 1 month [39]. Moreover, there are several case reports on the occurrence of intraoral ulceration after administration of propylthiouracil [55].

19.2.11 Nicorandil

Nicorandil is a nicotinamide nitrate ester, which is used for the treatment of patients with angina pectoris. The substance has the characteristics of nitrates but acts in addition as an activator of ATP-dependent potassium channels. The opening of potassium channels leads to hyperpolarization of the cell membrane and to a decrease in intracellular calcium. This causes relaxation of smooth muscle cells and vasodilation. Nicorandil is a peripheral and coronary vasodilator, lowers systolic blood pressure, and increases heart rate reflex.

A 73-year-old woman took nicorandil twice daily for 2 years, until for the first time leg ulcers over her Achilles' tendon occurred. At the same time, there was also an onset of perianal ulcerations. After discontinuation of nicorandil, all ulcers healed after 5 months [30]. For example, in a case series of 10 patients in an average of 26.6 months after starting a therapy with nicorandil, it came to the occurrence of ulcers. After discontinuation of the drug, the ulceration healed after 12 weeks (median) [56]. In a report from the French Pharmacovigilance Network, 148 patients were described in whom nicorandil-induced ulcers occurred. The wounds occurred mainly on the mucosal, oral, and anal sites. The median time between the start of nicorandil use and the appearance of the ulcer was 23.4 months [32]. The occurrence of ulcers located intraorally or on the penis and perianal region is a well-documented side effect when taking nicorandil [29, 31].

19.2.12 Levamisole

Levamisole is the levo-isomer of tetramisole and belongs to the group of imidazothiazole. It is an anthelmintic agent which is clinically employed as an immunomodulating drug in particular in the treatment of children with nephrotic syndrome. In addition, levamisole is also used for the adjuvant treatment of patients with colon carcinoma. In addition, cocaine is often contaminated with levamisole.

In a 67-year-old woman with rheumatoid arthritis, already healed venous leg ulcers were described. After she started taking levamisole, the leg ulcer recurred. At the same time, livid erythema on the arms and intraoral ulcerations occurred. After discontinuation of the drug, all ulcers healed within 1 month completely [24]. In another case report, an 11-year-old boy with heterozygous factor V Leiden mutation and nephrotic syndrome developed leg ulcers after he had already taken levamisole for the last 3 years. Furthermore, at the same time, livid erythema and ulcers on the forearms, hands, and ears could be observed. After discontinuation of levamisole and initiation of therapy with cyclophosphamide, the ulcerations healed after about 4 weeks [25]. The occurrence of lesions in the form of purpura and/or lichenoid papules 12–44 months after initiation of systemic therapy with levamisole has been repeatedly described in particular on the ears. Although the underlying pathogenic mechanism is unclear, a potential connection between the levamisole intake and an infection was discussed. In some patients, the formation of autoantibodies such as antineutrophil cytoplasmic antibodies (ANCAs) and lupus anticoagulant with an immune complex vasculitis or an occlusive vasculopathy could be shown [57].

The occurrence of pyoderma gangrenosum has been repeatedly described after ingestion of cocaine [58]. Since levamisole is often added as a adulterant, it was discussed whether levamisole might be the substance responsible for the induction of this ulcerative neutrophilic disease [26].

19.2.13 Pentazocine

Pentazocine is a benzomorphan derivative from the group of opioids which are used as highly potent analgesic drugs. It is not only a strong analgesic but also a sedative and respiratory depressant.

Several case reports have been published in which the appearance of wounds on the skin occurred after ingestion of pentazocine.

These occur frequently on the buttocks, thighs, or shins [36, 37] [34]. A case report series described a total of 10 patients with ulcers after taking pentazocine. There were 4 men and 6 women aged between 20 and 43 years. Prior to the first occurrence of the ulcers, the patient had been taking pentazocine for 10 days to 7 years. Most of the patients had multiple ulcerations on the lower extremities [35].

19.2.14 Tyrosine Kinase Inhibitors

Tyrosine kinase inhibitors are synthetically produced drugs that inhibit various enzymes from the tyrosine kinase group. These enzymes have important functions in the activation of cellular signal transduction pathways. As drugs, they are predominantly used for targeted therapies in oncology. Other indications include chronic inflammatory diseases, for example in rheumatology.

For various medications from the group of tyrosine kinase inhibitors, it has already been described that necroses, erosions, or even ulcerations occurred. For example, an 82-year-old female patient experienced repeated ulcerations around a stoma 18 weeks after initiation of therapy with cetuximab [41]. Leg ulcers have been described in association with the use of sunitinib, nilotinib [42], or pazopanib [43]. In another case report, chronic sores on the feet occurred and were discussed with the use of ruxolitinib [44]. The association of pyoderma gangrenosum with drug use has been repeatedly described in association with the use of various tyrosine kinase inhibitors. In addition to imatinib, sunitinib, ibrutinib, gefitinib, pazopanib, dabrafenib, and trametinib have also been described as cases [45]. However, it must also be critically discussed here that pyoderma gangrenosum is a potentially paraneoplastic disease, so that the oncological underlying disease of these patients can also be seen as a trigger [58].

19.3 Therapy

There is no standardized therapy for patients who have developed necrosis or ulcers as a result of systemically given medications. Once the causal relationship has been clarified, discontinuation of medication is usually recommended. Thereafter, local therapy follows the principles of modern moist wound therapy oriented to the phases of wound healing. For systemic therapies, it should be discussed in interdisciplinary terms whether immunosuppressive therapy is necessary in individual cases, for example in patients with severe inflammation [59]. Rheological therapy concepts should be considered for vasculopathies [60]. Moderate compression therapy also often supports the success of treatment when the wounds are localized to the lower extremities [61].

19.4 Conclusion

The pathophysiological relevance of the systemic intake of medication on the onset of necrosis or ulcers of the skin is not always clear. For most of the medications, there exist only a few case reports which describe an association with skin necrosis or ulcerations. Several of these patients took multiple medications and suffered from various underlying diseases that could potentially also cause ulcers. Necrosis and ulcers from the intake of medications are therefore usually a diagnosis of exclusion that can be discussed because of a temporal relationship. An exception with greater case report series is medications that contain the drug hydroxyurea or coumarins.

In summary, it is important that all healthcare professionals recognize medications as a rare but potentially relevant factor for skin necrosis or ulcers. If this correlation is not recognized early, this can lead to severe and prolonged problems for the patients.

References

1. Dissemond J. Ulcus cruris—Grundlagen, Diagnostik und Therapie. 4th ed. Bremen/London/Boston: UNI-MED Verlag; 2012.
2. Kitano Y, Nomura S, Saiki T, Osawa G. Leg ulceration during amezinium methylsulfate therapy for hypotension in a hemodialyzed patient with generalized vascular calcification. Nephron. 1995;71:115.
3. Rappoport L, Körber A, Grabbe S, Dissemond J. Auftreten von Ulcera crurum durch Anagrelid. Dtsch Med Wochenschr. 2007;132:319–21.
4. Oskay T, Özen M. Leg ulcers associated with anagrelide. Turk J Haematol. 2021;38:338–40.
5. Oberste-Lehn H, Kaulen-Becker L. Necroses after barbituric acid and nodular poisoning. Z Haut Geschlechtskr. 1969;44(5):169–74.
6. Chan Y, Valenti D, Mansfield AO, Stansby G. Warfarin induced skin necrosis. Br J Surg. 2000;87:266–72.
7. Ellbrück D, Wankmüller H, Rasche H, Seifried E. The clinical course of coumarin-induced necrosis. Dtsch Med Wochenschr. 1991;116:1307–12.
8. Franson TR, Rose HD, Spivey MR, Maroney J, Libnoch JA. Late-onset, warfarin-caused necrosis occurring in a patient with infectious mononucleosis. Arch Dermatol. 1984;120:927–31.
9. Muniesa C, Marcoval J, Moreno A, Giménez S, Sánchez J, Ferreres JR, Peyrí J. Coumarin necrosis induced by renal insufficiency. Br J Dermatol. 2004;151:502–4.
10. Morán-Mariños C, Corcuera-Ciudad R, Velásquez-Rimachi V, Nieto-Gutierrez W. Systematic review of warfarin-induced skin necrosis case reports and secondary analysis of factors associated with mortality. Int J Clin Pract. 2021;75:15001.
11. Carmichael AJ, Paul CJ. Vasculitic leg ulcers associated with diltiazem. BMJ. 1988;297(6647):562.
12. Gibson A, Gardner J, O'Donnell J. Erythropoietin and painful leg ulcers: thrombosis or vasculitis? Arthritis Rheum. 2005;53:792.
13. Siregusa M, Alberti A, Schepis C. Skin ulcers in a young woman on low-dose estrogen-combination pill. Int J Dermatol. 1997;36:317–8.

14. Siddiqui MA, Zaman MN. Recurrent and chronic leg ulcers secondary to furosemide-induced bullous pemphigoid. J Am Geriatr Soc. 1995;43:1183–4.
15. Helbig D, Hillen U, Grabbe S, Dissemond J. Haut- und Schleimhautulzerationen bei Heparin-induzierter Thrombozytopenie (HIT) II. Hautarzt. 2007;58:774–80.
16. Leblanc M, Roy LF, Legault L, Dufresne LR, Morin C, Thuot C. Severe skin necrosis associated with heparin in hemodialysis. Nephron. 1994;68:133–7.
17. Kissin MW, Williamson RC. Hydralazine-induced SLE-like syndrome presenting as a leg ulcer. Br Med J. 1979;2:1330.
18. Best PJ, Daoud MS, Pittelkow MR, Petitt RM. Hydroxyurea-induced leg ulceration in 14 patients. Ann Intern Med. 1998;128:29–32.
19. Eming SA, Peters T, Hartmann K, Scharffetter-Kochanek K, Mahrle G. Lichenoid chronic graft-versus-host-disease-like acrodermatitis induced by hydroxyurea. J Am Acad Dermatol. 2001;45:321–3.
20. Sirieix ME, Debure C, Baudot N, Dubertret L, Roux ME, Morel P, Frances C, Loubeyres S, Beylot C, Lambert D, Humbert P, Gauthier O, Dandurand M, Guillot B, Vaillant L, Lorette G, Bonnetblanc JM, Lok C, Denoeux JP. Leg ulcers and hydroxyurea: forty-one cases. Arch Dermatol. 1999;135:818–20.
21. Holm EA, Balslev E, Jemec GBE. Vasculitis occurring during leflunomide therapy. Dermatology. 2001;203:258–9.
22. Jakob A, Porstmann R, Rompel R. Skin ulceration after leflunomide treatment in two patients with rheumatoid arthritis. J Dtsch Dermatol Ges. 2006;4:324–7.
23. Knab J, Goos M, Dissemond J. Successful treatment of a leg ulcer occurring in a rheumatoid arthritis patient under leflunomide therapy. J Eur Acad Dermatol Venereol. 2005;19:243–6.
24. El-Ghobarey M, Maurikasis M, Morgan R, Mathieu J. Delayed healing of varicose ulcer with levamisole. Br Med J. 1977;1:616–7.
25. Powell J, Grech H, Holder J. A boy with cutaneous necrosis occurring during treatment with levamisole. Clin Exp Dermatol. 2002;27:32–3.
26. Martínez-Gómez M, Ramírez-Ospina JA, Ruiz-Restrepo JD, Velásquez-Lopera MM. Pyoderma gangrenosum associated to the use of cocaine/levamisole. Series of three cases and literature review. An Bras Dermatol. 2021;96:188–95.
27. Berna R, Rosenbach M, Margolis DJ, Mitra N, Baumrin E. Methotrexate cutaneous ulceration: a systematic review of cases. Am J Clin Dermatol. 2022;23(4):449–57. https://doi.org/10.1007/s40257-022-00692-1.
28. Del Pozo J, Martínez W, García-Silva J, Almagro M, Peña-Penabad C, Fonseca E. Cutaneous ulceration as a sign of methotrexate toxicity. Eur J Dermatol. 2001;11:450–2.
29. Birnie A, Dearing N, Littlewood S, Carlin E. Nicorandil-induced ulceration of the penis. Clin Exp Dermatol. 2008;33:215–6.
30. McKenna DJ, Donnelly J, Armstrong DK. Nicorandil-induced leg ulceration. Br J Dermatol. 2007;156:394–6.
31. Yap T, Philippou P, Perry M, Lam W, Corbishley C, Watkin N. Nicorandil-induced penile ulcerations: a case series. BJU Int. 2011;107:268–71.
32. Babic V, Petitpain N, Guy C, Trechot P, Bursztejn AC, Faillie JL, Vial T, Schmutz JL, Gillet P. Nicorandil-induced ulcerations: a 10-year observational study of all cases spontaneously reported to the French pharmacovigilance network. Int Wound J. 2018;15(4):508–18.
33. Luca S, Romeo S. Edema and skin ulcers of the lower limbs as a collateral effect of nifedipine. A clinical case report. Minerva Cardioangiol. 1999;47:219–22.
34. De D, Dogra S, Kanwar AJ. Pentazocine-induced leg ulcers and fibrous papules. Indian J Dermatol Venereol Leprol. 2007;73:112–3.
35. Prasad HR, Khaitan BK, Ramam M, Sharma VK, Pandhi RK, Agarwal S, Dhawan A, Jain R, Singh MK. Diagnostic clinical features of pentazocine-induced ulcers. Int J Dermatol. 2005;44:910–5.
36. Kathuria S, Ramesh V, Singh A. Pentazocine induced ulceration of the buttocks. Indian J Dermatol Venereol Leprol. 2012;78:521.
37. Sahu KK, Sawatkar GU, Sahu SA, Mishra AK, Lal A. Pentazocine-induced skin ulcers. Am J Med Sci. 2020;359:182–3.
38. Gottlieb JR, Lewis VL Jr, Bashioum RW. Care of pentamadine ulcers in AIDS patients. Plast Reconstr Surg. 1985;76:630–2.
39. Hong SB, Lee MH. A case of propylthiouracil-induced pyoderma gangrenosum associated with antineutrophil cytoplasmic antibody. Dermatology. 2004;208:339–41.
40. Houston BD, Crouch ME, Brick JE, DiBartolomeo AG. Apparent vasculitis associated with propylthiouracil use. Arthritis Rheum. 1979;22:925–8.
41. Tsuboi K, Kawase Y, Okochi O, Hattori M, Takami Y, Takeda S, Mizuno A, Sato Y, Uno Y, Hayashi T, Sasada Y, Takamura S, Kozaki K. Cetuximab-associated skin ulceration in patient with metastatic colorectal cancer: a case report. Gan To Kagaku Ryoho. 2011;38:1549–52.
42. Roger A, Sigal M-L, Bagan P, Sin C, Bilan P, Dakhil B, Fargeas C, Couffinhal JC, Mahé E. Leg ulcers occurring under tyrosine kinase inhibitor therapy (sunitinib, nilotinib). Ann Dermatol Venereol. 2017;144:49–54.
43. Fujita H, Oda K, Sato M, Wada H, Aihara M. Pazopanib-induced leg ulcer in a patient with malignant fibrous histiocytoma. J Dermatol. 2014;41:1022–3.
44. Del Rosario M, Tsai H, Dasanu CA. Persistent foot ulcer due to ruxolitinib therapy for primary myelofibrosis. J Oncol Pharm Pract. 2018;24:226–8.

45. Khoshnam-Rad N, Gheymati A, Jahangard-Rafsanjani Z. Tyrosine kinase inhibitors-associated pyoderma gangrenosum, a systematic review of published case reports. Anticancer Drugs. 2022;33:1–8.
46. Dissemond J, Höft D, Knab J, Franckson T, Kröger K, Goos M. Leg ulcer in a patient associated with hydroxyurea therapy. Int J Dermatol. 2006;45:158–60.
47. Dissemond J, Körber A. Hydroxyurea-induced ulcers on the leg. CMAJ. 2009;180:1132.
48. Blum AE, Tsiaras WG, Kemp JM. Hydroxyurea-induced genital ulcers and erosions: two case reports. J Tissue Viability. 2021;30:462–4.
49. Weinlich G, Schuler G, Greil R, Kofler H, Fritsch P. Leg ulcers associated with long-term hydroxyurea therapy. J Am Acad Dermatol. 1998;8:372–4.
50. Kikuchi K, Arita K, Tateishi Y, Onozawa M, Akiyama M, Shimizu H. Recurrence of hydroxyurea-induced leg ulcer after discontinuation of treatment. Acta Derm Venereol. 2011;91:373–4.
51. Tamir A, Wolf R, Brenner S. Leukocytoclastic vasculitis: another coumarin-induced hemorrhagic reaction. Acta Derm Venereol. 1994;74:138–9.
52. Pearce HP, Wilson BB. Erosion of psoriatic plaques: an early sign of methotrexate toxicity. J Am Acad Dermatol. 1996;35:835–8.
53. Rozman B. Clinical pharmacokinetics of leflunomide. Clin Pharmacokinet. 2002;41:421–30.
54. McCoy CM. Leflunomide-associated skin ulceration. Ann Pharmacother. 2002;336:1009–11.
55. Tsuboi K, Ishihara Y, Ishikawa M, Tsuchida Y, Nagasawa K, Watanabe N, Ueshiba H, Yoshino G. Unusual oral ulceration, skin rash, and fever in a patient receiving propylthiouracil. Thyroid. 2009;19:421–2.
56. Cooke NS, Tolland JP, Dolan OM. Nicorandil-associated perianal ulceration: a case series of 10 patients. Br J Dermatol. 2006;154:199–200.
57. Rongioletti F, Ghio L, Ginevri F, Bleidl D, Rinaldi S, Edefonti A, Gambini C, Rizzoni G, Rebora A. Purpura of the ears: a distinctive vasculopathy with circulating autoantibodies complicating long-term treatment with levamisole in children. Br J Dermatol. 1999;140:948–51.
58. Maverakis E, Marzano AV, Le ST, Callen JP, Brüggen MC, Guenova E, Dissemond J, Shinkai K, Langan SM. Pyoderma gangrenosum. Nat Rev Dis Primers. 2020;6:81.
59. Dissemond J, Romanelli M. Inflammatory skin diseases and wounds. Br J Dermatol. 2022;187(2):167–77. https://doi.org/10.1111/bjd.21619.
60. Mufti A, Maliyar K, Syed M, Pagnoux C, Alavi A. Approaches to microthrombotic wounds: a review of pathogenesis and clinical features. Adv Skin Wound Care. 2020;33:68–75.
61. Dissemond J, Assenheimer B, Bültemann A, Gerber V, Gretener S, Kohler-von Siebenthal E, Koller S, Kröger K, Kurz P, Läuchli S, Münter C, Panfil EM, Probst S, Protz K, Riepe G, Strohal R, Traber J, Partsch H. Compression therapy in patients with venous leg ulcers. J Dtsch Dermatol Ges. 2016;14:1072–87.

Open Access This chapter is licensed under the terms of the Creative Commons Attribution-NonCommercial-NoDerivatives 4.0 International License (http://creativecommons.org/licenses/by-nc-nd/4.0/), which permits any non-commercial use, sharing, distribution and reproduction in any medium or format, as long as you give appropriate credit to the original author(s) and the source, provide a link to the Creative Commons license and indicate if you modified the licensed material. You do not have permission under this license to share adapted material derived from this chapter or parts of it.

The images or other third party material in this chapter are included in the chapter's Creative Commons license, unless indicated otherwise in a credit line to the material. If material is not included in the chapter's Creative Commons license and your intended use is not permitted by statutory regulation or exceeds the permitted use, you will need to obtain permission directly from the copyright holder.

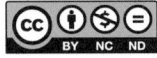

Toxic Syndromes

20

Shota Suda, Sho Yamakawa, and Kenji Hayashida

20.1 Epidemiology and Clinical Features

20.1.1 Staphylococcal Toxic Shock Syndrome

S. aureus is a ubiquitous and virulent pathogen. It colonizes the skin and mucous membranes in 30–50% of healthy adults and children, most commonly in the anterior nares, skin, vagina, and rectum [1]. The organism causes many infections, including folliculitis, skin abscesses, bacteremia, and endocarditis. The Centers for Disease Control and Prevention (CDC) proposed a revised clinical case definition of TSS in 1981, which currently remains in use (Table 20.1).

There are two types of TSS: menstrual and nonmenstrual. Menstrual TSS occurs during menstruation and is associated with absorbent tampons. However, the number of menstrual TSS cases has been greatly reduced in recent years. Previously, menstrual and nonmenstrual TSS were observed in equal numbers in young women; however, a recent study in the United Kingdom showed that the incidence of nonmenstrual TSS has remained unchanged, while the number of cases of menstrual TSS has decreased [2]. Nonmenstrual TSS may result from any primary staphylococcal infection or

Table 20.1 Staphylococcal toxic shock syndrome clinical case definition

Clinical criteria
1. Fever: Temperature $\geq$ 38.9 °C
2. Rash: Diffuse macular erythroderma
3. Desquamation: 1–2 weeks after the onset of rash
4. Hypotension: For adults: Systolic blood pressure $\leq$ 90 mmHg; for children <16 years of age: Systolic blood pressure less than fifth percentile by age
5. Multisystem involvement (three or more of the following):
A. Gastrointestinal: Vomiting or diarrhea at the onset of illness
B. Muscular: Severe myalgia or creatine phosphokinase elevation >2 times the upper limit of normal
C. Mucous membrane: Vaginal, oropharyngeal, or conjunctival hyperemia
D. Renal: Blood urea nitrogen or serum creatinine >2 times the upper limit of normal or pyuria (>5 leukocytes/high-power field) in the absence of urinary tract infection
E. Hepatic: Bilirubin or transaminases >2 times the upper limit of normal
F. Hematological: Platelets $\leq 100 \times 10^9$/L
G. Central nervous system: Disorientation or alterations in consciousness without focal neurologic signs when fever and hypotension are absent
Laboratory criteria
1. Cultures (blood or cerebrospinal fluid) negative for alternative pathogens (blood cultures may be positive for *Staphylococcus aureus*)
2. Serologic tests negative (if obtained) for Rocky Mountain spotted fever, leptospirosis, or measles
Case classification
Probable case: a case which meets the laboratory criteria and four of the five clinical criteria

(continued)

S. Suda · S. Yamakawa · K. Hayashida (✉)
Division of Plastic and Reconstructive Surgery, Shimane University, Shimane, Japan
e-mail: s.suda@med.shimane-u.ac.jp

Table 20.1 (continued)

Confirmed case: a case which meets the laboratory criteria and all five of the clinical criteria, including desquamation (unless the patient dies before desquamation occurs)

colonization by a toxin-producing strain of *S. aureus*, including methicillin-resistant *S. aureus* (MRSA), which occurs after physical or chemical damage to the epidermis. Therefore, TSS should be considered in patients presenting with both shock and skin damage. The focus of a nonmenstrual infection is more likely to be superficial and may complicate burns, surgical wounds, or foreign bodies. Postoperative TSS usually occurs within 48 h of surgery, and in many cases, evidence of a clinically significant surgical site infection is lacking at the time of presentation.

20.1.2 Skin Manifestation

A variety of skin manifestations are observed in TSS. Initial erythroderma involves both the skin and mucous membranes and is characterized by a diffuse, red, macular rash resembling sunburn and involving the palms and soles. In postoperative TSS, erythema may instead be more intense around the surgical wound site. Late-onset skin manifestations include a pruritic maculopapular rash that may occur 1 to 2 weeks after disease onset, and desquamation of the palms and soles that characteristically begins from 1 to 3 weeks after the onset of illness. Since desquamation occurs late, it is often difficult to identify TSS as a differential diagnosis, and thus the acute diagnosis of TSS may not take advantage of this clinical feature (Figs. 20.1, 20.2, 20.3, and 20.4).

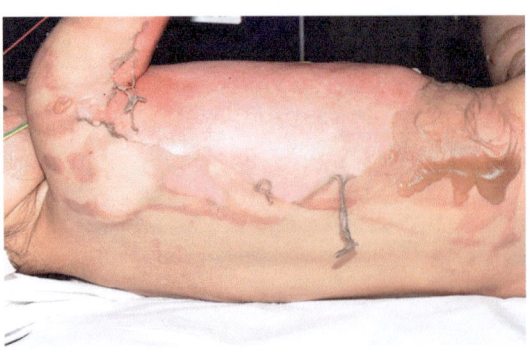

Fig. 20.1 At the time of hospitalization

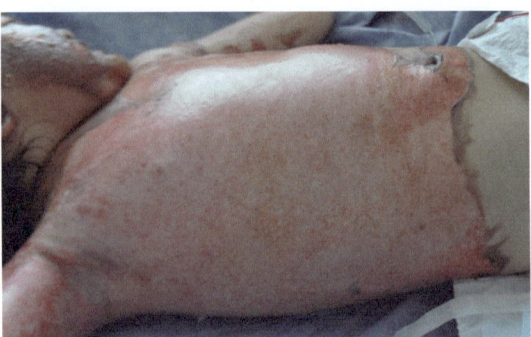

Fig. 20.2 Day 3. Diffuse erythroderma appeared in the burned area

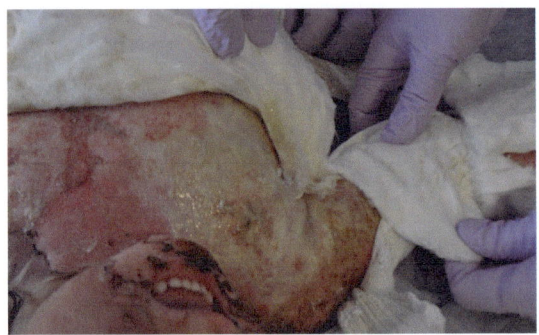

Fig. 20.3 Day 8. Infected necrotic tissue adhered to the burn site, and erythema spread to the entire body

20.1.2.1 Streptococcal Toxic Shock Syndrome

Streptococcal TSS occurs as a complication of invasive group A streptococcus (GAS, e.g., *Streptococcus pyogenes*) disease and is characterized by shock and multiorgan failure due to capillary leakage and tissue damage caused by the release of inflammatory cytokines induced by streptococcal toxins. Severe invasive GAS infections are defined as bacteremia, pneumonia, or any other infection along with the isolation of GAS from a normally sterile body site [3]. Invasive infections include necrotizing fasciitis and spontaneous gangrenous myositis.

The diagnosis of streptococcal TSS was established based on clinical criteria and culture findings. GAS TSS is defined as any GAS infection associated with acute onset of shock and organ failure (Table 20.2).

The most common portals of entry for streptococcal infections are the skin, vagina, or

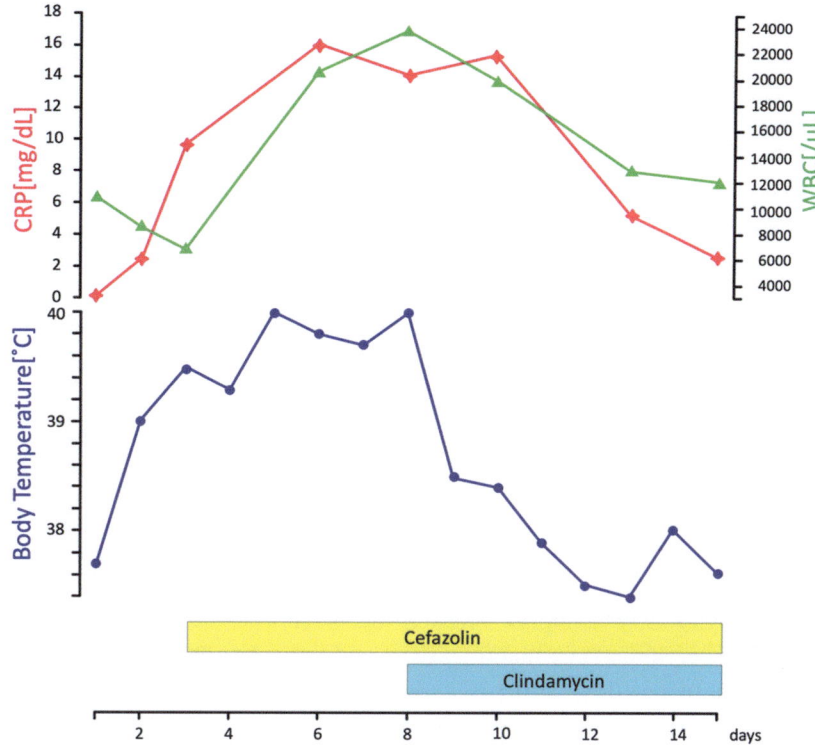

Fig. 20.4 Clinical course of the patient. After admission, the patient was managed without antibiotics. On the third day, the patient developed a fever of over 39 °C, and treatment with cephazolin was initiated. Although antipyretics were also administered, the patient still had a fever of nearly 40 °C. Clindamycin was introduced on the eighth day, and the fever gradually resolved the following day

Table 20.2 Streptococcal toxic shock syndrome clinical case definition

Clinical criteria
1. Hypotension: For adults: Systolic blood pressure ≤ 90 mmHg; for children <16 years of age: Systolic blood pressure less than the fifth percentile by age
2. Multi-organ involvement characterized by two or more of the following:
A. Renal impairment: Creatinine >2 mg/dL (177 µmol/L)
B. Coagulopathy: Platelets ≤100 × 10⁹/L or disseminated intravascular coagulation
C. Liver involvement: Alanine aminotransferase, aspartate aminotransferase, or total bilirubin twice the upper limit of normal
D. Acute respiratory distress syndrome
E. A generalized erythematous macular rash that may desquamate
F. Soft tissue necrosis, including necrotizing fasciitis or myositis, or gangrene
Laboratory criteria for diagnosis
Isolation of group A streptococcus
Case classification
Probable: a case that meets the clinical case definition in the absence of another identified etiology for the illness and with isolation of group A streptococcus from a non-sterile site
Confirmed: a case that meets the clinical case definition and with isolation of group A streptococcus from a normally sterile site

pharynx. However, among patients who develop GAS TSS, the portal of entry remains unidentified in 45% of cases [4]. These patients frequently develop deep-seated infections, such as necrotizing fasciitis or myositis, within 24–72 h of minor trauma at the exact site of injuries such as bruises, strained muscles, or sprained ankles, frequently without a visible break in the skin. Pain may be more severe and relentless than that of staphylococcal TSS and is a common reason for seeking medical attention. Hypotension and organ dysfunction progress rapidly in GAS TSS.

20.1.2.2 Skin Manifestation

Clinical signs of soft tissue infection typically include localized swelling and erythema followed by ecchymoses and sloughing of the skin, which progress to necrotizing fasciitis or myositis. A variety of clinical presentations may be observed in patients without soft tissue findings. The most common initial symptom of GAS TSS is diffuse or localized pain, which develops aggressively and is commonly preceded by other physical symptoms.

20.2 Pathophysiology

Superantigens are a group of staphylococcal and streptococcal exotoxins that are involved in host immune responses in the human body, as in TSS [5]. More than 20 different superantigens have been identified in *S. aureus* isolates, including staphylococcal enterotoxins, enterotoxin-like proteins, and TSS toxin-1 (TSST-1) [4] [6] [7]. More than 60% of clinical *S. aureus* isolates carry at least one superantigen; these superantigens can activate T lymphocytes and antigen-presenting cells (APCs). As a result, activated T cells and APCs induce a massive release of cytokines and chemokines, causing the symptoms observed in TSS.

The mechanism of action of superantigens is as follows: superantigens bind to the major histocompatibility complex (MHC) class II molecules of APCs (i.e., macrophages) and the Vβ region of T-cell receptors in a non-antigen-specific manner, which leads to a massive release of cytokines and chemokines as well as the clonal expansion of certain clonal types of T cells.

Patients with TSS have inadequate antibody responses to exotoxins from staphylococcus and streptococcus that act as superantigens; in a study of burn patients with MRSA infections, those who developed TSS showed lower levels of antibodies to TSST-1 than those who did not [8]. In addition, children between 6 months and 2 years of age have been shown to be at a high risk of developing TSS as passive immunity from their mothers is declining and active immunity has not yet been developed during this age range. One study found that children aged 0–6 months had antibody levels of 76% against TSST-1, whereas those aged 7–24 months had only about 30% [9] (Fig. 20.5).

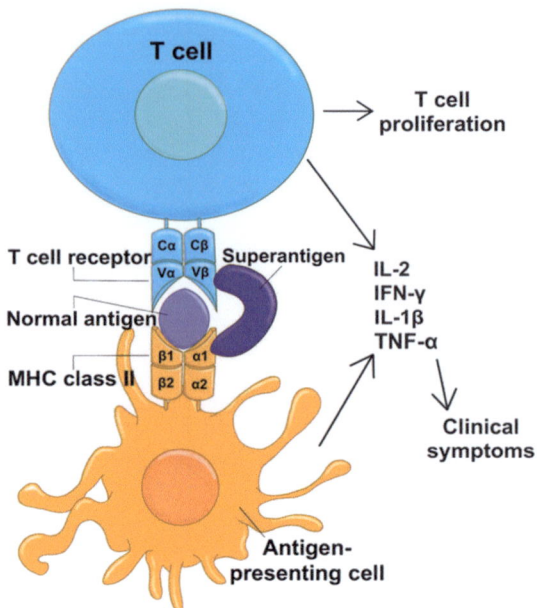

Fig. 20.5 The mechanism of action of superantigens

20.3 Treatment

20.3.1 Antibiotic Therapy

To the best of our knowledge, no randomized studies have evaluated antibiotic regimens for the treatment of TSS thus far. In patients with TSS originating from methicillin-susceptible *S. aureus* or MRSA, our hospital administers empiric therapy with clindamycin plus vancomycin. Once the diagnosis of GAS TSS is established, we recommend a combination therapy of clindamycin and penicillin G until hemodynamics have stabilized. In cases of resistance to clindamycin treatment, linezolid may be considered as an alternative drug candidate. Clindamycin and linezolid are considered effective TSS treatments because these bacteriostatic antimicrobial agents have the ability to inhibit staphylococcal exotoxin production.

Additionally, no clinical trials have been conducted to determine the duration of antimicrobial therapy for staphylococcal TSS. In our hospital, we administer antibiotics for 10–14 days in patients with an absence of bacteremia or a distinct focus of infection.

20.3.2 Intravenous Immune Globulin

Intravenous immune globulin (IVIG) treatment may be considered for patients with severe staphylococcal TSS that does not respond to other therapies, and IVIG therapy may be effective in patients with low antibody levels to exotoxins. However, few studies have shown the benefits of IVIG therapy for TSS, and decisions regarding its use should be carefully considered.

20.3.3 Surgical Therapy

For TSS, drainage and debridement of any identified infectious focuses are essential. Lesions should be examined for the presence of foreign bodies, and if present, these bodies should be removed surgically. In postsurgical patients, surgical wounds may appear uninfected because of a decreased inflammatory response; however, if the patient meets the clinical criteria for TSS, examination and debridement are still necessary.

In GAS TSS, prompt and aggressive exploration and surgical debridement are mandatory. It is critically important that surgeons are involved early in GAS TSS as a surgical intervention may be impossible later in the course of the disease because the general condition of the patient often deteriorates rapidly, with the infectious lesion extending to vital areas that are difficult to debride (e.g., the head and neck, thorax, or abdomen).

References

1. Centers for Disease Control and Prevention. Case definitions for infectious conditions under public health surveillance. MMWR Recomm Rep. 1997;46(RR-10):1.
2. Sharma H, Smith D, Turner CE, Game L, Pichon B, Hope R, Hill R, Kearns A, Sriskandan S. Clinical and molecular epidemiology of Staphylococcal toxic shock syndrome in the United Kingdom. Emerg Infect Dis. 2018;24(2):258–66.
3. Working Group on Severe Streptococcal Infection. Defining the group a streptococcal toxic shock syndrome. Rationale and consensus definition. JAMA. 1993;269:390–1.
4. Stevens DL, Tanner MH, Winship J, Swarts R, Ries KM, Schlievert PM, Kaplan E. Severe group a streptococcal infections associated with a toxic shock-like syndrome and scarlet fever toxin a. N Engl J Med. 1989;321:1–7.
5. Schlievert PM. Role of superantigens in human disease. J Infect Dis. 1993;167(5):997–1002.
6. Murray RJ. Recognition and management of Staphylococcus aureus toxin-mediated disease. Intern Med J. 2005;35(Suppl 2):S106–19.
7. Emma L, Andrew JF. Gram-positive toxic shock syndromes. Lancet Infect Dis. 2009;9:281–90.
8. Matsushima A, Kuroki Y, Nakajima S, Sakai T, Kojima H, Ueyama M. Low level of TSST-1 antibody in burn patients with toxic shock syndrome caused by methicillin-resistant Staphylococcus aureus. J Burn Care Res. 2015;36(3):e120–4.
9. Quan L, Morita R, Kawakami S. Toxic shock syndrome toxin-1 (TSST-1) antibody levels in Japanese children. Burns. 2010;36(5):716–21.

Open Access This chapter is licensed under the terms of the Creative Commons Attribution-NonCommercial-NoDerivatives 4.0 International License (http://creativecommons.org/licenses/by-nc-nd/4.0/), which permits any non-commercial use, sharing, distribution and reproduction in any medium or format, as long as you give appropriate credit to the original author(s) and the source, provide a link to the Creative Commons license and indicate if you modified the licensed material. You do not have permission under this license to share adapted material derived from this chapter or parts of it.

The images or other third party material in this chapter are included in the chapter's Creative Commons license, unless indicated otherwise in a credit line to the material. If material is not included in the chapter's Creative Commons license and your intended use is not permitted by statutory regulation or exceeds the permitted use, you will need to obtain permission directly from the copyright holder.

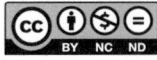

Skin Necrosis Due to Snakebites

Masaki Fujioka

21.1 Introduction

About 5.4 million people are bitten by venomous snakes, resulting in 2.7 million envenomings, almost 138,000 deaths, and 400,000 cases of sequelae or disability, mostly in Asia, Africa, and Latin America every year. Many patients survive, but most victims suffer from local complications such as skin necrosis if blisters are present [1, 2]. In 2019, the World Health Organization (WHO) launched a program to prevent and control snakebite incidents, thereby aiming to reduce snakebite mortality and morbidity by 50% by 2030 [3]. This chapter presents a review of published reports on the incidence, pathology, and treatment of snakebites; focuses on the prevalence of necrotic wounds; and discusses surgical treatment.

21.2 Systemic and Local Complications After Envenomation

Snake venom contains more than ten enzymes, several nonenzymatic proteins, and peptides, which can be a combination of many toxins, including cytotoxins, hemotoxins, neurotoxins, and myotoxins. Systemic clinical manifestations encompass a wide variety of problems including pain, weakness, dizziness, nausea, vomiting, hypotension, thrombocytopenia, tachycardia, and anuria. On envenomation, the enzyme hyaluronidase catalyzes the hydrolysis of the main interstitial constituents, increasing tissue permeability. Proteolytic enzymes destroy the endothelium and basal membrane of capillaries. Phospholipase A acts directly on erythrocyte membranes, which leads to intravascular hemolysis. Local edema with pain and swelling, which can progress rapidly and may involve the entire extremity, can be attributed to the phospholipase A2 and metalloproteinases. Serous or hemorrhagic blisters appear around the fang marks (Fig. 21.1a). Some enzymes destroy tissue, resulting in necrosis (Fig. 21.1b, c) [4].

M. Fujioka (✉)
Department of Plastic and Reconstructive Surgery, National Hospital Organization Nagasaki Medical Center, Nagasaki, Japan

© The Author(s) 2024
L. Téot et al. (eds.), *Skin Necrosis*, https://doi.org/10.1007/978-3-031-60954-1_21

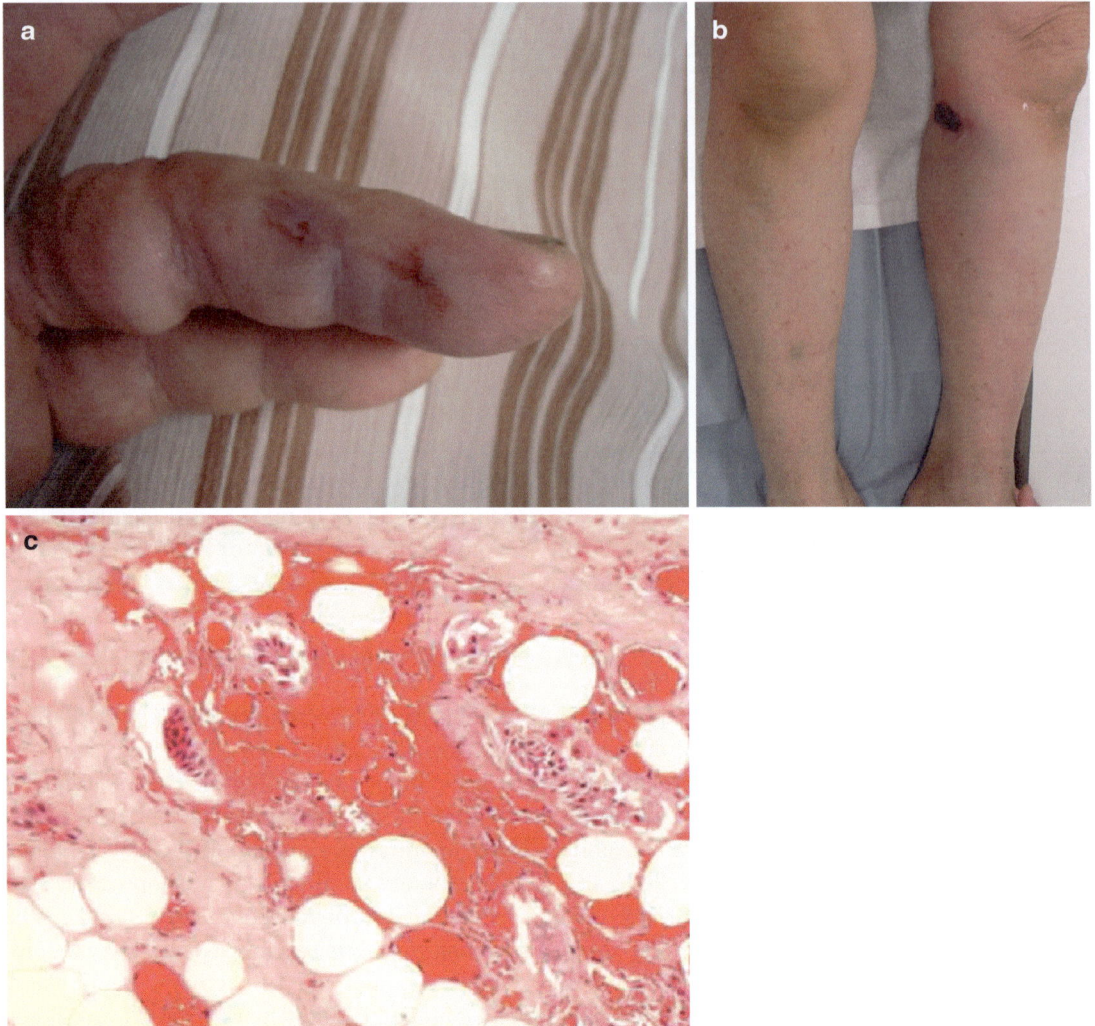

Fig. 21.1 (a) The picture shows two fang marks on the left ring finger. Swelling and tissue necrosis are visible around the fang marks. (b) The picture shows that the left knee was swollen with an area of soft tissue necrosis measuring 3.5 × 2.0 cm around the fang marks. (c) Histopathological findings of the fang mark site immediately after injury. The image shows red cell extravasation, vessel fibrinoid necrosis, and subcutaneous hemorrhagic necrosis with neutrophil infiltration

21.3 Dry Bite

The severity of a snakebite depends on the size of the snake and severity of envenomation. Venomous snakes sometimes bite without injecting venom. Such "dry bites" are known to occur in a number of venomous snake species. A study conducted over 3 years demonstrated that in over 776 snakebite admissions, 86% of the patients had received a bite in which no venom had been injected; thus, dry bite may account for in excess of 50% of bites in some species [5–7]. It can be difficult to determine whether a bite is "dry" or not, as a snakebite itself will often cause inflammation and swelling, which makes it more difficult to determine early if a victim of a snakebite needs antivenom [6].

21.4 First Aid

"Guidelines for the Management of Snakebites" by the World Health Organization (2010) [8] recommend the following: the victim must avoid physical activity, and the bite site should be immobilized and kept below heart level to prevent venom absorption and systemic spread. Tourniquet application, incision, excision, or mouth suction should not be performed. Many organizations, including the American Medical Association and the American Red Cross, recommend washing the bite with soap and water. The use of a compression bandage is generally as effective; however, some guidelines state that nonprofessionals should not apply a pressure bandage (Fig. 21.2) [9].

21.5 Antivenom Treatment

Antivenom is still the only effective treatment for envenomation. It is indicated to reduce convalescence time in moderate to severe cases and prevent death in severe cases. The British National Formulary suggested that antivenom should be given whenever there is any evidence of systemic envenoming or when local symptoms of envenoming are severe if, within 4 h of a bite on the hand or foot, swelling extends beyond the wrist or ankle [7]. There is evidence that antivenoms limit the spread of necrosis by inhibiting protease activity and reducing edema, leading to decreased risk of compartment syndrome.

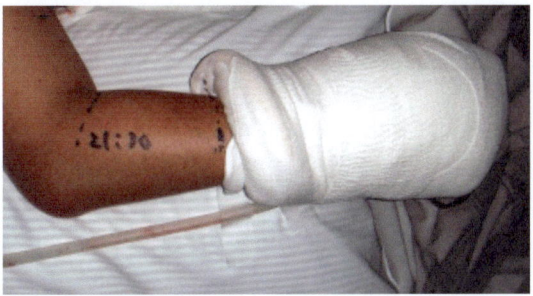

Fig. 21.2 Pressure immobilization using a compression bandage

21.6 Allergic Reactions to Antivenom

Allergic reactions to antivenom are possible. The most common reaction to antivenom is an anaphylactoid reaction, in 3–54% of patients. Ismail et al. reported that 40% of patients showing early reactions develop systemic anaphylaxis.

Serum sickness-type reactions have been reported to occur in 10–75% of patients receiving equine antivenin. The onset of delayed serum sickness usually occurs within 3 weeks after antivenin treatment and consists of fatigue, itching, urticaria, arthralgia, lymphadenopathy, periarticular swelling, albuminuria, and, rarely, encephalopathy [10].

Patients who have had prior reactions to horse serum and those who have had previous antivenin treatments can develop severe, delayed hypersensitivity reactions.

21.7 Surgical Treatment

Most of the literature is focused on snakebite mortality. However, many patients survive and suffer from local complications. Although snakebites are most commonly treated with specific antivenoms, surgical management has also been practiced. Urgent fasciotomy may be required if there is a sudden swelling of the limbs immediately after the injury. About 10% of all cases were in need of fasciotomy when compartment syndrome was diagnosed by measuring the intracompartmental pressure [11]. A meta-analysis reported an incidence of 5.5% sequelae and 3% amputations. Snakebite patients with skin necrosis require serial wound debridement, followed by reconstructive surgery using skin grafting and/or a flap. Chattopadhyay et al. reported that 28% of 58 patients required debridement to treat local necrosis. Maintenance of necrotic tissue in the wounds will certainly aggravate the local and general conditions of patients [12]. Surgery plays an important role in the management of snakebite patients with tissue necrosis. However, this involves late debridement, performed after skin necrosis has occurred.

21.8 Immediate Debridement of Fang Marks

If a snakebite is intracutaneous, the venom slowly spreads through lymphatic and superficial venous vessels, but there has to be a sufficient venom concentration to reach the systemic circulation in a few hours.

Recent guidelines for first aid against viper envenomation call for avoiding incision and recommend the administration of antivenom. However, antivenom carries the risk of an anaphylactic reaction, so its usage should be approached with extreme caution.

Since the snakebite severity depends on the amount of venom injected into the victim, if even a small part of it can be removed, patients should present milder symptoms.

Even in the case of perfectly performed incision and suction, only 20% of venom can be removed. Also, since snake fangs are curved, the venom is not directly under the bite marks; therefore, only a very deep incision can reach it [9]. To prevent later sequela, snakebites are best treated acutely by surgical debridement to remove as much venom as possible, which consequently decreases inflammatory responses and the necessity of antivenom [13].

In dry bite cases, radical ablation of fang marks should not be performed until local signs of envenomation appear. Since the aim of this procedure is the removal of injected venom, all necrotic soft tissue and inflamed skin must be debrided.

The standard method of wound management was presented in 2003 as a guideline for woundbed preparation, stating that "efficient debridement is an essential step in acute and chronic wound management. Regular debridement is necessary to reduce the necrotic burden and achieve healthy granulation tissue. Debridement also reduces wound contamination." Furthermore, it is well known that all animal bites present a high risk of infection. Once tissue undergoes necrotic changes, it cannot survive. Thus, the removal of necrotic tissue as soon as possible is a reasonable option from the viewpoint of wound management and infection control. Moreover, this procedure ensures the removal of the remaining venom in necrotic tissue [14].

Although immediate radical ablation can reduce the volume of injected venom, total removal is impossible. Continuous observation is indispensable after ablation, and if severe systemic symptoms of envenomation occur, antivenom treatment should be indicated with no hesitation [15].

21.9 Case Reports

The Japanese viper (*Gloydius b. blomhoffii, Japanese mamushi*) is responsible for the majority of venomous snakebites in Japan, and more than 1000 cases of Japanese viper bites are believed to occur annually. I present successful cases of immediate radical ablation of fang marks due to Japanese viper bites.

21.9.1 Case 1

The left index finger of a 74-year-old man was bitten by a Japanese viper. About 30 min after the injury, the victim arrived at our emergency unit, where the initial examination revealed that the finger was swollen with an area of soft tissue necrosis measuring 1.5 × 0.6 cm around the fang marks (Fig. 21.3a). Immediate ablation was performed of the damaged skin, including the surrounding inflamed surface, covering a total area of 2.0 × 1.0 cm (Fig. 21.3b). Antivenom was not administered, since the general condition and laboratory data of the patient indicated stability. Treatment with ointment was performed, and the wound healed within 2 months with no sensory or functional impairment (Fig. 21.3c).

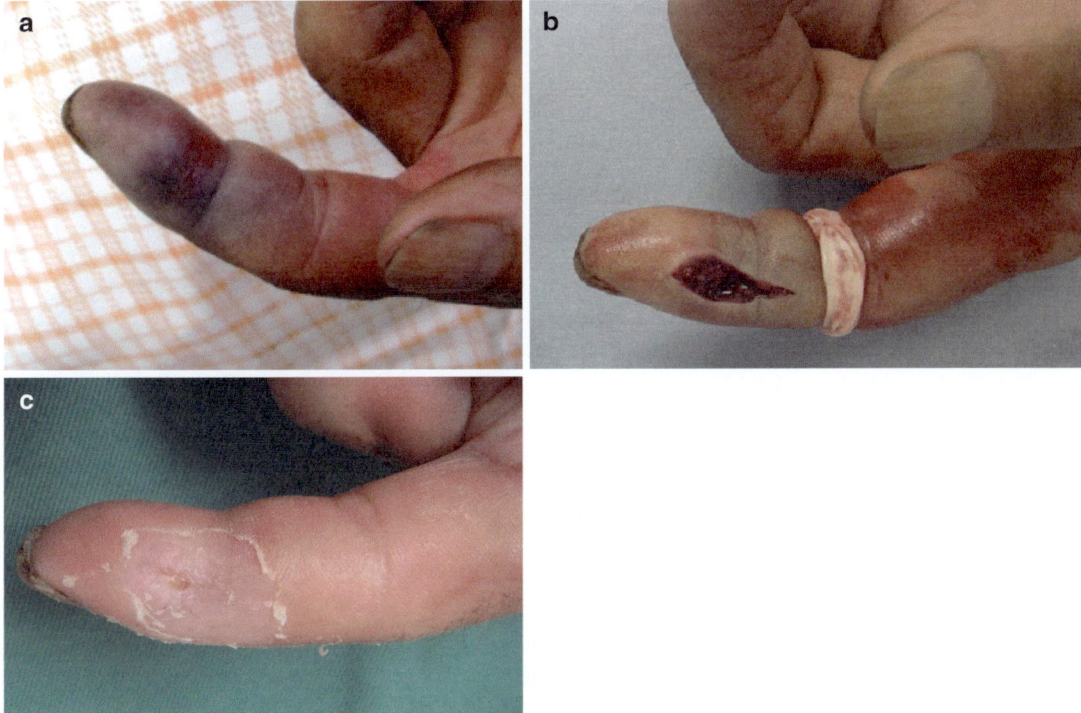

Fig. 21.3 (**a**) Case 1: At 30 min after being bitten, the finger was swollen with tissue necrosis. (**b**) The picture shows the wound after the removal of a 2.0 × 1.0 cm area of soft tissue. (**c**) Two months after injury, the picture shows that the wound has completely healed

21.9.2 Case 2

A 72-year-old woman was bitten on her left leg by a Japanese viper and arrived at our unit 50 min after the injury. The left knee was swollen, with an area of ecchymosis and necrotic soft tissue measuring 3.5 × 2.0 cm (Fig. 21.4a). Surgical debridement of the ecchymotic surface, as well as necrotic tissue, including the surrounding inflamed skin (total of 8.5 × 7.0 cm), was immediately performed (Fig. 21.4b). Antivenom was not administered as severe systemic symptoms were not observed. Two weeks later, the patient received a split-thickness skin graft. Six months after the injury, the patient could return to work without any complications (Fig. 21.4c).

21.9.3 Case 3

A 78-year-old man was bitten on his left index finger by a Japanese viper and transferred to our emergency unit 1 h later. The finger was swollen with ecchymosis as well as ischemic soft tissue around the fang marks (Fig. 21.5a). The necrotic tissue and inflamed skin were ablated (Fig. 21.5b). The wound healed with no sensory or functional impairment within 2 months (Fig. 21.5c).

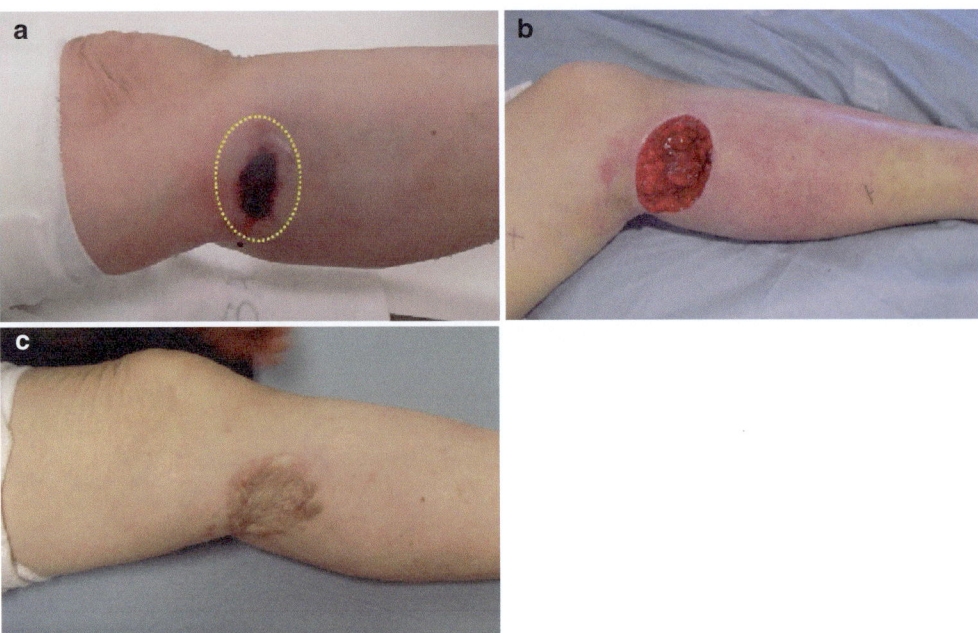

Fig. 21.4 (**a**) Case 2: At 30 min after being bitten, the left knee was swollen with an area of soft tissue necrosis measuring 3.5 × 2.0 cm around the fang marks. The dotted line indicates the debridement area. (**b**) The picture shows the wound immediately after surgical debridement of the ecchymotic surface, as well as ischemic and necrotic tissue, including the surrounding inflamed skin. (**c**) Six months after injury, the picture shows that the wound has completely healed

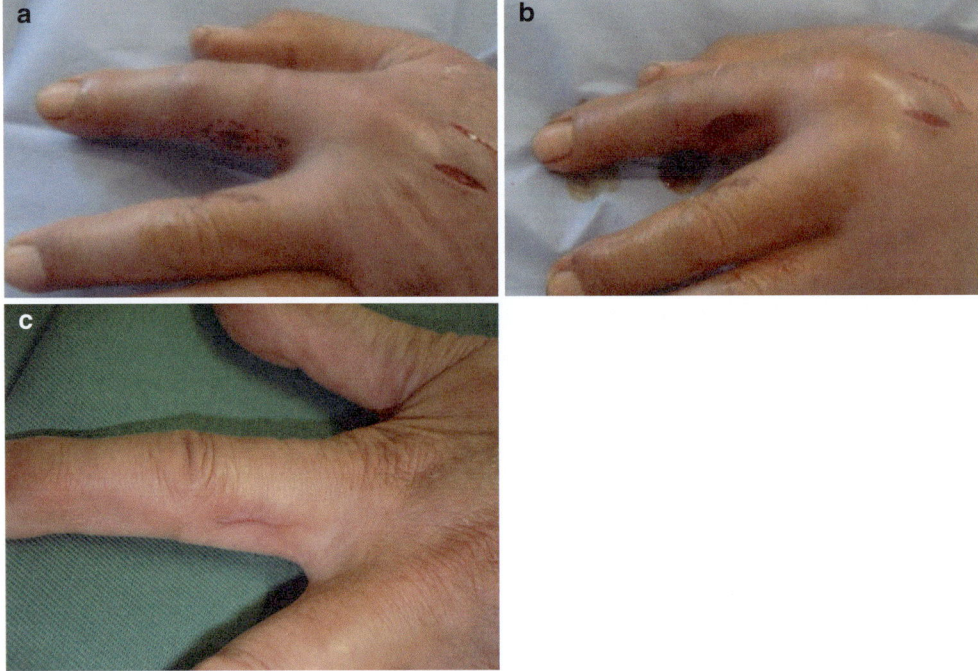

Fig. 21.5 (**a**) Case 3: At 1 h after being bitten, the left index finger was swollen with tissue necrosis. (**b**) The picture shows the wound after the removal of a 2.5 × 0.6 cm area of soft tissue. (**c**) The photograph shows the wound 2 months after injury, with favorable resurfacing

21.10 Conclusion

Although surgery is not as important as antivenom therapy for snakebites, surgical intervention will minimize functional loss [13]. Immediate radical ablation is a useful procedure that can reduce the amount of venom in tissue, which, consequently, decreases inflammatory reactions and reduces the necessity of antivenom usage.

Acknowledgments None.

References

1. Rojnuckarin P, Mahasandana S, Intragumthornchai T, Sutcharitchan P, Swasdikul D. Prognostic factors of green pit viper bites. Am J Trop Med Hyg. 1998;58(1):22–5.
2. WHO. Snakebite envenoming—key facts. 2019. https://www.who.int/news-room/fact-sheets/detail/snakebite-envenoming. Accessed 22 Apr 2020.
3. WHO Snakebite: WHO targets 50% reduction in deaths and disabilities. https://www.who.int/news-room/detail/23-05-2019-who-launches-global-strategy-for-prevention-and-control-of-snanebite-envenoming. Accessed 23 Apr 2020.
4. Chotenimitkhun R, Rojnuckarin P. Systemic antivenom and skin necrosis after green pit viper bites. Clin Toxicol. 2008;46:122–5.
5. Kularatne K, Budagoda S, Maduwage K, Naser K, Kumarasiri R, Kularatne S. Parallels between Russell's viper (*Daboia russelii*) and hump–nosed viper (*Hypnale* species) bites in the central hills of Sri Lanka amidst the heavy burden of unidentified snake bites. Asian Pac J Trop Med. 2011;4:564–7.
6. Pucca MB, Knudsen C, Oliveira SI, Rimbault C, Cerni AF, Wen FH, Sachett J, Sartim MA, Laustsen AH, Monteiro WM. Current Knowledge on Snake Dry Bites. Toxins (Basel). 2020;12(11):668. https://doi.org/10.3390/toxins12110668.
7. Reading CJ. Incidence, pathology, and treatment of adder (Vipera berus L.) bites in man. J Accid Emerg Med. 1996;13(5):346–51.
8. Warrel DA. Guidelines for the management of snakebites. World Health Organization; 2010. p. 61–5. http://apps.searo.who.int/PDS_DOCS/B4508.pdf.
9. Adukauskienė D, Varanauskienė E, Adukauskaitė A. Venomous snakebites. Medicina (Kaunas). 2011;47(8):461–7.
10. Ismail M, Memish ZA. Venomous snakes of Saudi Arabia and the Middle East: a keynote for travellers. Int J Antimicrob Agents. 2003;21:164–9.
11. Kim YH, Choi JH, Kim J, Chung YK. Fasciotomy in compartment syndrome from snakebite. Arch Plast Surg. 2019;46(1):69–74. https://doi.org/10.5999/aps.2018.00577.
12. Chattopadhyay A, Patra RD, Shenoy V, Kumar V, Nagendhar Y. Surgical implications of snakebites. Indian J Pediatr. 2004;71(5):397–9.
13. Mehmet B, Yalcin K, Fatih Z, Emin K. The management of pit viper envenomation of the hand. Hand (N Y). 2008;3(4):324–31.
14. Fujioka M. Although surgery should not be used as first-line treatment, immediate ablation should be performed when necrotic change around the fang mark is recognized. J Venom Anim Toxins Incl Trop Dis. 2010;16(3):5–6.
15. Fujioka M, Oka K, Yakabe A, Kitamura R. Immediate radical fang mark ablation may allow treatment of Japanese viper bite without antivenom. J Venom Anim Toxins Incl Trop Dis. 2009;15(1):68–178.

Open Access This chapter is licensed under the terms of the Creative Commons Attribution-NonCommercial-NoDerivatives 4.0 International License (http://creativecommons.org/licenses/by-nc-nd/4.0/), which permits any non-commercial use, sharing, distribution and reproduction in any medium or format, as long as you give appropriate credit to the original author(s) and the source, provide a link to the Creative Commons license and indicate if you modified the licensed material. You do not have permission under this license to share adapted material derived from this chapter or parts of it.

The images or other third party material in this chapter are included in the chapter's Creative Commons license, unless indicated otherwise in a credit line to the material. If material is not included in the chapter's Creative Commons license and your intended use is not permitted by statutory regulation or exceeds the permitted use, you will need to obtain permission directly from the copyright holder.

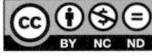

Stonefish Necrosis

Jan Dirk Harms, Cyril D'Andréa, and Nadia Fartaoui

The marine environment is rich in poisonous and venomous animals and plants. Among them, the stonefish is responsible for wounds with poisoning, which sometimes evolve towards necrosis. The geographical distribution of such fish is widespread, and it usually lives in shallow water; as a result, the stings are not rare among the human population. The wounds of stings are at risk of extensive necrosis.

22.1 The Stonefish [3, 4]

22.1.1 Identification

Stonefishes are of the family Scorpaenidae (according to ITIS[1]) or Synanceiinae (according to FishBase[2]). There are several species among which *Synanceia verrucosa* (Figs. 22.1 and 22.2) is the one present in La Réunion.

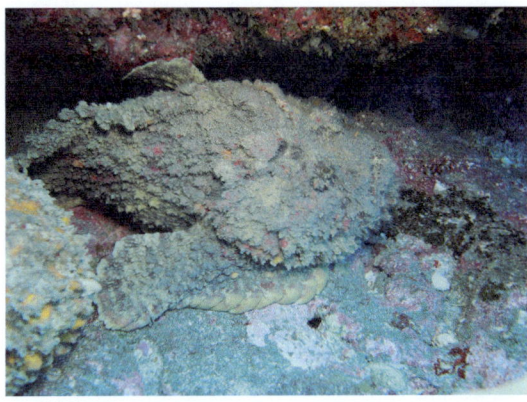

Fig. 22.1 Stonefish (Courtesy of Olivier Allart, Diony-Bulles, Réunion Island)

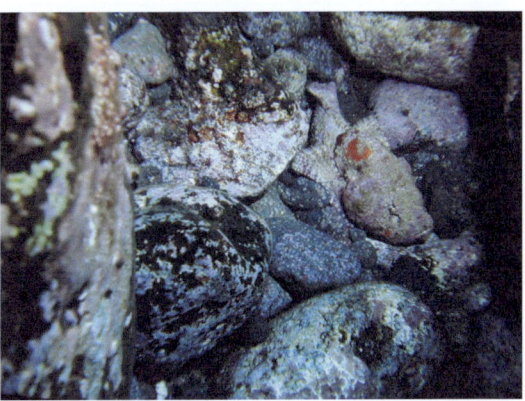

Fig. 22.2 Example of mimetized stonefish on seabed

---

[1] ITIS: Integrated Taxonomic Information System (Joined)
[2] FishBase: Consortium since 2000, established (constituted) by AfricaMuseum; Aristotle University of Thessaloniki; Chinese Academy of Fisheries; Fisheries Centre, University of British Columbia; United Nations Organization for Food (supply) and Agriculture (farming); IFM-GEOMAR; National Natural History Museum; Swedish Museum of Natural History; and WorldFish Center

---

J. D. Harms (✉) · C. D'Andréa
Unité de Médecine Hyperbare—Plaies et Cicatrisation, CHU de la REUNION-GHSR, Saint-Pierre (Réunion), France
e-mail: jan-dirk.harms@chu-reunion.fr

N. Fartaoui
Département Universitaire de Médecine Générale, Bobigny, France

© The Author(s) 2024
L. Téot et al. (eds.), *Skin Necrosis*, https://doi.org/10.1007/978-3-031-60954-1_22

22.1.2 Habitat

Stonefishes are found on coral reefs, muddy waters or sandblasters of the Indian Ocean, Red Sea, Indonesia, Australia, New Caledonia and the Pacific [5].

22.1.3 Venomous Apparatus

22.1.3.1 Thorns and Glands with Venom

The stonefish has 13 thorns on its dorsal fin, which rise in case of danger. Every thorn is covered with a verrucose tegumental envelope and has a pair of glands with venom in its base. Every gland has a canal filled with poison leading to the top of the thorn. If someone walks on or tries to seize the stonefish, its thorns penetrate into the skin and the tegumental envelope is then pushed downward causing the compression of the gland, which if sufficient will launch the release of the poison. The stinging and poisoning are a defensive mechanism.

The venom: its composition is complex: substances such as histamine, adrenalin, norepinephrine and dopamine as well as enzymes such as hyaluronidase, protease and lipase. The main toxin is the verrucotoxin: it inhibits the calcic canals, and it activates the potassium canals. The venom is myotoxic, neurotoxic and haemolytic. It is inactivated at 54 °C [3].

22.2 Stings by Stonefish

22.2.1 General Ideas

Stonefishes were notorious for being among the most venomous animals of the world, and its stings were thought to be lethal. In fact, the sting by stonefish provokes an extremely intense pain that can possibly result in a faint fit. Also, if it happens to a scuba diver, it may cause an accident if the diver is unable to control his ascent (barotraumatism) or to make the required decompression stops (desaturation accident).

22.2.2 Circumstances

The stonefish is a sedentary and benthic fish. It favours rocky areas or lays buried under sand or mud. It feeds on small fishes and shrimps, which it swallows with its mouth. The stonefish can survive several hours out of the water, and its venom remains active from 24 to 48 h after its death. Stings by stonefishes mostly occur during activities such as bathing, fishing, snorkelling and scuba diving.

22.2.3 Wound Location

The wounds are mainly seen on the feet of people who accidentally walked on a stonefish. They can also be seen on hands due to an attempt to touch or seize the fish.

22.2.4 Clinical Evidence

The pain is immediate and very intense. It can cause a person to faint. The pain is quoted between 8 and 10 on the visual analogic pain scale. It often results in restlessness and aggressiveness.

There are one or several wounds, mostly in the foot or in the hand.

An oedema quickly develops, sometimes limited around the wound, often wider and spreading. Not rarely, it might extend to the whole limb up to its base.

General symptoms are often noticed: sweats, nauseas, arterial hypotension, tachycardia, heart rhythm disorders, myasthenia and pulmonary oedema.

22.2.5 Diagnosis

The diagnosis is easy when the victim saw the fish and clearly identified it. It is often the case with fishermen and scuba divers. In many other cases, it is about a person who was bathing and suddenly felt an excruciating pain without seeing the cause of such pain. Thus, there is a doubt that it could also be a wound by a piece of coral or shell or a sting by another marine animal (*Pterois volitans*, ray, poisonous shell, etc.).

The diagnosis is then based on assumption. If the stonefish is not clearly identified, the elements which allow to incriminate the stonefish are the following:

- The pain which is of maximum intensity at once and resists to painkillers, including level 3 analgesics. The pain remains at highest intensity during 12–18 h and then gradually decreases within 2–3 days.
- The examination of the wound allows identifying the origin of the sting: if there are several stings by several thorns, they are distributed at equal distance. Every sting presents a small wound with clear edges from 1 to 2 mm in length with an inflammatory area and a bluish halo (Fig. 22.3) and sometimes a small blood and fluid flow.

Often, the delay is more important and thus the inflammation has further extended with oedema and phlyctenas around the wound.

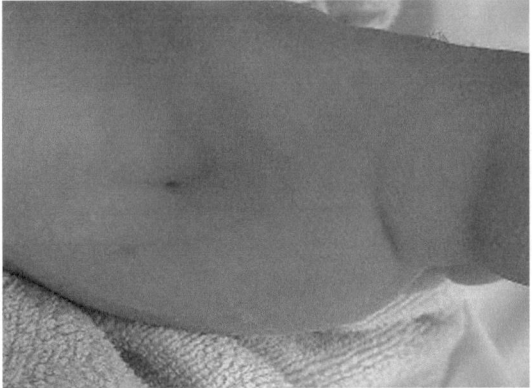

Fig. 22.3 Typical aspect of a sting with punctiform lesion and bluish halo

The association of a sudden, intense pain and these local aspects allows evoking the diagnosis of sting by stonefish.

22.2.6 Severity of the Wound Depends on Several Factors

The size of the fish: the bigger the stonefish is, the more venom is injected and the more serious is the wound.

The wound: the number and depth of the stings.

The victim: his (or her) age, weight and medical history.

The time period until medical care is given.

22.2.7 Medical Complications

Presence of a foreign body which will have to be removed: a piece of thorn that would have broken into the wound. Medical imaging might be necessary if there is a doubt, though this is rare since the *Synanceia verrucosa* thorns are very resistant.

Superinfection of wounds: the marine environment is rich in bacteria of all kinds, and any wound by marine animals may become infected.

Extended infection: the risk of a spread infection is real, possibly leading to cellulitis, fasciitis or gas gangrene.

Thromboembolic complications are also possible.

The necrosis of wounds is the most frequently met complication, though rather infrequent. If necrosis is observed, medical supervision of the wound and its course is required. The bluish halo around the sting usually evolves within a few days towards a small lesion: a superficial necrosis which only requires simple dressing. However, the necrosis sometimes extends reaching the dermis, hypodermis and the muscle and tendon underneath. This necrosis continues to extend in spite of local care, and from the initial, limited lesion, the wound extends to its neighbouring structures. This is serious and worrisome for both the patient and physician.

22.2.8 Treatment

Treatment of the pain from the beginning is an absolute priority due to its intensity:

- Grade 1 (paracetamol) or 2 (tramadol) analgesics are often ineffective. Morphine must be tried, but in a number of cases and in spite of important doses, it remains ineffective too.
- Heat is used because the venom is inactivated at 54 °C. It is necessary to dip the limb in a 45 °C water tub and let it soak until the pain decreases. This "hot-water technique" is sometimes very effective, sometimes not. The duration of the soaking is important which exposes the patient to a risk of burn. It seems that the sooner the technique is used, the better the result is. However, the disparities observed in the results are important. In all, some disadvise this technique because of the potential burns, whereas others use it. In our personal experience, we used it with sometimes dramatic results and often failures or poor improvements, in particular the outbreak of the pain as soon as the hot water is removed [1, 2].
- The equimolar gas oxygen/nitrous oxide (Entonox®) can be used, but it is often insufficient since the relief only lasts while the gas is given and it cannot be given for a prolonged duration. It can be helpful then while waiting for the analgesics to become efficient.
- The local injection of lidocaine can be used.
- Locoregional anaesthesia is the most effective method for the treatment of the pain. We implemented an epidural anaesthesia using bupivacaine and continuous administration through a catheter during 12 h for a patient whose pain was unbearable and resistant to the drugs. C. Maillaud in New Caledonia successfully realised several truncal locoregional anaesthesias on patients [6]. This requires anaesthesiologist availability, and in our hospital, we have set up a protocol for locoregional anaesthesia made by anaesthesiologists in our operating unit preparation room: "single shot" (no indication of nervous catheter) with naropeine in a sciatic block in the lower limb or axillary, infraclavicular or humeral block in the upper limb. The patient must stay at hospital for 1 day.

22.2.9 Other Used Treatments

The antivenom serum for stonefish is made by the Commonwealth Serum Laboratories in Australia by immunisation of horse with some venom of *Synanceia trachynis* and would be effective according to its manufacturer on the venom of *Synanceia verrucosa*. This serum is expensive; it must be kept between 2 and 8 °C, and its duration of use is limited. It is not available in Réunion Island, but it is in Mauritius. S. Hansrod, in her report of interuniversity diploma of physiology and hyperbaric and underwater medicine, studied the Mauritian experience: the injection of "serum anti-stonefish" would have a very fast effect on the decrease of pain especially if the intramuscular injection can be prematurely made. The intravenous route can be exceptionally used. The risk of anaphylactic shock and serum disease must be taken into account [1–3].

Steroids as anti-inflammation medication: their efficacy has not been demonstrated by any study, and their effect is not recommended because of the risk of infection.

The antibiotic therapy is often prescribed, especially if one or several wounds were not prematurely disinfected. Amoxicillin/clavulanate potassium or a third-generation cephalosporin is prescribed for 3 in 5 days [3].

The tetanus prevention must be considered and implemented depending on the vaccine status of the subject.

Low-molecular-weight heparins are prescribed if there is an important oedema or to patients at risk.

The treatment of the wound requires the earliest possible disinfection and dressings.

The surgery is sometimes necessary, secondly, for the treatment of complicated wounds.

The hyperbaric oxygen therapy (HBOT) is used for the treatment of wounds evolving unfavourably as an adjuvant therapy to improve the healing. It becomes essential in case of infection such as cellulitis or gas gangrene [2].

22.3 Our Experience in Réunion Island

In 2008, we made a retrospective study in Réunion Island. We had listed the suspicions of sting by stonefish in the Emergency Unit of the Groupe Hospitalier Sud Réunion from 2000 until 2005: 51 cases had been counted. It was 11 females and 40 males (average age 30, 6 years/extremes: 3 and 63 years). The stings concerned the feet in 78% of the cases and the hands in 22%. In all the cases, we found a very intense pain, a local oedema (57%) or extended (in cases involving the whole limb) (16%), an ecchymosis (16%), an inflammation (20%) and an early local necrosis (16%). Analgesics were used in 70% of the cases with an association of different grades in 33% and using morphine in 43%. The hot-water soaking was used in 65% of the cases and the local injection of lidocaine in 9%. An antibiotic therapy was prescribed in 43% of the cases. The patients were hospitalised in 46% of the cases. The extension of the necrosis occurred in four cases, and the surgery was necessary in two cases. HBOT was used in three cases [2].

22.4 Clinical Cases

22.4.1 Case 1

It is an old report from 2001. A 63-year-old fisherman caught a stonefish of a beautiful size, estimated at 2 kg. By picking it up, his right-hand middle finger got wounded. He came to the emergency unit to consult a physician only the next day. Figure 22.4 was taken on the 13th of February 2001 at his admission in the emergency unit. There is a necrosis of the pulp of the third phalanx, while there was initially a phlyctena. Figure 22.5 was taken on the 21st, and later evolution of the wound is seen in Fig. 22.6: the

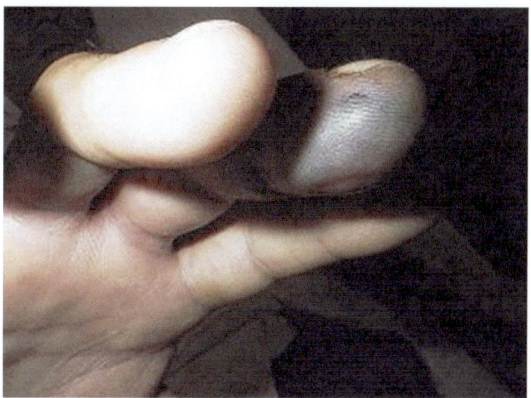

Fig. 22.4 Case 1: Pulp necrosis of the finger the day after the sting

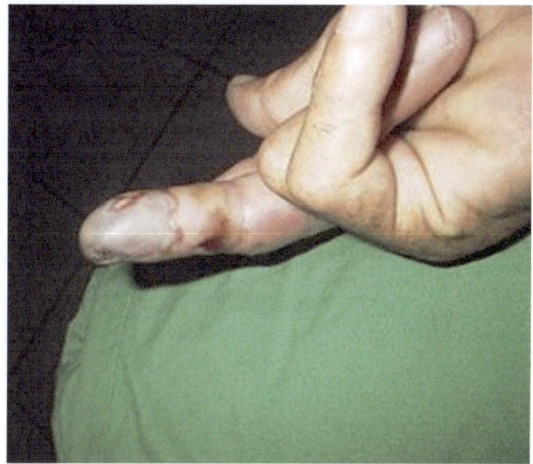

Fig. 22.5 Case 1: Aspect after 3 weeks

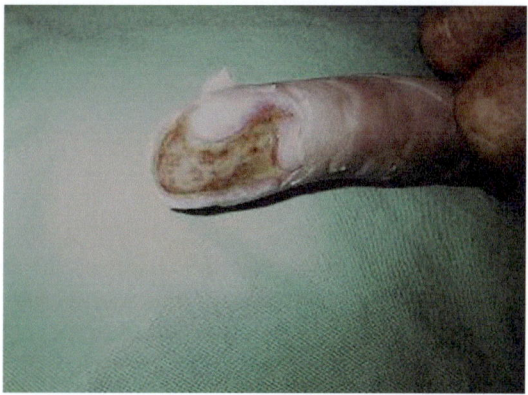

Fig. 22.6 Case 1: Later evolution

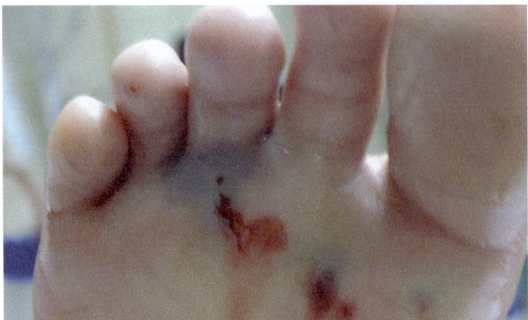

Fig. 22.7 Case 2: Typical early aspect with three points of sting

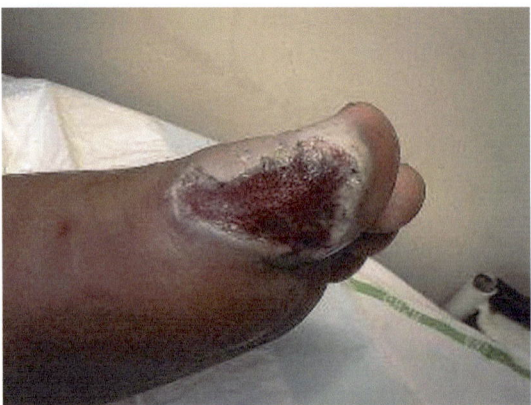

Fig. 22.8 Case 3: Intermediate aspect after use of hydrocolloid dressings

examination of the wound suggested the necessity of a distal amputation. This patient was treated by dressings and HBOT sessions (Fig. 22.6). The healing of a good quality will be obtained after 5 months of care.

22.4.2 Case 2

It is about a 12-year-old boy who was stung while bathing in a rocky area. We saw him approximately half an hour after the sting (Fig. 22.7). The pain was extreme with a state of agitation. The aspect is characteristic because we see three stings made by three thorns: they are regularly spaced out. We clearly distinguish the stings, with blood and an ecchymosis which is spread on the most external lesion. The internal injury has a small halo: the penetration of the thorn was superficial at this level. The soaking associated with analgesics was effective and the course simple.

22.4.3 Case 3

An 8-year-old girl was stung, and we saw her a month later. Her mother was very worried. We gave her explanations onto the usual evolution of these wounds and our project for dressings with stop of the daily use of povidone-iodine disinfection, and use of dressings changed all the 3 or 4 days. The evolution was quickly positive, and healing was obtained a month and a half later (Fig. 22.8).

The stings by stonefish are frequent in all the tropical zones of Indian and Pacific seas because of the presence of the fish in shallow water. The severe pain monopolises the immediate care. The risk of evolution in extensive necrosis, difficult and long to be treated, should impose a particular surveillance after initial care.

Acknowledgements Thanks to Elodie Couture for help in translation.

References

1. Hansrod. Utilisation du sérum anti-stonefish dans les accidents par piqûre de poisson-pierre (Expérience mauricienne). Mémoire du DIU de physiologie et médecine hyperbare et subaquatique Université de Lille II Session de la Réunion 06 novembre 2001.
2. Harms JD, D'Andréa C, Grandcolas N, Staïkowsky F. Piqûres par poisson-pierre à la Réunion. J Plaies et Cicatrisations. 2009;68(XIII):66–8.
3. Leuteritz A. La piqûre de poisson-pierre : quoi de neuf en 2009? Mémoire du DIU de physiologie et médecine hyperbare et subaquatique. Université de Lille II, Session de la Réunion, 03 mars 2010.
4. Levêque Y. Risques naturels des récifs coralliens de l'archipel des Mascareignes. Thèse de doctorat en médecine. Université de Poitiers. 2001.
5. Louis-François C, Mathoulin C, Halbswahs C, Grivois JP, Bricaire F, Caumes E. Complications cutanées des envenimations par poisson-pierre chez 6 voyageurs au retour de la région maritime indo-pacifique. Bul Soc Pathol Exot. 2003;96(5):415–9.
6. Maillaud C, Maillard A. Prise en charge des envenimations par poissons-pierres et autres scorpénidés. Intérêt de l'anesthésie locorégionale JEUR. 2004;17:192–7.

Open Access This chapter is licensed under the terms of the Creative Commons Attribution-NonCommercial-NoDerivatives 4.0 International License (http://creativecommons.org/licenses/by-nc-nd/4.0/), which permits any non-commercial use, sharing, distribution and reproduction in any medium or format, as long as you give appropriate credit to the original author(s) and the source, provide a link to the Creative Commons license and indicate if you modified the licensed material. You do not have permission under this license to share adapted material derived from this chapter or parts of it.

The images or other third party material in this chapter are included in the chapter's Creative Commons license, unless indicated otherwise in a credit line to the material. If material is not included in the chapter's Creative Commons license and your intended use is not permitted by statutory regulation or exceeds the permitted use, you will need to obtain permission directly from the copyright holder.

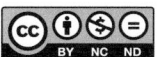

Skin Necrosis from Coma Blister

Masayuki Kashiwagi and Shin-ichi Kubo

23.1 Introduction

Skin lesions in forensic autopsy cases are mainly injuries such as skin discoloration, subcutaneous hemorrhage, and epidermal exfoliation. Pressure ulcers are often experienced as skin necrosis. In addition, there are many cases of death due to sepsis caused by decubitus ulcers.

On the other hand, in forensic autopsy cases, skin lesions may be useful to know antemortem conditions and causes of death. A typical example is coma blister. Coma blisters, as the name suggests, are skin lesions observed associated with coma. Therefore, the finding of this skin lesion at autopsy or postmortem examination suggests that the deceased had coma prior to death and that an overdose of sleeping pills was the cause. Coma blisters are important skin lesions in forensic autopsies and autopsies. However, the details of the generating mechanism of the coma blister, such as drug eruption, necrosis, or some other mechanism, are still unclear.

This chapter introduces the coma blister.

In forensic autopsy cases, when there are spiloplaxia and vesicles on the body surface, those regions are suspected as having thermal trauma or frostbite congelation [1]. Although traditionally associated with barbiturate overdose, they can be seen in the setting of coma due to other etiologies. The vesicles observed by Holzer in cases of barbiturate intoxication have been known for a long time [2].

The erythematous patches and vesicles that are observed in coma patients, usually from an overdose of medication, are known in the dermatology field as coma blisters [3–5]. Recently, it had been reported that a similar spiloplaxia and vesicles are also observed in non-coma cases [6, 7]. Therefore, the pathogenesis of those skin lesions is unclear. It is unknown whether the degenerated sweat gland is a necrosis or apoptosis.

We examined the skin lesions such as spiloplaxia and vesication histologically and immunohistochemically, observed in forensic autopsy cases, to investigate the characteristics and pathogenesis of the coma blister. We also investigated the histological and immunohistological characteristics of the coma blister, especially sweat gland degeneration.

In our study, the apoptosis might be involved in the sweat gland degenerations of coma blisters. There are not so many forensic autopsy cases of the coma blister. Further prospective studies would be useful to further elucidate the underlying pathogenesis.

M. Kashiwagi · S.-i. Kubo (✉)
Department of Forensic Medicine, Faculty of Medicine, Fukuoka University, Fukuoka, Japan
e-mail: kuboshin@fukuoka-u.ac.jp

23.2 Case Examination

Skin samples: Skin region samples of bullae and/or discoloration from a forensic autopsy case and normal skin were collected from other autopsy cases, as follows:

Case outline: A female in her 30 s was caring for her bedridden mother. One day in November, the mother's care manager visited their house; however, there was no response, and none of the doors were locked. The care manager notified the police, and the policeman entered the house and found the daughter dead on her back in her bedroom. *Autopsy findings:* The decedent was 159.7 cm in height and 43.0 kg in weight. Postmortem lividity was intense on the back. Spiloplaxia with excoriation and spiloplaxia with a red halo were observed in the precordial region. The spiloplaxia with the red halo was observed in the left femoral region. Blisters surrounded by rims of erythema were observed in the left femoral region, the lower left thigh, and the right knee (Fig. 23.1). The blister on the right knee was 1.0 cm in diameter (Fig. 23.2). Obvious abnormalities, such as hemorrhages, were not observed in the subcutaneous region of these wounds. Five hundred and fifty milliliters of urine had been collected in the bladder. There was no fatal trauma or disease observed. Autopsy also revealed that postmortem interval (PMI) was suspected for 4 days.

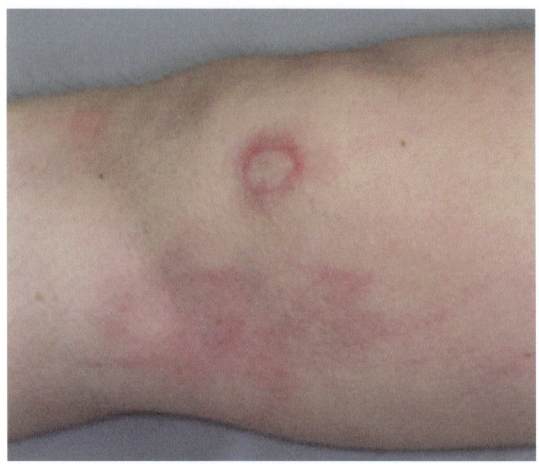

Fig. 23.2 Blister surrounded by rims of erythema on the right knee

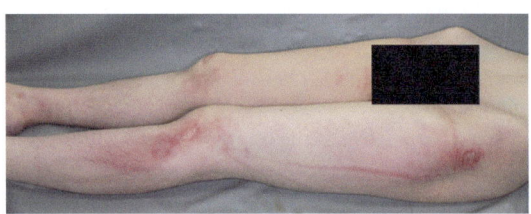

Fig. 23.1 Blisters surrounded by rims of erythema were observed in the left femoral region, the lower left thigh, and the right knee

Toxicological analysis: Caffeine, ibuprofen, bromovalerylurea, bromoisovaleric acid, and ethoxybenzoic acid were detected in the blood. Caffeine, ibuprofen, bromovalerylurea, ethenzamide, ethoxybenzoic acid, and salicylamide were detected in the urine. Quantitative analysis revealed that ibuprofen, bromovalerylurea, and caffeine were 26, 11, and 52 μg/g in the blood, respectively.

23.2.1 Immunohistochemical Examinations

Histological and immunohistochemical examinations of the skin lesions were performed. The samples were fixed in 10% phosphate-buffered

23 Skin Necrosis from Coma Blister

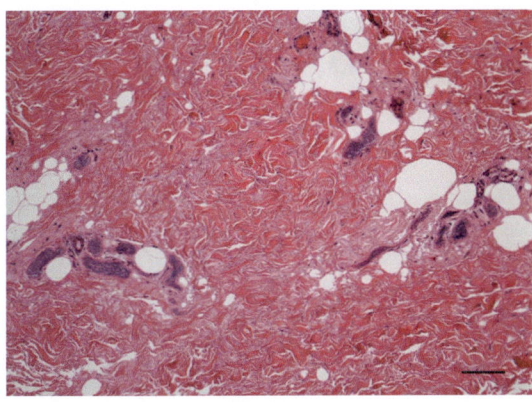

Fig. 23.3 In the secretory cells of the eccrine sweat glands, eosinophilic homogenization of the cytoplasm and pyknosis or absence of nuclei were observed (right knee). Length of bar indicates 50 μm

Table 23.1 Immunoreactivities in the degenerated sweat glands

Antigens	Lesion	Control
Inflammatory cell markers		
CD3	−	−
CD8	−	−
CD45RO	+	−
Keratin markers		
CK-W	+	+
CK-H	+	+
CK-L	±	+
Stress markers		
HSP70	−	−
Ub	−	−
ORP150	−	−
Apoptosis markers		
M30	+	−
TUNEL	−	−

formalin and embedded in paraffin. Sections of 4 μm thickness were stained with hematoxylin-eosin (HE). Immunohistochemically, CD3 (Dako, Japan); CD8 (Leica Microsystems, Germany); CD45RO (Dako, Japan); Cytokeratin, Wide Spectrum Screening (CK-W) (Dako, Japan); Cytokeratin, High Molecular Weight (keratin 34βE12) (CK-H) (Dako, Japan); Cytokeratin 8, Low Molecular Weight (CK-L) (Dako, Japan); 70 kD heat-shock protein (HSP70) (Amersham, USA); ubiquitin (Ub) (DAKO, Japan); 150 kD oxygen-regulated protein (ORP150) (Abcom, UK); and caspase-cleaved keratin 18 neo-epitope M30 (M30) (Previa AB, Sweden) were observed using a labeled streptavidin biotin (LSAB)/horseradish peroxidase (HRP) technique (Histofine SAB-PO kit, Nichirei, Japan), following the manufacturer's instructions. Staining specificity was checked using negative control slides omitting the primary antibody. Additionally, tissue specimens other than positive control tissues were used in a negative control study. To detect the apoptosis, skin samples were stained by the terminal deoxynucleotidyl transferase-mediated deoxyuridine triphosphate nick end labeling (TUNEL) method with ApopTag peroxidase in situ Apoptosis Detection Kit (Takara Bio Inc., Japan), also according to the manufacturer's instructions.

Histological examination of the skin lesions from the right knee showed necrosed keratinocytes and the epidermis was thin in some areas. Subepidermal vesicles were observed in the blister. In the secretory cells of the eccrine sweat glands, eosinophilic homogenization of the cytoplasm and pyknosis or absence of nuclei were observed (Fig. 23.3). Summary of the immunoreactivities in the degenerated sweat glands is shown in Table 23.1. The degenerated sweat glands showed good immunoreactivities for CK-W and CK-H just like the control. However, the typical immunoreactivity for CK-L decreased (Figs. 23.4). Weak CD45RO immunoreactivity was observed (Fig. 23.5). However, no immunoreactivities for HSP70, Ub, or ORP 150 were observed. Further, apoptosis was not detected by the TUNEL method. Otherwise, mild degenerated sweat glands showed partial M30 immunoreactivity (Fig. 23.6).

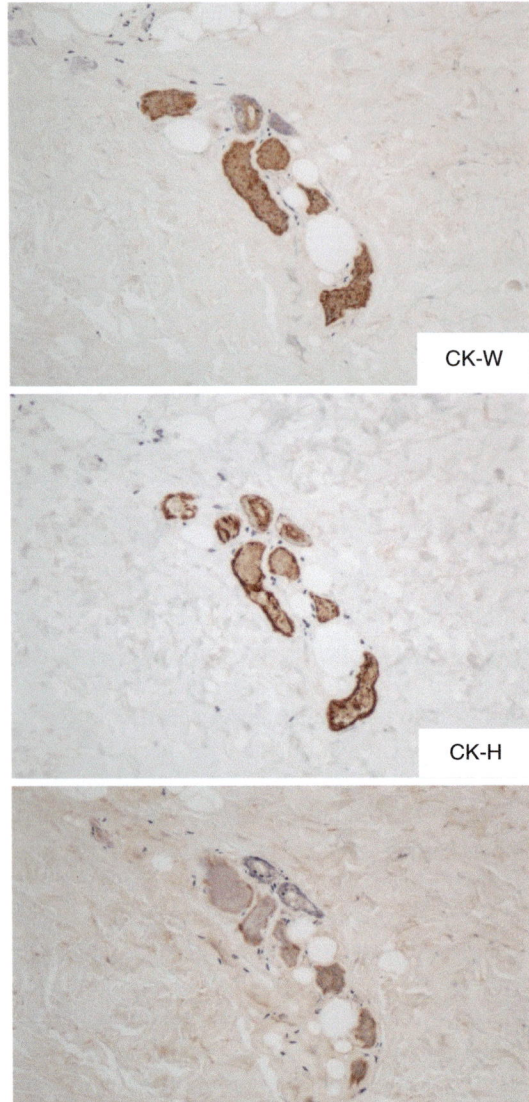

Fig. 23.4 The degenerated sweat glands showed good immunoreactivities for CK-W and CK-H just like the control, but decreased the typical immunoreactivity for CK-L

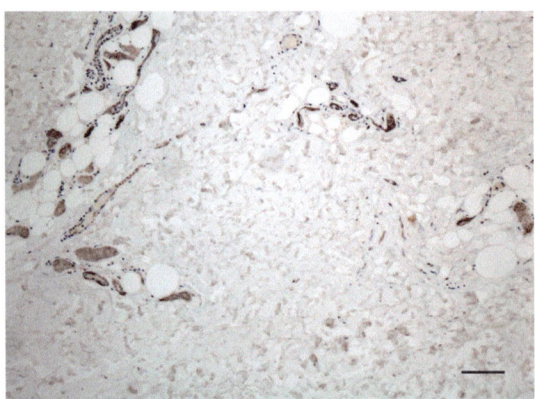

Fig. 23.5 The degenerated eccrine sweat glands showed weak CD45RO immunoreactivity (right knee). Length of bar indicates 50 μm

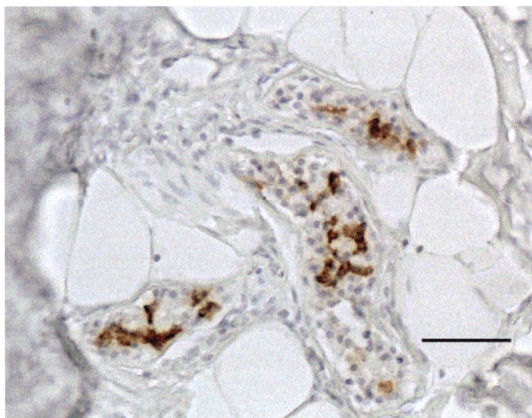

Fig. 23.6 The mild degenerated sweat glands showed partial M30 immunoreactivity (chest). Length of bar indicates 50 μm

23.3 Features of Coma Blister

Skin blisters with underlying sweat gland necrosis were first reported by Larrey in 1812 occurring in comatose patients after carbon monoxide intoxication [8]. Since then, most previously reported cases with characteristic bullous skin lesions and sweat gland necrosis were comatose secondary to an overdosage of drugs [3–5, 9], carbon monoxide poisoning [10], alcohol toxicity [11], or central nervous system disorders [12] such as hypoglycemia [13] or diabetic ketoacidosis [14]. Similar clinical and histopathologic features can also be observed in cases with nondrug-induced coma [6, 15] and, in such cases, can be interpreted as a drug side effect in the absence of coma [7]. Therefore, local pressure, hypoxia, and/or drug toxicity are contributing factors to the formation of coma blisters and sweat gland necrosis [10, 16–20]. However, the underlying pathogenesis remains unclear. Histochemical analysis revealed features similar to those reported in the literature [6, 7, 15, 18]. However, inflammatory infiltration, often reported to be observed around the vessels in drug-induced coma [18], was not observed in this case. In this study, immunohistochemical analysis revealed that sweat gland degeneration was CK-W positive. This result agrees with Setterfield's report [21]. CK-L is known to be immunopositive in secretory cells, such as eccrine gland [22–24]. Degenerated sweat gland was shown to decrease immunoreactivity for CK-L. In addition, CD45RO immunoreactivity might suggest a connection between sweat gland degeneration and inflammatory infiltration participation of monocytes, macrophages, and/or granulocytes [25]. CD3 and CD8 immunoreactivities were not observed in sweat gland regions, suggesting less relation to T-cell filtration [26, 27]. Degenerated epidermis and sweat gland degeneration observed in coma blisters were described as necrosis in almost all previous literature [4, 5, 7, 11], and it was the same even after the apoptosis was defined [28]. However, a coma blister was observed in a case of DNA fragmentation in one report [29]. During epithelial cell apoptosis, intermediate filaments are reorganized, and keratin 18 is cleaved by caspases to liberate M30, one of the most specific and earliest detected indications of apoptosis [30–32]. The TUNEL method detects single-stranded [33] and double-stranded breaks associated with apoptosis. Drug-induced DNA damage is not identified by the TUNEL assay unless it is coupled to the apoptotic response [34]. In addition, this technique can detect early-stage apoptosis in systems where chromatin condensation has begun and strand breaks are fewer, even before the nucleus undergoes major morphological changes [34, 35]. In this study, the apoptosis was detected by M30 but not by the TUNEL method. This result was not contradicted, because the nucleus had undergone severe morphological changes in the degenerated sweat gland, and the skin legions were obtained from drug intoxication cases. Therefore, the apoptosis might be involved in the sweat gland degenerations of coma blisters. In this study, no sweat gland degenerations were observed except the regions of coma blister. And sweat gland degeneration was not observed in other cases, which were suspected in the same PMI. So, the sweat gland degeneration was considered as specific for coma blister. Immunohistochemical staining for CD45RO, CK-L, and M30 might be useful in observing the sweat gland degeneration in coma blisters. There are not so many forensic autopsy cases of the coma blister. Before this study, we found only one case of coma blisters in a case of a female in her 20 s with barbiturate intoxication. Prospective studies would be useful to further elucidate the underlying pathogenesis.

23.4 Conclusion

We investigated the characteristic bullous skin lesions without local pressure after overdosage of drugs. Microscopically, sweat gland degeneration was observed. Immunohistochemical examination of CD45RO, CK-L, and M30 might be useful for the diagnosis of coma blisters. Further, apoptosis might be involved in coma blisters and sweat gland degenerations [36].Conflicts of InterestWe declare that the presenting authors have no conflicts of interest.

References

1. Di Maio DJ, VJM DM. Foresic pathology. Deaths due to fire. Florida: CRC Press LLC; 1993. p. 327–41.
2. Holzer FJ. Leichenbefunde nach Schlafmittelvergiftung. Dtsch Z Gesamte Gerichtl Med. 1940;34:307–21.

3. Beveridge GW, AAH L. Occurrence of bullous lesions in acute barbiturate intoxication. Br Med J. 1965;1(5438):835–7.
4. Varma AJ, Fisher BK, Sarin MK. Diazepam-induced coma with bullae and eccrine sweat gland necrosis. Arch Intern Med. 1977;137(9):1207–10.
5. Herschthal D, Robinson MJ. Blisters of the skin in coma induced by amitriptyline and clorazepate dipotassium. Report of a case with underlying sweat gland necrosis. Arch Dermatol. 1979;115(4):499.
6. Kato N, Ueno H, Mimura M. Histopathology of cutaneous changes in non-drug-induced coma. Am J Dermatopathol. 1996;18(4):344–50.
7. Ferreli C, Sulica VI, Aste N, Atzori L, Pinna M, Biggio P. Drug-induced sweat gland necrosis in a non-comatose patient : a case presentation. J Eur Acad Dermatol Venereol. 2003;17(4):443–5.
8. Larrey DJ. Memoires de Chirurgie Militaire et Campagnes, vol. 3. Paris: Smith and Buisson; 1812. p. 13.
9. Holten C. Cutaneous phenomena in acute barbiturate poisoning. Acta Derm Venereol Suppl (Stockh). 1952;32(29):162–8.
10. Mandy S, Ackerman AB. Characteristic traumatic skin lesions in drug-induced coma. JAMA. 1970;213(2):253–6.
11. You MY, Yun SK. Ihm W : bullae and sweat gland necrosis after an alcoholic deep slumber. Cutis. 2002;69(4):265–8.
12. Arndt KA, Mihm MC Jr, Parrish JA. Bullae : a cutaneous sign of a variety of neurologic diseases. J Invest Dermatol. 1973;60(5):312–20.
13. Raymond LW, Cohen AB. "Barbiturate blisters" in a case of severe hypoglycaemic coma. Lancet. 1972;2(7780):764.
14. Mehregan DR, Daoud M, Rogers RS 3rd. Coma blisters in a patient with diabetic ketoacidosis. J Am Acad Dermatol. 1992;27(2 Pt 1):269–70.
15. Kim KJ, Suh HS, Choi JH, Sung KJ, Moon KC, Koh JK. Two cases of coma-associated bulla with eccrine gland necrosis in patients without drug intoxication. Acta Derm Venereol. 2002;82(5):378–80.
16. Wenzel FG, Horn TD. Nonneoplastic disorders of the eccrine glands. J Am Acad Dermatol. 1998;38(1):1–17.
17. Adebahr G. Hautveranderungen bei schlafmittelvergiftung. Landarzt. 1963;30:130–8.
18. Sánchez Yus E, Requena L, Simón P. Histopathology of cutaneous changes in drug - induced coma. Am J Dermatopathol. 1993;15:208–16.
19. Achten G, Ledoux-Corbusier M, Thys JP. Carbon monoxide poisoning and cutaneous lesions. Ann Dermatol Syphiligr (Paris). 1971;98(4):421–8.
20. Sorensen BF. Skin symptoms in acute narcotic intoxication. Dan Med Bull. 1963;10:130–1.
21. Setterfield JF, Robinson R, MacDonald D, Calonje E. Coma-induced bullae and sweat gland necrosis following clobazam. Clin Exp Dermatol. 2000;25(3):215–8.
22. Bártek J, Vojtesek B, Stasková Z, Bártková J, Kerekés Z, Rejthar A, Kovarík J. A series of 14 new monoclonal antibodies to keratins : characterization and value in diagnostic histopathology. J Pathol. 1991;164(3):215–24.
23. Tsubura A, Okada H, Sasaki M, Dairkee SH, Morii S. Immunohistochemical demonstration of keratins 8 and 14 in benign tumours of the skin appendage. Virchows Arch A Pathol Anat Histopathol. 1991;418(6):503–7.
24. Antley CM, Carrington PR, Mrak RE, Smoller BR. Grover's disease (transient acantholytic dermatosis): relationship of acantholysis to acrosyringia. J Cutan Pathol. 1998;25(10):545–9.
25. Sewell WA, Cooley MA, Hegen M. CD45 workshop panel report. In: Kishimoto T, et al., editors. Leucocyte typing VI, white cell differentiation antigens. New York: Garland Publishing Inc; 1997. p. 499–502.
26. Chetty R, Gatter K. CD3 : structure, function, and role of immunostaining in clinical practice. J Pathol. 1994;173(4):303–7.
27. Mason DY, Cordell JL, Gaulard P, Tse AG, Brown MH. Immunohistological detection of human cytotoxic/suppressor T cells using antibodies to a CD8 peptide sequence. J Clin Pathol. 1992;45(12):1084–8.
28. Kerr JF, Wyllie AH, Currie AR. Apoptosis: a basic biological phenomenon with wide-ranging implications in tissue kinetics. Br J Cancer. 1972;26(4):239–57.
29. Sato K, Kon S. A case of coma blister with DNA fragmentation in the malpighian layer. JPN J Dermatol. 1996;106(6):905–11.
30. Caulín C, Salvesen GS, Oshima RG. Caspase cleavage of keratin 18 and reorganization of intermediate filaments during epithelial cell apoptosis. J Cell Biol. 1997;138(6):1379–94.
31. Leers MP, Kölgen W, Björklund V, Bergman T, Tribbick G, Persson B, Björklund P, Ramaekers FC, Björklund B, Nap M, Jörnvall H, Schutte B. Immunocytochemical detection and mapping of a cytokeratin 18 neo-epitope exposed during early apoptosis. J Pathol. 1999;187(5):567–72.
32. Bantel H, Ruck P, Gregor M, Schulze-Osthoff K. Detection of elevated caspase activation and early apoptosis in liver diseases. Eur J Cell Biol. 2001;80(3):230–9.
33. Stratos I, Madry H, Rotter R, Weimer A, Graff J, Cucchiarini M, Mittlmeier T, Vollmar B. Fibroblast growth factor-2-overexpressing myoblasts encapsulated in alginate spheres increase proliferation, reduce apoptosis, induce adipogenesis, and enhance regener-

ation following skeletal muscle injury in rats. Tissue Eng Part A. 2011;17(21–22):2867–77.
34. Wang L, Ohishi T, Shiraki A, Morita R, Akane H, Ikarashi Y, Mitsumori K, Shibutani M. Developmental exposure to manganese chloride induces sustained aberration of neurogenesis in the hippocampal dentate gyrus of mice. Toxicol Sci. 2012;127(2):508–21.
35. Hori T, Gardner LB, Chen F, Baine AM, Hata T, Uemoto S, Nguyen JH. Impact of hepatic arterial reconstruction on orthotopic liver transplantation in the rat. J Investig Surg. 2012;25(4):242–52.
36. Kashiwagi M, Ishigami A, Hara K, MatsusueA WB, Takayama M, Tokunaga I, Nishimura N, Kubo S. Immunohistochemical investigation of the coma blister and its pathogenesis. J Med Investig. 2013;60:256–61.

Open Access This chapter is licensed under the terms of the Creative Commons Attribution-NonCommercial-NoDerivatives 4.0 International License (http://creativecommons.org/licenses/by-nc-nd/4.0/), which permits any non-commercial use, sharing, distribution and reproduction in any medium or format, as long as you give appropriate credit to the original author(s) and the source, provide a link to the Creative Commons license and indicate if you modified the licensed material. You do not have permission under this license to share adapted material derived from this chapter or parts of it.

The images or other third party material in this chapter are included in the chapter's Creative Commons license, unless indicated otherwise in a credit line to the material. If material is not included in the chapter's Creative Commons license and your intended use is not permitted by statutory regulation or exceeds the permitted use, you will need to obtain permission directly from the copyright holder.

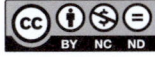

Part IV

Skin Necrosis of Medical Origin

Introduction of Skin Necrosis of Medical Origin

Véronique Del Marmol and Sylvie Meaume

It is essential to define the origin and the therapeutic attitude according to the origin, location, extent, and type of necrosis. Although the origin of necrosis is generally ischemic, because it is correlated with a lack of tissue oxygenation, the etiology remains very diverse: the cause guides the treatment, especially for the necrosis of medical origin. The goal of this chapter is to review some of the medical causes of necrosis.

Cutaneous and other vasculitis are specific inflammations of the blood vessel wall that can take place in any organ system of the body including the skin. Vasculitis has been traditionally divided according to the size of the vessel involved (small, medium, and large). Vasculitis is more of a reaction pattern rather than a specific disease entity. Therefore, the clinical presentation of vasculitis (most commonly palpable purpura on the lower extremities) dictates a thorough history, review of systems, and a meticulous physical examination. The diagnosis of vasculitis also relies on histopathology and immunofluorescence.

The clinical topography, age of the patient, or specific symptoms such as loss of vision or jaw claudication may be essential in the case of giant cell arteritis or Horton's disease.

Extremely painful ulcers located on the lower part of the legs in women over 60 with uncontrolled hypertension are important diagnostic features related to Martorell's ulcers or necrotic angiodermatitis. In this condition, local therapeutic management is essential.

Another ulceration site suggestive of vasculitis with a clinically quite specific aspect is livedoid vasculitis. This type of vasculitis is most often found in the lateral areas of the foot or ankle with white atrophy.

In the context of necrosis of inflammatory origin, pyoderma gangrenosum does not present any specific localization, but in a large proportion of cases, it occurs in a clinical context (hematological disease, IBD, etc.). Since anatomopathological diagnosis is usually noncontributory, the diagnosis of pyoderma gangrenosum is based on all the clinical elements and requires very specific local and systemic immunosuppressive therapy.

Cryoglobulin and calciphylaxis are in a medical context which may determine either the origin of a pathology (in the case of cryoglobulin) or a

V. Del Marmol (✉)
Hôpital Erasme—HUB, Université Libre de Bruxelles, Bruxelles, Belgium
e-mail: veronique.delmarmol@hubruxelles.be; v.marmol@drvdm.be

S. Meaume
Department of Geriatrics, Wound Healing and Dermatology, Hôpital Rothschild, Assistance Publique Hôpitaux de Paris (AP HP), Sorbonne University, Paris, France
e-mail: sylvie.meaume@aphp.fr

much more severe prognosis in the case of calciphylaxis. The identification of necrosis, particularly of calciphylaxis, may lead to very specific medical management (phosphor/calcium balance and parathyroidectomy), as well as surgical debridement.

In conclusion, this chapter does not cover all the medical causes of necrosis but highlights the essential role of identifying necrosis to manage a complex pathology.

Open Access This chapter is licensed under the terms of the Creative Commons Attribution-NonCommercial-NoDerivatives 4.0 International License (http://creativecommons.org/licenses/by-nc-nd/4.0/), which permits any non-commercial use, sharing, distribution and reproduction in any medium or format, as long as you give appropriate credit to the original author(s) and the source, provide a link to the Creative Commons license and indicate if you modified the licensed material. You do not have permission under this license to share adapted material derived from this chapter or parts of it.

The images or other third party material in this chapter are included in the chapter's Creative Commons license, unless indicated otherwise in a credit line to the material. If material is not included in the chapter's Creative Commons license and your intended use is not permitted by statutory regulation or exceeds the permitted use, you will need to obtain permission directly from the copyright holder.

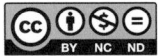

Rheumatoid and Systemic Collagenosis Vasculitis

25

Masaki Fujioka

25.1 Introduction

Rheumatoid arthritis (RA) and systemic collagenosis vasculitis affect all the systems of the body, causing neurological, cardiovascular, pulmonary, hematological, endocrine-metabolic, and dermatological disorders [1]. Among them, ulceration in RA is a difficult clinical problem and a common cause of morbidity. Patients with RA and systemic collagenosis vasculitis appear to be at increased risk of developing chronic ulcers, and it was believed that 66% of them had erosive skin disease [2].

Wound bed preparation has allowed uncomplicated wounds to heal quickly without surgery. However, ulcers induced by RA and other inflammatory connective tissue disorders are hard to heal because of the combination of rheumatoid vasculitis (RV), venous stasis disease, and chronic glucocorticoid use.

This chapter focuses on the prevalence of complex wounds among patients with RA and systemic collagenosis vasculitis and shows effective and successive treatments of these wounds.

25.2 How Do Ulcers Develop in Patients with RA and Systemic Collagenosis Diseases?

Many inflammatory diseases affect the skin and joints. RA and several connective tissue diseases are considered to be rheumatic conditions with secondary skin involvement, which commonly result in ulcers or necrosis [2]. The frequency of leg ulcer in patients with RA may be up to 10%. Ulcers in RA are usually multifactorial in etiology, including cutaneous vasculitis, peripheral arterial disease, venous insufficiency, skin fragility due to poor nutrition and corticosteroids, minor trauma, foot deformity, peripheral neuropathy, and peripheral edema [3].

25.2.1 Vasculitis

Ulcers are mainly attributed to vasculitis, which can be identified by histology and direct immunofluorescence [2]. Formerly, it was estimated that vasculitis had an ethological role in 18–37% of leg ulcers in patients with RA; however, the prevalence of RV is now decreasing because of improved control of RA in the era of biologic therapy [4]. The ulcers secondary to vasculitis are painful and deep and showed well-demarcated or punched-out appearance (Fig. 25.1). The medium-vessel vasculitis can also lead to digital ischemia and necrosis (Fig. 25.2a, b).

M. Fujioka (✉)
Department of Plastic and Reconstructive Surgery, National Hospital Organization Nagasaki Medical Center, Ohmura, Nagasaki, Japan

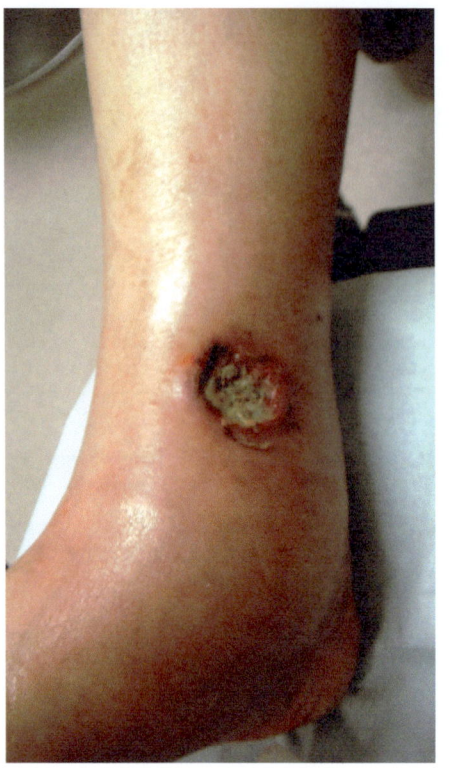

Fig. 25.1 Deep ulcer with necrotic eschar was found on the medial malleolus in patient with RA

Pathologic features of rheumatoid vasculitis include mononuclear cells or neutrophilic infiltration of the vessel wall of small and medium vessels.

25.2.2 Neutrophilic Dermatoses

Neutrophilic dermatoses are the conditions that have an inflammatory infiltrate consisting of mature polymorphonuclear leukocytes with no evidence of infection; these include Sweet's syndrome and pyoderma gangrenosum. The pathogenesis of neutrophilic dermatoses shows that these disorders represent a state of altered immunologic reactivity because they generally respond to systemic glucocorticoids and other immunomodulatory therapies [5].

25.2.3 Venous Stasis

Ulcerative lesions may also result from venous stasis. Ankle joint dysfunction caused by RA reduces ankle movement, which is responsible

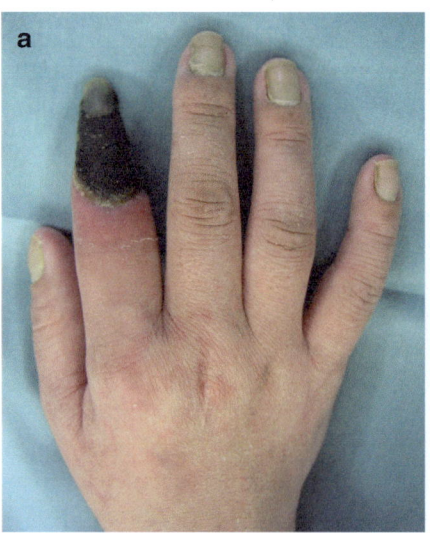
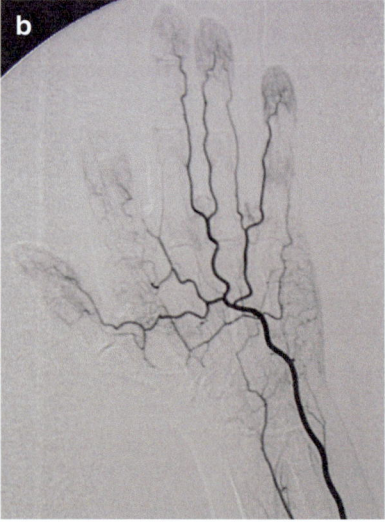

Fig. 25.2 (a) Right-finger necrosis due to ischemia was found in patient with RA. (b) Angiography showed the obstruction of digital artery due to vasculitis of medium peripheral vessel

25 Rheumatoid and Systemic Collagenosis Vasculitis

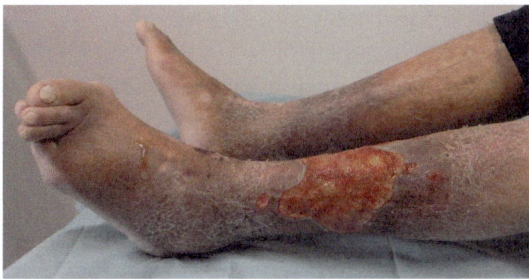

Fig. 25.3 Venous stasis ulcer located at the lower leg surrounded by varicosis. Toe and ankle deformities caused by RA were also found

for impairment of the normal venous pump function and leads to venous hypertension [6]. This unfavorable state leads to increased tissue fibrosis and decreases the diffusion of oxygen to the skin, producing skin fragility and resulting in venous ulceration [5] (Fig. 25.3). Leg ulcers in RA are associated with venous disease in as many as 45% [4].

25.2.4 Arterial Disease

Arterial insufficiency is one of the reasons to develop ulcer, especially in the toes or feet of patients with RA and several connective tissue diseases, such as systemic sclerosis and scleroderma. Pun et al. found arterial insufficiency in 36% of ulcerated legs in 26 patients with RA, and Baker et al. did found ischemia in 41% of those in 27 patients with RA [4].

25.2.5 Corticosteroid Therapy

Medications used to treat RA can cause skin changes [7]. It is a common clinical practice to use systemic glucocorticoids to suppress RV and other connective tissue diseases. Glucocorticoids are administrated to about half of the patients with RA leg ulcers. Effects of glucocorticoids inhibiting wound healing include stabilization of lysosomal membranes which inhibits the release of chemical mediators, suppression of fibroblasts and immunity,

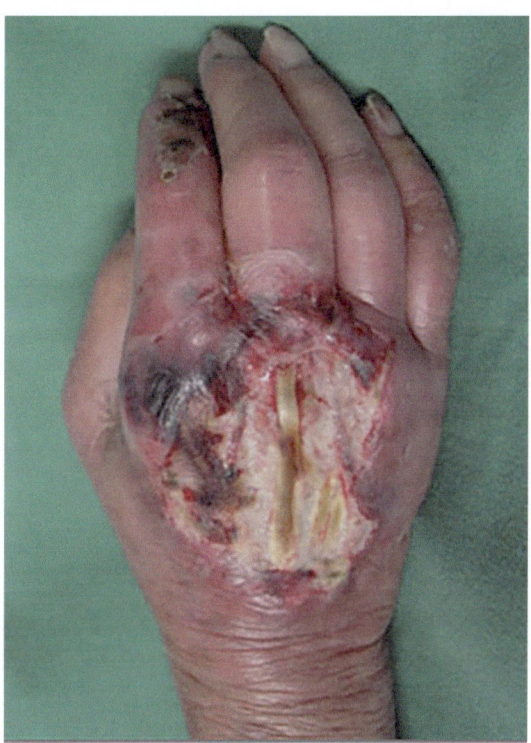

Fig. 25.4 Small wound of the hand of SLE patients has become more severe because infections occurred

and inhibition of collagen fiber synthesis causing skin atrophy [8]. Atrophic skin of RA patients treated with continuous glucocorticoids can be easily torn and develop lacerations, which are likely to be more severe because infections are common (Fig. 25.4).

25.3 Ulcers in Other Connective Tissue Diseases

25.3.1 Systemic Lupus Erythematosus (SLE)

Ten to twenty percent of patients with SLE develop cutaneous vasculitis and show purpuric papules, which sometimes cause ulceration [4]. The lower extremity is a common site, and leg ulcer caused by leukocytoclastic vasculitis or necrotizing arteritis was found in 5–6% of patients with SLE (Fig. 25.5).

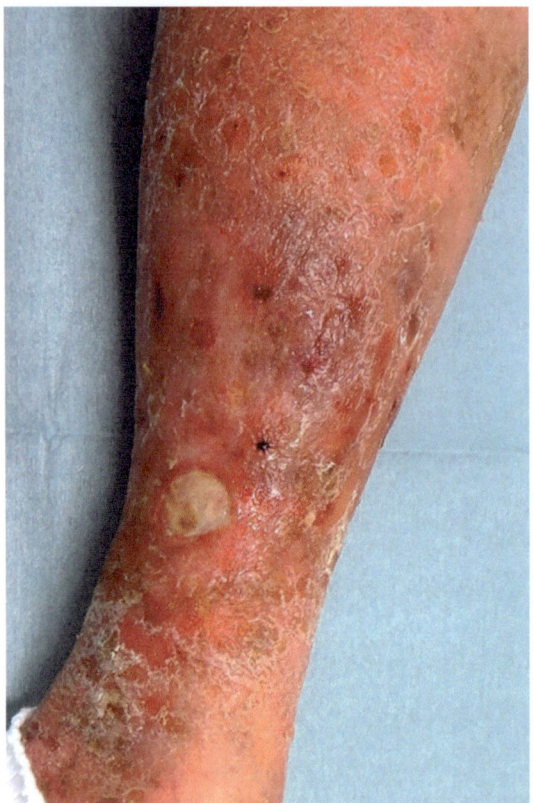

Fig. 25.5 A patient with SLE had a leg ulcer for 2 years

25.3.2 Systemic Sclerosis

Sclerodermatous change develops usually in the feet and legs, which sometimes results in ischemic necrosis and ulceration of the toes. Early skin changes in systemic forms may include edematous change, which lasts or is replaced by thickening and tightening of the skin. Painful ulcerations appear, especially on the area of the skin overlying bony prominence. These lesions are hard to heal [7].

25.3.3 Dermatomyositis

A small-vessel vasculitis and calcinosis in the subcutaneous tissue cause ulceration usually on the feet. Healing is slow, and ulcer often requires debridement of calcinotic material surgically [7].

25.3.4 Sjögren's Syndrome

Sjögren's syndrome is associated with RA, SLE, and some inflammatory connective tissue disease. Cutaneous magnifications include Raynaud's phenomenon (in 33% of patients), dryness of skin, purpura, and vasculitic ulcers of the legs [7].

25.3.5 Scleroderma

Although scleroderma (SSc) is a clinically heterogeneous disorder, the loss of cutaneous elasticity and accompanying tightness followed by thickening and hardening of the skin is an almost universal manifestation. Painful digital ulcers that occur on the fingertips as a result of local ischemia and vascular insufficiency are a frequent complication. While some SSc patients have skin lesions that remain largely confined to the extremities, others exhibit skin thickening that extends progressively from the extremities to the trunk [7].

25.3.6 Behcet's Syndrome

Behcet's syndrome develops arthritis, and pustule cutaneous ulcers are one of the classical triad features. The small ulcers are due to vasculitis of small vessels and tend to relapse [7].

25.4 Treatments of Ulcers in Patients with RA and Other Connective Tissue Diseases

25.4.1 Systemic Approach

Treatment for rheumatoid vasculitis is determined by the degree of organ system involvement, and systemic vasculitis requires aggressive therapy. In general, this treatment regimen consists of the combination of high doses of glucocorticoids and a cytotoxic agent [6, 9]. Mild rheumatoid vasculitis involving the skin can be treated with prednisone (30–200 mg/day orally or IV) and methotrexate (MTX) (10–25 mg/week orally or IM) or azathioprine (50–150 mg/day orally). More serious organ system involvement may require treatment with higher dose steroids and cyclophosphamide or biologic agents [9]. Since the latter half of 1990, synthetic and biological disease-modifying antirheumatic drugs (DMARDs) such as monoclonal antibodies against TNFα have been developed, and their indications have been expanded not only for rheumatism treatment but also for various collagen diseases. Furthermore, small-molecule target compounds such as JAK inhibitors and these biosimilar DMARDs are also being used in daily treatment. These are expected to have clinical effects when used in RA patients with inadequate MTX effects. However, these efficacy assessments have been evaluated for joint symptoms, and there is insufficient evidence for their efficacy on skin ulcers [10].

25.4.2 Topical Wound Treatment

Chronic ulcers have a complex, inflammatory nature and produce exudates, which interfere with the healing process. Essentially, effective strategies to heal the chronic ulcers in association with RA can be developed by the principle of wound bed preparation [4].

25.4.3 Occlusive Dressings

Occlusive dressings may be beneficial in some respects, such as preventing crust formation and encouraging migration of inflammatory cells into the wounds. An appropriate wound dressing changing can remove excess exudates while retaining a moist environment that can accelerate wound healing. Hydrogels, polyurethane foams, hydrocolloids, and hydrofibers are usually used to control the wound exudates.

25.4.4 Approach for the Wound Infection

Generally, open wounds have bacteria, and many wounds involve colonization. The amount of bacteria can be minimized through adequate cleaning of the wound, absorption of drainage, and debridement if necessary [4]. When considering bacteriological findings, it is important to differentiate between colonization and infection. When infectious signs are noted, cleansing, wet-to-dry dressing or irrigation, and surgical debridement if necessary should be performed.

25.4.5 Several Adjuvant Devices in the Management of Hard-to-Heal Wounds

In this section, several adjuvant devices are presented, including growth factor, bioengineered tissues, and a negative-pressure system, which are combined to improve the complex wounds. It was found that dermal wounds treated with collagen sponges seeded with fibroblasts or coated with bFGF show an increased degree of reepithelialization, indicating that this method facilitates early dermal and epidermal wound healing [11]. Combination treatment with bFGF and artificial dermis promotes proliferation and recruitment of fibroblasts, neovascularization, and synthesis of collagen fibers. Consequently, this method improves complex wounds and quickly prepares a favorable wound bed. We usually perform wound bed preparation with a combination of these therapies for the improvement of complex wounds (Fig. 25.6a–c).

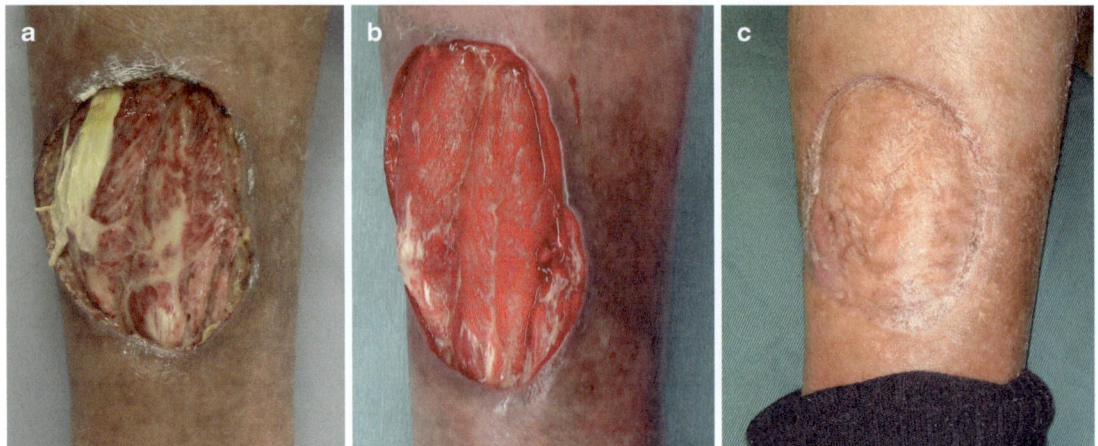

Fig. 25.6 (a) The photograph shows the unsatisfactory wound bed in patient with SLE at initial examination. The tendon was exposed, and infection had occurred. (b) The wound became clean, and a favorable wound bed had developed 2 weeks after the start of combination treatment with bFGF and artificial dermis. (c) The photograph shows the resurfaced wound 3 years after skin grafting, showing no relapse of ulcer

25.5 Surgical Wound Closure for Patients with RA

The resurfacing of wounds is one of the most important procedures because such wounds will cause further infection, exudates, odors, and bleeding, which decrease the patient's quality of life. When a wound is covered with suitable granulation and no contamination is observed, split-thickness autologous skin grafts should be performed as soon as possible (Fig. 25.7a, b). In cases of bone- or tendon-exposed wounds, some vascularized flaps are required to resurface the wounds because grafted skin will not take directly on the tendon or bone (Fig. 25.8a–c).

25 Rheumatoid and Systemic Collagenosis Vasculitis

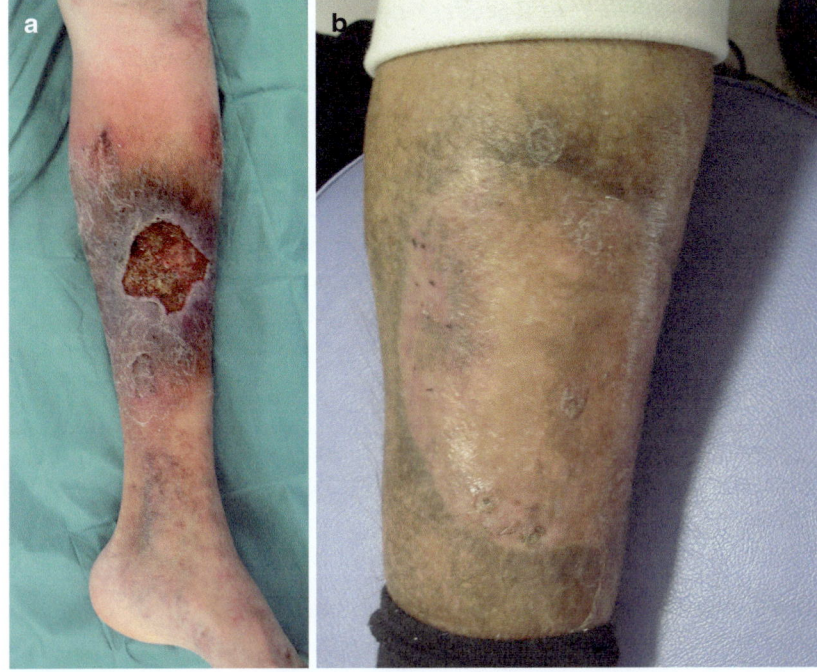

Fig. 25.7 (**a**) The photograph shows the unsatisfactory wound bed with infection in patient with pyoderma gangrenosum. (**b**) A photograph 6 months after skin grafting shows favorable wound resurfacing without relapse

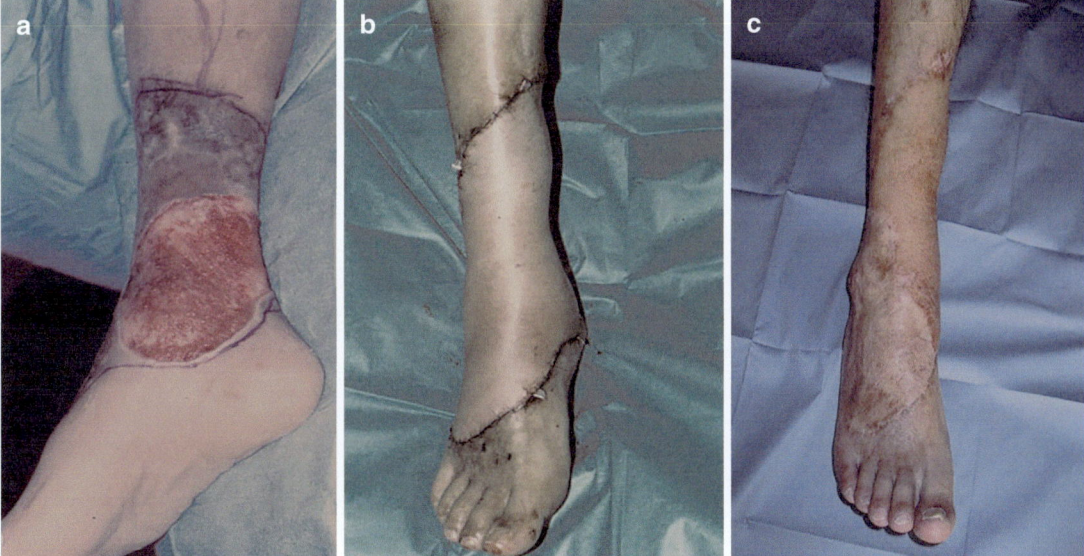

Fig. 25.8 (**a**) The photograph shows the venous stasis ulcer located at the lower leg in patient with RA. The patient underwent immediate debridement, and consequently tendons were exposed. (**b**) The photograph taken immediately after the surgery. The wound was resurfaced with a free groin flap. (**c**) A photograph 6 months after the surgery shows favorable wound resurfacing without relapse

25.6 Prevention of Recurrence

Once the ulcer has healed, the patients should be aware of the risk of recurrence. If venous insufficiency is present, compression bandaging should be considered. If there is peripheral arterial disease, cessation of smoking and lowering of the serum cholesterol are important. Besides, adequate nutrition and appropriate footwear will reduce the risk of recurrence of leg ulcers [2].

Acknowledgments None.

References

1. Scott DG, Bacon PA, Tribe CR. Systemic rheumatoid vasculitis: a clinical and laboratory study of 50 cases. Medicine (Baltimore). 1981;60:288.
2. McRorie ER. The assessment and management of leg ulcers in rheumatoid arthritis. J Wound Care. 2000;9(6):289–92.
3. McRorie ER, Jobanputra P, Ruckley CV, Nuki G. Leg ulceration in rheumatoid arthritis. Br J Rheumatol. 1994;33(11):1078–84.
4. Pun YL, Barraclough DR, Muirden KD. Leg ulcers in rheumatoid arthritis. Med J Aust. 1990;153(10):585–7.
5. Foster CS, Forstot SL, Wilson LA. Mortality rate in rheumatoid arthritis patients developing necrotizing scleritis or peripheral ulcerative keratitis. Effects of systemic immunosuppression. Ophthalmology. 1984;91:1253.
6. Helliwell PS, Cheesbrough MJ. Arthropathica ulcerosa: a study of reduced ankle movement in association with chronic leg ulceration. J Rheumatol. 1994;21(8):1512–4.
7. Kaminski MJ. Skin disorders associated with rheumatic disease. Clin Podiatr Med Surg. 1996;13(1):139–53.
8. Kirsner AB, Diller JG, Sheon RP. Systemic lupus erythematosus with cutaneous ulceration. Correlation of immunologic factors with therapy and clinical activity. JAMA. 1971;217(6):821–3.
9. Scott DG, Bacon PA. Intravenous cyclophosphamide plus methylprednisolone in treatment of systemic rheumatoid vasculitis. Am J Med. 1984;76:377.
10. Smolen JS, Landewé RBM, Bijlsma JWJ, Burmester GR, Dougados M, Kerschbaumer A, McInnes IB, Sepriano A, van Vollenhoven RF, de Wit M, Aletaha D, Aringer M, Askling J, Balsa A, Boers M, den Broeder AA, Buch MH, Buttgereit F, Caporali R, Cardiel MH, De Cock D, Codreanu C, Cutolo M, Edwards CJ, van Eijk-Hustings Y, Emery P, Finckh A, Gossec L, Gottenberg JE, Hetland ML, Huizinga TWJ, Koloumas M, Li Z, Mariette X, Müller-Ladner U, Mysler EF, da Silva JAP, Poór G, Pope JE, Rubbert-Roth A, Ruyssen-Witrand A, Saag KG, Strangfeld A, Takeuchi T, Voshaar M, Westhovens R, van der Heijde D. EULAR recommendations for the management of rheumatoid arthritis with synthetic and biological disease-modifying antirheumatic drugs: 2019 update. Ann Rheum Dis. 2020;79(6):685–99. https://doi.org/10.1136/annrheumdis-2019-216655.
11. Fujioka M. Combination treatment with basic fibroblast growth factor and artificial dermis improves complex wounds caused by collagen diseases with steroid use. Dermatologic Surg. 2009;35(9):1422–5.

Open Access This chapter is licensed under the terms of the Creative Commons Attribution-NonCommercial-NoDerivatives 4.0 International License (http://creativecommons.org/licenses/by-nc-nd/4.0/), which permits any non-commercial use, sharing, distribution and reproduction in any medium or format, as long as you give appropriate credit to the original author(s) and the source, provide a link to the Creative Commons license and indicate if you modified the licensed material. You do not have permission under this license to share adapted material derived from this chapter or parts of it.

The images or other third party material in this chapter are included in the chapter's Creative Commons license, unless indicated otherwise in a credit line to the material. If material is not included in the chapter's Creative Commons license and your intended use is not permitted by statutory regulation or exceeds the permitted use, you will need to obtain permission directly from the copyright holder.

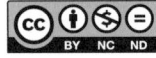

Giant Cell Arteritis

Pauline Lecerf and Sophie Golstein

26.1 Introduction/Physiopathology

Giant cell arteritis (GCA) or Horton's disease is a systemic granulomatous vasculitis. According to the Chapel Hill classification, it affects large vessels, namely, the aorta and its main branches. This is an antigen-driven disease with local T-cell and macrophage activation in the vessel wall and with an important role of proinflammatory cytokines. GCA is also called "temporal arteritis" because it involves often the superficial temporal arteries. The condition affects especially the extracranial branches of the carotid artery, but GCA has been recognized to also affect limb arteries and the aorta [1, 2].

GCA typically affects adults older than 50 years of age with a peak incidence at the eighth decade of life [1]. Most patients will have laboratory evidence of acute inflammation (elevation of erythrocyte sedimentation rate and C-reactive protein).

26.2 Diagnosis

26.2.1 Medical Context

- GCA is the most common vasculitis in the elderly.
- Incidence increases with aging of the population.
- GCA affects mainly white individuals over 50 years of age, with a peak incidence in the 70–79-year-old age group (Figs. 26.1, 26.2 and 26.3).
- Women are mostly affected (sex ratio 3:1) [3, 4].

P. Lecerf (✉) · S. Golstein
Department of Dermatology, University Hospital Brugmann and Saint-Pierre, Université Libre de Bruxelles, Brussels, Belgium

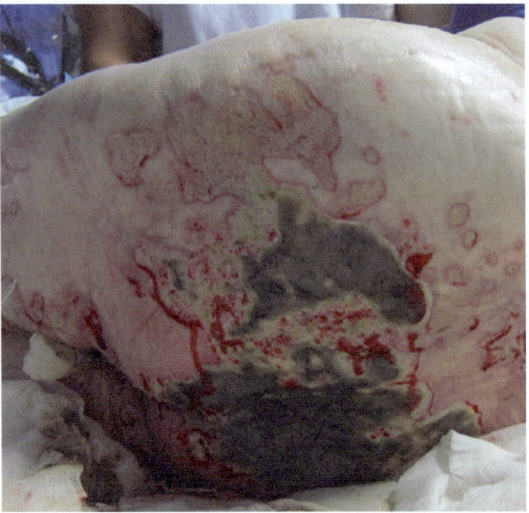

Fig. 26.1 Vast ulceration and necrosis of the buttock due to giant cell arteritis in a 76-year-old female, with associated signs: jaw claudication, temporal artery pulseless, weight loss, visual manifestations, and amputations of the left forefoot weeks before. Improvement of the ulcerations of the seat after initiation of glucocorticoid therapy

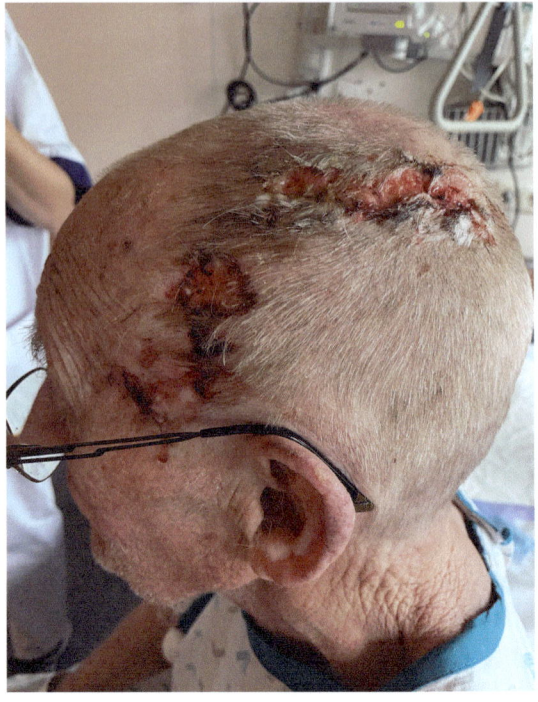

Fig. 26.3 Same patient with giant cell arteritis, left side of the scalp

26.2.2 Semiology

Symptoms are correlated with the localization of the vasculitic involvement of the arteries.

Classical form of GCA, with involvement of the extracranial branches of the carotid artery	
Early	Headache, jaw claudication, purpuric lesions and tender nodules in temporal region, temporal artery pain, temporal artery pulseless, weight loss, fever, visual manifestations, polymyalgia rheumatica (in 30–50% of the cases) [5]
Late	Ulceration and/or gangrene of frontotemporal scalp or tongue
Involvement of limb arteries [6–8]	
Early	Swelling, pain, claudication
Late	Ulceration, necrosis (Fig. 26.1), gangrene of the distal parts of the limbs
Major complications	
Ischemic optic neuritis/blindness, stroke (mainly vertebrobasilar territory), aortic complications (aneurysms, dissection) [6]	

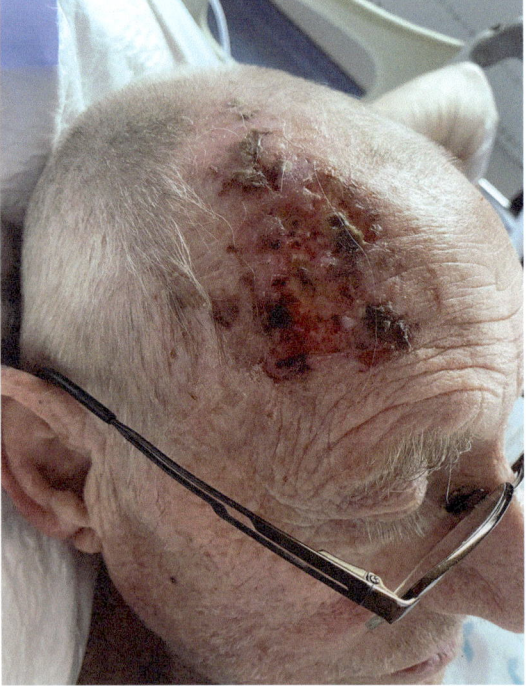

Fig. 26.2 Patient with giant cell arteritis, right side of the scalp

26.2.3 Criteria (Table 26.1)

Table 26.1 ACR classification criteria for giant cell arteritis

Age ≥ 50 years at disease onset
New onset of localized headache
Temporal artery tenderness or decreased temporal artery pulse
ESR ≥50 mm/h
Biopsy: Necrotizing arteritis; mononuclear cell infiltrates, or a granulomatous process with multinucleated giant cells
Presence of ≥ 3/5: Sensitivity of 93% and specificity of 91% for distinguishing GCA from other primary vasculitis syndromes

American College of Rheumatology (ACR), 1990

26.2.4 Routine Evaluation

(a) *Biology*
   - Elevated C-reactive protein (CRP), erythrocyte sedimentation rate (ESR).
   - Thrombocytosis.
   - Anemia.
   - Abnormal liver function tests, particularly raised alkaline phosphatase.
   - Raised $\alpha 1$ and $\alpha 2$ globulins on serum electrophoresis.
   - No autoimmune disorders [2].

(b) *Histology*

- *Temporal artery biopsy (TAB)*
   - Recommended in all suspected cases.
   - Should be performed soon after the onset of treatment.
   - The sensitivity and specificity of TAB have been reported to be around 75% and 90%, respectively.
   - Histological features: inflammation of the vessel wall by infiltration of T cells and macrophages, presence of giant cells, granulomatous lesions, intimal hyperplasia and destruction of elastic fibers, and arterial lumen partially or completely occluded.
   - Histologic signs of inflammation may be missed in TABs performed in arteritis-free segments because GCA affects vessels focally and segmentally.

- *Skin biopsies*

   - Histological features from limb ulcer edge, nodule, and purpuric patch show nonspecific ulceration if the biopsy is superficial and do not include deep medium or large vessels. The extracranial large vessel had similar histopathologic features to those seen in the temporal arteries and showed a lymphocytic panarteritis with a variable number of giant cells. Direct immunofluorescence is negative [9].

(c) *Imaging*

The prevalence of limb arteries' involvement in GCA is clinically underestimated. Imaging studies are useful in identifying the involvement of the latter [2]:

- Ultrasonography.
- Positron-emission tomography (PET).
- Computed tomography angiography (CTA).
- Magnetic resonance angiography (MRA).

It is also recommended to perform a screening for aortic aneurysms and for extra-aortic large-vessel involvement.

26.3 Treatment

High-dose glucocorticosteroid therapy is the first-line therapy as soon as the diagnosis has been established or if there is a strong clinical suspicion of GCA to prevent visual loss [10, 11].

1. Recommended starting dosages of glucocorticosteroids are:

Uncomplicated GCA (no jaw claudication or visual disturbance)	40–60 mg prednisolone daily
Evolving visual loss or amaurosis fugax (complicated GCA)	500 mg to 1 g of i.v. methylprednisolone for 3 days before oral glucocorticosteroids
Established visual loss	60 mg prednisolone daily to protect the contralateral eye

Do not forget bone protection and proton pump inhibitors for gastrointestinal protection.
2. Symptoms of GCA should respond rapidly to high-dose glucocorticosteroid treatment, followed by resolution of the inflammatory response. Failure to do so should raise the question of an alternative diagnosis.
3. Glucocorticosteroid reduction:
   (a) Should be considered only in the absence of clinical symptoms, signs, and laboratory abnormalities suggestive of active disease.
   (b) Introduction of MTX or alternative immunosuppressants should be considered as adjuvant therapy for recurrent relapse.

26.4 Tocilizumab

Tocilizumab is an anti-interleukin-6 receptor monoclonal antibody. Recent American recommendations propose to use a combination of prednisone and tocilizumab as first-line therapy in new-onset GCA.

It can be used in newly diagnosed GCA patients already presenting corticosteroid-related adverse events (AE) or at high risk for such AE [10–13].

26.5 Methotrexate

Methotrexate is initially associated with systemic corticosteroids in patients presenting or at high risk of corticosteroid-related AE (as an alternative to tocilizumab) and allows the gradual tapering of the systemic corticosteroid treatment. Although stronger clinical evidence supports the use of tocilizumab compared to methotrexate, the latter can be considered if the patient is at risk of recurrent infections or for cost reasons [14].

References

1. Kesten F, Aschwanden M, Gubser P, Glatz K, Daikeler T, Hess C. Giant cell arteritis—a changing entity. Swiss Med Wkly. 2011;28:141.
2. Borchers AT, Gershwin ME. Giant cell arteritis: a review of classification, pathophysiology, geo-epidemiology and treatment. Autoimmun Rev. 2012;11(6–7):A544.
3. Gonzalez-Gay MA, Vazquez-Rodriguez TR, Lopez-Diaz MJ, Miranda-Filloy JA, Gonzalez-Juanatey C, Martin J, et al. Epidemiology of giant cell arteritis and polymyalgia rheumatica. Arthritis Rheum. 2009;61(10):1454–61.
4. Salvarani C, Cantini F, Boiardi L, Hunder GG. Polymyalgia rheumatica and giant-cell arteritis [review]. N Engl J Med. 2002;347:261–71.
5. Weyand CM, Goronzy JJ. Giant-cell arteritis and polymyalgia rheumatica. Ann Intern Med. 2003;139:505–15.
6. Assie C, Janvresse A, Plissonier D, Levesque H, Marie I. Long-term follow-up of upper and lower extremity vasculitis related to giant cell arteritis: a series of 36 patients. Medicine (Baltimore). 2011;90:40–51.
7. Kermani TA, Matteson EL, Hunter GC, Warrington KJ. Symptomatic lower extremity vasculitis in giant cell arteritis: a case series. J Rheumatol. 2009;36:2277–83.
8. Kermani TA, Warrington KJ. Lower extremity vasculitis in polymyalgia rheumatica and giant cell arteritis. Curr Opin Rheumatol. 2011;23(1):38–42. https://doi.org/10.1097/BOR.0b013e3283410072.
9. Klein RG, Campbell RJ, Hunder GG, Carney JA. Skip lesions in temporal arteritis. Mayo Clin Proc. 1976;51:504–10.
10. Maz M, Chung SA, Abril A, et al. 2021 American College of Rheumatology/Vasculitis Foundation guideline for the management of giant cell arteritis and Takayasu arteritis. Arthritis Rheumatol. 2021;73:1349–65.
11. Gonzalez-Gay M. The diagnosis and management of patients with giant cell arteritis. J Rheumatol. 2005;32:1186–8.
12. Greigert H, Ramon E, Tarris G, Martin L, Bonnotte B. Temporal artery vascular diseases. J Clin Med. 2022;11:275.
13. Unizony SH, Dasgupta B, Fisheleva E, Rowell L, Schett G, Spiera R, Zwerina J, Harari O, Stone JH. Design of the tocilizumab in giant cell arteritis trial. Int J Rheumatol. 2013;2013:912562. https://doi.org/10.1155/2013/912562.
14. Golstein S, Delguste T, Lesage V, Vandergheynst F, Debusscher C. Rapid-onset bilateral scalp ulceration with visual loss. JAAD Case Rep. 2022;28:97–9.

Open Access This chapter is licensed under the terms of the Creative Commons Attribution-NonCommercial-NoDerivatives 4.0 International License (http://creativecommons.org/licenses/by-nc-nd/4.0/), which permits any non-commercial use, sharing, distribution and reproduction in any medium or format, as long as you give appropriate credit to the original author(s) and the source, provide a link to the Creative Commons license and indicate if you modified the licensed material. You do not have permission under this license to share adapted material derived from this chapter or parts of it.

The images or other third party material in this chapter are included in the chapter's Creative Commons license, unless indicated otherwise in a credit line to the material. If material is not included in the chapter's Creative Commons license and your intended use is not permitted by statutory regulation or exceeds the permitted use, you will need to obtain permission directly from the copyright holder.

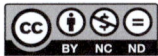

Hidradenitis Suppurativa

27

Kian Zarchi, Véronique Del Marmol, and Gregor B. E. Jemec

27.1 Introduction

Hidradenitis suppurativa is a chronic inflammatory skin disease affecting approximately 1% of the adult population [1, 2]. It presents clinically as painful inflammatory nodules, draining sinuses, and abscesses, causing considerable pain, suppuration, and malodor. It has a substantial negative impact on the quality of life, more so than many other skin diseases, such as eczema and psoriasis [3]. The disease is associated with physical and psychological morbidity, such as depression, metabolic syndrome, and an increased risk of skin cancer.

The typical age of onset is the early 20 s, but the disease may present in younger ages, and occasionally affection of prepubertal children is seen. Symptoms persist for years to decades, characterized by periods of flares and remission. The disease activity often diminishes with age, as the prevalence decreases among adults aged 50 years and older. The sex ratio is 3:1, female to male. Family history is reported by one in three patients, and an autosomal dominant pattern of inheritance has been described [1, 2]. Other risk factors include obesity and smoking, both being associated with severe disease.

27.2 Diagnosis

Patients with hidradenitis suppurativa are usually diagnosed several years after the onset of symptoms, mostly due to failure on the part of healthcare professionals to recognize the disease. The diagnosis is primarily clinical, based on the presence of recurring noninflammatory and inflammatory nodules, abscesses, and sinus tracts. The inflammatory nodules and abscesses are erythematous, tender, and not uncommonly painful. They may persist for weeks to months without any considerable change, or they may rupture, yielding purulent discharge. In moderate and severe disease, drainage also occurs through sinus tracts, causing malodorous suppuration. The lesions are distributed characteristically with predilection sites being the axillary, inguinofemoral, and anogenital regions. Extensions beyond these areas are occasionally seen.

The most commonly used classification system for hidradenitis suppurativa is that of Hurley (stages I–III), stage I representing solitary or multiple nodules and abscesses, stage II recurrent abscesses with sinus tract formation and scarring (Fig. 27.1), and stage III diffuse involvement of the area with mul-

---

GB Jemec and V Del Marmol are part of ERN skin network.

K. Zarchi (✉) · G. B. E. Jemec
Department of Dermatology, Roskilde Hospital, Faculty of Health and Medical Sciences, University of Copenhagen, Roskilde, Denmark

V. Del Marmol
Department of dermatology, Hopital Erasme HUB, Univesité Libre de Bruxelles, Bruxelles, Belgium
e-mail: Veronique.delmarmol@hubruxelles.be

Secondary lesions include cutaneous ulcerations, pyogenic granulomas, and hypertrophic scars, with the latter appearing as indurated plaques or linearly ropelike scars. In contrast to closed comedones, which never occur in HS-affected areas, multiple, big, open comedones (the so-called tombstone comedones) may be seen in previously active areas.

Biopsies are rarely needed as the diagnosis is based on the clinical presentation; nonetheless, in some cases, differentiation from other skin diseases, such as pyoderma gangrenosum and cutaneous Crohn's disease, might be difficult and require histopathological investigations. The characteristic histological findings include follicular hyperplasia and hyperkeratosis, local infiltration of inflammatory cells, formation of sinus tracts, and presence of necrosis. Microbiological examinations most frequently fail to identify pathogens [2].

27.3 Pathophysiology

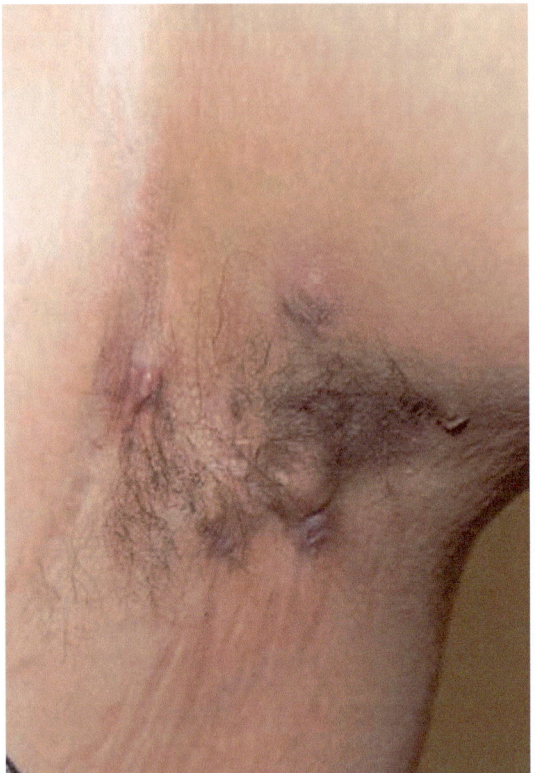

Fig. 27.1 Hurley stage II characterized by recurrent nodules and abscesses, formation of sinus tracts, and scarring. At this stage, zone with normal skin remains

The folliculo-pilosebaceous unit is the primary focus of the pathologic processes involved in hidradenitis suppurativa. The etiology of HS is multifactorial, encompassing genetic and environmental factors, lifestyle, hormonal status, and microbiota. These factors lead to immune activation around the terminal hair follicles and hyperkeratosis (thickening of the horny layer) in the infundibulum. Different theories have been proposed to explain the pathogenesis. These include the suggestion of an immune response dysfunction, as it has been proposed that the disease is a result of an inappropriate immunologic response to the normal skin flora, similar to the pathogenic processes involved in Crohn's disease. Indeed, elevated levels of proinflammatory cytokines, including tumor necrosis factor-α and interleukin-1β, and involvement of the interleukin-12–interleukin-23 pathway have been shown [2, 5].

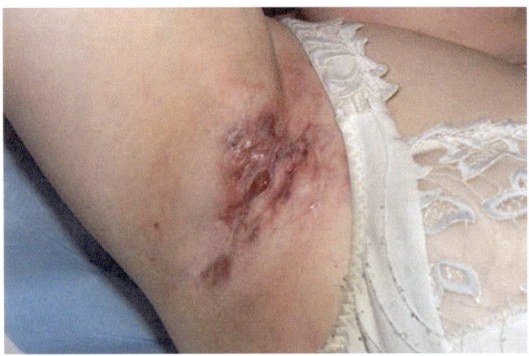

Fig. 27.2 Hurley stage III characterized by diffuse involvement of the area with multiple interconnected sinus tracts

tiple interconnected sinus tracts (Fig. 27.2) [4]. The majority of patients suffer from mild disease corresponding to stages I and II, while a smaller proportion progresses to severe disease which usually predominates in hospital populations.

Further, the lack of expression of human beta-defensin-2, an important antimicrobial peptide of the innate immune system against Gram-negative bacteria, in HS lesions supports this theory.

However, the histopathological findings in early disease and investigations of basal membrane zone in the folliculo-pilosebaceous unit point towards a structural defect in the sebofollicular junction as the possible main cause [6]. It is hypothesized that mechanical trauma makes the structurally defective folliculo-pilosebaceous unit release keratin and other mediators, thereby triggering inflammation and inducing tissue destruction and necrosis.

The possibility of HS being a defect in wound healing has also been discussed. It has been hypothesized that whereas breaches of the follicular epithelium are common following infections or physical trauma, the perpetuation of the subsequent inflammatory process which could lead to HS is not. It may, therefore, be speculated that a disturbed wound-healing process following the inflammatory stage occurs as a major factor in HS. This theory is supported by the detection of highly elevated levels of matrix metalloproteinase-2 in keratinocytes, fibroblasts, sweat glands, and hair follicles in lesional HS skin, indicating dysregulated tissue repair and reconstruction following unspecific tissue damage [7].

27.4 Treatment

Treatment of hidradenitis suppurativa is often a challenge [8]. By the time the diagnosis is made, most patients have been treated with short-term antibiotic regimens for several years without experiencing any effect, as the lesions are commonly misinterpreted as furunculosis or common abscesses. Establishing a strong alliance with the patient, attempting to restore the patient's faith in the doctor-patient relationship, and explaining the fluctuating nature of the disease are highly beneficial in minimizing the risk of low patient compliance. This is especially important in the case of resistant disease, where several therapeutic approaches might be carried out until the one or the combination inducing sufficient improvement is found.

Mild disease is often managed with topical therapy, such as topical clindamycin, or occasional intralesional glucocorticoid injections. However, in case of moderate to severe disease, topical agents are inadequate and systemic therapy is usually indicated. Systemic treatment options include oral antibiotics with immunomodulatory properties such as tetracycline, doxycycline, clindamycin, and rifampicin; antiandrogenic therapies; and systemic immunosuppressive therapy, including tumor necrosis factor-α inhibitors [1, 2]. Adalimumab was the first FDA- and EMA-licensed biologic agent for the management of moderate to severe HS. Immunomodulation targeting IL-1, IL-12/Th1, and IL-23/Th17 pathways is rapidly becoming the cornerstone of therapy for moderate to severe HS.

In elements refractory to medical treatment and in the presence of scarred lesions, surgery, nonetheless, is a mainstay of therapy. Surgical approaches include exteriorization ("deroofing" of sinus tract, abscesses, and cysts [Fig. 27.3]) and surgical excision of lesional skin, with radical excisions being associated with lower recurrence rates. Alternatively, destruction of lesional hair-bearing skin is achieved using ablative CO_2 laser [9]. The surgical and ablative laser approaches are based on the removal/destruction of the cutaneous structures involved in the disease, thereby causing open wounds requiring closure or management.

Primary suture, skin graft, or flap reconstruction can be used to close the wounds depending on the extent of procedure, or closure may be achieved by secondary intention. Generally, sec-

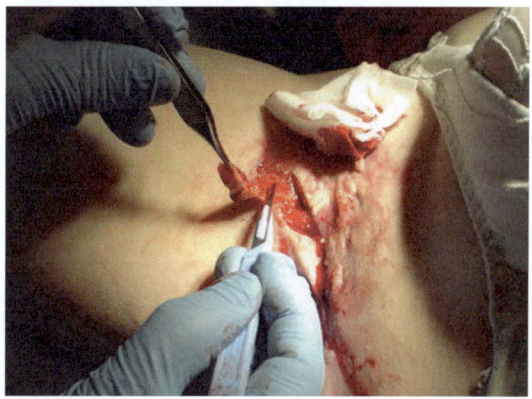

Fig. 27.3 "Deroofing" of a sinus tract

ondary intention healing is recommended for all but the smallest excisions. A comparison of skin grafting versus closure by secondary intention using foam dressing in patients undergoing bilateral excision revealed that skin grafting led to more rapid healing; however, closure by secondary intention provided good cosmetic results and avoided the need for immobilization and a painful donor side and was preferred by the patients [10]. Long-term evaluation of healing by secondary intention suggests acceptable to excellent outcome qualities.

Secondary healing requires suitable bandaging for periods of up to 12 weeks. Since the disease affects concave surfaces of the body, it presents a practical challenge. Appropriate nonadherent dressings, such as foams, silicone-coated dressings, alginates, and hydrocolloids, are generally better suited to convex surfaces. Bandage type may be adjusted during the healing process as per normal practice; for example, the initial combination of a saline gel and a silicone dressing may be gradually replaced by silicone dressing and ultimately a simple bandage to protect the final epithelialization of the wound. Individual adjustments may need to be performed, and once the wound is fully covered by granulation tissue, some patients prefer to avoid bandages all together. This non-recommended patient behavior most likely reflects the patients' experience with chronic suppurating preoperative lesions.

Vacuum-assisted closure (VAC) may be used to promote angiogenesis of the underlying subcutaneous tissue, reduce bacterial counts, and stabilize skin grafts. VAC has been successfully used in the treatment of large postoperative wounds.

27.5 Adjuvant Therapy

Although the primary aim of therapy remains the elimination or a substantial reduction in the inflammatory activities and the excision of severely involved lesional skin, providing adjuvant therapy throughout the disease course is necessary to improve the patients' quality of life. The disease presents many practical problems to the patients such as pain, tenderness, visible scars, suppuration, and malodor; hence, therapeutic decisions should address all those issues. Effective bandaging represents one of the challenges. Bandages should provide a secure and comfortable barrier against malodorous leakage and be absorbent to prevent maceration of the skin, easy to use, and inexpensive [11, 12]. Currently, no bandage meets all these requirements, and the available solutions are, therefore, combinations of products that are both expensive and difficult to apply to inverse area. As a consequence, patients are often forced to turn towards alternative and inexpensive solutions such as sanitary pads, which are not designed for this purpose (Fig. 27.4). The morbidity due to HS is such that this issue of adjuvant therapy warrants more attention by healthcare providers than it currently receives. It is strongly recommended to address the practical problems of this hitherto neglected group of patients by providing appropriate attention to improved adjuvant therapy.

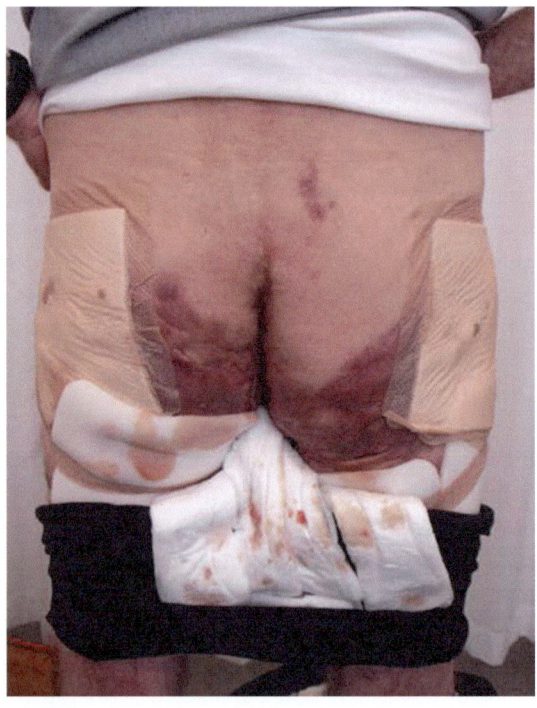

Fig. 27.4 Many HS patients are forced to use sanitary pads due to the lack of inexpensive appropriate dressings

27.6 Conclusion

Although HS is an inflammatory skin disease, wound care is important in the treatment. Adjuvant therapy is an important aspect of this highly disturbing disease, because it provides both safe symptom management and patient empowerment. Most patients are left to their own initiatives due to lack of appropriate dressing materials, and when patients present in wound care clinics for treatment, they constitute a challenge for many.

References

1. Jemec GB. Clinical practice. Hidradenitis suppurativa. N Engl J Med. 2012;366(2):158–64.
2. Sabat R, Jemec GB, Matusiak L, Kimbal AB, Prens E, Wolk K. Hidradenitis Suppurativa. Nat Rev. 2020;6:18.
3. Von der Werth JM, Jemec GB. Morbidity in patients with hidradenitis suppurativa. Br J Dermatol. 2001;144:809–13.
4. Hurley H. Dermatologic surgery, principles and practice. In: Roenigk RK, Roenigk HH, editors. Dermatologic surgery, principles and practice. New York: Marcel Dekker; 1989. p. 729–39.
5. van der Zee HH, de Ruiter L, van den Broecke DG, Dik WA, Laman JD, Prens EP. Elevated levels of tumour necrosis factor (TNF)-α, interleukin (IL)-1β and IL-10 in hidradenitis suppurativa skin: a rationale for targeting TNF-α and IL-1β. Br J Dermatol. 2011;164(6):1292–8.
6. Danby FW, Jemec GB, Marsch WC, von Laffert M. Preliminary findings suggest hidradenitis suppurativa may be due to defective follicular support. Br J Dermatol. 2013;168(5):1034–9.
7. Mozeika E, Pilmane M, Nürnberg BM, Jemec GB. Tumour necrosis factor-alpha and matrix metalloproteinase-2 are expressed strongly in hidradenitis suppurativa. Acta Derm Venereol. 2013;93(3):301–4.
8. Zarchi K, Dufour DN, Jemec GB. Successful treatment of severe hidradenitis suppurativa with anakinra. JAMA Dermatol. 2013;149(10):1192–4.
9. Hazen PG, Hazen BP. Hidradenitis suppurativa: successful treatment using carbon dioxide laser excision and marsupialization. Dermatologic Surg. 2010;36(2):208–13.
10. Morgan WP, Harding KG, Hughes LE. A comparison of skin grafting and healing by granulation, following axillary excision for hidradenitis suppurativa. Ann R Coll Surg Engl. 1983;65(4):235–6.
11. Chopra D, Anand N, Brito S, Coutts P, George R, Kimball A, Kirsner RS, Alavi A and Lev-Tov Hadaar. Wound Care for patients with hidradenitis suppurativa : recommendations of an international panel of experts, J Am Acad Dermatol. 2023;89(6):1289-1292.
12. Ragozo NM, Masson R, Gillenwater TJ, Hsiao JL SVY. Emerging treatment and the clinical trial landscape for hidradenitis suppurativa—Part II: procedural and wound care therapies. Dermatol Ther (Heidelb). 2023;13:1699–720.

Open Access This chapter is licensed under the terms of the Creative Commons Attribution-NonCommercial-NoDerivatives 4.0 International License (http://creativecommons.org/licenses/by-nc-nd/4.0/), which permits any non-commercial use, sharing, distribution and reproduction in any medium or format, as long as you give appropriate credit to the original author(s) and the source, provide a link to the Creative Commons license and indicate if you modified the licensed material. You do not have permission under this license to share adapted material derived from this chapter or parts of it.

The images or other third party material in this chapter are included in the chapter's Creative Commons license, unless indicated otherwise in a credit line to the material. If material is not included in the chapter's Creative Commons license and your intended use is not permitted by statutory regulation or exceeds the permitted use, you will need to obtain permission directly from the copyright holder.

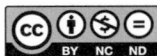

Martorell Hypertensive Ischemic Ulcer

Sylvie Meaume and Hester Colboc

Martorell hypertensive ischemic ulcer, also called necrotic angiodermatitis (NA), represents a particular type of leg ulcer with a specific clinical presentation, histopathological appearance, and therapeutic management. Its origin is independent of an underlying venous or arterial pathology, but, on the other hand, it is linked to the deleterious action of arterial hypertension on the cutaneous microvascularization. NA was mentioned for the first time in 1945 by Martorell, a Spanish cardiologist who described the first clinical cases and observed the relationship with arterial hypertension [1].

28.1 Epidemiology

NA is not an exceptional condition (9–15% of leg ulcers) [2–4] but is often overlooked and poses problems of differential diagnosis with calciphylaxis, pyoderma gangrenosum, and certain vasculitis. The female sex seems predominant (61–70%) [2, 3] with an age usually above 60 years [2, 4]. Hypertension is present in nearly 100% of cases, diabetes in 30–50%, and chronic smoking in 20% of cases [4].

28.2 Etiopathogenesis

The pathophysiology of NA is not fully elucidated at present. The in vivo vascularization of NA was compared to that of arterial ulcers using a scintigraphic method [5]. Lower tissue perfusion than in patients with arterial disease has been identified and explained by increased arteriolar resistance. This hypoperfusion would be responsible for local ischemia and necrosis.

In another pathogenetic hypothesis, NA would be a "cutaneous vascular accident" caused by hypotensive episodes in patients on polymedicated therapy for their arterial hypertension and with a pathological arteriolar network [6].

Finally, other authors put forward a hypothesis of paradoxical hypercoagulation phenomena, in a context of anticoagulation with antivitamin K [4].

28.3 Clinical Diagnosis

NA has a characteristic monomorphic clinical expression, but there is a diagnostic delay of several weeks. It has a sudden post-traumatic onset in 25–50% of cases [3, 4]. The onset is a purplish macula, a bulla, or a hemorrhagic crust with a purpuric periphery, which rapidly transforms into a superficial necrotic plaque with characteristic jagged and livedoid inflammatory edges of variable sizes between 10 and 20 cm^2 (Fig. 28.1). The extension of this superficial ulcer is rapid

S. Meaume (✉) · H. Colboc
Department of Geriatric and wound care, Rothschild University Hospital, Assistance Publique Hôpitaux de Paris, Sorbonne Université, Paris, France
e-mail: sylvie.meaume@aphp.fr

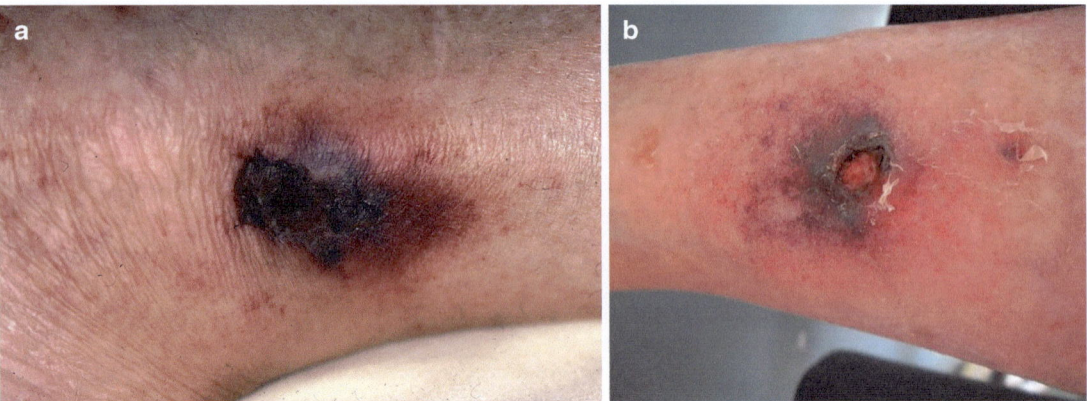

Fig. 28.1 (a) NA in the early stage of necrosis (b) NA with central wound and peripheric necrosis

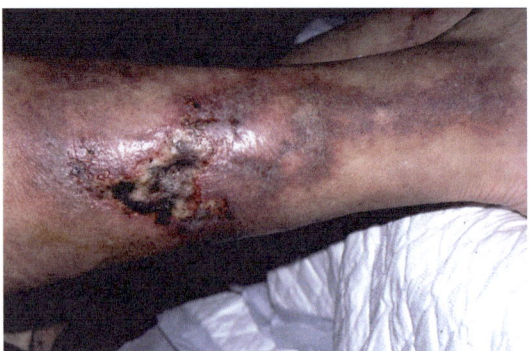

Fig. 28.2 Characteristic livedoid skin around NA necrosis

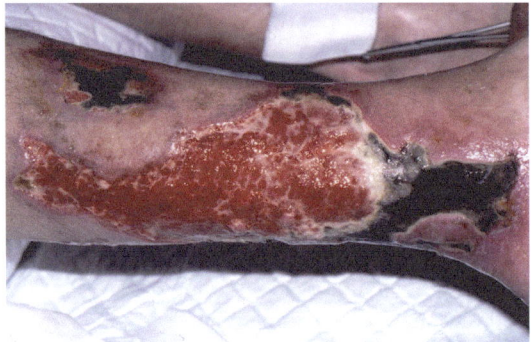

Fig. 28.3 NA : extensive superficial necrosis

(Figs. 28.2 and 28.3). The ulcers are spontaneously hyperalgic and usually require quick transfer to a hospital to manage pain. The painful character with paroxysms is an essential element of the diagnosis.

The preferential location of the NA is the lower third of the leg. The lesions can be single or multiple, and sometimes bilateral and symmetrical. Variable inflammatory outbreaks with serpiginous ulcerative extension may follow one another with the appearance of satellite elements. Changes in position, lowering of the limb, rest, or elevation, do not relieve the pain, which is an important semiological element. A deep evolution with necrosis of the subcutaneous tissues down to the muscle fascia and exposure of the tendons is possible but rare, mainly the Achilles' tendon (13% of patients) [3]. Distal arteriopathy is not usually hemodynamically significant but can accompany NA in 40% of cases as comorbidity. Chronic venous insufficiency can be associated in 25–40% of cases and has to be managed with compression bandages if ankle-brachial pressure index is correct [4]. Spontaneous evolution of NA is towards stabilization and then regression centripetal. A scar is sometimes visible after spontaneous regression of the lesions.

28.4 Histopathology

Biopsy is not mandatory if the clinical diagnosis is certain [2]. The histological picture is not specific but allows a diagnostic orientation. Above all, it makes it possible to eliminate a differential diagnosis. It is recommended to perform a skin biopsy in an area of normal skin at the periphery

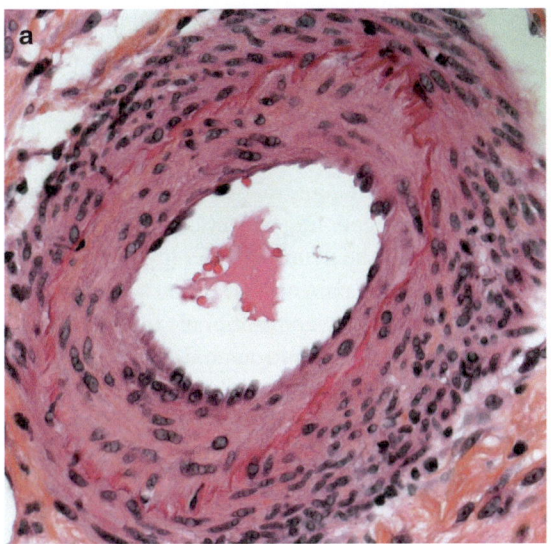 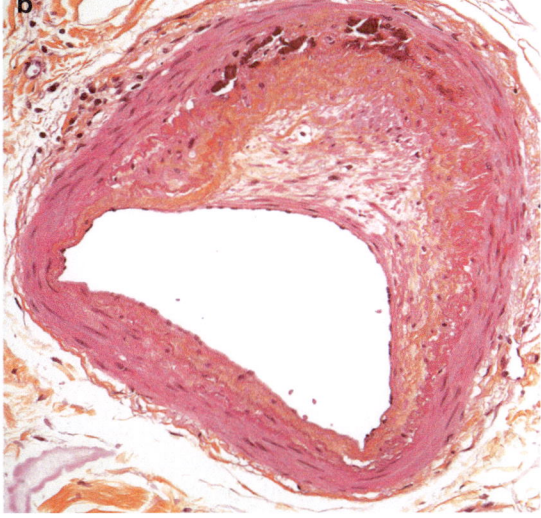

Fig. 28.4 Histopathology of NA, hematoxylin–eosin–saffron stained: (**a**) arteriolosclerosis with reduction of lumen of subcutaneous arterioles in NA. (**b**) Arteriolosclerosis with asymmetrical fibrous intimal thickening, here associated to calcification of the internal elastic lamina and media (courtesy of Dr Moguelet)

of the ulceration and at the level of the area of necrosis. If a biopsy is performed in the necrosis, deep and extensive hemorrhagic crust associated with arteriolar and venular thrombosis can be observed. If a peri-ulcer biopsy is performed, it shows unspecific thickening of the media of small-caliber arterioles and muscular arteries in the dermis and hypodermis (arteriolosclerosis of dermal vessels) (Fig. 28.4).

28.5 Differential Diagnoses

NA poses problems of differential diagnosis with other vascular diseases. Diagnosis is usually based on the characteristic clinical appearance in the absence of underlying venous or arterial etiology, except in cases where these conditions may be associated. Extreme pain and skin necrosis exclude the diagnosis of venous ulcer, and the absence of claudication and superficial trophic disorders is not in favor of an arterial ulcer.

Pyoderma gangrenosum is differentiated from NA by the presence of peripheral purulent pits, sunken "mined" edges, and cribriform scars, as well as a characteristic histopathological examination with neutrophil-rich dermal infiltration and signs of vasculitis. Any mechanical cleansing is prohibited due to the phenomena of pathergy.

Calciphylaxis, also called calcium arteriolopathy, is a rare pathology associated with high morbidity that most often appears in the context of end-stage chronic renal failure in a dialysis or transplant patient. It is characterized by the association of vascular calcifications related to a phosphocalcic imbalance, with cutaneous necrosis. The clinic is marked by the appearance of indurated and painful livedoid plaques with livedoid purpura and deep central necrosis within the plaques. Cutaneous lesions have a predilection for regions rich in adipose tissue such as the abdomen and the root of the thighs in the proximal form of uremic calciphylaxis. Less commonly, they appear on the legs, constituting the distal form of uremic calciphylaxis [3]. A variant of non-uremic calciphylaxis has been described, in the absence of renal or parathyroid pathology, but is on the other hand often associated with two cardiovascular risk factors: arterial hypertension and diabetes. Patients may have other serious comorbidities such as cancers or hepatic cirrhosis. The clinic is also marked by extensive, deep, and hyperalgesic necrotic lesions of the abdomen, breasts, or thighs. Treatment is difficult, and mortality is high: 40–60% of cases [3].

The other differential diagnoses are thrombosing conditions (cryoglobulinemia, antiphospholipid syndrome, thrombophilia, etc.), cutaneous vasculitis, and infectious or drug-induced ulcers.

28.6 Evolution

The evolution can be marked by successive outbreaks with recurrences in 60–80% of cases. These occur in other territories or on the contralateral limb. The local prognosis is on the other hand rather favorable, with the rate of amputation being less than 1%.

28.7 Treatment of NA

1. *The use of analgesics is essential* not only for the comfort of the patient but also for a better realization of the care. Although skin grafting remains the main means of relieving the patient, the patient should generally be administered WHO level II or III analgesics as soon as possible. The use of morphine is often necessary and must be quickly instituted. Neuropathic analgesic treatments can be associated (pregabalin, tricyclic antidepressants) because of the neuropathic component associated with the pain of NA. Faced with pain that is resistant to conventional medical treatments, the use of nitrous oxide at the time of care and the use of nerve blocks via a perineural catheter may be necessary.

2. *Skin grafts* (Figs. 28.5 and 28.6) currently represent the "gold standard" of NA treatment. This beneficial therapeutic effect of skin grafting was described in 1995 [7]. This involves pinch skin graft or mesh graft, performed after mechanical or autolytic debridement of necrotic tissue. They must be carried out as soon as possible when the diagnosis is evoked. The common results obtained on the grafts in the NA confirm the effectiveness on pain with analgesic withdrawal in 8 days, disappearance of the peripheral pur-

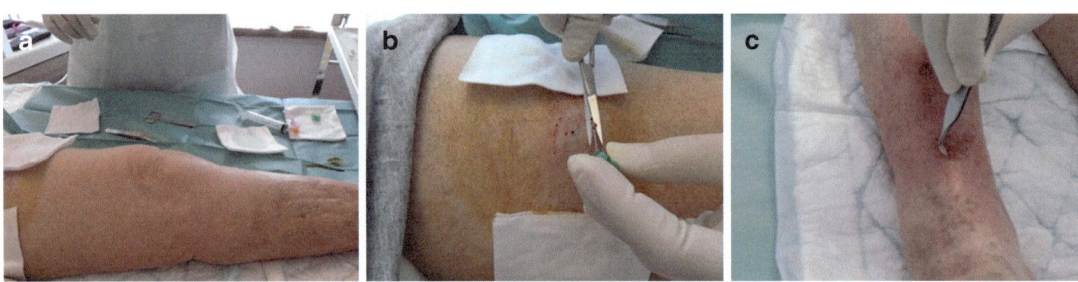

Fig. 28.5 Pinch graft procedure: (**a**) preparation of the donor site (inner side of the thigh) and of the material. (**b**) Grafts harvesting. (**c**) Grafts placement

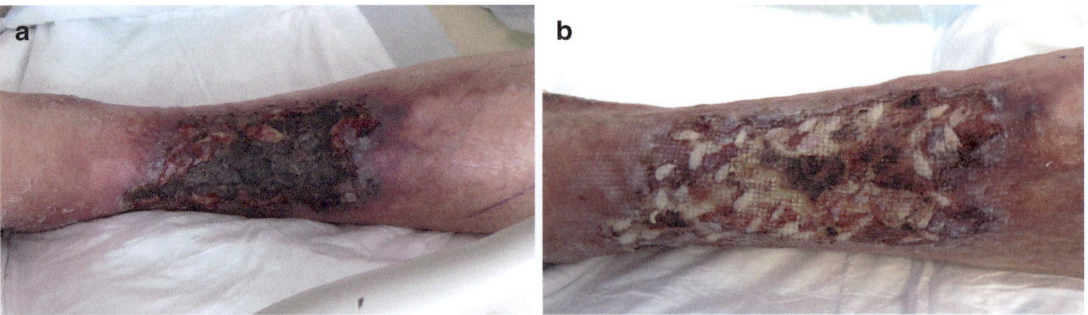

Fig. 28.6 Evolution of pinch graft on a typical NA. (**a**) Before pinch graft. (**b**) Day 4 pinch grafts

plish halo in 8 days, and complete healing in 30–45 days on average. This effectiveness is demonstrated if the transplants are early and repeated (ref à ajouter) [3, 8, 9].

3. *Wound care*, as an alternative treatment of NA, is centered on the autolytic debridement of the cutaneous necrosis, and using suitable dressings such as hydrogels, irrigoabsorbents, alginates, or hydrofibers, depending on the degree of exudate and the quality of the surrounding skin of the wound, can be proposed. *Strong to very strong local topical corticosteroids* used around the ulcer on the inflamed areas in the absence of signs of local infection are prescribed in order to reduce the extension of the lesion. *Electrostimulation* techniques have been proposed in the NA. They allow a debridement of necrotic and fibrinous wounds and above all have an analgesic effect [10]. *Negative-pressure therapy* has been proposed pre- or post-skin graft [3]. However, medical measures alone only allow healing in 6% of cases according to Hafner et al. [3] and 10–25% of cases according to Senet [11], which underlines the fundamental role of skin grafting in the treatment of NA.

28.8 Other Treatments

The preventive measures of NA essentially concern the control of arterial pressure, which should not vary too much over time. In case of association with venous insufficiency, compression bandage must be associated. It also stabilizes the grafts and often allows faster healing. Cessation of smoking and nonselective beta-blockers is often recommended [2].

28.9 Conclusion

NA is a non-exceptional cause of leg ulcer but too often overlooked and often leads to late diagnosis. It is a very painful arteriolar ulcer, difficult to treat and which has a negative impact on the patient's quality of life. Management is based on pain management, blood pressure control, and mechanical or autolytic debridement followed by skin grafting.

References

1. Martorell F. Las ulceras supramaleolares por arteriolitis de las grandes hipertensas. Actas (Reunion Cientifica Cuerpo Facultad). Instituto Policlinico Barcelona. 1945;1(1):6–9.
2. Vuerstaek JDD, Reeder SWI, Henquet CJM, H. a. M. Neumann. Arteriolosclerotic ulcer of Martorell. J Eur Acad Dermatol Venereol. 2010;24(8):867–74.
3. Hafner J, Nobbe S, Partsch H, Läuchli S, Mayer D, Amann-Vesti B, Speich R, Schmid C, Burg G, French LE. Martorell hypertensive ischemic leg ulcer: a model of ischemic subcutaneous arteriolosclerosis. Arch Dermatol. 2010;146(9):961–8.
4. Nicol P, Bernard P, Nguyen P, Durlach A, Perceau G. Retrospective study of hypertensive leg ulcers at Reims university hospital: epidemiological, clinical, disease progression data, effects of vitamin K antagonists. Ann Dermatol Venereol. 2017;144(1):37–44.
5. Duncan HJ, Faris IB. Martorell's hypertensive ischemic leg ulcers are secondary to an increase in the local vascular resistance. J Vasc Surg. 1985;2(4):581–4.
6. Saadallah S, Couillet D, Richard M, Vaisse B, Guillaume JC, Grob JJ, et al. L'angiodermite nécrotique, un « accident vasculaire cutané » par hypotension brutale sur une artériolopathie hypertensive ? Étude ouverte prospective preliminaire. Annales de Dermatologie et Venereologie. 2000;127:4S8-9.
7. Lazareth I, Priollet P. Necrotic angiodermatitis: treatment by early cutaneous grafts. Ann Dermatol Venereol. 1995;122(9):575–8.
8. Dagregorio G, Guillet G. A retrospective review of 20 hypertensive leg ulcers treated with mesh skin grafts. J Eur Acad Dermatol Venereol. 2006 Feb;20(2):166–9.
9. El Khatib K, Danino A, Rzin A, Malka G. Necrotic angiodermatitis: evaluation of an early skin graft treatment. Ann Chir Plast Esthet. 2009;54(6):567–70.
10. Leloup P, Toussaint P, Lembelembe JP, Célérier P, Maillard H. The analgesic effect of electrostimulation (WoundEL®) in the treatment of leg ulcers. Int Wound J. 2015;12(6):706–9.
11. Senet P, Vicaut E, Beneton N, Debure C, Lok C, Chosidow O. Topical treatment of hypertensive leg ulcers with platelet-derived growth factor-BB: a randomized controlled trial. Arch Dermatol. 2011;147(8):926–30.

Open Access This chapter is licensed under the terms of the Creative Commons Attribution-NonCommercial-NoDerivatives 4.0 International License (http://creativecommons.org/licenses/by-nc-nd/4.0/), which permits any non-commercial use, sharing, distribution and reproduction in any medium or format, as long as you give appropriate credit to the original author(s) and the source, provide a link to the Creative Commons license and indicate if you modified the licensed material. You do not have permission under this license to share adapted material derived from this chapter or parts of it.

The images or other third party material in this chapter are included in the chapter's Creative Commons license, unless indicated otherwise in a credit line to the material. If material is not included in the chapter's Creative Commons license and your intended use is not permitted by statutory regulation or exceeds the permitted use, you will need to obtain permission directly from the copyright holder.

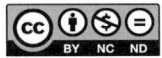

Vasculitis

Nicolas Kluger

29.1 Diagnosis of Cutaneous Vasculitis Is Made on Histology

Physical cutaneous signs of vasculitis are wide and nonspecific. Cutaneous vasculitis (CV) affects the skin with varying intensity, depth, and distribution. Even though a certain number of syndromes have been described, a patient may present with symptoms that overlap with another clinical diagnosis making a diagnosis "at first sight" impossible. Most of all, vasculitis has a histopathologic definition; therefore, its confirmation comes only from the microscopic examination of the lesion [1–5].

The diagnosis of CV is made by microscopic examination of hematoxylin-eosin-stained biopsies. A list of criteria allows a trained pathologist to diagnose and distinguish an active vasculitis from chronic and healed lesions of vasculitis and changes that are adjacent to vasculitis and may help to define a subtype or the etiology of the CV. Inflammatory infiltrates within and around the vessel walls associated with intramural and/or intraluminal fibrin deposition (fibrinoid necrosis) confirm the diagnosis of vasculitis. Some changes are suggestive of active vasculitis such as red blood cell extravasation, perivascular nuclear dust (leukocytoclasia), eccrine gland necrosis, ulceration, and necrosis/infarction. In the absence of fibrinoid necrosis, the diagnosis of CV becomes more difficult. Lamination of the adventitia, media, and/or intima; perivascular nuclear dust (leukocytoclasia) without fibrinoid necrosis; loss of the elastic lamina with acellular scar tissue; or subendothelial intramuscular and/or adventitial inflammatory cells in large vessels are all other indications for vessel wall damages [1–5].

A direct immunofluorescence (DIF) examination is also recommended in case of CV. It does not confirm the diagnosis of CV but allows to orient for one or another diagnosis.

- Absence of immune complex is in favor for pauci-immune vasculitis: granulomatosis with polyangiitis (Wegener's, GPA), eosinophilic granulomatosis with polyangiitis (Churg-Strauss syndrome, EGPA), and microscopic polyangiitis (MPA).
- Immunoglobulin (Ig) G, IgM, IgA, and/or C3 in or around the vessels may be found in immune-mediated vasculitis like cryoglobulinemia.
- In all cases of CV, immune depositions of Ig and complement may be found, especially C3 and IgM.

N. Kluger (✉)
Departments of Dermatology, Allergology and Venereology, Helsinki University Hospital and University of Helsinki, Helsinki, Finland
e-mail: nicolas.kluger@hus.fi

However, the older the biopsied lesion is, the less immunoglobulin is found. After 72 h, only C3 is detected. Therefore, a negative DIF does not rule out the diagnosis of CV [1–5].

- Predominance of IgA is highly in favor for IgA vasculitis (Henoch-Schönlein purpura) without being constant or specific.
- IgM depositions are observed, especially in case of circulating rheumatoid factor or cryoglobulinemia. IgA deposits are absent in case of cryoglobulinemia.

Of note, positive DIF without pathological assessment of CV is not relevant.

After confirmation of the diagnosis of CV itself, vasculitis may be defined more accurately by vessel size involvement (small, small and medium, and medium to large vessel), extent of the lesions (superficial perivascular to dermal and/or subcutaneous), and predominant inflammatory cell infiltration. The finding of small-vessel vasculitis with predominance of neutrophilic infiltrate and positive DIF is indicative of cutaneous leukocytoclastic vasculitis, IgA vasculitis, urticarial vasculitis, or erythema elevatum diutinum. More rarely, other cells may predominate such as eosinophils or lymphocytes. Presence of both small- and medium-sized vasculitis favors ANCA-associated/pauci-immune vasculitis (with negative DIF): EGPA, MPA, GPA or cryoglobulinemia, connective tissue disease (lupus, rheumatoid arthritis, etc.), or hypocomplementemic vasculitis if DIF is positive. Polyarteritis nodosa is characterized by a neutrophilic infiltration associated with a medium-vessel artery vasculitis [1–5].

It is considered that biopsy of CV is not of help to determine its cause [6]. Tissue eosinophilia could point out towards drug-induced vasculitis [7]. Some extravascular histologic pattern found in the surrounding tissue may be helpful to indicate a specific disease. Thus, palisading granulomatous dermatitis ("Winkelmann granuloma") is in favor for GPA, EGPA, rheumatoid arthritis, or systemic lupus erythematosus. Presence of eosinophils and flame figures associated with such granulomas is found in EGAP while neutrophils and basophilic debris in PGA and rheumatoid vasculitis. Vacuolar interface dermatitis with sometimes dermal mucin deposition is associated with lupus erythematosus and dermatomyositis. Intraepidermal or dermal pustules with neutrophil small-vessel vasculitis are related to an infectious related vasculitis. Skin biopsy allows excluding pseudovasculitic disorder, a wide group of heterogeneous diseases that may mimic cutaneous vasculitis [8] (Table 29.1).

Table 29.1 Approach to the diagnosis of cutaneous vasculitis and its differential diagnosis [1, 6]

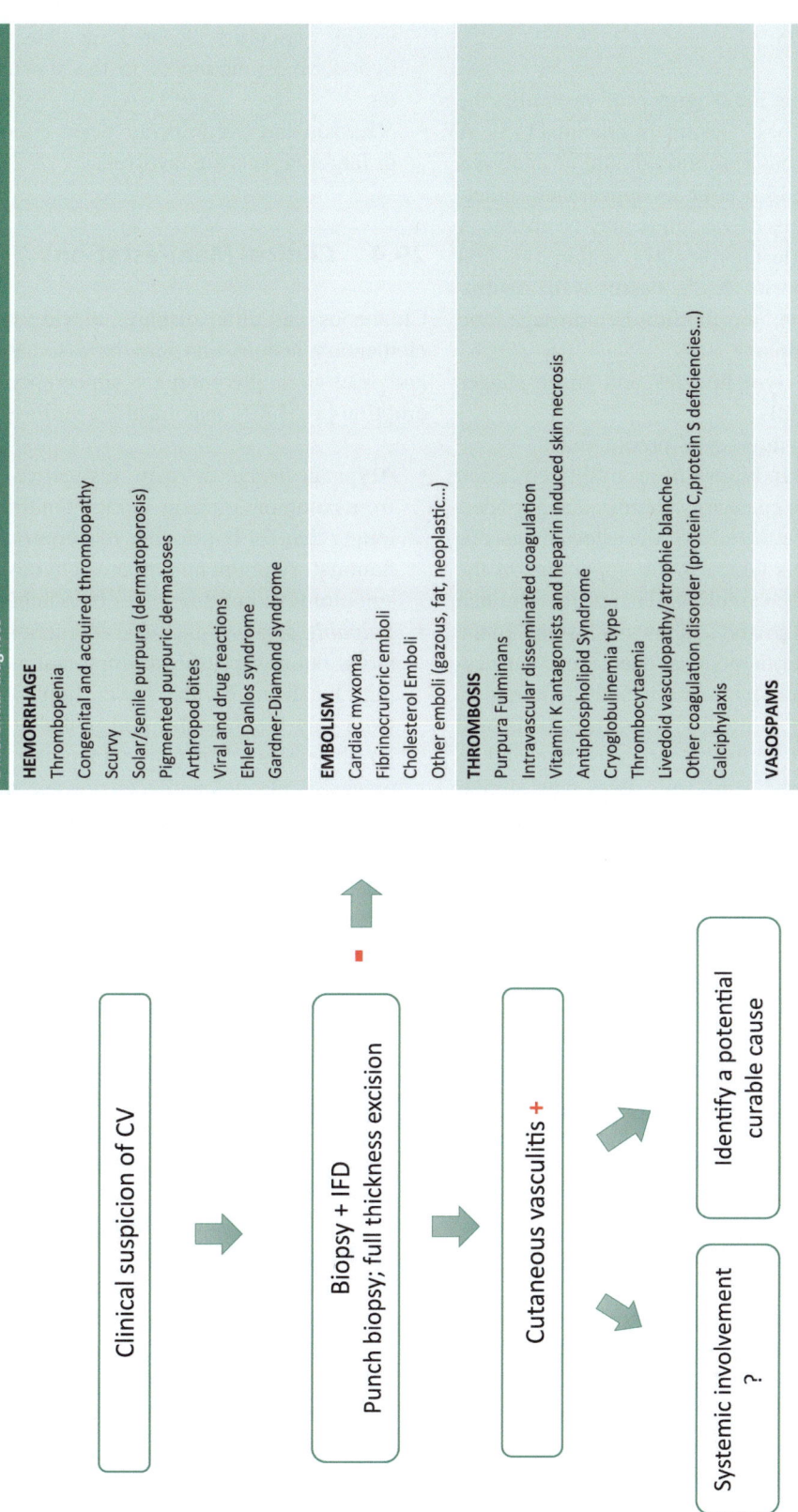

29.2 Pitfalls

In order to enable the diagnosis of vasculitis, the choice of the "best" lesion is crucial [1–5]. A lesion of cutaneous vasculitis should be analyzed within the first 48 h after its appearance; otherwise, typical signs of vasculitis may be absent. A fresh purpuric lesion displays within the first 24-h fibrin deposits in the vessel wall, neutrophilic infiltration, surrounding hemorrhage, and intranuclear debris.

After 24 h, lymphocytes and macrophages replace neutrophils.

After 48 h, lymphocytes predominate.

Moreover, skin biopsy of an infiltrated lesion must include the epidermis, dermis, and hypodermis to determine the size of the affected vessels. Some CV affects typically the upper part of the dermis like IgA vasculitis. Therefore, a punch skin biopsy will permit to show the lesions. In the case of polyarteritis nodosa, deep muscular vessels of the dermis-hypodermis and the hypodermis are affected, which implies a deep incisional biopsy. Similarly, a livedo should be biopsied on its most infiltrated or necrotic areas with similar deep biopsy [9].

In some specific cases, an *incidental vasculitis* may be found on the skin biopsy. This pathologic statement should not mislead to diagnose a vasculitis:

- Biopsy performed on an ulcer.
- Biopsy in lesions related to neutrophilic dermatoses (Sweet's syndrome).

29.3 Clinical Pathologic Correlation

The cutaneous lesions correlate sometimes with the size of the affected vessels [1–5].

- Palpable purpura, infiltrated erythema, urticaria, vesicles, and blisters are mainly related to small-vessel vasculitis of the dermis.
- Subcutaneous nodules, ulceration, and gangrene are frequently related to medium-sized vessel vasculitis located at the dermohypodermal junction or in the subcutaneous fat.
- Necrosis and livedo occur when either small or larger vessels are involved.

29.4 Clinical Manifestations

Cutaneous vasculitis displays a wide range of elementary lesions that may be associated with and lead to a pleomorphic appearance of the eruption [1–5]. CV may manifest variously as:

- Atypical *urticaria*, with distinctive feature from common urticaria: duration of the lesions longer than 24 h, presence of purpura, postinflammatory pigmentation or ecchymoses, and symptoms of burning rather than itching.
- *Palpable purpura*: the most frequent manifestation but nonspecific; asymptomatic or burning; localized on the lower limbs, ranging from tiny red macules and pinhead to coin-sized petechia, but also sometimes to more extensive plaques and ecchymoses; may disclose a necrotic evolution leading to vesicles, blisters, erosions, ulcerations, and ulcer. It is often an association of different lesions in a same patient simultaneously: erythematous to purpuric macules, papules, and necrotic lesions.
- *Retiform purpura* is a peculiar clinical form of branching purpuric lesions in a fishnet pattern for which a distinction from an infiltrated or necrotic livedo is difficult. Retiform purpura implies the performance of a skin biopsy like any infiltrated purpura or livedo.
- *Other manifestations*: infiltrated erythema; hemorrhagic vesicles; ulcers; inflammatory, tender, or painful dermal or hypodermal nodules; livedo racemosa, infarcts, and digital gangrene. Lesions affect primarily the lower limbs. Upper extremity, trunk, and head and neck involvement are not usual and may be considered as a sign of severity and/or of a systemic vasculitis (Figs. 29.1, 29.2, 29.3, and 29.4).

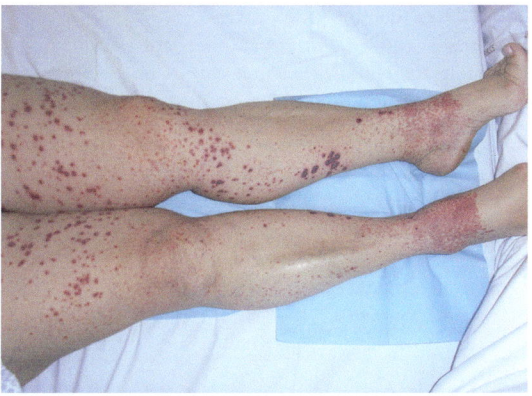

Fig. 29.1 Vasculitis of the lower limbs associated with different clinical lesions of purpura: macules, papules, and vesiculous lesions. Notice the absence of lesions on the dorsum of the feet due to the compression of the shoes

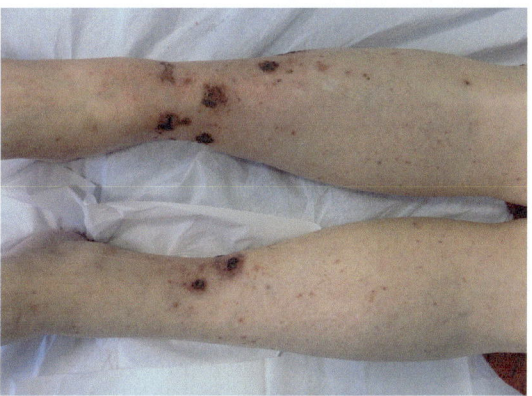

Fig. 29.2 Necrotic lesions of the lower legs during cutaneous vasculitis

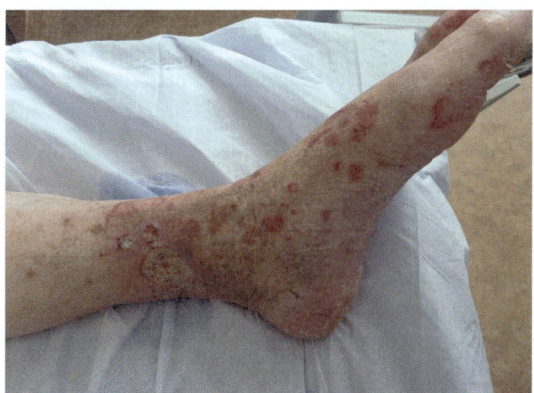

Fig. 29.3 Cryoglobulinemic vasculitis with purpura and leg ulcer

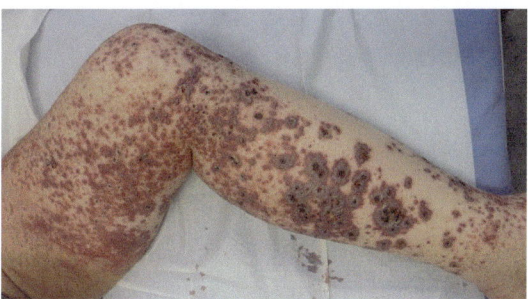

Fig. 29.4 Extensive necrotizing vasculitis of the leg

Other skin manifestations are associated with systemic vasculitis, but they do not display vasculitis upon histology [1]:

- *Extravascular necrotizing granuloma*: occurs during Churg-Strauss syndrome especially, red to purple papules or nodules involving symmetrically the extensor aspects of the elbows and the fingers, but other localizations have also been reported.
- *Panniculitis:* recurrent crops of erythematous, edematous, and tender subcutaneous nodules; usually of symmetrical distribution on the thighs and the lower legs; spontaneous regression with hypopigmentation and atrophic scar due to fat necrosis (lobular panniculitis) or the extensor aspects of the lower limbs with a spontaneous regression without atrophic scar (septal panniculitis).
- *Pyoderma gangrenosum.*
- *Granuloma*: granulomatous lesions with neither vasculitis nor central necrosis may be observed in systemic vasculitis, especially WG with a highly variable presentation ranging from papules, nodules, subcutaneous infiltration, and pseudotumor to chronic ulcers and affecting any site of the body.
- *Superficial thrombophlebitis.*
- *Gangrene*: resulting from arterial occlusion and may be observed in all vasculitis involving medium- or large-sized arteries.
- *Raynaud's phenomenon*: classically associated with all types of vasculitis. However, its prevalence is unknown in many vasculitis, and its diagnostic value is very low.

29.5 Classification

Classification of vasculitis is a real brainteaser [1]. Existence of overlapping clinical features, lack of knowledge regarding precise etiopathogenetic process of each vasculitis, and lack of "pathognomonic" clinical, laboratory, or radiologic findings make it almost impossible to have a perfect classification. Several classifications have been proposed, each of them presenting advantages and weaknesses. Most commonly used criteria for classification of vasculitis are of the American College of Rheumatology (ACR) established in 1990 [10] and the Chapel Hill Consensus Conference (CHCC) that was revised in 2012 [11]. The latter is a nomenclature system of vasculitis providing names and definitions (Table 29.2). Of note, a dermatologic addendum was published to standardize the name and definitions for cutaneous vasculitis [12]. Classification criteria should be restricted to their primary use, i.e., stratify uniform populations who carry a diagnosis. In clinical practice, a final diagnosis should rely on the interpretation of clinical, laboratory, radiologic, and pathological findings.

Table 29.2 Names and definitions for vasculitides adopted by the 2012 International Chapel Hill Consensus Conference on the Nomenclature of Vasculitides [11]

Large-vessel vasculitis (LVV)
Vasculitis affecting the aorta and its major branches more often than other vasculitides
Takayasu arteritis (TAK)
Giant cell arteritis (GCA)
Medium-vessel vasculitis (MVV)
Vasculitis that predominantly affects medium arteries defined as the main visceral arteries and their branches
Polyarteritis nodosa (PAN)
Kawasaki disease (KD)
Small-vessel vasculitis (SVV)
Antineutrophil cytoplasmic antibody (ANCA)-associated vasculitis (AAV)
Microscopic polyangiitis (MPA)
Granulomatosis with polyangiitis (Wegener's) (GPA)
Eosinophilic granulomatosis with polyangiitis (Churg-Strauss) (EGPA)
Immune complex SVV
Anti-glomerular basement membrane (anti-GBM) disease
Cryoglobulinemic vasculitis (CV)
IgA vasculitis (Henoch-Schönlein) (IgAV)
Hypocomplementemic urticarial vasculitis (HUV) (anti-C1q vasculitis)
(continued)
Variable vessel vasculitis (VVV)
Vasculitis with no predominant type of vessel involved. Can affect vessels of any type and size
Behcet's disease (BD)
Cogan's syndrome (CS)
Single-organ vasculitis (SOV)
Vasculitis in a single organ that has no features indicating that it is a limited expression of a systemic vasculitis
Cutaneous leukocytoclastic angiitis
Cutaneous arteritis
Primary central nervous system vasculitis isolated aortitis
Others
Vasculitis associated with systemic disease
Lupus vasculitis
Rheumatoid vasculitis
Sarcoid vasculitis
Others
Vasculitis associated with probable etiology
Hepatitis C virus-associated cryoglobulinemic vasculitis
Hepatitis B virus-associated vasculitis
Syphilis-associated aortitis
Drug-associated immune complex vasculitis
Drug-associated ANCA-associated vasculitis
Cancer-associated vasculitis
Others

29.6 Approach to the Diagnosis of Cutaneous Vasculitis

- The first step being completed—having proved by a skin biopsy the presence of cutaneous vasculitis and analyzed its precise subtype (cell infiltration, size of the involved vessel, DIF)—the physician collects all the relevant data that will help him (1) to establish the severity of the CV by the absence or presence of systemic involvement that will prompt to initiate immunosuppressive treatment and (2) to identify a potential curable cause [1] (Table 29.3).
- The precise diagnosis is made by the combination of clinical history and clinical, laboratory, and radiologic findings. Therefore, patients' precise past medical data, history

Table 29.3 Approach to the diagnosis of isolated, biopsy-proven, cutaneous vasculitis [1]

Establish the Severity : Systemic Involvement ?
  Complete physical examination
  General manifestations : fever, night sweats, weight loss
  Joint (arthralgias), muscles (myalgias), lung (hemoptysis, cough, shortness of breath, wheezing), heart (chest pain, murmur)
gastrointestinal tract (abdominal pain, gastro-intestinal bleeding), ear, nose, throat (sinusitis, rhinitis) and ocular symtoms
(scleritis, sicca syndrome), peripheral (paresthesia, numbness) and central (cephalagia, seizures) nervous system, urologic and
genital symptoms (hematuria, testicular pain)
  Laboratory studies
  Kidney function every 3 months : urinalysis, proteinuria, blood urea/creatinine
  Electrocardiography
  Chest X-ray
Identify a Potential Cause
Recently introduced drug ?
Laboratory studies recommended in the absence of clinical relevant symptoms
  Blood cell count, C-reactive protein,
  Serum electrophoresis
  Liver tests: transaminases, hepatitis B and C virus serologies
  Cryoglobulins
  Antinuclear antibodies, anti-dsDNA, anti-extractable nuclear antigens (Ro/Ssa, La/SSb, RNP, Sm…), rheumatoid factors
  Antineutrophils cytoplasmic antibodies (ANCA)
  Complement levels (CH50, C3, C4)
  Anti-streptolysin O titers
Complementary exams according to medical history and clinical findings
  HIV test
  Blood culture
  Lumbar puncture
  Echocardiography
  Viral serologies (parvovirus B19, Epstein Barr virus, CMV, COVID-19…), proposed in case of clinical suspicion, pregnancy or in immunocompromised hosts
  Sinus CT scan and teeth examination

of the disease including newly introduced drugs, and episode evocative for acute infection are mandatory. Indeed, any cutaneous vasculitis occurring in a patient with a known systemic vasculitis should prompt to look for the intercurrent triggering factor like infection or a newly introduced drug before diagnosis or flare-up of the disease.

Physical examination must be complete and extensive. Of note, peculiar attention should be brought on relapsing retiform purpura in young adults as it can disclose the abuse of levamisole-adulterated cocaine. The patients do present a striking involvement of the ear that could be a clue to suspect such diagnosis [1].

- Physicians should not lose from sight and warn the patients that in 50% of all cases of cutaneous vasculitis, no specific cause is found.

29.7 Management of Cutaneous Vasculitis

Management of biopsy-proven CV includes the following [1]:

- Looking for the presence of systemic involvement (heart, lung, kidney).
- Identifying a potential curable cause.
- However, complementary explorations should be oriented by clinical context.
- Any patient with a known underlying disease that may be responsible for CV should be asked about any new drug intake and infectious like episode and carefully examined to rule out another potential cause of vasculitis.

In most of the cases, CV remains restricted to a single, self-limited, and short-lived episode of purpura of the lower limbs without any visceral involvement and any relapse. In this frequent situation, treatment is not compulsory. However, support stockings or panty hose as well as bed rest and leg elevation are recommended. Topical corticosteroids or anti-inflammatory agents can be given for symptomatic relief [13]. Conversely, there is to date no indication for heparin therapy or antivitamin K treatment for the management of vasculitis, except if additional thrombotic factors are found concomitantly (i.e. circulating anti-phospholipids) (Table 29.4).

If the disease persists, worsens, or is symptomatic (burning sensation, pain) with a restriction to the skin, various drugs can be given,

Table 29.4 Treatment of cutaneous vasculitis according to severity [13]

Severity	Treatment
Single, self-limited and short-lived episode of purpura of the lower limbs without any visceral involvement and any relapse,	• Treatment is not compulsory • Bed rest, elevated legs, support stockings or panty hose • Topical corticosteroids, anti-inflammatory agents for symptomatic relief
If the disease persists, worsen or is symptomatic (burning sensation, pain) with a restriction to the skin	• Colchicine (1mg/day) for one to three months • Dapsone (50-100 mg/day) • Pentoxyphililine (400 mg, 3 times a day). • Combination
Extensive, recurrent skin disease with persistent lesions, vesicles, ulcers, nodules; intractable symptoms or systemic vasculitis with other organ involvement	• Corticosteroids • Methotrexate, azathioprine, cyclosporine, cyclophosphamide • Intravenous immunoglobulins, rituximab • TNF alpha antagonists (Behcet,...); tocilizumab (giant cell arteritis)

usually colchicine at a dose of 1 mg/day for 1–3 months. Alternatives include dapsone (50–100 mg/day), alone or in combination with colchicine [13], and pentoxifylline (400 mg × 3/day), alone or in combination with other treatments [1–5]. Longer treatments can be given in case of relapse after withdrawal.

Extensive, recurrent skin disease with persistent lesions, vesicles, ulcers, and nodules; intractable symptoms; or systemic vasculitis with other organ involvement may prompt initiation of immunosuppressive therapies such as corticosteroids, methotrexate, azathioprine, mycophenolate mofetil, cyclosporine, or cyclophosphamide. Rituximab may be of interest in case of severe vasculitis, in the ANCA-related group especially. The place of anti-tumor necrosis factor remains to be established. Indeed, several cases of severe cutaneous vasculitis have been treated successfully with infliximab. Besides, infliximab does have a clear-cut indication for Behcet's disease. However, cases of vasculitis induced by infliximab or other TNF alpha inhibitors, in patients with psoriasis especially, nuance the place of this class in carefully selected cases.

Besides, management includes pain control and standardized care for necrotic and fibrous ulcers along with the control of the underlying process [1].

References

1. Kluger N, Francès C. Cutaneous vasculitis and their differential diagnoses. Clin Exp Rheumatol. 2009;27:S124–38.
2. Carlson JA, Cavaliere LF, Grant-Kels JM. Cutaneous vasculitis: diagnosis and management. Clin Dermatol. 2006;24:414–29.
3. Carlson JA, Chen KR. Cutaneous vasculitis update: small vessel neutrophilic vasculitis syndromes. Am J Dermatopathol. 2006;28:486–506.
4. Crowson AN, Mihm MC Jr, Magro CM. Cutaneous vasculitis: a review. J Cutan Pathol. 2003;30:161–73.

5. Fiorentino DF. Cutaneous vasculitis. J Am Acad Dermatol. 2003;48:311–40.
6. Jung AJ, Schaeffer M, Mitcov M, Scrivener Y, Cribier B, Lipsker D. Clinicopathological study of purpura: is a skin biopsy necessary for palpable purpura? Ann Dermatol Venereol. 2016;143:347–53.
7. Bahrami S, Malone JC, Webb KG, Callen JP. Tissue eosinophilia as an indicator of drug-induced cutaneous small-vessel vasculitis. Arch Dermatol. 2006;142:155–61.
8. Carlson JA, Chen KR. Cutaneous pseudovasculitis. Am J Dermatopathol. 2007;29:44–55.
9. Kluger N, Molinari E, Francès C. Livedo in adults. Ann Dermatol Venereol. 2005;132:710–7.
10. Hunder GG, Arend WP, Bloch DA, et al. The American College of Rheumatology 1990 criteria for the classification of vasculitis. Introduction. Arthritis Rheum. 1990;33:1065–7.
11. Jennette JC, Falk RJ, Bacon PA, et al. 2012 revised international Chapel Hill consensus conference nomenclature of Vasculitides. Arthritis Rheum. 2013;65:1–11.
12. Sunderkötter CH, Zelger B, Chen KR, et al. Nomenclature of cutaneous Vasculitis: dermatologic addendum to the 2012 revised international Chapel Hill consensus conference nomenclature of Vasculitides. Arthritis Rheumatol. 2018;70:171–84.
13. Goeser MR, Laniosz V, Wetter DA. A practical approach to the diagnosis, evaluation, and management of cutaneous small-vessel vasculitis. Am J Clin Dermatol. 2014;15:299–306.

Open Access This chapter is licensed under the terms of the Creative Commons Attribution-NonCommercial-NoDerivatives 4.0 International License (http://creativecommons.org/licenses/by-nc-nd/4.0/), which permits any non-commercial use, sharing, distribution and reproduction in any medium or format, as long as you give appropriate credit to the original author(s) and the source, provide a link to the Creative Commons license and indicate if you modified the licensed material. You do not have permission under this license to share adapted material derived from this chapter or parts of it.

The images or other third party material in this chapter are included in the chapter's Creative Commons license, unless indicated otherwise in a credit line to the material. If material is not included in the chapter's Creative Commons license and your intended use is not permitted by statutory regulation or exceeds the permitted use, you will need to obtain permission directly from the copyright holder.

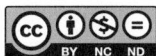

Necrobiosis Lipoidica

Miruna Negulescu

30.1 Introduction

Necrobiosis lipoidica (NL) is a rare chronic granulomatous skin disease usually associated with diabetes mellitus, especially type 1 [1].

In 1930, Oppenheim first described and called it dermatitis atrophicans lipoidica diabetica [2]. It was then named necrobiosis lipoidica diabeticorum (NLD) by Urbach in 1932 [3]. The several cases of NLD described in nondiabetic patients led to deletion of "diabetes" word from the denomination [2].

The relationship between NL and diabetes mellitus is still debated. First, the link has been established by studies from the 1960s, which showed diabetes or abnormal glucose metabolism in over 60% of patients with NL [4]. Since the 1960s, no prevalence-based studies on NL have been conducted. Thereby, most studies are based on the 65% incidence in their work [4].

Despite the increased prevalence of NL in diabetics, NL has also been met in patients with normal glycemia, autoimmune thyroiditis, rheumatoid arthritis, sarcoidosis, inflammatory bowel disease, and monoclonal gammopathy [4].

M. Negulescu (✉)
Department of Dermatology, Hôpital Erasme,
Université Libre de Bruxelles, Brussel, Belgium
e-mail: miruna.negulescu@ulb.ac.be

30.2 Epidemiology

This pathology affects 0.3–1.2% of the diabetic population with a female predominance (female-to-male ratio 3:1) [1, 4]. The early symptoms start typically in type 1 diabetic adults during the third decade of life and the fourth decade in type 2 or nondiabetic people [4]. In up to 14% of cases, diagnosis of diabetes is realized after NL lesions, in up to 24% is simultaneously made, and in 62% of cases occurs before NL lesions [4].

30.3 Pathogenesis and Histology

The pathogenesis of NL is still controversial. The diabetic microangiopathy has been involved [1, 4, 5]. An initial immune complex-mediated vasculitis is suggested by the presence of immunoglobulin M deposits, C3, and fibrin in the vessel walls in direct immunofluorescence [1, 2].

Histologically, a collagen degeneration, granulomatous formation, fat deposition, and thickening of blood vessel walls are described [2, 4, 5].

30.4 Clinical Findings and Complications

Initial alterations present as papules and nodules matching to form yellow-brown, nonpainful patches, with active raised and erythematous borders (Figs. 30.1 and 30.2). The center is atrophic,

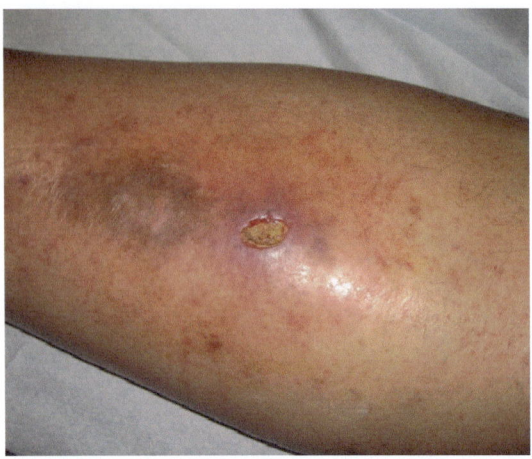

Fig. 30.1 Two lesions. The first one in the left side on the picture is atrophic, white center surrounded by brown borders. The second one showed ulcerative center containing fibrin, surrounded by erythematous, active borders

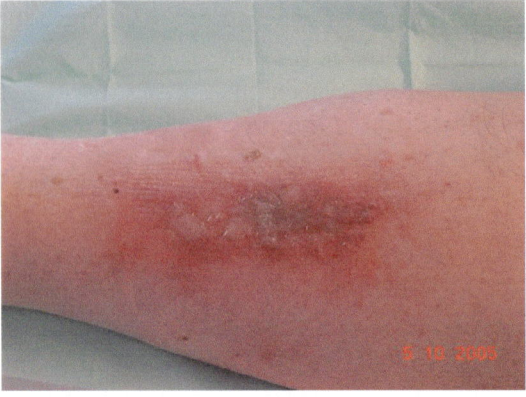

Fig. 30.2 Waxy, smooth, white plaque surrounded by erythematous borders

first appearing red-brown and becoming yellow-orange and smooth. Sometimes, telangiectasia may occur [1, 4, 5].

As mentioned, the lesions are mostly painless due to nerve damage, but ulcerated lesions may cause pain. These ones may occur following minor trauma in up to 35% of cases [4].

In 90% of patients, NL arises on legs, bilaterally and symmetrically [1]. Less frequently, lesions may appear on the scalp, face, trunk, forearms, and penis, which are less considered associated with diabetes mellitus [1, 5].

The progression is slow, and sometimes regression of lesions may happen in 20% of cases [1]. The main complication is ulceration [1, 4] with secondary infection [6]. Some exceptional cases of squamous cell carcinoma have been reported in long-standing NL [1, 4]. The origin of malignant transformation is even unclear [4].

30.5 Treatment

The first step is to prevent lesions by avoidance of trauma [2]. Indeed, NL may also occur by Koebner effect, in addition to ulceration risk [2, 4]. Control of diabetes seems to be without any improvement [1, 4, 5].

Several treatments have been tested with random results. Most of them are based on case reports.

Treatment by topical corticosteroids is effective to prevent progression and reduce inflammatory process, especially on the active borders [1, 2, 4, 5].

Wound care is highly important in NL. Infected wounds must be treated by antiseptics and adapted dressings [2]. Sometimes, systemic antibiotics are helpful [4].

Ulcerated NLs are improved by granulocyte-macrophage colony-stimulating factor [4].

An association of aspirin and dipyridamole was suggested as NL treatment, but no trial has showed any improvement [2, 4]. The use of low-dose aspirin did not suggest any benefit in another trial [4].

The use of stanozolol, ticlopidine, inositol nicotinate, pentoxifylline, and prostaglandin E1 seemed to have beneficial effects [2, 4].

Psoralen plus ultraviolet A (PUVA) therapy also seems to be successful. One study of ten patients with NL showed 100% healing rate after 47 sessions [4].

Tests with methyl aminolevulinate photodynamic therapy have been unsuccessful [4].

Some immunomodulatory drugs like oral cyclosporine and mycophenolate mofetil have been tested on ulcerating NL and showed improvement of lesions. In both cases, recurrence occurred after cessation of treatment [2, 4]. Infliximab, thalidomide, and etanercept also have been tested, with beneficial results [2, 4].

Surgery is not recommended in the NL treatment because of Koebnerized lesions on surgical scars [2, 4]. Usually, lesions are excised down to deep fascia or periosteum to prevent recurrences [2, 4]. The defect is filled by skin graft. Cosmetic results after removal of lesions in these areas are substantial [2].

Occasionally, pulse dye lasers have been tested to treat telangiectasia, with mixed results [4].

References

1. Bessis D, et al. Manifestations dermatologiques des maladies d'organes, vol. 4. France: Springer-Verlag, Paris. Chap. 76-4-5
2. Kota SK, et al. Necrobiosis lipoidica diabeticorum: a case-based review of literature. Indian J Endocrinol Metab. 2012;16(4):614–20.
3. Sehgal VN, Bhattacharya SN, Verma P. Juvenile, insulin-dependent diabetes mellitus, type 1-related dermatoses. J Eur Acad Dermatol. 2011;25:625–36.
4. Reid SD, et al. Update on necrobiosis lipoidica: a review of etiology, diagnosis, and treatment options. J Am Acad Dermatol. 2013;63:783–91.
5. Callen JP, Jorizzo JL. Dermatological signs of internal disease. 4th ed. Philadelphia: W.B. Saunders.
6. Behm B, Schreml S, Landthaler M, Babilas P. Skin signs in diabetes mellitus. J Eur Acad Dermatol. 2012;26:1203–11.

Open Access This chapter is licensed under the terms of the Creative Commons Attribution-NonCommercial-NoDerivatives 4.0 International License (http://creativecommons.org/licenses/by-nc-nd/4.0/), which permits any non-commercial use, sharing, distribution and reproduction in any medium or format, as long as you give appropriate credit to the original author(s) and the source, provide a link to the Creative Commons license and indicate if you modified the licensed material. You do not have permission under this license to share adapted material derived from this chapter or parts of it.

The images or other third party material in this chapter are included in the chapter's Creative Commons license, unless indicated otherwise in a credit line to the material. If material is not included in the chapter's Creative Commons license and your intended use is not permitted by statutory regulation or exceeds the permitted use, you will need to obtain permission directly from the copyright holder.

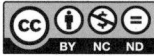

Purpura Fulminans

31

Nancy Hajjar and Véronique Del Marmol

31.1 Introduction

Purpura fulminans is a rare life-threatening condition often associated with disseminated intravascular coagulation leading to vast skin necrosis and tissue thrombosis [1–3].

It is generally seen in neonates with homozygous protein C or S deficiency. An acquired form of protein C deficiency in the context of infection and septicemia can also trigger this condition [1–3].

31.2 Epidemiology

There are three main subtypes of purpura fulminans:

1. The neonatal form with a prevalence of 1:1,000,000 births [3].
2. The infectious form with variable prevalence and a predilection to some bacteria. It mainly occurs in meningococcal infections where PF complicates in 10–20% of cases, followed by streptococcal pneumonia. Varicella is the most common viral infection causing PF, but cases remain very rare. Fewer publications report relatively less virulent germs.

   COVID-19 infection was also reported as a triggering infectious agent of PF [3–5]. In addition, one case of purpura fulminans associated with COVID-19 vaccination was described, manifesting 6 weeks after the vaccine [6].
3. The idiopathic form is very exceptional with only a few cases reported [3, 7].

31.3 When to Suspect Purpura Fulminans

- Neonates who develop extensive ecchymoses especially in the first days of life followed by diffuse arterial and venous thrombosis. Later presentation in infancy is also reported.
- Retiform purpuric skin lesions in the context of sepsis (mainly severe meningococcal infection) associated with severe cutaneous pain out of proportion with the physical exam.

31.4 Pathogenesis

In the three forms of purpura fulminans, the coagulation balance is disrupted in favor of procoagulant factors [1–3].

1. Neonatal: Inherited deficiency of protein C/S or antithrombin III, which are anticoagulant

N. Hajjar (✉)
Department of Dermatology, CHU Henri Mondor, Créteil, France

V. Del Marmol
Department of Dermatology, Université libre de Bruxelles (ULB), Hôpital Universitaire de Bruxelles (H.U.B.), CUB Hôpital Erasme, Brussels, Belgium

factors, will lead to microvascular thrombosis and hemorrhagic necrosis [3, 8].
2. Infectious: In this form, secondary consumption of protein C is the speculated process [3, 9].
3. Idiopathic: A postinfectious autoimmune mechanism is suspected in this entity during which mainly a relative insufficiency of protein S is observed due to anti-protein S antibody formation [3, 7].

31.5 Clinical Presentation

PF usually starts with ill-defined painful erythema centered by bluish necrosis. Sometimes, bullous lesions can be seen. In advanced stages, sensitivity is lost, and necrosis becomes very extensive [1–3].

The patient is often septic with signs of shock (hypotension, tachycardia, altered mental status, weak peripheral pulses) and/or signs of end-organ damage.

Since DIC often complicates PF, bleeding from intravenous lines and mucous membranes can be seen [1–3].

31.5.1 Workup

In the neonatal form: The dosage of protein C and protein S activity is the recommended diagnostic tool. If feasible, genetic testing allows the confirmation of this entity [8, 10].

In the infectious form: Complete sepsis workup is important to treat the causative agent, with sometimes the need for extensive laboratory exams, imaging, and repeated cultures.

This conventional workup is not satisfactory in all cases. Bacterial polymerase chain reaction (PCR) on skin biopsy is now practicable and allows etiological diagnosis rapidly. Thus, biopsy of a purpura lesion with direct examination, culture, and PCR is now recommended [2].

A DIC workup is mandatory including platelet count, PT, PTT, D-dimer, fibrinogen, and blood smear [3].

31.5.2 Management

Hydration and supportive care are very important in all the forms of PF to avoid end-organ damage. In addition, frequent assessment of necrosis status for early surgical debridement is necessary.

1. In the neonatal form: The mainstream of treatment consists of protein C/S supplementation in addition to fresh frozen plasma (FFP) [3, 10, 11].
2. In the infectious form: Broad-spectrum antibiotics are used (generally carbapenem or vancomycin + beta-lactam-beta-lactamase inhibitor +/− clindamycin).

    Intravenous immunoglobulin therapy and activated protein C supplementation can be beneficial.

    Anticoagulation is discussed in every case based on the occurrence of DIC [1–3].
3. In the idiopathic form: In addition to the previously mentioned strategies, systemic corticosteroids can be discussed [3, 7].

31.5.3 Differential Diagnosis

In front of a necrotic skin process and an ill patient, one should consider the following main differential diagnoses: [3]

- Vasculitis
- Coumadin-induced skin necrosis
- Meningococcemia
- Calciphylaxis
- Necrotizing fasciitis

31.6 Long-Term Sequelae of Purpura Fulminans

Many patients with purpura fulminans require extensive debridement, fasciotomy, or even amputation. Thus, qualitative rehabilitation is very important to decrease neurological and psychological long-term outcomes.

In neonates, severe protein C deficiency is associated with neurological and ophthalmological complications, mainly epilepsy, cerebral palsy, delayed psychomotor development, and blindness. It also requires long-term protein C supplementation and/or anticoagulation. Liver transplantation can be a curative option in some cases [1].

Take Home Messages

- PF is a life-threatening condition with high morbidity and mortality.
- PF can begin very subtly: bruising in neonates and petechial rash in an infectious context should lead to PF consideration.
- Early diagnosis is crucial to avoid end-organ damage.
- A multidisciplinary approach is necessary with adequate supportive care, etiological treatment, as well as surgical consultation early in the necrotic process.

References

1. Chalmers E, Cooper P, Forman K, Grimley C, Khair K, Minford A, Morgan M, Mumford AD. Purpura fulminans: recognition, diagnosis and management. Arch Dis Child. 2011;96(11):1066–71. https://doi.org/10.1136/adc.2010.199919. Epub 2011 Jan 12.
2. Contou D, de Prost N. Purpura fulminans de l'adulte [Purpura fulminans in adult patients]. Rev Prat. 2023;73(1):71–8.
3. Perera TB, Murphy-Lavoie HM. Purpura fulminans. In: StatPearls. Treasure Island (FL): StatPearls Publishing; 2023.
4. Watanabe Y, Abe T. Purpura fulminans due to pneumococcal infection. J Gen Fam Med. 2017;18(6):458–9. https://doi.org/10.1002/jgf2.105.
5. Khan IA, Karmakar S, Chakraborty U, Sil A, Chandra A. Purpura fulminans as the presenting manifestation of COVID-19. Postgrad Med J. 2021;97(1149):473. https://doi.org/10.1136/postgradmedj-2020-139202. Epub 2021 Feb 9. PMID: 33563711; PMCID: PMC7878050.
6. Griss J, Eichinger S, Winkler S, Weninger W, Petzelbauer P. A case of COVID-19 vaccination-associated forme fruste purpura fulminans. Br J Dermatol. 2022;186(1):e1. https://doi.org/10.1111/bjd.20744. Epub 2021 Sep 28. PMID: 34585371; PMCID: PMC8652590.
7. Bektas F, Soyuncu S. Idiopathic purpura fulminans. Am J Emerg Med. 2011;29(4):475.e5–6.
8. Irfan Kazi SG, Siddiqui E, Habib I, Tabassum S, Afzal B, Khan IQ. Neonatal purpura fulminans, a rare genetic disorder due to protein C deficiency: a case report. J Pak Med Assoc. 2018;68(3):463–5.
9. Colling ME, Bendapudi PK. Purpura fulminans: mechanism and management of dysregulated hemostasis. Transfus Med Rev. 2018;32(2):69–76.
10. Price VE, Ledingham DL, Krümpel A, Chan AK. Diagnosis and management of neonatal purpura fulminans. Semin Fetal Neonatal Med. 2011;16(6):318–22. https://doi.org/10.1016/j.siny.2011.07.009. Epub 2011 Aug 11.
11. Kizilocak H, Ozdemir N, Dikme G, Koc B, Celkan T. Homozygous protein C deficiency presenting as neonatal purpura fulminans: management with fresh frozen plasma, low molecular weight heparin and protein C concentrate. J Thromb Thrombolysis. 2018;45(2):315–8.

Open Access This chapter is licensed under the terms of the Creative Commons Attribution-NonCommercial-NoDerivatives 4.0 International License (http://creativecommons.org/licenses/by-nc-nd/4.0/), which permits any non-commercial use, sharing, distribution and reproduction in any medium or format, as long as you give appropriate credit to the original author(s) and the source, provide a link to the Creative Commons license and indicate if you modified the licensed material. You do not have permission under this license to share adapted material derived from this chapter or parts of it.

The images or other third party material in this chapter are included in the chapter's Creative Commons license, unless indicated otherwise in a credit line to the material. If material is not included in the chapter's Creative Commons license and your intended use is not permitted by statutory regulation or exceeds the permitted use, you will need to obtain permission directly from the copyright holder.

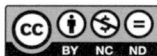

Protein C and Protein S Deficiencies

32

Sébastien Humbert and Philippe Humbert

32.1 Physiopathology

Protein C and protein S are vitamin K-dependent proteins with natural anticoagulant properties that play a major role in the coagulation pathway. Protein C is activated by the thrombin/thrombomodulin complex. Activated protein C cleaves membrane-bound active factors V and VIII and inactivates them. Protein C inhibitor and α-1 antitrypsin are the main inhibitors of protein C. Protein S is a cofactor of activated protein C and can also directly bond to activated factors V and X.

Protein C and protein S deficiencies manifest usually as recurrent venous thromboembolism with an annual incidence of recurrent venous thromboembolism of 6.0% and 8.4%, respectively. A severe deficiency can cause skin necrosis, especially in newborns as a purpura fulminans. The cause of protein C and protein S can be genetically determined or acquired (Table 32.1).

Table 32.1 Causes of protein C and protein S acquired deficiency

Acquired protein C deficiency	Acquired protein S deficiency
Vitamin K antagonist, vitamin K deficiency	Vitamin K antagonist, vitamin K deficiency
Hepatic insufficiency	Hepatic insufficiency
Disseminated intravascular coagulation	Disseminated intravascular coagulation
Autoimmune syndrome	Pregnancy
L-Asparaginase therapy	Autoimmune syndrome
	AIDS, varicella zoster virus
	Nephrotic syndrome

32.2 Diagnosis

- *Medical context*:

  – In newborns, homozygote protein C or protein S deficiency manifests in fatal purpura fulminans.
  – In adults with heterozygous protein C or protein S deficiency, introduction of vitamin K antagonist can induce skin necrosis within 3–5 days.

- *Semiology*
  – A massive thrombosis of the dermic vascular network can lead to large ecchymotic

S. Humbert
Department of Internal Medicine, University Hospital, Besancon, France
e-mail: shumbert@chu-besancon.fr

P. Humbert (✉)
Department of Dermatology, University Hospital, Besancon, France

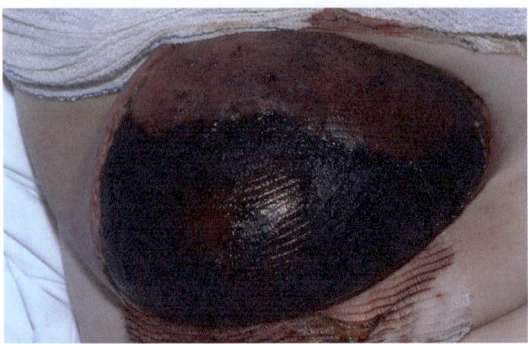

Picture 32.1 Skin necrosis of the breast after introduction of VKA

patches that can evolve to hemorrhagic bullae and then irreversible necrosis.
- When vitamin K antagonists are involved, lesions are located in areas where the fat layer is the thickest: breast, thighs, abdomen, and buttocks. Genital involvement is also possible in men (Picture 32.1).

- *Biology*: Increase in INR (international normalized ratio) and prothrombin time (if vitamin K antagonist), decrease or even collapse in protein C or protein S.
- *Histology*: We can observe obstructive thrombosis of capillaries and venules, vascular fibrin deposition, and dermal and fat tissue diffuse necrosis.

32.3 Treatment

- Prevent pain (morphines)
- Prevent infection
- Stop vitamin K antagonist and vitamin K administration
- Heparin therapy
- Protein C concentrate
- Adapted local treatment: surgical excision of necrotic tissue and transplant

Open Access This chapter is licensed under the terms of the Creative Commons Attribution-NonCommercial-NoDerivatives 4.0 International License (http://creativecommons.org/licenses/by-nc-nd/4.0/), which permits any non-commercial use, sharing, distribution and reproduction in any medium or format, as long as you give appropriate credit to the original author(s) and the source, provide a link to the Creative Commons license and indicate if you modified the licensed material. You do not have permission under this license to share adapted material derived from this chapter or parts of it.

The images or other third party material in this chapter are included in the chapter's Creative Commons license, unless indicated otherwise in a credit line to the material. If material is not included in the chapter's Creative Commons license and your intended use is not permitted by statutory regulation or exceeds the permitted use, you will need to obtain permission directly from the copyright holder.

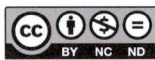

Renal Insufficiency and Necrosis

Elia Ricci

Renal insufficiency in itself is found to be correlated indirectly to cutaneous necroses. In fact, renal insufficiency may cause complications, which in turn lead to the formation of gangrenous cutaneous pathologies.

Renal insufficiency is classified into five progressive stages based on the values of glomerular filtration. Table 33.1 shows the KDOQI classification [1]. Alterations at the cutaneous level begin from stage III onward and become progressively more severe until they become evident in the so-called final stage. Renal disease itself leads to cutaneous alterations that may be summarised as follows:

- Xerosis: Beginning with dehydration and reddening, prevalently in the areas of the extensor muscles of the limbs, progressively evolving into oedema and fissures. In the most advanced stages, there may be areas of lichenification and/or contact erythema. The fissured areas may allow bacteria to enter with consequent cutaneous infections. This form afflicts from 50 to 70% of patients in dialysis.
- Pigmentary disorders: These are directly correlated to the duration of the renal insufficiency. They range from hyperpigmentation to a yellowish colouring, prevalently in the areas exposed to the sun. Pallor is associated with frequent anaemia in such patients. This form afflicts from 20 to 70% of patients in dialytic treatment.
- Itching: Frequent in some patients and may be minimal, but in 8% of cases, it is found to be non-remittent and serious. It leads to a net deterioration in the quality of life.

Another clinical situation of a dermatological type is nephrogenic dermal fibrosis (NDF), described in 2000 [2] and currently classified as systemic [3]. It is a pathology that is prevalently cutaneous and characterised by being associated with renal damage. Patients present oedemas and retractions prevalently in the lower limbs; the main symptoms are burning pain and itching. On a cutaneous level, there is the appearance of papules or plaques that are red or brown in colour and which, on rare occasions, may become ulcerous (Fig. 33.1). Around 5% of these forms may exhibit aggressive and sudden worsening with the involvement of muscles, possibly leading to paralysis. As of now, the cause remains poorly defined: possible causes may include the use of gadolinium as a means of contrast [4], erythropoietin, and stages of hypercoagulability. Under X-ray inspection, diffuse calcifications are noted on a subcutaneous level (Fig. 33.2).

End-stage renal insufficiency (ESRD) in itself behaves as a form of comorbidity in preexisting situations causing complications that lead to the formation of necrotic tissues, as well as exacerbation in the appearance of cutaneous ulcerous lesions. Lastly, as a direct cause, it leads to complications that progress to ulcers.

E. Ricci (✉)
Difficult Wound Healing Unit, Clinica Eporediese Monza"s Policlinic Group, Ivrea, Italy
e-mail: eliaricci@tin.it

Table 33.1 KDOQI classification

Stage	GFR*	Description	Treatment stage
1	90+	Normal kidney function but urine findings or structural abnormalities or genetic trait point to kidney disease	Observation, control of blood pressure. More on management of Stages 1 and 2 CKD.
2	60-89	Mildly reduced kidney function, and other findings (as for stage 1) point to kidney disease	Observation, control of blood pressure and risk factors. More on management of Stages 1 and 2 CKD.
3A 3B	45-59 30-44	Moderately reduced kidney function	Observation, control of blood pressure and risk factors. More on management of Stage 3 CKD.
4	15-29	Severely reduced kidney function	Planning for endstage renal failure. More on management of Stages 4 and 5 CKD.
5	<15 or on dialysis	Very severe, or **endstage** kidney failure (sometimes call **established renal failure**)	Treatment choices. More on management of Stages 4 and 5 CKD.

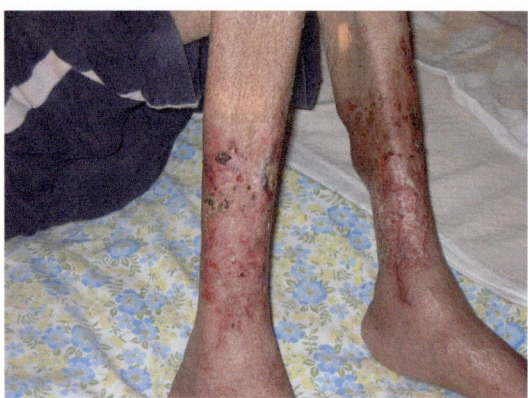

Fig. 33.1 Nephrogenic dermal fibrosis (NDF)

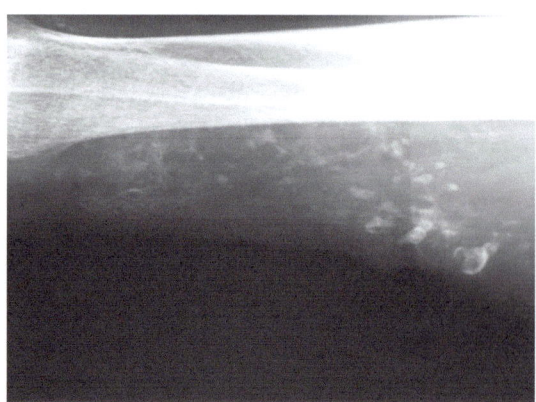

Fig. 33.2 Subcutaneous calcification in NDF

33.1 Comorbidity

ESRD in itself leads to a state of fragility in the patient, with reduction of the immune system defences and consequently a greater incidence of infective phenomena. The reduction in renal clearing leads to an accumulation of catabolites that in themselves have an inflammatory action. A situation of increased phlogosis means healing times are lengthened, with a slowing down both of the retraction and the re-epithelialisation phenomena. Some examples are the following: the frequent association with diabetes leads to a prognostic deterioration with an increase in the number of amputations and the evolution in a necrotic direction of the diabetic foot [5, 6]. Patients who have been in dialysis for long periods present a high rate of arterial disease which, with the phenomena of vascular calcinosis, may lead to the development of cutaneous necrotic ulcers of an arterial type [7]. Al Ghazal [8] also suggests a correlation with the development of forms such as pyoderma gangrenosum. Yates [9] has noted an increase in infections from MRSA in patients who have ulcers with ESRD. The cutaneous blood flow is significantly reduced in dialysis patients compared with healthy control group [10]. Tercercedor [11] suggests that the frequency of malignant skin tumours is increased in dialysis patients; he describes skin carcinomatous lesions in 2.4% of patients. In severe case, kidney transplantation can reverse the skin lesions and overcome the symptoms improving the quality of life [12, 13].

33.2 Exacerbation

The forms in which we may define ESRD as exacerbation are forms in which there is a net increase in the incidence of cutaneous ulcerous disease in the presence of the combination. These are not actual syndromes, because there is no direct cause-effect relationship, but the frequent association, besides complicating the situation, leads to a therapeutic approach that must be combined.

The antiphospholipid antibody form, of itself, besides the cutaneous damage involved, may lead to renal damage. There is therefore an effect on negative synergic terms between the two forms [14], which on the one hand can lead to a worsening of the nephrological situation while on the other, in patients with ESRD and cutaneous damage, the form of hypercoagulability facilitates the development of ulcers [15] (Fig. 33.3) (see Chap. 18).

Ulcers from anticoagulants, or cutaneous necrosis from anticoagulants, are particularly frequent in patients with renal insufficiency. The increase in the coagulation time, combined with the reduced capacity for elimination of the medicine, facilitates the development of haematomas. The skin, modified in the presence of ESRD to become more rigid and fragile, tends to be damaged more easily in the case of even minor traumas. A haematoma, which itself tends to compress the skin, can easily lead to the onset of necrotic phenomena (see Chap. 13). The same mechanism is involved in the use of heparin, especially in patients subjected to dialytic treatment.

Some vasculitic forms are characterised by contemporaneous damage at the level of the renal glomerular, such as in the antiphospholipid antibody form, involving a synergic effect. The coagulative disorders, damage on a cutaneous level secondary to ESRD, lead to a vicious circle that moves beyond the simple situation of underlying comorbidity (see Chap. 20).

33.3 Direct Cause

Patients with systemic vasculitis may simultaneously develop necrotising skin lesions and kidney injury in the form of acute glomerulonephritis [16]. A broad spectrum of autoimmune disorders may be responsible for the above manifestations, including systemic lupus erythematosus, antineutrophil cytoplasmic antibody (ANCA) vasculitis, cryoglobulinaemia, cryofibrinogenaemia, and polyarteritis nodosa.

The ulcerous form directly linked to ESRD is the so-called calciphylaxis or calcified uraemic arteritis (CUA). This is a rare ulcerous form often with an inauspicious prognosis, which begins with necrotic cutaneous ulcerations with undefined edges (Fig. 33.4) and can spread extensively (see Chap. 14). Recognised risk factors for CUA include diabetes mellitus, poorly controlled secondary hyperparathyroidism along with the use of calcium-based phosphorus binders, obesity, female gender, history of RRT, white ethnicity, low albumin level, and impairment of the vitamin K pathway because of warfarin use [17]. CUA leads to substantial morbidity, prolonged hospitalisation, and mortality rates as high as 80%. The clinical presentation is frequently characterised by the development of proximal (and often symmetrical) lesions on the buttocks, thighs, and abdomen with less common involvement of the acral regions. Nonhealing wounds provide an opportunity for infection with multiple microorganisms and sepsis.

In a patient with ESRD, it is necessary to carry out a differential diagnosis, especially for the

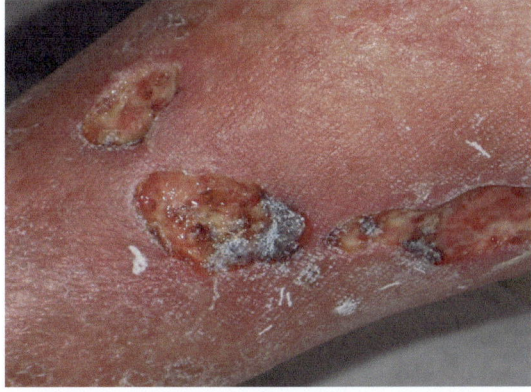

Fig. 33.3 Antiphospholipid antibody syndrome with ESRD V stage with skin ulcers

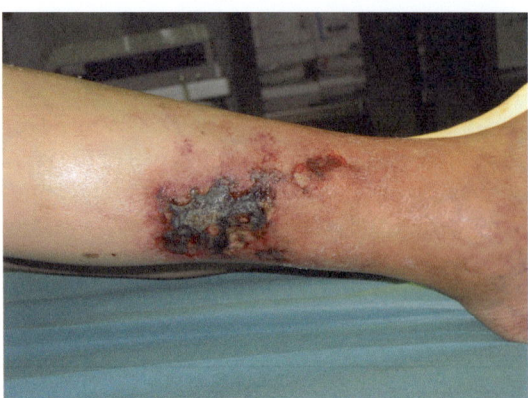

Fig. 33.4 Calciphylaxis, typical skin lesion

Table 33.2 Differential diagnosis of necrotic lesion on lower limb (from Dean, Vasc Med, 2008)

Antiphospholipid antibody syndrome
Calciphylaxis
Vasculitis
Atheroembolic disease
Warfarin skin necrosis
Heparin skin necrosis
Spider bites

atypical forms that affect the lower limbs [18]. The differential diagnosis in terms of pathologies that must be considered is illustrated in Table 33.2.

33.4 Treatment

Treatment is based on the re-equilibration of the renal situation through diet, diuretics, corticosteroids and/or immunosuppressants, dyalitic treatment, or transplant if indicated. The specific treatment of the various forms involves a correct diagnostic approach, with identification of the diverse pathological situation that has led to the cutaneous necrosis; for such treatments, see the specific paragraphs. Milas [19] suggests that an early recognition of calciphylaxis and multidisciplinary treatment, including wound debridement, parathyroidectomy, and appropriate arterial revascularisation, can lead to improved wound healing and limb salvage. Intravenous administration of sodium thiosulfate has shown some beneficial effects in terms of pain reduction and wound regression. Sodium thiosulfate increases the solubility of calcium deposits and possesses antioxidant and chelating properties, which alleviate systemic inflammation and increase the synthesis of inhibitors of extra-osseous calcification [20, 21].

References

1. http://www.kidney.org/professionals/kdoqi.
2. Cowper SE, Robin HS, Steinberg SM, Su LD, Gupta S, LeBoit PE. Scleromyxoedema-like cutaneous diseases in renal-dialysis patients. Lancet. 2000;356(9234):1000.
3. Swartz RD, Crofford LJ, Pam SH, Ike RW, Su LD. Nephrogenic fibrosing dermopathy: a novel cutaneous fibrosing disorder in patients with renal failure. Am J Med. 2003;114:563.
4. Grobner T. Gadolinium—a specific trigger for the development of nephrogenic fibrosing dermopathy and nephrogenic systemic fibrosis? Nephrol Dial Transplant. 2006;21:1104.
5. Venermo M, Biancari F, Arvela E, Korhonen M, Soderstrom M, Halesmaki K, Alback A, Lepantalo M. The role of chronic kidney disease as predictor of outcome after revascularization of the ulcerated diabetic foot. Diabetologia. 2011;54(12):2971.
6. Ndip A, Rutter MK, Vileikyte L, Vardhan A, Asari A, Jameel M, Tahir HA, Lavery LA, Boulton AJ. Dialysis treatment is an independent risk factor for foot ulceration in patients with diabetes and stage 4 or 5 chronic kidney disease. Diabetes Care. 2010;33(8):1811.
7. Chan YL, Mahony JF, Turner JJ, Posen S. The vascular lesions associated with skin necrosis in renal disease. Br J Dermatol. 1983;109(1):85.
8. Al Ghazal P, Korber A, Klode J, Dissemond J. Investigation of new co-factors in 49 patients with pyoderma gangrenosum. J Dtsch Dermatol Res. 2012;10(4):251.
9. Yates C, May K, Hale T, Allard B, Rowling N, Freeman A, Harrison J, McCan J, Wraight P. Wound chronicity, inpatients care, and chronic kidney disease predispose to MRSA infection in diabetic foot ulcers. Diabetes Care. 1907;32(10):2009.
10. Taylor JE, Belch JJ, Henderson I, Steward WK. Peripheral microcirculatory blood flow in haemodialysis patients treated with erythropoietin. Int Angiol. 1996;15:33–8.
11. Tercercedor J, Lopez-Hernandez B, Rodenas JM, Delgado-Rodriguez M, Cerezo S, Serrano-Ortega SA. Multivariate analysis of cutaneous markers

of aging in chronic hemodialyzed patients. Int J Dermatol. 1995;34:546–50.
12. Avermaete A, Altmeyer P, Bacharach-Bhules M. Skin changes in dialysis patients: a review. Nephrol Dial Transplant. 2001;16:2293–6.
13. Maroz N, Simman R. Wound healing in patients with impaired kidney function. J Am Coll Clin Wound Spec. 2014;5:2–7.
14. Griffiths MH, Papadaki L, Neild GH. The renal pathology of primary antiphospholipid syndrome: a distinctive form of endothelial injury. QJM. 2000;93(7):457.
15. Rollino C, Boero R, Elia F, Montaruli B, Massara C, Beltrame G. Antiphospholipid antibodies and hypertension. Lupus. 2004;13:769.
16. Floege J, Johnson RJ, Feehally J. Comprehensive clinical nephrology. 4th ed. Elsevier; 2010. p. 292–307.
17. Sethi S, Sethi N. Wound healing in renal impairment. Int J Curr Res. 2017;9(6):52029–34.
18. Dean SM. Atypical ischemic lower extremity ulcerations: a differential diagnosis. Vasc Med. 2008;13:47.
19. Milas M, Bush RL, Lin P, Brown K, Mackay G, Lumsden A, Weber C, Dodson TF. Calciphylaxis and nonhealing wounds: the role of the vascular surgeon in a multidisciplinary treatment. J Vasc Surg. 2003;37(3):501–7.
20. Ross E. Evolution of treatment strategies for calciphylaxis. Am J Nephrol. 2011;34:460–7.
21. Hayden M, Goldsmith D. Sodium thiosulfate: new hope for the treatment of calciphylaxis. Semin Dial. 2010;23(3):258–62.

Open Access This chapter is licensed under the terms of the Creative Commons Attribution-NonCommercial-NoDerivatives 4.0 International License (http://creativecommons.org/licenses/by-nc-nd/4.0/), which permits any non-commercial use, sharing, distribution and reproduction in any medium or format, as long as you give appropriate credit to the original author(s) and the source, provide a link to the Creative Commons license and indicate if you modified the licensed material. You do not have permission under this license to share adapted material derived from this chapter or parts of it.

The images or other third party material in this chapter are included in the chapter's Creative Commons license, unless indicated otherwise in a credit line to the material. If material is not included in the chapter's Creative Commons license and your intended use is not permitted by statutory regulation or exceeds the permitted use, you will need to obtain permission directly from the copyright holder.

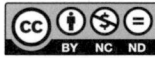

Calciphylaxis

Mariam Kabbani, Véronique Del Marmol, and Farida Benhadou

34.1 Introduction

Calciphylaxis is a rare cause of skin ischemia and necrosis with an estimated 6-month mortality rate of 57% [1, 2]. Although the exact pathogenesis remains unclear, calcification of dermal and subcutaneous capillaries and arterioles plays an integral role, as suggested by the histology [3]. End-stage renal disease is the main risk factor [4]. Since therapeutic modalities are extrapolated from observational retrospective studies, case series, and expert opinion, management is yet to be standardized [5, 6].

34.2 Risk Factors

The main risk factor of calciphylaxis is end-stage renal disease (ESRD). Therefore, most other predictive risk factors were studied in ESRD patients on hemodialysis, and they include female sex, diabetes mellitus, obesity, hypercalcemia, hyperphosphatemia, hyperparathyroidism, nutritional vitamin D, vitamin K deficiency, and warfarin treatment [4]. Additional risk factors were observed in patients with normal renal function comprising malignancies, chemotherapy, connective tissue disease, hepatic cirrhosis, protein C or S deficiency, rapid weight loss, hypoalbuminemia, systemic corticosteroid use, and infection [7, 8]. However, most patients with these risk factors do not develop calciphylaxis; therefore, it has been suggested that some events such as repetitive skin trauma might act as a trigger. This is supported by the observation that the risk of calciphylaxis is augmented not only in diabetic patients receiving insulin injections compared to those not getting any injections, but also with the increase in daily injections received [4]. Nonetheless, in most patients, no trigger can be found.

34.3 Clinical Manifestation

Calciphylaxis presents with painful skin lesions starting usually as indurated plaques with overlying livedo racemosa. Pain is often out of proportion with the clinical picture, and it might even precede the appearance of the skin lesions. The presence of a dusky skin discoloration is a sign of imminent necrosis. The plaques then progress to satellite-shaped nonhealing ulcers with black eschars [1, 9]. Calciphylaxis can be classified as central or peripheral. Central calciphylaxis involves central body regions rich in adipose tissue such as the abdomen and thighs, whereas peripheral calciphylaxis is confined to peripheral areas with limited adipose tissue such as the fingers. Furthermore, it can be classified as uremic or nonuremic. Although both latter subtypes have

M. Kabbani · V. Del Marmol · F. Benhadou (✉)
Université libre de Bruxelles (ULB), Hôpital Universitaire de Bruxelles (H.U.B.), CUB Hôpital Erasme, Brussels, Belgium
e-mail: Farida.BENHADOU@erasme.ulb.ac.be

the same clinical presentation, uremic patients more likely have central calciphylaxis [1].

34.4 Pathophysiology

The pathogenesis of calciphylaxis remains unclear, but the reduced blood flow is thought to firstly result from the calcification of dermal and subcutaneous arterioles. Medial calcification is caused by ectopic bone formation by vascular smooth muscle cells. These cells transform, in response to hyperphosphatemia, hypercalcemia, and hyperglycemia, into osteoblast-like cells capable of producing hydroxyapatite crystals. Moreover, there also exists a relative deficiency of calcification inhibitors including matrix gla protein, whose carboxylation is vitamin K dependent, and fetuin-A, which is decreased in chronic inflammatory conditions such as chronic kidney disease [1, 5]. Finally, thrombosis develops in the lumens of these vessels leading to tissue ischemia and infarction. Thrombosis could be promoted by a local prothrombotic state due to endothelial dysfunction and intimal fibrosis, but it can also be explained by systemic hypercoagulable conditions. It has been demonstrated that calciphylaxis patients have high prevalence of protein C and S deficiency, lupus anticoagulant, and antithrombin deficiency [10].

34.5 Diagnosis

There are no universally accepted diagnostic criteria for calciphylaxis. Clinical suspicion is critical, and skin biopsy is the standard confirmational method, especially in early stages of the disease and in nonuremic patients. Nonetheless, taking into account the risk of infection and provoking new nonhealing ulcers, a biopsy is often not needed for an ESRD patient presenting with painful necrotic ulcers covered by an eschar. The biopsy of an active margin by the double-punch technique is the preferred procedure in which a 4–6 mm punch is inserted in the center of the defect produced by an 8 mm punch in order to retrieve deep subcutaneous tissue. A single punch has a high risk for false-negative results, while an excisional biopsy carries the risk of ulceration and necrosis [1, 5].

Histopathological features vary with the different clinical stages of the disease. Prior to the development of purpuric plaques, biopsies of indurated tender lesions demonstrate trace calcifications in capillaries and extravascular structures highlighted by von Kossa or Alizarin Red stains. However, when tissue necrosis is clinically visible, histopathological examination shows microthrombi and frank calcification of subcutaneous and dermal vessels. Other findings include intimal hyperplasia, extravascular soft tissue calcification, panniculitis, and epidermal necrosis with dermal–epidermal separation [3].

No laboratory test is specific for calciphylaxis, and even though hypercalcemia, hyperphosphatemia, and hyperparathyroidism are common, their absence does not exclude the diagnosis. Nonetheless, workup should include evaluation for the previously mentioned risk factors. Additionally, the role for imaging studies including radioactive bone scans remains unclear, but they may provide supportive findings in atypical cases with nondiagnostic biopsies [1, 5].

34.6 Treatment

Treatment is challenging and not standardized due to the lack of double-blind placebo-controlled clinical trials. Thus, it is advised to form a multidisciplinary team consisting of a dermatologist, nephrologist, surgeon, anesthesiologist specialized in pain management, and dietician with the goal of optimizing wound management, reducing the risk factors, and stopping the progression of vascular calcification [5].

Wound care centers on lesion protection with appropriate nonadhesive dressings and debridement of devitalized tissue to prevent infection and promote tissue regeneration. Early surgical debridement in calciphylaxis patients has been shown to increase survival at 6 months [2]. The use of adjunctive hyperbaric oxygen therapy is controversial; it is supported by positive outcomes from small observational studies, but a recent meta-analysis did not find any significant mortality benefit [6, 11]. Moreover, nutritional management and correction of anemia are required for optimal wound healing [6]. Furthermore, given the extremely painful nature of calciphylaxis lesions, pain control becomes integral with many patients requiring high doses of opioids [6].

Metabolic abnormalities should be corrected to maintain normal serum levels of calcium and phosphate. In addition to optimizing dialysis, this can be achieved by stopping calcium and vitamin D supplements and using non-calcium-based phosphate binders as sevelamer and lanthanum. The optimal level of parathyroid hormone is debated, but most experts agree on maintaining the level between 150 and 300 ng/mL. The use of cinacalcet, a calcimimetic that decreases parathyroid hormone levels, has been shown to decrease the incidence of calciphylaxis in dialysis patients and is thus recommended over parathyroidectomy. The latter treatment modality is controversial due to the risk of infection and hungry bone syndrome and is thus reserved for patients with hyperparathyroidism refractory to medical treatment [1, 5, 6].

Attention should be given to stopping any triggering medication including warfarin and systemic corticosteroids. If anticoagulation is deemed necessary, the use of apixaban or unfractionated heparin is recommended [5, 6].

The most commonly used first-line treatment in calciphylaxis is sodium thiosulfate. It is a calcium chelator and antioxidant that acts by decalcifying blood vessels, decreasing inflammation, and promoting vasodilation [5]. In hemodialysis patients, it is usually given during the last hour of the session according to a weight-based regimen wherein patients weighing more than 60 kg receive 25 g and those weighing less than 60 kg receive half the dose [5]. The duration of treatment depends on the clinical response, but usually lasts 3–6 months [1, 5, 6]. Regular electrocardiogram monitoring is advised due to the risk of QT prolongation. Intralesional sodium thiosulfate may be an alternative treatment in patients who cannot tolerate the medication systemically, albeit it is painful [6]. Although the efficacy of intravenous sodium thiosulfate is supported by case reports and a systematic review [12], a recent meta-analysis did not find a significant benefit on mortality [11]. Two clinical trials are ongoing to better study the efficacy and safety of sodium thiosulfate in calciphylaxis (Current Controlled Trials ISRCTN73380053 and ClinicalTrials.gov NCT03150420).

Finally, given the role of vitamin K deficiency in the pathogenesis of calciphylaxis by decreasing the levels of carboxylated matrix gla protein, a calcification inhibitor, vitamin K supplementation has been successfully used alone in the treatment of calciphylaxis [13]. Currently, a study of proof of concept for vitamin K1 is underway (ClinicalTrials.gov NCT02278692).

References

1. Nigwekar SU, Thadhani R, Brandenburg VM. Calciphylaxis. N Engl J Med. 2018;378(18):1704–14. https://doi.org/10.1056/NEJMra1505292.
2. McCarthy JT, el-Azhary RA, Patzelt MT, et al. Survival, risk factors, and effect of treatment in 101 patients with calciphylaxis. Mayo Clin Proc. 2016;91(10):1384–94. https://doi.org/10.1016/j.mayocp.2016.06.025.
3. Bahrani E, Perkins IU, North JP. Diagnosing calciphylaxis: a review with emphasis on histopathology. Am J Dermatopathol. 2020;42(7):471–80. https://doi.org/10.1097/DAD.0000000000001526.
4. Nigwekar SU, Zhao S, Wenger J, et al. A nationally representative study of calcific uremic arteriolopathy risk factors. J Am Soc Nephrol. 2016;27(11):3421–9. https://doi.org/10.1681/ASN.2015091065.
5. Chang JJ. Calciphylaxis: diagnosis, pathogenesis, and treatment. Adv Skin Wound Care. 2019;32(5):205–15. https://doi.org/10.1097/01.ASW.0000554443.14002.13.
6. Rick J, Rrapi R, Chand S, et al. Calciphylaxis: treatment and outlook-CME part II. J Am Acad Dermatol. 2022;86(5):985–92. https://doi.org/10.1016/j.jaad.2021.10.063.
7. Kalajian AH, Malhotra PS, Callen JP, Parker LP. Calciphylaxis with normal renal and parathyroid function: not as rare as previously believed. Arch Dermatol. 2009;145(4):602. https://doi.org/10.1001/archdermatol.2008.602.
8. Nigwekar SU, Wolf M, Sterns RH, Hix JK. Calciphylaxis from nonuremic causes: a systematic review. Clin J Am Soc Nephrol. 2008;3(4):1139–43. https://doi.org/10.2215/CJN.00530108.

9. Ghosh T, Winchester DS, Davis MDP, el-Azhary R, Comfere NI. Early clinical presentations and progression of calciphylaxis. Int J Dermatol. 2017;56(8):856–61. https://doi.org/10.1111/ijd.13622.
10. el-Azhary RA, Patzelt MT, McBane RD, et al. Calciphylaxis: a disease of pannicular thrombosis. Mayo Clin Proc. 2016;91(10):1395–402. https://doi.org/10.1016/j.mayocp.2016.06.026.
11. Udomkarnjananun S, Kongnatthasate K, Praditpornsilpa K, Eiam-Ong S, Jaber BL, Susantitaphong P. Treatment of calciphylaxis in CKD: a systematic review and meta-analysis. Kidney Int Rep. 2018;4(2):231–44. https://doi.org/10.1016/j.ekir.2018.10.002.
12. Peng T, Zhuo L, Wang Y, et al. Systematic review of sodium thiosulfate in treating calciphylaxis in chronic kidney disease patients: sodium thiosulphate and calciphylaxis. Nephrology. 2018;23(7):669–75. https://doi.org/10.1111/nep.13081.
13. Wajih Z, Singer R. Successful treatment of calciphylaxis with vitamin K in a patient on haemodialysis. Clin Kidney J. 2022;15(2):354–6. https://doi.org/10.1093/ckj/sfab209.

Open Access This chapter is licensed under the terms of the Creative Commons Attribution-NonCommercial-NoDerivatives 4.0 International License (http://creativecommons.org/licenses/by-nc-nd/4.0/), which permits any non-commercial use, sharing, distribution and reproduction in any medium or format, as long as you give appropriate credit to the original author(s) and the source, provide a link to the Creative Commons license and indicate if you modified the licensed material. You do not have permission under this license to share adapted material derived from this chapter or parts of it.

The images or other third party material in this chapter are included in the chapter's Creative Commons license, unless indicated otherwise in a credit line to the material. If material is not included in the chapter's Creative Commons license and your intended use is not permitted by statutory regulation or exceeds the permitted use, you will need to obtain permission directly from the copyright holder.

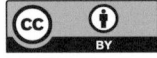

Livedo(id) Vasculitis

35

Farida Benhadou and Jean-Claude Wautrecht

35.1 Introduction [1]

Livedoid vasculitis (LV) is a rare vasculopathic disorder. Different names are used in the literature to define LV, and one of them is "atrophie blanche." Atrophie blanche is a confusing term because it is a sign that is frequently observed in chronic venous insufficiency and not specific for LV.

LV can occur at any age but is most commonly a disease of adulthood. LV can be divided into a primary or idiopathic form and a secondary form, which has been associated with other diseases.

Data in the literature concerning LV are limited and mainly based on the review of case reports.

35.2 Histology [1]

Usually, deposition of fibrinoid material in dermal vessels with secondary ischemic change of the overlying epidermis leads to ulceration.

F. Benhadou (✉)
Department of Dermatology, Hôpital Erasme,
Université Libre de Bruxelles, Brussels, Belgium

J.-C. Wautrecht
Department of Vascular Diseases, Hôpital Erasme,
Université Libre de Bruxelles, Brussels, Belgium

35.3 Pathogenesis [1, 2]

Pathogenesis is not fully elucidated. Several hypotheses have been proposed:

- Defective endothelial cell synthesis of tissue plasminogen activator and/or prostacyclin
- Dysregulation of coagulation and fibrinolysis
- Dysfunction of platelets or erythrocytes
- Vasospasm and changes in hydrostatic pressure

35.4 Clinical Presentation

35.4.1 Signs and Symptoms [1–3]

- Persistent livedo with purpuric macules and papules that progress to small, tender, irregular, and extremely *painful* ulcerations.
- In our experience, we have observed in the early stage of the disease that the patients are experiencing severe pain even before the development of the ulceration.
- Ulcerations may recur and heal with stellate, ivory-white atrophic plaques, sometimes with surrounding hyperpigmentation and telangiectases.
- Atrophie blanche represents the end-stage lesions and is characterized by irregular, white/ivory, depressed scars. Atrophie blanche can also be observed in the context of venous

© The Author(s) 2024
L. Téot et al. (eds.), *Skin Necrosis*, https://doi.org/10.1007/978-3-031-60954-1_35

insufficiency and requires separate diagnostic and therapeutic approaches [1].
- Seasonal exacerbations are described [1].
- Neurological symptoms are rarely described (mononeuropathy multiplex) [2, 3].

35.4.2 Location

- Lower legs, ankles, and/or dorsal surface of the feet.

35.4.3 Possible Associated Conditions [4, 5]

- Connective tissue diseases (systemic lupus erythematosus)
- Cryoglobulinemia
- Antiphospholipid antibody syndrome
- Vasculitis (polyarteritis nodosa)
- Abnormalities of the coagulation system (protein C deficiency, abnormalities of the tissue plasminogen activator system, antithrombin III deficiency, elevated homocysteine levels, prothrombin G201210A gene mutation, and factor V Leiden)
- Venous insufficiency

35.5 Diagnosis [2, 3]

- Clinical presentation and evolution help for the diagnosis.
- Skin biopsy has to be performed in case of doubt:
  - *Early stage*: Fibrin deposition in the vessel wall and/or lumen in early lesions. A lymphocytic infiltrate and infarction with hemorrhages may be present.
  - *End stage*: Epidermal atrophy with sclerosis of the dermis and a minimal cellular infiltrate. Vessel walls may have segmental thickening and hyalinization of the intima. Recanalized thrombotic vessels may be noted. Superficial or deep vessels may be involved.

35.6 Treatment [6–11]

Many treatment modalities have been attempted to control the disease process.

Unfortunately, many cases remain difficult to treat. Suggested therapeutical options are often based on the experience from a few case reports.

35.6.1 General Management

- Be sure of the diagnosis!
- Diagnose and treat the associated conditions (connective tissue disease, venous insufficiency, etc.)
- Avoid pain (analgesics).
- Adapt topical wound care.
- Avoid infection.
- Check risk factors for wound healing impairment (malnutrition, smoking, etc.).
- Compression therapy can be suggested.

35.6.2 Therapeutic Modalities

- Antiplatelet agents (aspirin, dipyridamole)
- Fibrinolytic agents (danazol, tissue plasminogen activator)
- Anticoagulant agents (subcutaneous low-molecular-weight heparin or antivitamin K agents)
- Vasodilating agents (nifedipine, nicotinic acid)
- Pentoxifylline (enhances the blood flow and decreases the blood viscosity)
- Doxycycline is used for its anti-inflammatory properties
- Immunosuppressive therapies (prednisone, methotrexate, cyclosporin, etc.)
- PUVA therapy
- Intravenous immunoglobulins
- Hyperbaric oxygen therapy (Figs. 35.1, 35.2, 35.3 and 35.4)

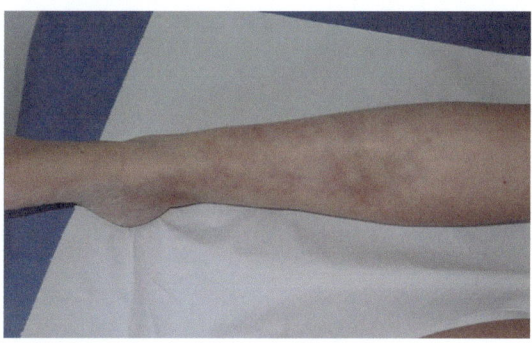

Fig. 35.1 Livedo

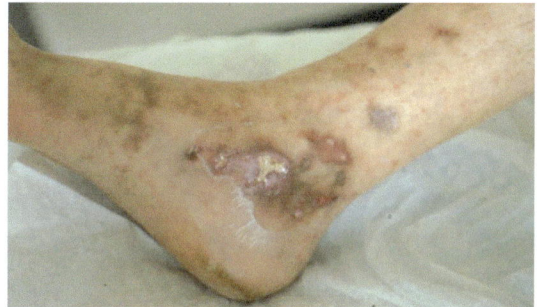

Fig. 35.2 Ulceration and livedoid aspect

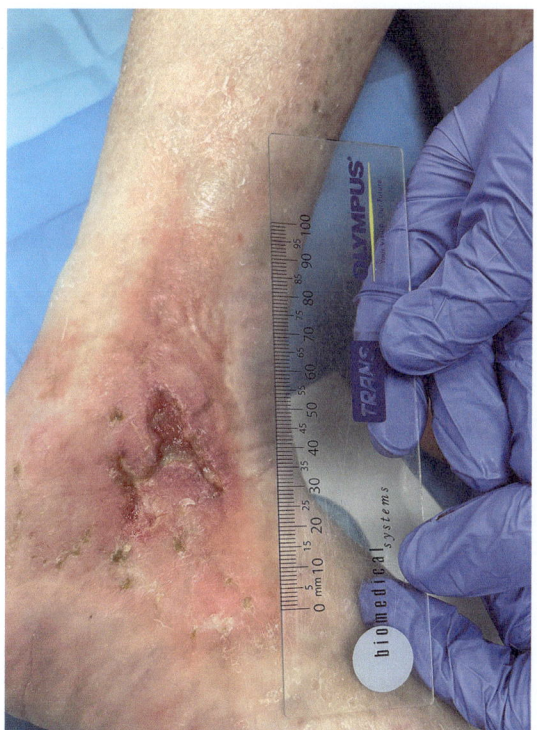

Fig. 35.3 Chronic ulcerations surrounded by atrophie blanche aspect

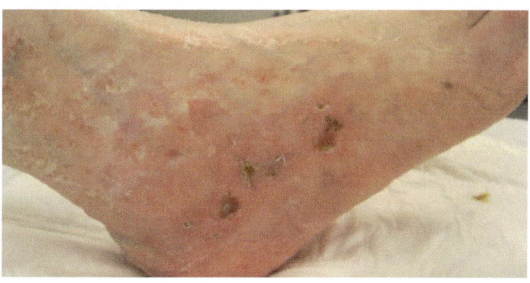

Fig. 35.4 Healing with white atrophic surrounding plaques and telangiectases

35.6.3 Perspectives

- The "CHAP" regimen combines calcium channel blockade, hydroxychloroquine, aspirin, and pentoxifylline. The CHAP regimen has been assessed in 12 patients with a very good tolerance. This combination targets the pathogenic mechanisms of LV by acting on vasodilation, decreased platelet aggregation, prevention of thrombus formation, and immunomodulation. Complete or partial remission has been observed in all patients occurring within 3–6 months.
- The use of anti-TNF-α agents and Janus kinase inhibitors may represent an interesting therapeutic strategy in refractory cases, but the lack of evidence and the small number of reported observations represent limiting factors for their use.

References

1. Alavi A, Hafner J, Dutz JP, Mayer D, Sibbald RG, Criado PR, Senet P, Callen JP, Phillips TJ, Romanelli M, Kirsner RS. Livedoid vasculopathy: an in-depth analysis using a modified Delphi approach. J Am Acad Dermatol. 2013;69(6):1033–1042.e1. https://doi.org/10.1016/j.jaad.2013.07.019.
2. Khenifer S, Thomas L, Balme B, Delle S. Livedoid vasculopathy: thrombotic or inflammatory disease? Clin Exp Dermatol. 2009;35:693–8.
3. Hairston B, Davis MD, Pittelkow MR, Ahmed I. Livedoid vasculopathy: further evidence for procoagulant pathogenesis. Arch Dermatol. 2006;142(11):1413–8.
4. Lefebvre P, Motte S, Wautrecht JC, Cornez N, Delplace J, Dereume JP. Livedoid vasculitis. J Mal Vasc. 1996;21(1):50–3.

5. Mimouni D, Rencic A, Nikolskaia OV, Bernstein BD, Nousari HC. Cutaneous polyarteritis nodosa in patients presenting with atrophie blanche. Br J Dermatol. 2003;148(4):789–94.
6. Kim JE, et al. Ischemic neuropathy associated with livedoid vasculitis. J Clin Neurol. 2011;7:233–6.
7. Camille F, Stéphane B. Difficult management of livedoid vasculopathy. Arch Dermatol. 2004;140:1011.
8. Ravat F, Evans A, Russell-Jones R. Response of livedoid vasculitis to intravenous immunoglobulin. Br J Dermatol. 2002;147(1):166–9.
9. Jetton R, Lazazrus G. Minidose heparin therapy for vasculitis atrophie blanche. JAAD. 1983;8:23–6.
10. Choi H, Hann S. Livedo reticularis and livedoid vasculitis responding to PUVA. JJAD. 1999;40(2):204–7.
11. Keller M, Lee J, Webster G. Livedoid thrombotic vasculopathy responding to doxycycline therapy. J Clin Aesthet Dermatol. 2008;1(4):22–4.

Open Access This chapter is licensed under the terms of the Creative Commons Attribution-NonCommercial-NoDerivatives 4.0 International License (http://creativecommons.org/licenses/by-nc-nd/4.0/), which permits any non-commercial use, sharing, distribution and reproduction in any medium or format, as long as you give appropriate credit to the original author(s) and the source, provide a link to the Creative Commons license and indicate if you modified the licensed material. You do not have permission under this license to share adapted material derived from this chapter or parts of it.

The images or other third party material in this chapter are included in the chapter's Creative Commons license, unless indicated otherwise in a credit line to the material. If material is not included in the chapter's Creative Commons license and your intended use is not permitted by statutory regulation or exceeds the permitted use, you will need to obtain permission directly from the copyright holder.

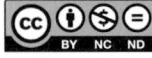

Pyoderma Gangrenosum

Hiroshi Yoshimoto

36.1 Introduction

Pyoderma gangrenosum (PG) is a very rare ulcerative neutrophilic inflammatory skin disease. The clinical manifestations of PG are pain, tenderness, an erythematous nodule, or a sterile pustule in the early stage, which progress to deep ulcers with a purulent base and undermined margin [1]. The ulcers heal with characteristic cribriform scars; however, sometimes multiple relapses occur. The patients with PG have frequently an associated systemic disease including inflammatory bowel disease, arthritis, hepatitis, or malignancy [2, 3].

The cause of PG remains unknown, although suggested causes include immune complex-mediated neutrophilic vascular reactions [4].

PG has no definite diagnostic criteria and is a diagnosis of exclusion. The diagnosis of PG is based primarily on the clinical history, clinical manifestation, and biopsy result. Although the histopathology of PG is nonspecific, the pathological findings are useful in differential diagnosis [3].

It is difficult to get cured completely by local wound management alone. If the patients have a systemic disease, the systemic disease should be preferentially treated [4]. The severe PG is commonly treated with steroids or other immunomodulators. More recently, tumor necrosis factor-alpha blockers and other biologic agents have been used with some success for PG patients [5, 6].

Therefore, the diagnosis of PG can be difficult, and misdiagnosis might lead to serious complications [7].

36.2 Etiopathogenesis

The cause of PG remains unknown, although suggested causes include immune complex-mediated neutrophilic vascular reactions [4].

The incidence of PG is very low. PG commonly affects women aged 30–50 on the lower limbs, although it occurs in all age groups and any other site including the peristomal area. The histopathology of PG is nonspecific, and the ulcers of PG show necrotic tissue surrounded by neutrophil infiltrates with monocytes and giant cells. About 50% of PG patients have an associated systemic disease including inflammatory bowel disease, arthritis, HIV infection, hematologic disease, hepatitis, and malignancy [3].

36.3 Clinical Detailing

The clinical manifestations of PG are pain, tenderness, an erythematous nodule, or a sterile pustule in the early stage, which progress to deep

H. Yoshimoto (✉)
Department of Plastic and Reconstructive Surgery, Nagasaki University Hospital, Nagasaki, Japan
e-mail: hy671117@nagasaki-u.ac.jp

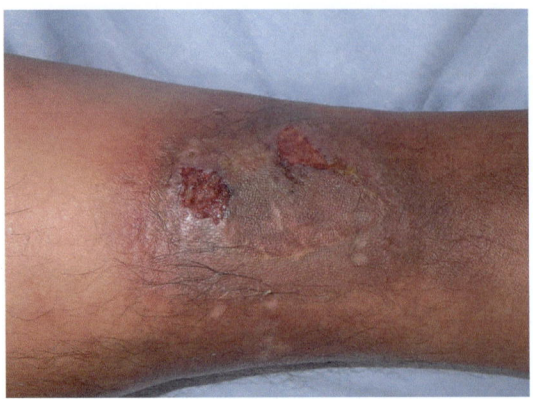

Fig. 36.1 A right leg ulcer in a 20-year-old male that originated from initial abrasion. He has no systemic disease

Table 36.1 Causes of ulcers mimicking PG

Infection
Fungal
Mycobacterial
Necrotizing fasciitis
Vascular occlusive disease
Antiphospholipid-antibody syndrome
Venous stasis ulceration
Vasculitis
Wegener's granulomatosis
Polyarteritis nodosa
Neoplasms
Lymphoma
Leukemia cutis
Drug reactions
Hydroxyurea-induced ulcer

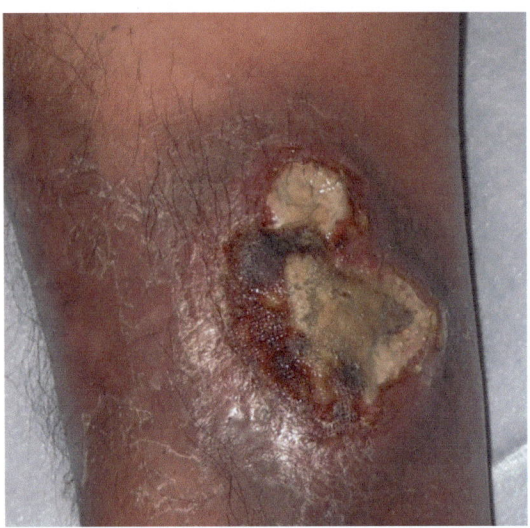

Fig. 36.2 The ulcer expanded with a purulent and necrotic base even though ointment was used

ulcers with a purulent base and undermined margin. The ulcers heal with characteristic cribriform scars; however, sometimes multiple relapses occur (Figs. 36.1 and 36.2) [2].

Pathergy is a specific but not sensitive finding of PG. The lesion sites expand radically, especially if the borders of the lesion site are traumatized by debridement or by other mechanical trauma [2]. No laboratory finding is diagnostic of PG. PG has no definite diagnostic criteria and is a diagnosis of exclusion. The diagnosis of PG is very difficult and based primarily on the clinical history, clinical manifestation, and biopsy result while being careful about misdiagnosis (Table 36.1) [1, 3, 5].

36.4 Treatments

If the patients have a systemic disease, the systemic disease should be preferentially treated. It is difficult to get cured completely by local wound management alone. Topical treatments are chosen depending on the purpose such as the prevention of secondary bacterial infection or the promotion of reepithelialization. Some topical agents such as tacrolimus, strong corticosteroids, and cyclosporine have reported efficacy in small case series. PG is commonly treated with systemic corticosteroids and/or cyclosporine [4].

Other immunomodulators have reported efficacy in case reports (Table 36.2).

Tumor necrosis factor-alpha blockers have reported to be very effective in the treatment of PG patients with inflammatory bowel disease or rheumatoid arthritis. Infliximab (tumor necrosis factor-alpha blocker) is the only systemic agent to have demonstrated efficacy for PG in a randomized, double-blind, placebo-controlled trial [6]. The patient's level of pain and signs of inflammation help guide response to treatment. The inflammatory component of PG is assessed by the border elevation and lesion expansion. We must give a diagnosis and choose treatment care-

Table 36.2 Systemic treatments for PG

Nonbiological treatments
Prednisone, cyclosporine, dapsone, thalidomide, methotrexate, tacrolimus, mycophenolate mofetil, azathioprine, granulocyte apheresis, intravenous immunoglobulin

Biological treatments
Infliximab, etanercept, alefacept, adalimumab, efalizumab

fully since PG has no definite diagnostic criteria and no standard protocol for treatment (Figs. 36.3 and 36.4).

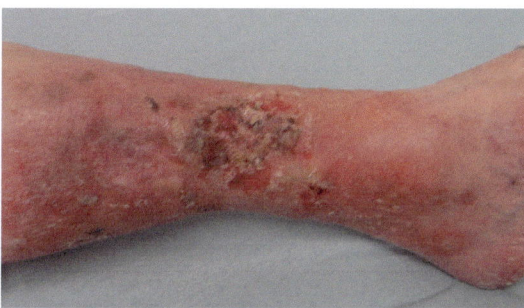

Fig. 36.3 A left leg ulcer in a 58-year-old female with systemic lupus erythematosus (SLE): bizarre configuration of ulceration rims, undermined edges, and soft edematous ulcerated area (this photo is provided by Dr. Fujioka)

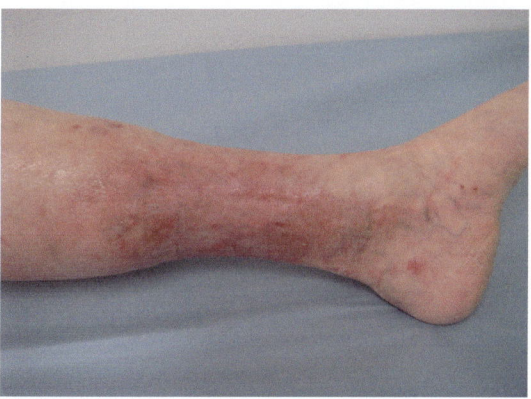

Fig. 36.4 There is no recurrence on 8 months after skin graft. SLE has been treated with prednisone 5 mg/day (this photo is provided by Dr. Fujioka)

References

1. Kari HN, Jeffrey JM, Klaus FH. Case reports and a review of the literature on ulcers mimicking pyoderma gangrenosum. Int J Dermatol. 2003;42(2):84–94.
2. Hadi A, Lebwohl M. Clinical features of pyoderma gangrenosum and current diagnostic trends. J Am Acad Dermatol. 2011;64(5):950–4.
3. Powell FC, Su WP, Perry HO. Pyoderma gangrenosum: classification and management. J Am Acad Dermatol. 1996;34(3):395–409.
4. Reichrath J, Bens G, Bonowitz A, Tilgen W. Treatment recommendations for pyoderma gangrenosum: an evidence-based review of the literature based on more than 350 patients. J Am Acad Dermatol. 2005;53(2):273–83.
5. Miller J, Yentzer BA, Clark A, Jorizzo JL, Feldman SR. Pyoderma gangrenosum: a review and update on new therapies. J Am Acad Dermatol. 2010;62(4):646–54.
6. Brooklyn TN, Dunnill MG, Shetty A, Bowden JJ, Williams JD, Griffiths CE, Forbes A, Greenwood R, Probert CS. Infliximab for the treatment of pyoderma gangrenosum: a randomised, double blind, placebo controlled trial. Gut. 2006;55(4):505–9.
7. Weenig RH, Davis MD, Dahl PR, Su WP. Skin ulcers misdiagnosed as pyoderma gangrenosum. N Engl J Med. 2002;347(18):1412–8.

Open Access This chapter is licensed under the terms of the Creative Commons Attribution-NonCommercial-NoDerivatives 4.0 International License (http://creativecommons.org/licenses/by-nc-nd/4.0/), which permits any non-commercial use, sharing, distribution and reproduction in any medium or format, as long as you give appropriate credit to the original author(s) and the source, provide a link to the Creative Commons license and indicate if you modified the licensed material. You do not have permission under this license to share adapted material derived from this chapter or parts of it.

The images or other third party material in this chapter are included in the chapter's Creative Commons license, unless indicated otherwise in a credit line to the material. If material is not included in the chapter's Creative Commons license and your intended use is not permitted by statutory regulation or exceeds the permitted use, you will need to obtain permission directly from the copyright holder.

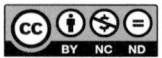

Cryoglobulinemia

Alessandra Michelucci, Salvatore Panduri, Valentina Dini, and Marco Romanelli

37.1 Physiopathology

Cryoglobulinemia (CR) is a disease characterized by the presence, in the serum, of abnormal proteins that precipitate reversibly at low temperatures, and generally the cryoglobulins lead to a systemic inflammatory syndrome characterized by myalgia, arthralgia, purpura (Meltzer's triad), neuropathy, and glomerulonephritis [1]. According to immunochemical characteristic, cryoglobulins have been classified into three distinct groups:

- *Type I* with monoclonal immunoglobulin (Ig) (IgG, IgA, IgM): This type is associated with lymphoproliferative malignancies or hematologic disorders.
- *Type II* with monoclonal or polyclonal Ig.
- *Type III* with polyclonal immune complex.

In 25% of cases, an involvement of the skin is present, and the most frequent cutaneous manifestations are palpable purpura, Raynaud's phenomenon, cutaneous ulcers, skin rash, livedo reticularis, and acrocyanosis. Only in 2% of cases with skin involvement is it possible to observe digital ischemia and gangrene. Renal, neurological, and joint involvement occur in 21–38% of the patients [2]. The cause of the precipitation of the immunoglobulins is still unclear, but it has been hypothesized that abnormalities of the carbohydrates decrease the solubility of the cryoglobulins [3]. It has been suggested that various interactions between immunoglobulins at low temperatures cause the precipitation of this protein [4]. Mixed cryoglobulinemia type II or III represents the most common manifestation of CR. There are only few cases in the literature of type I cryoglobulinemia. Mixed cryoglobulinemia is frequently associated with hepatitis C virus (HCV) infection, and this creates a doubt on the existence of essential cryoglobulinemia. The clinical manifestations of type I cryoglobulinemia are essentially due to self-aggregation through complement fraction fragment of monoclonal immunoglobulin that causes hyperviscosity, thrombosis, ischemia, and vasculopathy, involving the skin and kidney. The clinical presentation of type II or III is determined by the cryoglobulinemic vasculitis (leukocytoclastic vasculitis), which is able to determine various cutaneous lesions and multisystem involvement [2].

37.2 Diagnosis

- *Laboratory*: Determination of the cryoglobulins (blood drawn into warmed syringe, red blood cells (RBCs) removed via warmed centrifuge, plasma refrigerated in a Wintrobe tube at 4 °C for 24–72 h and then centrifuged, and cryocrit determined).

A. Michelucci · S. Panduri · V. Dini ·
M. Romanelli (✉)
Department of Dermatology, University of Pisa, Pisa, Italy

Table 37.1 Skin manifestations

Ischemic necrosis (40% in type I, 0–20% in mixed types)
Palpable purpura (15% in type I, 80% in mixed types)
Livedoid vasculitis (1% in type I, 14% in type III)
Cold-induced urticaria (15% in type I, 10% in type III)
Hyperkeratotic spicules in areas exposed to cold
Scarring of the tip of the nose, pinnae, fingertips, and toes
Acrocyanosis
Nail-fold capillary abnormalities

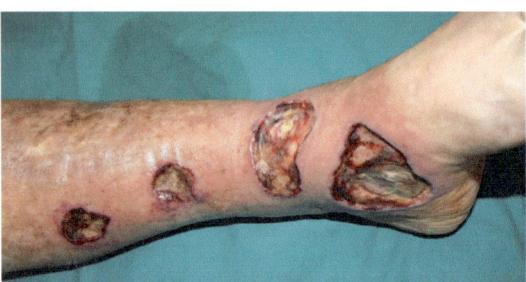

Fig. 37.1 Multiple punched-out ulcers, extremely painful, on the lower leg. Necrotic tissue and adherent fibrin on the wound bed in the absence of arterial disease

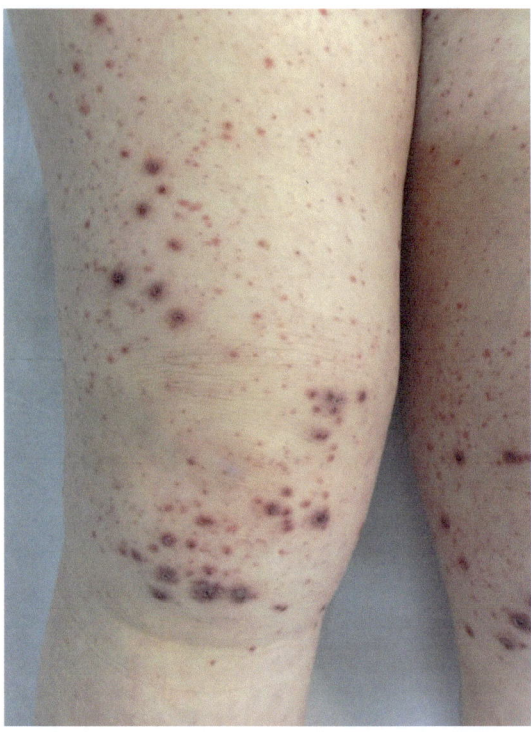

Fig. 37.2 Palpable purpura with hemorrhagic crusts

- *Semiology*: The course is characterized by cyclic eruptions induced by cold or fluctuations of the activity of underlying disease (Table 37.1). The skin involvement in type I is represented by livedoid vasculitis, cold-induced acrocyanosis, leg ulcers, and cold urticaria. Types II and III are associated with vascular palpable purpura and leg ulcers (Figs. 37.1 and 37.2) [3].
- *Biology*: Presence or absence of disorders related to underlying conditions.
- *Histology*: In cryoglobulinemia type I, it is evident that there is the presence of an eosinophilic pink coagulum filling dermal venules. In mixed cryoglobulinemia, there are the classical aspects of leukocytoclastic vasculitis (fibrinous degeneration of the vascular endothelium along with other signs of vasculitis: nuclear dust, perivascular hemorrhage, and vascular destruction).

It is necessary to perform a differential diagnosis with other vasculitides affecting small- and medium-caliber vessels:

- Antineutrophil cytoplasmic antibody (ANCA)-associated vasculitis, microscopic polyangiitis, and eosinophilic granulomatosis with polyangiitis (Churg-Strauss).
- IgA vasculitis (Henoch-Schönlein purpura).
- Other vasculitis: drug-induced small-vessel vasculitis (hypersensitivity vasculitis), cutaneous small-vessel vasculitis, infection-related vasculitis, connective tissue disorder-associated vasculitis [5].

37.3 Treatment

37.3.1 Systemic Treatment

The therapy is often directed to the underlying condition.

- For patients with chronic HCV infection, antiviral therapy is indicated [6].
- In patients with organ involvement or recalcitrant disease, immunosuppressive or immuno-

modulatory therapy is indicated: steroids, plasmapheresis, and cytotoxic agents.
- Rituximab, a mouse/human chimeric monoclonal anti-CD 20 antibody, in monotherapy is more effective than standard immunosuppressive therapy over the long term, where therapy with antiviral agent is not indicated [7].
- Cyclophosphamide can be used in patients who failed or cannot tolerate rituximab therapy.
- In patients treated with steroids or other immunosuppressive drugs, a prophylaxis against opportunistic infection should be performed: trimethoprim-sulfamethoxazole (TMP/SMZ) is employed in order to avoid *Pneumocystis pneumonia* infection.
- All patients should receive supportive measures: control of pain is necessary [5].

37.3.2 Local Treatment

- Corticosteroids (purpura)
- Moist wound dressing
- Compression bandages
- Bed rest

Disease control also includes the prevention of arising complications that can decrease the patient's survival rate, such as kidney failure and other organ involvement.

References

1. Takada S, Shimizu T, Hadano Y, et al. Cryoglobulinemia (review). Mol Med Rep. 2012;6(1):3–8.
2. Krishnaram AS, Geetha T, Pratheepa AS. Primary cryoglobulinemia with cutaneous features. Indian J Dermatol Venereol Leprol. 2013;79:427–30.
3. Levo Y. Nature of cryoglobulinemia. Lancet. 1980;1:285–7.
4. Grey HM, Kohler PF. Cryoimmunoglobulins. Semin Hematol. 1973;10:87–112.
5. Roccatello D, Saadoun D, Ramos-Casals M, Tzioufas AG, Fervenza FC, Cacoub P, Zignego AL, Ferri C. Cryoglobulinaemia. Nat Rev Dis Primers. 2018;4(1):11.
6. Dammacco F, Sansonno D. Therapy for hepatitis C virus-related cryoglobulinemic vasculitis. N Engl J Med. 2013;369(11):1035–45.
7. De Vita S, Quartuccio L, Isola M, et al. A randomized controlled trial of rituximab for the treatments of severe cryoglobulinemic vasculitis. Arthritis Rheum. 2012;64(3):843–53.

Open Access This chapter is licensed under the terms of the Creative Commons Attribution-NonCommercial-NoDerivatives 4.0 International License (http://creativecommons.org/licenses/by-nc-nd/4.0/), which permits any non-commercial use, sharing, distribution and reproduction in any medium or format, as long as you give appropriate credit to the original author(s) and the source, provide a link to the Creative Commons license and indicate if you modified the licensed material. You do not have permission under this license to share adapted material derived from this chapter or parts of it.

The images or other third party material in this chapter are included in the chapter's Creative Commons license, unless indicated otherwise in a credit line to the material. If material is not included in the chapter's Creative Commons license and your intended use is not permitted by statutory regulation or exceeds the permitted use, you will need to obtain permission directly from the copyright holder.

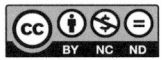

Hand Necrosis

38

Yasser Farid, Nicolas Cuylits, Farida Benhadou, and Véronique Del Marmol

38.1 Introduction

Loss of fingers represents an important aesthetic and functional handicap. Finger ischemia is a rare pathology but can have several different etiologies and needs to be closely managed to limit the extension of necrosis. The management of finger ischemia is dependent on the etiological factors and type of necrosis. This is why a close collaboration between the surgical and medical specialties is mandatory for limiting extension of necrosis and amputation of the fingers. When necrosis occurs and is delimiting, optimization of clinical assessment and conservative treatment often decreases the need of surgical shortening of the finger and can sometimes save some important functional parts of the hand. We will discuss in this chapter the way to diagnose and how to manage necrosis of the fingers.

38.2 Vascularization

The hand and the wrist are supplied by four arteries linked together at the level of the carpus by four anastomotic arcades. Those arteries are the radial, ulnar, anterior, and posterior interosseous arteries. Each long finger is vascularized by a pair of digital arteries running about 1 mm under the skin on the ulnar and radial sides of the finger. Those arteries are connected by means of several constant anastomoses able to compensate interruption of one digital artery. The thumb is also supplied by two additional short dorsal arteries, which can offer additional supply in case of ischemia. A dense capillary network nourished by those arteries is responsible for the excellent finger vascularization [1].

38.3 Mechanisms

The digital vascularization can be altered in different conditions.

The two main mechanisms of digital ischemia are due to an occlusive vascular process (thrombi, emboli, inflammation, vasospasm, external compression, etc.) and/or a decreased blood supply process (hemodynamic shock, trauma, etc.). The occlusive vascular process results from an obstruction of the digital arterial lumens, leading progressively to the interruption of the digital blood flow and finally to the ischemia of the extremities. A diameter reduction of 60% or a

Y. Farid · N. Cuylits (✉)
Department of Plastic Surgery, Hôpital Erasme, Université Libre de Bruxelles, Brussels, Belgium
e-mail: nicolas.cuylits@hubruxelles.be

F. Benhadou · V. Del Marmol
Department of Dermatology, Hôpital Erasme, Université Libre de Bruxelles, Brussels, Belgium
e-mail: Farida.BENHADOU@hubruxelles.be

cross-sectional area reduction of 70% represents a hemodynamically significant lesion, and these lesions produce a pressure drop across the stenotic area. The distal arterial bed is supplied by collateral blood vessels. In patients with acute arterial occlusions, collateral blood vessels are not formed, and perfusion decreases rapidly below a critical threshold level, which results in persistent pain and tissue necrosis [2].

38.4 Etiologies

Digital ischemia is an uncommon disorder reflecting diverse etiologies.

The main etiologies of digital ischemia have been classified in Table 38.1.

Each etiology will be discussed in the appropriate chapter [3–6].

Table 38.1 Etiologies of digital ischemia

Autoimmune diseases	Infection
Scleroderma and CREST syndrome	Hepatitis B and C
Lupus and antiphospholipid syndrome	HIV
Gougerot-Sjögren syndrome	Endocarditis
Sharp syndrome	Mycoplasma
Rheumatoid arthritis, Still's disease	Rickettsiosis
Dermatomyositis and polymyositis	
Primary biliary cirrhosis	
Inflammatory bowel disease	

Vasculitis	Inflammatory arteritis
Periarteritis nodosa	Horton
Micropolyangiitis	Takayasu
Wegener's granulomatosis	Kawasaki
Hypersensitivity vasculitis	Buerger
Rheumatoid purpura	
Cryoglobulinemia	

Atherosclerosis and aneurysms	Arteriopathy
Emboli	Hypothenar hammer syndrome
Atheromatosis	Vibration syndrome
Atherosclerosis and aneurysms	Arteriopathy
Cholesterol emboli	Radiotherapy
Calciphylaxis	Fibromuscular dysplasia

Cardiac embolism process	Endocrinopathy
Heart failure	Cushing
Endocarditis	Thyroidopathy
Cardiac rhythm trouble	Pheochromocytoma
Valvulopathy	
Myxoma	

Myeloproliferative syndrome and hematologic disorder	Cancers
Vaquez's disease	Solid cancers
Essential thrombocytosis	**Decreased blood flow**
Myeloid chronic leukemia	Trauma
Lymphoid chronic leukemia	Hemorrhage
Myeloma	Compression (carpal tunnel syndrome, thoracic outlet syndrome, etc.)
Waldenström	Heart failure
B lymphoma	Septic and hemodynamic shock, etc.
Hypereosinophilic syndrome	
Thrombophilia	

Cryoproteinemia	Toxic
Cryofibrinogen	Vinyl chloride
Cryoimmunoglobulin	Chromium
Cold agglutinin	Arsenic
	Epoxy resin
	Trichloroethylene
	Benzene
	Silica
	Silicone

Toxicomania	Drugs
Tobacco	Bleomycin
LSD	Vincristine
Cocaine	5-FU
	Cisplatin
	Tamoxifen
	Sympathicomimetics
	Vasoconstrictive drugs
	Ergotism
	Bromocriptine
	Beta-blockers
	Cyclosporine, etc.

38.5 Clinical Presentation of Digital Ischemia

The diagnosis of digital ischemia is easy at the stage of gangrene.

The clinical process is divided into three steps:

1. The early phase: pallor, poikilothermia, livedoid aspect, pulpar petechiae, periungual infarction, and splinter subungual hemorrhages.
2. The state phase: digital ulceration.
3. The late phase: distal gangrene.

The associated symptoms caused by the ischemia are the pain and the paresthesia.

The distal gangrene is a risk of complication including cutaneous and bone infection.

We can distinguish two classical types of digital necrosis presentations, the dry necrosis and the wet necrosis.

The dry necrosis (Fig. 38.1) is more often observed after arterial blood flow occlusion and is characterized by red-black dry necrotic tissue surrounded by painful red borders. The dry necrosis tissue spreads slowly and is often free of microbial infection resembling mummified flesh.

The wet necrosis has a less mummified aspect compared to dry necrosis due to microbiological load.

The wet necrosis results from a microbial critical colonization (*Clostridium perfringens*, *Bacillus fusiformis*, etc.), which causes the tissue to swell and emit a fetid smell. Wet necrosis usually develops rapidly due to blockage of venous and/or arterial blood flow. The affected part is saturated with stagnant blood, which promotes the rapid growth of bacteria and can lead to soft tissue infection and sepsis.

38.6 Diagnosis

The diagnosis is based on the clinical presentation as described above in a specific context.

The most important point is to investigate the etiological factors by doing a complete anamnesis and examination of the patient. Appropriate tests will be recommended according to the clinical findings.

- The *anamnesis* will highlight some important points:
    - Circumstances of occurrence (acute or chronic, trauma, etc.)
    - Aggravating factors (cold, etc.)
    - Medications
    - Smoking habits
    - A history of Raynaud's phenomenon
    - Exposure to chemicals or physical agents
    - Personal and familial medical history
    - History of surgical operation, interventional procedure, or intravenous use
    - The profession and occupational activities
    - The presence of systemic symptoms (cancer, vasculitis, endocrinopathy, etc.)
- The *clinical examination* will look for:
    - Ischemia signs (see above)
    - The extra-digital signs correlated with the underlying conditions: signs for arthritis, vasculitis, and connectivitis (scleroderma, lupus); signs of infection; signs of endocrinopathy; signs of cardiopathy, etc.

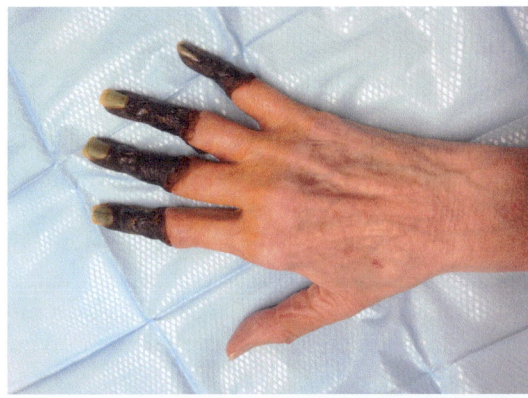

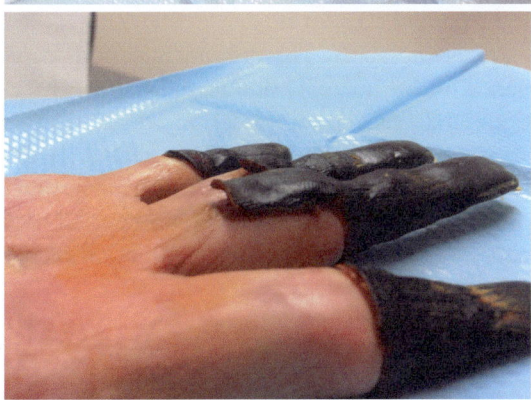

Fig. 38.1 Typical severe dry necrosis

- The *clinical testing:*
  - The venous refilling time
  - Arterial pulse
  - Allen's test
  - The blood pressure (right and left arms)
  - Cardiac auscultation
  - Phalen and Tinel maneuver
- The *complementary* testing:
  - Blood tests (hematology and coagulopathy, renal function, inflammatory syndrome, thyroid tests, antinuclear factors, lipids, serology, proteins and cryoproteins, etc.)
  - Capillaroscopy if Raynaud's phenomenon or suspicion of connective tissue diseases
  - Hand radiography if suspicion of CREST syndrome, rheumatoid arthritis, or calciphylaxis
  - Chest X-ray if scleroderma or compressive process is suspected
  - Cardiogram if arrhythmia is suspected
  - Echo Doppler of upper limbs
  - If asymmetric necrosis, an arteriography is recommended
  - The presence of systemic symptoms and clinical signs will help you to choose the appropriate tests [2]

38.7 Management

Up to date, the literature dealing with the clinical management of the necrotic finger is very poor.

Management of ischemic fingers should be divided into two stages, **the early ischemic stage** and **the late necrotic stage**.

In the early stage of ischemia of the fingers, we need to:

1. Identify the etiological factors(see Table 38.1)
2. Improve local perfusion by:
   - Vasodilators
   - Antiaggregants and anticoagulants
   - Hyperbaric oxygen
   - Surgical arteriolysis
3. Control the pain
4. *Avoid finger infection and adapt local treatment in each case*

If despite early ischemia management, we get to the late necrotic stage, we need to:

1. Define the type of necrosis (dry or wet)
2. Define its localization (proximal or distal)
3. Define the perfusion status of the different tissues, and in case of digit necrosis of frostbite origin, define the extent of necrosis (deep or superficial)

All of these factors will help in choosing between a more conservative treatment that involves mummification and auto-amputation or an early surgical treatment.

The type of necrosis: We can classify two types of digital necrosis presentations, the wet and dry necrosis.

If dry necrosis: As surgical amputation means often mandatory shortening, directed healing under the mummifying part gives the best length conservation. For this reason, dry dressings are recommended in an effort to keep the mummified part dry. The line of separation usually leads to a complete separation, with eventual falling off of the gangrenous tissue if it is not removed surgically; it is also called auto-amputation. Splinting is only recommended if finger retraction is occurring. Active finger motion is started early in all cases. Auto-amputation is a long process and is often not accepted by the patient. Anyway, waiting for a clear delimitation of the mummifying part often allows to limit the surgical shortening if the patient asks for it.

If wet necrosis: The prognosis is poor compared to dry necrosis due to the risk of infection and sepsis. Application of antiseptic dressing is recommended. The affected tissues have to be surgically removed. It is sometimes possible to convert the development of wet necrosis to dry necrosis by application of dry dressings (betadine gauze, alcohol-based dressing, etc.).

38.7.1 The Localization of Necrosis

The localization of necrosis demarcation is an important aspect of managing finger necrosis treatment, and we differentiate two main cases of finger necrosis linked to the anatomic blood supply of the fingers: necrosis of the fingertips and necrosis beyond the second phalange.

If necrosis is localized at the distal phalanx/fingertip, reperfusion can occur and conservative treatment is favored because of the rich and dense anastomosis network capable to compensate interruption of one digital artery.

If necrosis is localized at a trans-diaphysis location proximal to the distal phalange, then reperfusion is less frequent to occur, and evaluating the finger perfusion should be considered with the help of triple-phase bone scan. Triple-phase bone scan helps in assessing the extent of damaged tissue [7–10].

Three patterns are described to assess the extent of damaged tissue. In case we have a normal blood and bone pool images, then we should consider a conservative/auto-amputation treatment. In case we have an intermediate pattern with absent blood flow and absent early bone pool but with delayed bone blood flow, then demarcation and superficial debridement should be considered. When we have no or little blood flow in blood and bone pool, then a more aggressive attitude should be considered by early amputation (see Fig. 38.2).

38.7.2 The Perfusion Status and the Extent of Necrosis

In case of finger necrosis due to frostbite injuries, the mechanism of necrosis is different than when vascular obstruction occurs.

Tissue freezes slowly from outside to the inside in frostbite necrosis, whereas in necrosis due to vascular obstruction, necrosis starts from the inside and affects all layers of fingers at once. In frostbite injuries, there may be a wide discrepancy between the extent of damage to the skin versus that to the deeper structures, hence the need to evaluate the extent of necrosis with the help of triple-phase scan [7–10].

A triple-phase bone scan helps assess tissue perfusion to the different layers and affected area and should be used to better evaluate finger perfusion and hence helps in the decision-making (see Fig. 38.2).

Management of digital necrosis is summarized in Fig. 38.2 [7–13].

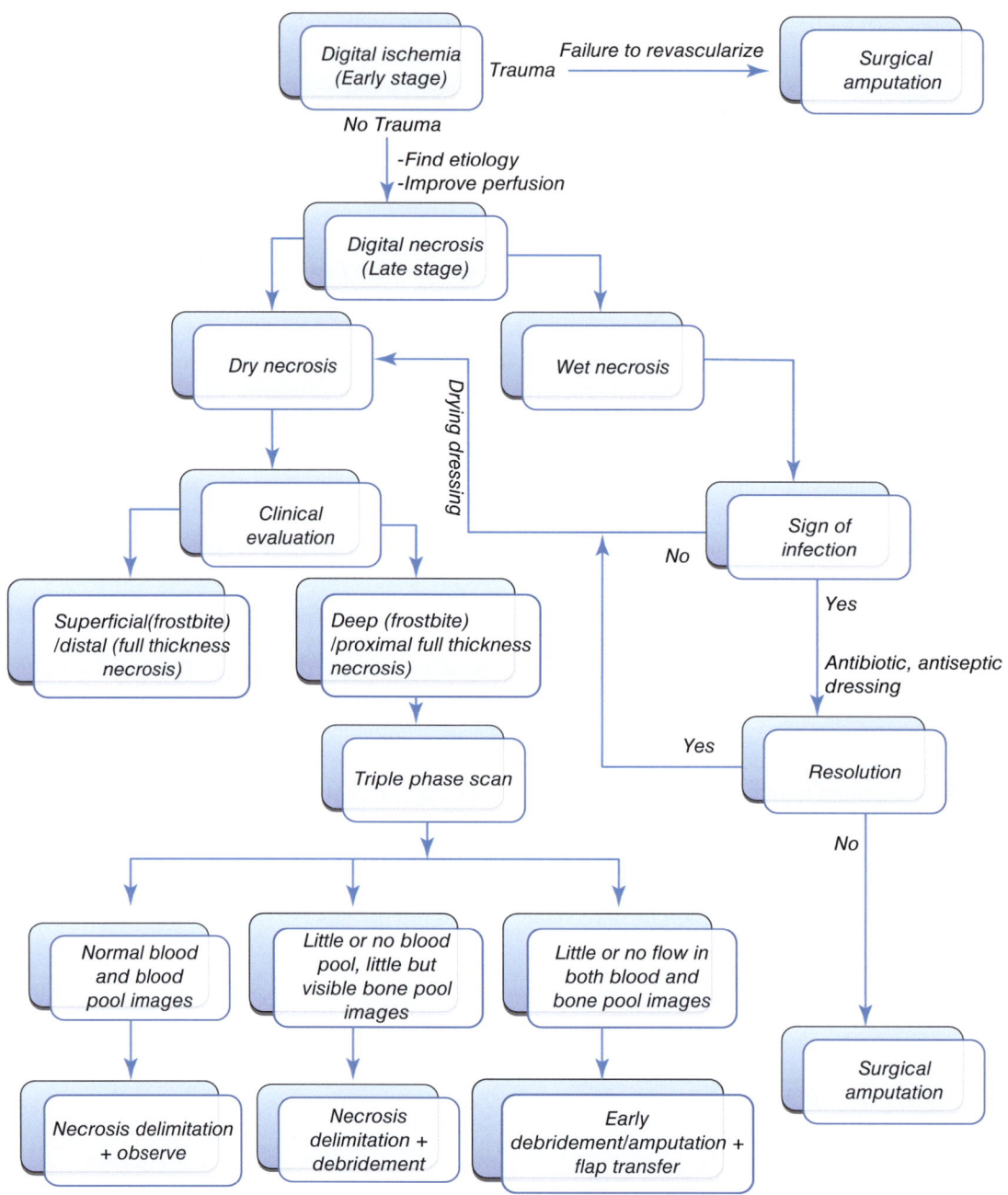

Fig. 38.2 Management of digital necrosis

References

1. Hand anatomy. www.medscape.com.
2. Jones NF. Acute and chronic ischemia of the hand: pathophysiology, treatment and prognosis. J Hand Surg Am. 1991;16(6):1074–83.
3. Esculier B, Barrier J, Bletry O, Malinsky M, Cabane J, Godeau P. Une cause rare d'artérite digitale avec phénomène de Raynaud et nécroses pulpaires: le virus b de l'hepatite-3 observations. Ann Med Interne. 1982;133:600–3.
4. Vayssairat M, Debure C, Cormier J, Bruneval P, Laurian C, Juillet Y. Hypothenar hammer syndrome; 17 cases with long term follow up. Vasc Surg. 1987;5:838–43.
5. Dompmartin A, Lemaitre M, Letessier D, Leroy D. Nécroses sous béta-bloquants? Ann Dermatol Vénéréol. 1988;115:593–6.
6. Werquin S, Kacet S, Caron J, et al. Phénomène de Raynaud et nécrose digitale après traitement d'un séminome ovarien par bléomycine, vinblastine et 5-FU. Ann Cardiol Angeiol (Paris). 1978;36:409–12.
7. Cauchy E, Chetaille E, Marchand V, Marsigny B. Retrospective study of 70 cases of severe frostbite lesions: a proposed new classification scheme. Wilderness Environ Med. 2001;12(4):248–55.
8. Cauchy E, Chetaille E, Lefevre M, Kerelou E, Marsigny B. The role of bone scanning in severe frostbite of the extremities: a retrospective study of 88 cases. Eur J Nucl Med. 2000;27(5):497–502.
9. Hutchison RL. Frostbite of the hand. J Hand Surg. 2014;39(9):1863–8.
10. Greenwald D, Cooper B, Gottlieb L. An algorithm for early aggressive treatment of frostbite with limb salvage directed by triple-phase scanning. Plast Reconstr Surg. 1998;102(4):1069–74.
11. Kaba A, Shoofs M, Leps P, Verlet E, Gstach JG, Mathevon H. Management of digital ischemia. 5 cases. Ann Chir Main Memb Super. 1991;10(4):364–72.
12. Pinede L, Ninet J. Les nécroses digitales du membre supérieur. Sang Thrombose Vaisseaux. 1995;7(5):323–32.
13. Batra M, Tandon P, Gupta N. Clinical approach to a patient with isolated digital ischaemia. JIACM. 2002;3(1):23–8.

Open Access This chapter is licensed under the terms of the Creative Commons Attribution-NonCommercial-NoDerivatives 4.0 International License (http://creativecommons.org/licenses/by-nc-nd/4.0/), which permits any non-commercial use, sharing, distribution and reproduction in any medium or format, as long as you give appropriate credit to the original author(s) and the source, provide a link to the Creative Commons license and indicate if you modified the licensed material. You do not have permission under this license to share adapted material derived from this chapter or parts of it.

The images or other third party material in this chapter are included in the chapter's Creative Commons license, unless indicated otherwise in a credit line to the material. If material is not included in the chapter's Creative Commons license and your intended use is not permitted by statutory regulation or exceeds the permitted use, you will need to obtain permission directly from the copyright holder.

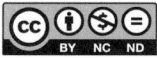

Factitious Disorders (Pathomimia) and Necrosis

39

Francoise Poot

39.1 Introduction

When facing a cutaneous necrosis of unknown origin, the clinician should always have in mind factitious disorder.

In this chapter, we will make clearer where to classify factitious disorders in the broader spectrum of self-inflicted skin lesions (SISLs). A clearer classification approach could result in better healthcare for these often difficult and "disarming" patients.

We will then describe the different clinical entities in factitious disorders.

In diagnosis and treatment, we will describe the comorbidities and the communication options adapted to the emotional structure of these patients. Finally, we will propose some specific therapeutic options and see what the prognosis can be.

39.2 Classification

In our paper published in 2013 with the European Society for Dermatology and Psychiatry [1], we proposed the utilization of the diagnostic category of self-inflicted skin lesion (SISL) as synonymous to "pathological SISL", to restrict this classification to dermatological lesions whose cause implies pathological behaviour.

There are three questions that are helpful for the classification of abnormal behaviour that potentially leads to somatic damage (Fig. 39.1):

- Is the behaviour responsible for the somatic damage denied or kept "secret" by the patient? A "yes" answer points to a factitious disorder1.
- If the answer to the first question is "yes", are there any external incentives? A "yes" answer indicates malingering, and a "no" answer points to factitious disorder.

Obviously, clinicians should refrain from asking patients with suspicious skin lesions direct and confronting questions: "Are you responsible for the lesions on your skin?" Rather, open-ended questions should be formulated: "How did these lesions appear?" Answers such as "I don't know!" or "I have no idea!" or "It is certainly not me!" point to a possible underlying pathological behaviour, denied or kept secret by the patient. On the other hand, answers like "When it itches, I can't stop picking my skin" or "When I am tired, I pull my hair without realizing it" confirm patients' responsibility for their lesions, even though they refer to mitigating circumstances.

If the answer to the first question is "yes", are there any external incentives? A "yes" answer indicates malingering, and a "no" answer points to factitious disorders.

F. Poot (✉)
HUB Erasme Hospital, Department of Dermatology, Brussels, Belgium

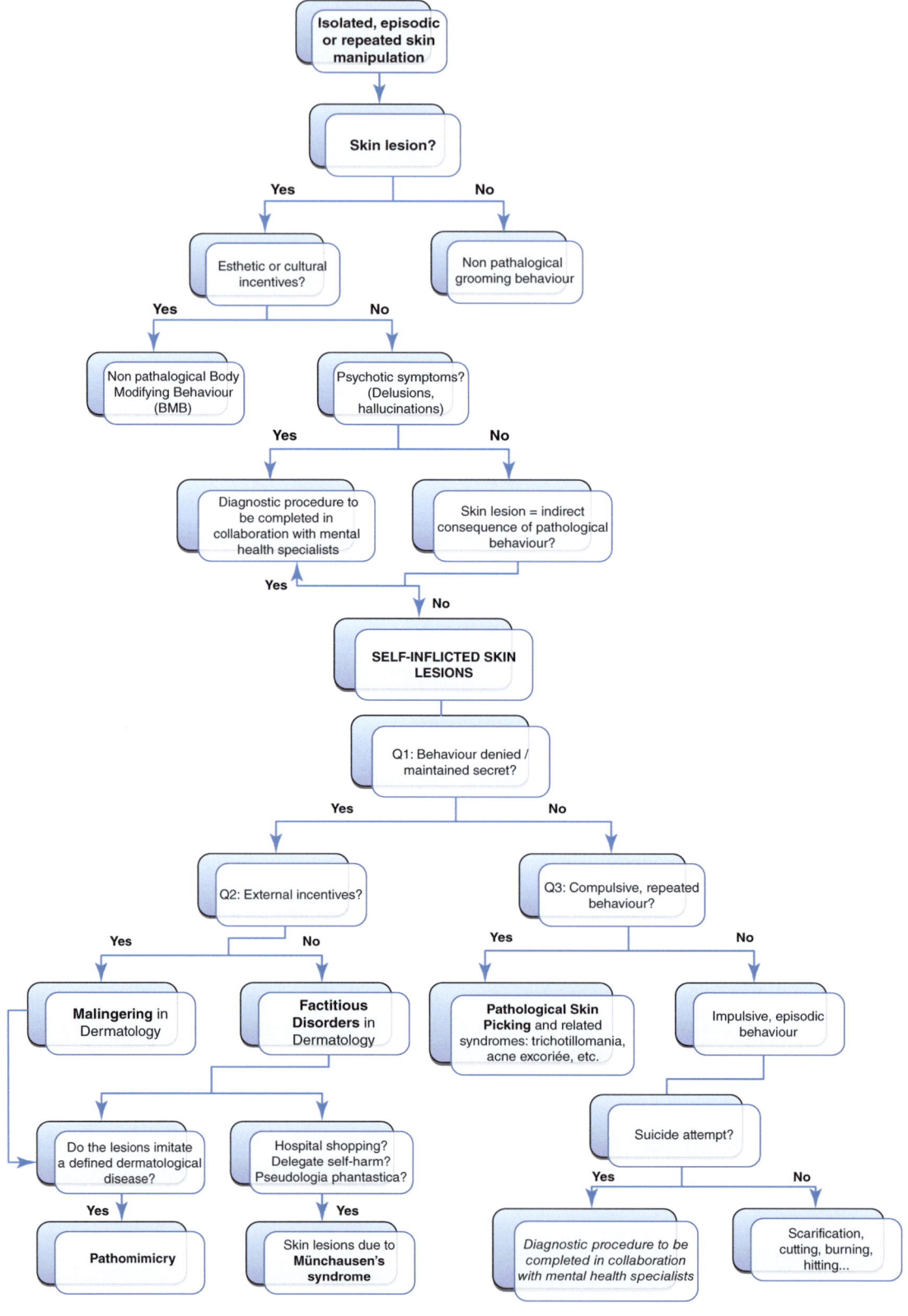

Fig. 39.1 Flow chart for the management of self-inflicted skin lesions Q1, Q2, and Q3

39.3 Syndromes Associated with a Denied or Hidden Pathological Behaviour

1. Factitious disorders: This expression refers to artificial or faked, self-provoked or alleged diseases, without clear external incentives, in the fields of internal medicine, psychiatry, and all somatic specialties [2–4]. It should be noted that an "external" trigger can precipitate, through emotional stress, the creation of the lesions, but the main contribution to the genesis must be found in internal, mainly unconscious, determinants. Child physical, sexual, or psychological abuse or neglect is quite frequent in the history of these patients.
2. Pathomimicry: This term has been used in a range of factitious disorders, referring to the resemblance with some genuine, natural diseases. In the dermatological context, this term can be used to signify the induction of lesions mimicking features of a recognized dermatological disorder [5], for example, atopic dermatitis-like lesions produced by contact with an irritating agent. Malingering may also underlie pathomimicry.
    (a) Munchausen syndrome: This syndrome, belonging to the factitious disorder category, is defined as the triad of (1) factitious symptoms, (2) hospital or doctor shopping and (3) pseudologia fantastica. Patients with Munchausen syndrome present, or claim, acute symptoms with demonstrative dramatic descriptions of complaints and false information on their medical history. It is also common for these patients to have a history of multiple hospitalizations and surgical procedures, sometimes with visible multiple sequels [6]. Self-harm is delegated to the care providers.
    (b) In Munchausen's syndrome by proxy, it is mainly children who are harmed by their caregivers in order to establish contact with health professionals.
3. Malingering: This term indicates the production or feigning of a symptom due to social (e.g. financial) incentives.
4. Simulation: This term is generally restricted to those cases of malingering or factitious disorders that simulate or mimic a known disease: general or dermatological (see the definition of pathomimicry above).

39.4 Diagnosis and Treatment

The diagnosis is not easy. However, usually these lesions do not mimic any of the known dermatosis and are associated with inconclusive skin biopsy. The history of the lesions, their chronic evolution, and cutaneous damages displayed on attainable areas of the body are characteristics [7]. In a review of atypical wounds [8], the authors found that factitious wounds were especially in young subjects. Differing markedly from other groups of atypical wounds in the present study, psychiatric comorbidities affected over 20% of the patients (Figs. 39.2, 39.3 and 39.4).

The basis for the management of all types of SISL is the patient-doctor relationship [9, 10].

1. Factitious disorders: The subject may be aware that he or she is driven to create the lesions, or in some instances, the activity may take place in a dissociative state outside the patient's awareness. The main motivation is assumed to be a method for coping with a severe psychological background and a pref-

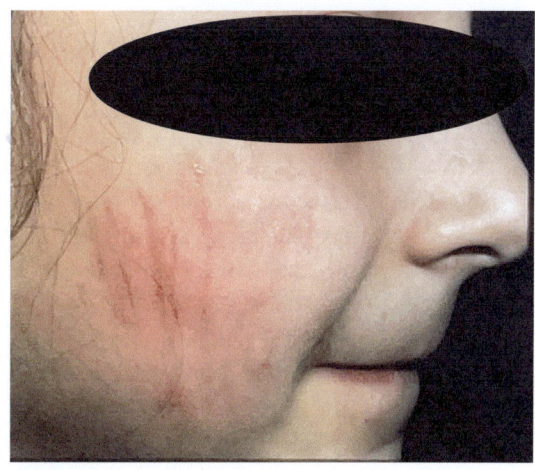

Fig. 39.2 Factitious disorder in a young girl

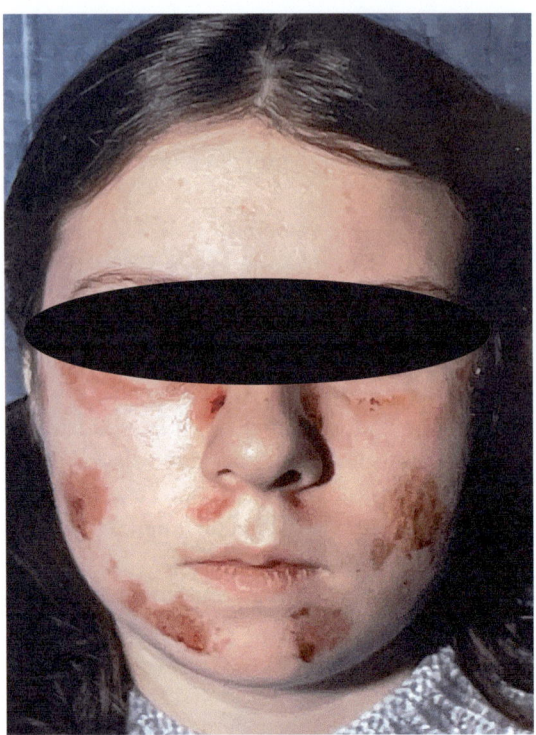

Fig. 39.3 Factitious disorder in an adolescent

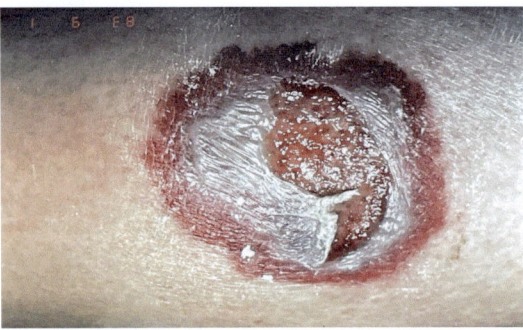

Fig. 39.4 Caustic wounds or burning as factitious disorders

complicate and delay the diagnosis, which is always difficult to establish. Borderline personality disorder, substance abuse, somatoform pain disorder, conversion disorders, sexual disorders, dysthymia and suicide attempts are frequently associated with factitious disorders [11]. Substance abuse, eating disorders and personality disorders are more frequently associated with factitious disorders consisting of direct self-harm (scratching, stabbing, burning) than in those consisting of indirect self-harm (using medications, chemicals or infectious substances) where anxiety disorders, adaptation disorders and somatoform disorders look more frequent.

(b) Communication between the patient and the healthcare providers

On the patient side: The relationship that the patient suffering from a factitious disorder establishes with the doctor is modelled on the relationship the patient may have had with his/her parental figures or relatives. Any close relationship or love bond, so vital and needed by patients with factitious disorders and on which these patients are dependent, is experienced as bearing a threat of betrayal, abandonment and even aggression. This may explain two things: first, the ambivalent attitude of patients with factitious disorders towards their physicians. Although initially a fusional relationship may develop between the physician and the patient, sooner or later, patients with a factitious disorder tend to show disappointment, snub and sometimes even develop an accusatory attitude towards their physicians. Secondly, the effects produced by the factitious skin disorder on the others will reproduce this ambivalence. The damaged skin represents a call for help, an appeal for care and love, and a means of distancing others, defying and aggressively manipulating others, who are perceived as unreliable and even dan-

erence for the sick role with no immediate tangible benefits. Factitious disorders in dermatology are at least twice more frequent in women than in men.

(a) Comorbidities

Cutaneous lesions can be accompanied by other factitious disorders; for example, a chronic fever can be associated, due to the manipulation of thermometer. These associations may gerous. It is a way to "control" people while keeping them at hand.

On the physician side: If the physician manages to think in terms of psychological suffering, he might find it easier to diagnose a factitious disorder and to follow up the patient. This would enable the diagnosis to be made initially, and not by elimination at the end of a long process, when the patient-physician relationship is already seriously deteriorated and no longer allows the psychological problems of the patient to be addressed serenely [12].

Attempts should be made to adhere to appointment schedules and limit investigations to a minimum and to create a safe and accepting environment during the consultation [13]. It is preferable to avoid any reference to the physical mechanisms causing the lesions, and instead focus on the "stress" as the probable mediator, which may be easier for the patient to accept and could be a rationale for the introduction of psychotherapy or a psychiatric consultation.

(c) Communication between the physician and healthcare teams

The whole healthcare team must function coherently, despite the patient's manipulation and ambivalence, to determine a common approach and to preserve the links between the various healthcare providers.

(d) Communication between the physician, patient's relatives and his/her general practitioner

Precautions must be taken when informing relatives, and even the patient's general practitioner, of the patient's condition. The dermatologist should insist on the seriousness of the psychological suffering expressed through the self-inflicted skin lesions [14]. It is important not to disclose to the relatives the patient's responsibility in provoking his/her lesions unless the relatives themselves proposed such a hypothesis. General practitioners should not transmit the suspicion to the patient and therefore jeopardize the further therapeutic approach.

(e) Specific therapeutic options

Most authors consider that confrontation is counterproductive and even dangerous [15]. Aggravating the cutaneous lesions, breaking off contact with the team, becoming delirious or committing suicide is reported when patients are confronted with the responsibility for the lesions.

Strictly occlusive dressings may be applied, and local treatments including antiseptic may be prescribed. As regards general treatment, antibiotics may be administered to treat secondary infections.

Surgical procedures should be avoided. Reparative plastic surgery should only be envisaged in collaboration with a psychiatrist-psychotherapist after a reasonable time has elapsed following healing of the skin and on condition that a marked improvement is observed in the patient's psychological frame of mind.

Regarding psychotropic drugs, antidepressants can be useful to treat an associated depressive syndrome and for making the patient accept a psychological approach without shocking or hurting him/her. Tranquillizers and antipsychotics should be used carefully, given the risk of abuse, for the first, and that of altering the trust towards the doctors, for the latter.

2. Prognostic aspects

In adolescents, factitious disorders represent more often than in adults "a call for help". More generally, an early onset of factitious disorders is of better prognosis than a late onset, as are the mild forms of factitious skin lesions, a shorter duration of the disease and the lesions produced in a dissociative state outside the patient's awareness. The quality of the psychotherapeutic relationship also contributes to a more favourable evolution. The prognosis is mostly worse, while the patients cannot be motivated into a specific therapy [16].

39.5 Conclusion

The clinician is often lacking efficient skills for facing patients with factitious disorders. This chapter aims to help deal with such patients. Moreover, if the clinician refuses to treat those patients or rejects them when the self-harm becomes obvious, this could lead to a repetitive behaviour, more and more difficult to treat.

References

1. Gieler U, Consoli SG, Tomás-Aragones L, Linder DM, Jemec GBE, Poot F, Szepietowski JC, de Korte J, Taube K-M, Lvov A, Silla M. Consoli self-inflicted lesions in dermatology: terminology and classification—a position paper from the European Society for Dermatology and Psychiatry (ESDaP). Acta Derm Venereol. 2013;93:4–12. https://doi.org/10.2340/00015555-1506.
2. Eisendrath SJ. Factitious physical disorders: treatment without confrontation. Psychosomatics. 1989;30:383–7.
3. Eckhardt A. Factitious disorders in the field of neurology and psychiatry. Psychother Psychosom. 1994;62:56–62.
4. Eisendrath SJ, McNiel D. Factitious physical disorders, litigation, and mortality. Psychosomatics. 2005;45:350–35.
5. Millard LG. Dermatological pathomimicry: a form of patient maladjustment. Lancet. 1984;2:969–71.
6. Robertson MM, Cervilla JA. Munchausen's syndrome. Br J Hosp Med. 1997;58:308–12.
7. Bouhamidi A, Mamouni Alaoui Y, Boui M, Hjira N. Cutaneous pathomimia in adults: a sign of psychiatric illness. Int J Adv Res. 2018;6:427–30. https://doi.org/10.21474/IJAR01/7379.
8. Virkkala J, Polet S, Jokelainen J, Huilaja L, Sinikumpu SP. Clinical characteristics and comorbidities of the most common atypical wounds in northern Finland in 1996–2019: a retrospective registry study. Health Sci Rep. 2022;5(5):e864. https://doi.org/10.1002/hsr2.864.
9. Poot F. Doctor-patient relations in dermatology: obligations and rights for a mutual satisfaction. J Eur Acad Dermatol Venereol. 2009;23(11):1233–9. https://doi.org/10.1111/j.1468-3083.2009.03297.x. Epub 2009 May 19.
10. Poot F, Sampogna F, Onnis L. Basic knowledge in psychodermatology. J Eur Acad Dermatol Venereol. 2007;21(2):227–34. https://doi.org/10.1111/j.1468-3083.2006.01910.x.
11. Stein DJ, Chamberlain SR, Fineberg N. An A–B–C model of habit disorders: hair-pulling, skin-picking, and other stereotypic conditions. CNS Spectr. 2006;11:824–7.
12. Mohandas P, Bewley A, Taylor R. Dermatitis artefacta and artefactual skin disease: the need for a psychodermatology multidisciplinary team to treat a difficult condition. Br J Dermatol. 2013;169:600–6.
13. Koblenzer CS. Dermatitis artefacta. Clinical features and approaches to treatment. Am J Clin Dermatol. 2000;1(1):47–55. https://doi.org/10.2165/00128071-200001010-00005.
14. Freyberger H, Nordmeyer JP, Freyberger HJ, Nordmeyer J. Patients suffering from factitious disorders in the clinico-psychosomatic consultation liaison service: psychodynamic processes, psychotherapeutic initial care and clinicointerdisciplinary cooperation. Psychother Psychosom. 1994;62(1–2):108–22. https://doi.org/10.1159/000288911.
15. Consoli SG. The case of a young woman with dermatitis artefacta: the course of the analysis. Dermatol Psychosom. 2001;2:26–32.
16. Feldman MD, Hamilton JC, Deemer HA. Factitious disorder. In: Philipps KA, editor. Somatoform and factitious disorders. Review of psychiatry, vol. 20. Washington, DC: American Psychiatric Press; 2001. p. 129–59.

Open Access This chapter is licensed under the terms of the Creative Commons Attribution-NonCommercial-NoDerivatives 4.0 International License (http://creativecommons.org/licenses/by-nc-nd/4.0/), which permits any non-commercial use, sharing, distribution and reproduction in any medium or format, as long as you give appropriate credit to the original author(s) and the source, provide a link to the Creative Commons license and indicate if you modified the licensed material. You do not have permission under this license to share adapted material derived from this chapter or parts of it.

The images or other third party material in this chapter are included in the chapter's Creative Commons license, unless indicated otherwise in a credit line to the material. If material is not included in the chapter's Creative Commons license and your intended use is not permitted by statutory regulation or exceeds the permitted use, you will need to obtain permission directly from the copyright holder.

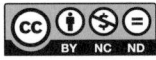

Part V

Skin Necrosis of Infectious Origin

Introduction to Necrosis with an Infectious Origin

Luc Téot

Infection leads to many types of skin necrosis, through various pathological mechanisms:

- Most of the time, germs directly induce toxicity in tissues through simple proliferation, and a massive accumulation of dead tissues will follow.
- In closed areas, like inside the foot of a patient with diabetes, an abscess forms and is surrounded by a large amount of inflammation, and the progression of this abscess will induce a level of hyperpressure that is capable of destroying tissues, such as in the case of an inverted-pressure ulcer. This mechanical process can be observed in other pathologies as generating an accumulation of pressure under the skin, like in dissecting haematomas or large eventrations when the mass of viscera applies excessive force beneath the skin, creating a devascularisation.
- In other cases, the germs may change their virulence in certain circumstances, such as a temporary decrease in immunological resistance (from a host resistance decrease from cancer, a severe infection, polytrauma, etc.). They also secrete necrotizing toxins. A series of well-known toxins, like Panton–Valentine leucocidin (PVL) and others, can destroy skin and muscles at a very large scale, require the amputation of limbs, and even be lethal.

L. Téot (✉)
Cicat Occitanie, Montpellier University Hospital, Montpellier, France
e-mail: l-teot@chu-montpellier.fr

Open Access This chapter is licensed under the terms of the Creative Commons Attribution-NonCommercial-NoDerivatives 4.0 International License (http://creativecommons.org/licenses/by-nc-nd/4.0/), which permits any non-commercial use, sharing, distribution and reproduction in any medium or format, as long as you give appropriate credit to the original author(s) and the source, provide a link to the Creative Commons license and indicate if you modified the licensed material. You do not have permission under this license to share adapted material derived from this chapter or parts of it.

The images or other third party material in this chapter are included in the chapter's Creative Commons license, unless indicated otherwise in a credit line to the material. If material is not included in the chapter's Creative Commons license and your intended use is not permitted by statutory regulation or exceeds the permitted use, you will need to obtain permission directly from the copyright holder.

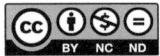

Necrosis and Infection

Farida Benhadou and Véronique Del Marmol

41.1 Introduction

Skin infection leading to cutaneous necrosis is a rare condition. The presence of an immunosuppressant state or an impaired vascular network is a risk factor associated with infection spreading and skin necrosis.

Numerous pathogens can cause skin necrosis, and some of them are associated with a high level of mortality.

This chapter reviews the various reported pathogens implicated in skin necrosis.

41.2 Bacteria

Necrotizing fasciitis, also known as the flesh-eating disease, is a progressively destructive bacterial infection of the skin, the subcutaneous tissues, and the deep fascia and carries a mortality rate of about 30%. Group A streptococcus, *Staphylococcus aureus*, *Clostridium perfringens*, *Bacteroides fragilis*, *Bacillus anthracis*, and *Aeromonas hydrophila* are the most reported bacteria causing necrotizing fasciitis [1].

Acinetobacter baumannii often with a multidrug-resistant phenotype is responsible for an increasing number of necrotizing fasciitis cases. *Acinetobacter baumannii* is a ubiquitous pathogen commonly found in water, soil, and the healthcare environment. Skin and soft tissue infections associated with *Acinetobacter* species are likely to be underrecognized. Clinicians should be aware of its potential as a multidrug-resistant pathogen causing hospital-acquired skin and soft tissue infections, particularly when associated with previous trauma or the use of invasive devices [2].

Another rare life-threatening infection is purpura fulminans characterized by cutaneous hemorrhage and necrosis associated with systemic symptoms. It usually occurs in children, but it has also been noted in adults. Infections reported to cause purpura fulminans include *Neisseria meningitidis*, *Streptococcus pneumoniae*, *Haemophilus influenzae*, *Haemophilus aegyptius*, *Staphylococcus aureus*, group A and other B-hemolytic streptococci, and *Pseudomonas aeruginosa*. Cases secondary to *Candida* and *Rickettsia* infection have also been reported [3] (Figs. 41.1 and 41.2).

Ecthyma gangrenosum (EG) is a well-recognized but rare case of cutaneous infection most often associated with a *Pseudomonas aeruginosa* bacteremia. Fungal and bacterial organisms, such as *Escherichia coli* and *Citrobacter freundii*, have been identified less often as the cause of EG. EG usually occurs in immunocompromised patients and is almost always a sign of pseudomonal sepsis. The characteristic lesions of EG are hemorrhagic pustules that evolve into necrotic ulcers. This clinical entity should be considered when otolaryngologists are asked to evaluate necrotic cutaneous lesions of the head and neck [4].

F. Benhadou (✉) · V. Del Marmol
Department of Dermatology, Hôpital Erasme, Université Libre de Bruxelles, Brussels, Belgium

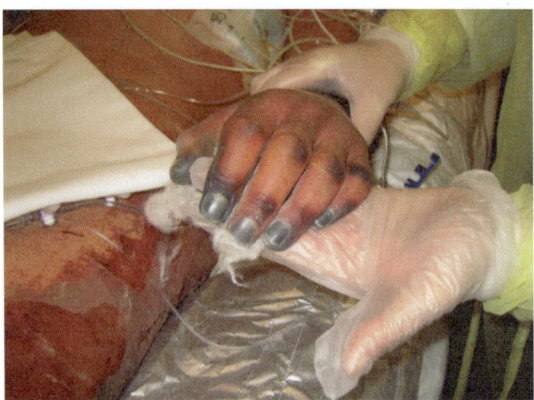

Fig. 41.1 *Acinetobacter baumannii* colonization and impaired blood flow

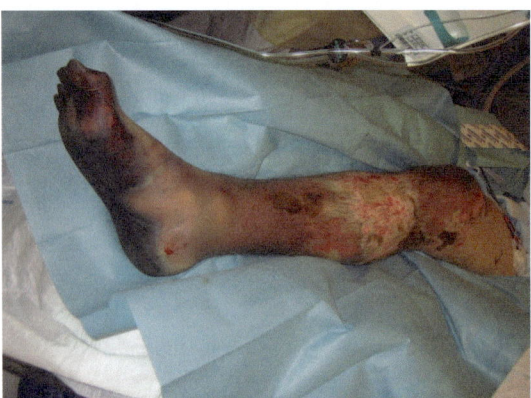

Fig. 41.2 *Acinetobacter baumannii* colonization and impaired blood flow

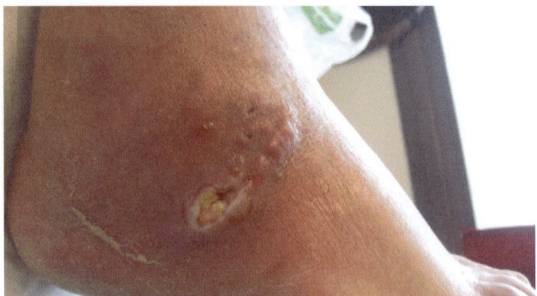

Fig. 41.3 Ulceration caused by mycobacterial infection

Syphilis is caused by a bacterium called *Treponema pallidum*. Syphilis remains a major health problem, and in spite of excellent methods for diagnosing and treating syphilis, the disease is still widespread. Syphilis is called the big faker because of its numerous and atypical clinical presentations. Cases of extensive necrotic plaques have been reported in patients with an HIV coinfection [5].

41.3 Mycobacteria

Mycobacteria affecting the skin like *Mycobacterium tuberculosis* or *marinum* are more frequently associated with chronic ulcers than with extensive skin necrosis (Fig. 41.3).

Mycobacterium ulcerans is the causative agent of Buruli ulcer. Buruli ulcer is a chronic debilitating skin and soft tissue infection that can lead to permanent disfigurement and disability. The bacterium is most prominent in tropical regions of Africa, Asia, Australia, and South America. Infection occurs through unknown environmental exposure; human-to-human infection is rare. The frequent clinical presentation is a deep, rapidly developing chronic ulcer associated with necrosis of subcutaneous fat. Bacteriological identification is not always possible. The pathogenic effect of the *Mycobacterium ulcerans* is due to the production of a necrotizing exotoxin with an immunosuppressive effect. Surgery is usually urgently required. The Buruli ulcer is now identified as a major public health problem in Africa [6].

Leprosy is caused by *Mycobacterium leprae*, an acid-fast, rod-shaped bacillus. The disease mainly affects the skin, peripheral nerves, mucosa of the upper respiratory tract, and eyes. It once affected every continent, and it has left behind a terrifying image in history and human memory—of mutilation, rejection, and exclusion from society. Lucio's phenomenon is a variant of type 2 leprosy reaction, and its clinical presentation is characterized by a necrotizing erythema. It is a rare condition that occurs in patients who were never treated or in those who have followed treatment irregularly. Lucio's phenomenon may reach severe proportions and cause death by disseminated intravascular coagulation and/or septicemia [7].

41.4 Viruses

The herpesvirus family and more specifically the herpes simplex and herpes zoster members are associated with cutaneous necrosis. Herpes simplex type 1 most commonly causes cold sores. It can also cause genital herpes. Herpes simplex type 2 is the usual cause of genital herpes, but it can also infect the mouth. Herpes zoster is the causal agent of varicella (chickenpox) and zona. The diagnosis of herpes infection has to be discussed in immunodeficient patients with extensive cutaneous necrosis [8].

Recently, cases of limited cutaneous necrosis have been described in young children who have been exposed to domestic rats. The necrosis was caused by the cowpox virus. Cowpox virus is part of the Orthopoxvirus genus, like variola virus, and is generally transmitted to humans by infected cats or rodents. The cowpox virus infection should be kept in mind when macular, vesicular, or necrotic cutaneous wounds do not improve with antibiotics [9].

Chronic hepatitis C infection is strongly associated with type II and III mixed cryoglobulinemia and occasionally associated with type I cryoglobulinemia.

Mixed cryoglobulinemia secondary to hepatitis C virus infection can involve the skin, and the development of a necrotizing vasculitis is observed in only 2–3% of patients with hepatitis C virus-related mixed cryoglobulinemia. The circumstances predisposing the infected patients to develop these manifestations remain unknown [10].

41.5 COVID-19 and Skin Necrosis

The COVID-19 pandemic is a global pandemic of coronavirus disease 2019 (COVID-19) caused by severe acute respiratory syndrome coronavirus 2 (SARS-CoV-2). The pandemic had caused more than 558 million cases and 6.36 million confirmed deaths. COVID-19 symptoms range from undetectable to deadly, but most commonly include fever, flu-like symptoms, and fatigue.

Nowadays, a wide spectrum of extrapulmonary manifestations in patients with COVID-19 have been documented. Rare cases of cutaneous leukocytoclastic vasculitis due to SARS-CoV-2 have been reported with fulminant necrosis. The mechanisms used by SARS-CoV-2 to induce leukocytoclastic vasculitis are not yet understood, but the hypotheses are that SARS-CoV-2 may induce endotheliitis, complement activation, and interleukin-6 release responsible for severe intra- and perivascular inflammation.

41.6 Yeast

Blastomycosis is an uncommon, chronic, granulomatous disease caused by the dimorphic fungus *Blastomyces dermatitidis*; blastomycosis has now been reported throughout Africa, in the Middle East, and in some parts of Europe. The skin is the most common site for dissemination, followed by bone, genitourinary tract, and central nervous system. Primary cutaneous blastomycosis is a rare illness occurring only after traumatic implantation of the fungus. The incidence of infection is highest in rural areas and in agricultural workers. Skin lesions in disseminated blastomycosis may be single or multiple, are often symmetrical, and are usually on the trunk rather than on the extremities. The primary cutaneous blastomycosis has a strong tendency for spontaneous recovery. Blastomycosis can be associated with necrotic skin lesions in immunodeficient patients [11].

There are fungal infections (*Aspergillus*, *Candida*, etc.) associated with a high level of mortality; therefore, prompt diagnosis and institution of antifungal therapy are vital, as is appropriate management of the underlying disease process. The mucormycosis usually affects the face or oropharyngeal cavity. The skin and the gastrointestinal tract can be affected. The immunocompromised patients are more prone to this fungal infection. The skin is rarely affected, and its clinical presentation is dominated by an erythema evolving into a necrosis [12] (Fig. 41.4).

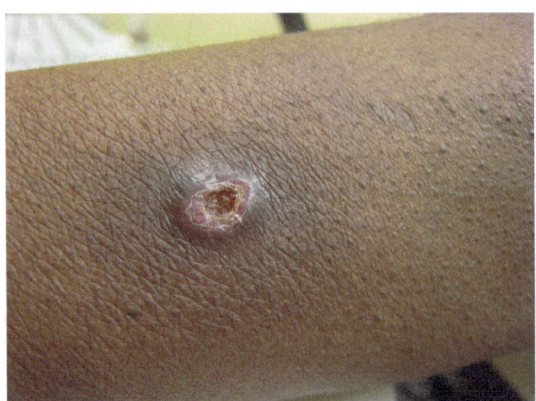

Fig. 41.4 Ulceration caused by candida infection in a renal graft recipient

41.7 Parasites

Leishmaniasis is caused by parasitic protozoan parasites transmitted by sandflies. Its clinical presentation is characterized by crusted papules or ulcers occurring several weeks to months after sandfly bite inoculation on exposed skin. Lesions may be associated with sporotrichotic spread and usually heal spontaneously. Leishmaniasis can also cause life-threatening widespread destructive ulcerations [13].

41.8 Pathological Mechanisms

Systemic activation of coagulation and dysregulation of the anticoagulation are the main pathways used by the pathogens to cause skin necrosis.

The interruption of the blood flow in the subcutaneous tissue causes ischemia and impedes oxidative destruction of bacteria by polymorphonuclear cells.

The pathogens can directly invade the blood vessel walls and injure endothelial cells, causing endothelial proliferation and decreasing the vascular lumen. Many factors help in the development of skin necrosis like decreased blood flow in the case of vasculopathy or diabetes, and an immunodeficiency gives the opportunity for the pathogens to proliferate.

Some pathogens are associated with skin necrosis secondary to the vasculitis process like the hepatitis C and the cryoglobulinemia vasculitis. The mechanisms used by the pathogens to induce skin necrosis are numerous and not completely understood.

References

1. Bellapianta JM, Ljungquist K, Tobin E, Uhl R. Necrotizing fasciitis. J Am Acad Orthop Surg. 2009;17(3):174–82.
2. Guerrero DM, Federico P, Conger NG, Solomkin JS, Adams MD, Rather PN, Bonomo RA. *Acinetobacter baumannii*-associated skin and soft tissue infections: recognizing a broadening spectrum of disease. Surg Infect. 2010;11(1):49–57.
3. Alvarez EF, Olarte KE, Ramesh MS. Purpura fulminans secondary to *Streptococcus pneumoniae* meningitis. Case Rep Infect Dis. 2012;2012:508503.
4. Chang AY, Carlos CA, Schuster M, Xu X, Rosenbach M. Nonpseudomonal ecthyma gangrenosum associated with methicillin-resistant *Staphylococcus aureus* infection: a case report and review of the literature. Cutis. 2012;90(2):67–9.
5. Jacobson M, Pollack RB, Maize JC Jr. Papulonecrotic eruption in a 44-year-old-man. S Med J. 2007;100(12):1221–2.
6. Doig K, et al. On the origin of mycobacterium ulcerans, the causative agent of Buruli ulcer. BMC Genomics. 2012;13:258.
7. Monteiro R. Lucio's phenomenon: another case reported in Brazil. An Bras Dermatol. 2012;87(2):296–300.
8. Peutherer F, Smith I, Roberston H. Necrotising balanitis due to a generalised primary infection with herpes simplex virus type 2. Br J Vener Dis. 1979;55:48–51.
9. Mancaux J, Vervela C, Bachoura N, Domartb Y, Emondc JP. Necrotic skin lesions caused by pet rats in two teenagers. Arch Pediatr. 2011;18:160–4.
10. Himoto T, Tsutomu M. Extrahepatic manifestations and autoantibodies in patients with hepatitis C virus infection. Clin Dev Immunol. 2012;2012:871401.
11. Dhamija A, D'Souza P, Salgia P, Meherda A, Kothiwala R. Blastomycosis presenting as solitary nodule: a rare presentation. Indian J Dermatol. 2012;57(2):133–5.
12. Zirak C, Brutus JP, De Mey A. Atypical cause of forearm skin ulceration in a leukaemic child: mucormycosis. A case report. Acta Chir Belg. 2005;105(5):551–3.
13. David CV, Craft N. Cutaneous and mucocutaneous leishmaniasis. Dermatol Ther. 2009;22(6):491–502.

Open Access This chapter is licensed under the terms of the Creative Commons Attribution-NonCommercial-NoDerivatives 4.0 International License (http://creativecommons.org/licenses/by-nc-nd/4.0/), which permits any non-commercial use, sharing, distribution and reproduction in any medium or format, as long as you give appropriate credit to the original author(s) and the source, provide a link to the Creative Commons license and indicate if you modified the licensed material. You do not have permission under this license to share adapted material derived from this chapter or parts of it.

The images or other third party material in this chapter are included in the chapter's Creative Commons license, unless indicated otherwise in a credit line to the material. If material is not included in the chapter's Creative Commons license and your intended use is not permitted by statutory regulation or exceeds the permitted use, you will need to obtain permission directly from the copyright holder.

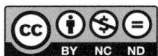

Fusarium solani

Raphael Masson

Fusarium solani is a filamentous ubiquitary yeast belonging to the *Fusarium* family, which includes several species. It is a pathogen that infects plants, but it can also infect immunodepressed patients [1]. The prognosis is severe [2]. Known risk factors are neutropenia and trauma. Sites of entry are the skin (cellulitis), nails (onychomycosis), lungs (sinuses, lungs), and eyes (keratitis) [3]. Dissemination is carried out via blood and induces fever in most cases.

Skin necrosis that looks like disseminated ecthyma gangrenosum may be observed in immunodepressed patients [4].

Negative prognosis factors are persisting neutropenia and long-term corticosteroid treatments [5, 6].

The check-up should include hemoccults and biopsies of the affected tissues to take histopathological samples, culture them, and later analyze the cultures.

The sensibility of *Fusarium solani* to antifungal therapies is demonstrated by a minimum inhibitory concentration (MIC) >8 in itraconazole, voriconazole, and posaconazole. MIC 50 and MIC 90 in amphotericin B are, respectively, at 1 to 7, which means that has amphotericin B exhibits the best in vitro activity on this yeast [6]. But MIC is not correlated to the efficacy of antifungal agents, and voriconazole may be an option in the treatment of cases of invasive fusariosis [7].

R. Masson (✉)
Wound Healing Unit, Montpellier University Hospital, Montpellier, France
e-mail: r-masson@chu-montpellier.fr

The antifungal therapeutic strategy aims to mitigate the risk factors and remove infected tissue through surgical debridement.

References

1. Venditti M, Micozzi A, Gentile G, Polonelli L, Morace G, Bianco P, et al. Invasive *Fusarium solani* infections in patients with acute leukemia. Rev Infect Dis. 1988;10(3):653–60.
2. Rabodonirina M, Piens MA, Monier MF, Guého E, Fière D, Mojon M. Fusarium infections in immunocompromised patients: case reports and literature review. Eur J Clin Microbiol Infect Dis. 1994;13(2):152–61.
3. Chang DC, Grant GB, O'Donnell K, Wannemuehler KA, Noble-Wang J, Rao CY, et al. Multistate outbreak of fusarium keratitis associated with use of a contact lens solution. JAMA. 2006;296(8):953–63.
4. Repiso T, García-Patos V, Martin N, Creus M, Bastida P, Castells A. Disseminated fusariosis. Pediatr Dermatol. 1996;13(2):118–21.
5. Nucci M, Anaissie EJ, Queiroz-Telles F, Martins CA, Trabasso P, Solza C, et al. Outcome predictors of 84 patients with hematologic malignancies and fusarium infection. Cancer. 2003;98(2):315–9.
6. Cuenca-Estrella M, Gomez-Lopez A, Mellado E, Buitrago MJ, Monzon A, Rodriguez-Tudela JL. Head-to-head comparison of the activities of currently available antifungal agents against 3378 Spanish clinical isolates of yeasts and filamentous fungi. Antimicrob Agents Chemother. 2006;50(3):917–21.
7. Lortholary O, Obenga G, Biswas P, Caillot D, Chachaty E, Bienvenu A-L, et al. International retrospective analysis of 73 cases of invasive fusariosis treated with voriconazole. Antimicrob Agents Chemother. 2010;54(10):4446–50.

Open Access This chapter is licensed under the terms of the Creative Commons Attribution-NonCommercial-NoDerivatives 4.0 International License (http://creativecommons.org/licenses/by-nc-nd/4.0/), which permits any non-commercial use, sharing, distribution and reproduction in any medium or format, as long as you give appropriate credit to the original author(s) and the source, provide a link to the Creative Commons license and indicate if you modified the licensed material. You do not have permission under this license to share adapted material derived from this chapter or parts of it.

The images or other third party material in this chapter are included in the chapter's Creative Commons license, unless indicated otherwise in a credit line to the material. If material is not included in the chapter's Creative Commons license and your intended use is not permitted by statutory regulation or exceeds the permitted use, you will need to obtain permission directly from the copyright holder.

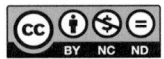

Fournier Gangrene

Tristan L. Hartzell and Dennis P. Orgill

43.1 Introduction and History

Fournier gangrene is a necrotizing soft tissue infection of the male perineum, although similar infections have been described in women. It is a type of necrotizing fasciitis, distinguished by its location of origin and with most cases being mixed infections of aerobic and anaerobic bacteria. It is characterized by a rapidly spreading soft tissue infection that travels along perineal subcutaneous fascial planes and obliterates perforating skin vessels but spares underlying muscle. High mortality rates have resulted in a heightened awareness by surgeons with a low threshold for intervention.

Severe, life-threatening soft tissue infections have been recognized throughout history. Hippocrates first described necrotizing fasciitis in the fifth century BC. It was not until 1764, however, that Baurienne first described a case of scrotal gangrene, characterized by a fast-spreading necrotizing infection. The disease ultimately took its name from Jean Alfred Fournier, a French venereologist who described five cases of perineal gangrene in clinical lectures in 1883 [1]. Even in this early practice of medicine and identification of a new disease process, academics recognized that diabetes and trauma were leading causes of Fournier gangrene. Fournier specifically described the ligation of the prepuce to control nighttime enuresis and archaic birth control regimens to prevent an adulterer from impregnating his married mistress as causes [1]. Herod the Great and Segundo Ruiz Belvis, a Puerto Rican abolitionist and independence leader, are suspected to have died from Fournier gangrene.

The number of annual cases of Fournier gangrene is difficult to ascertain, owing to inaccurate reporting, incorrect identification, and the many misnomers. Approximately 750 cases have been reported in the literature [2], and the prevalence has been estimated to be as high as 1 case in 7500 persons [3], although these numbers may be extremely inaccurate since Fournier gangrene is not a reportable disease.

The mortality rate has been reported to be between 14% and 80% [4]. The rate is on the high end in those who are older, have a rectal focus, and have diabetes [3]. The cornerstones of treatment continue to be early recognition, aggressive antibiotic coverage, prompt surgical debridement, and modern supportive care.

T. L. Hartzell
Faith Regional Physician Services Hand, Plastic and Reconstructive Surgery, Faith Regional Health System, Norfolk, NE, USA

D. P. Orgill (✉)
Division of Plastic Surgery, Brigham and Women's Hospital, Boston, MA, USA
e-mail: dorgill@bwh.harvard.edu

43.2 Physiopathogenesis

Fournier gangrene is no longer considered idiopathic in origin, as 95% of cases have a clearly identifiable cause [3]. For most cases, the triad of disruption to the skin barrier, location of the disruption in the perineum, and a decreased host response to bacterial invasion are present. The embryology and anatomy of this region that create multiple fascial planes that dissect reasonably easily, combined with the bacteriology of the perineum, undoubtedly contribute to the incidence of this disease.

Fournier gangrene starts as a routine infection in the anorectum, the urogenital tract, or the skin of the perineum caused by trauma, pressure necrosis, or conditions such as inflammatory bowel disease, rectal fistula, or hidradenitis suppurativa. In contrast to classical group A *Streptococcus* necrotizing fasciitis with a rapid onset in immunocompetent patients, Fournier gangrene has an indolent onset becoming fulminate due to a compromised immune system. Diabetes mellitus is by far the most common predisposing disease; however, numerous other predisposing comorbidities have been cited including chemotherapy, obesity, malignancy, alcoholism, intravenous drug use, malnutrition, cirrhosis, steroids and other immunosuppressant medications, cirrhosis, HIV infection, and Crohn disease [3].

In general, Fournier gangrene develops when an imbalance occurs between host immunity and virulence of the offending organism. The bacteria gain portal of entry from trauma (or one of the etiologic factors mentioned previously), the immunocompromised state of the individual allows these microorganisms to freely proliferate, and eventually the virulence of the bacteria leads to their rapid spread along fascial planes in the perineum (Fig. 43.1). Determining what virulent factors distinguish a routine, contained infection from uncontrolled necrotizing fasciitis has been the goal of researchers for decades.

Originally, Meleney reported in his 1924 series of Chinese men with necrotizing infections that streptococcal species were the responsible genus for this virulence [5]. Since this report, most cases of Fournier gangrene have been found to be polymicrobial and when streptococcal species is isolated, it is cultured alongside 2–5 other bacteria. Staphylococcal species, Enterobacteriaceae species, anaerobic organisms, and fungi are some of the more frequent causative organisms identified. In Fournier gangrene, it is believed that all of these organisms work in concert to create the final clinical picture. Macroscopically, necrotizing fasciitis produces rapid liquefactive necrosis of the subcutaneous fat and connective tissue, destroying skin perforators while sparing the overlying skin. This is in opposition to cellulitis and erysipelas, which affects the superficial layers of the skin and the lymphatics but spares the fat and fascia. With necrotizing fasciitis, liquefaction of fat leads to

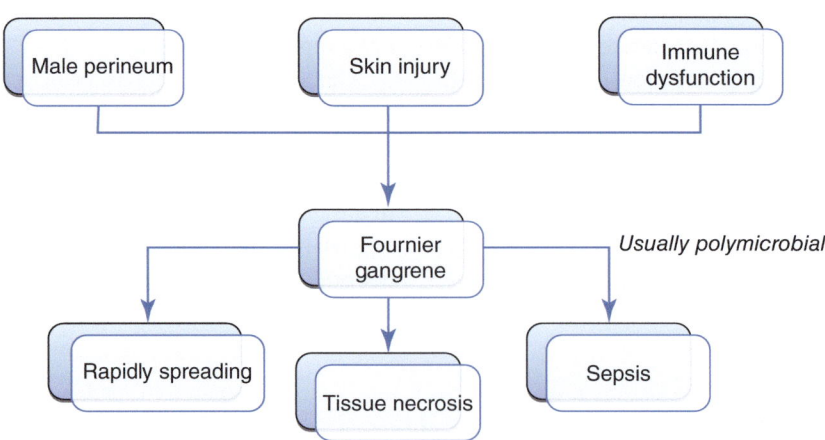

Fig. 43.1 Pathophysiology of Fournier gangrene

the development of a plane between the fascia and subcutaneous tissue that can easily be finger dissected. It also leads to massive edema and the pathognomonic "dishwater pus." Veins traversing the inflamed fat thrombose, and a vicious cycle of inflammation and necrosis propagates.

Researchers believe that a polymicrobial infection with a synergy of enzymes produces the macroscopic picture responsible for Fournier gangrene. For example, one organism may carry an enzyme that inflames vessels and leads to their thrombosis. Local tissue oxygen tension is decreased. This then allows an anaerobic bacterium to further propagate. This facultative anaerobe may have an enzyme such as collagenase in its arsenal that then digests fascial barriers and allows the infection to rapidly spread. Destructive proteases further destroy local tissue. A gram-negative bacterium then begins to propagate, releasing exotoxins and creating a cytokine storm and sepsis. Eventually, what started as a simple, indolent infection has become florid necrotizing fasciitis.

43.3 Diagnosis

A rapid diagnosis of Fournier gangrene reduces morbidity and mortality. However, the diagnosis is notoriously difficult and often missed until very late in the hospital course. Since there is no definitive test for Fournier gangrene, it is mandatory that the overall clinical picture be carefully considered. When there is doubt, early surgical treatment is preferred as the infection can progress to sepsis and death within hours. When unsure, a biopsy from normal-looking adjacent tissue, a fascial biopsy, and a gram stain can be performed before beginning with a disfiguring debridement.

A careful history can also aid in the diagnosis. Patients who are diabetics, obese, or immunocompromised should be of special concern. A history of recent trauma to the anogenital region, followed by an indolent infection, can usually be elicited. Patients often report weakness, low-grade fevers, and chills for a prodromal period of 2–7 days.

The examiner needs to be especially cautious in those patients who are unable to communicate pain or hesitant to allow a full examination. One should not hesitate to do an exam under anesthesia if necessary. A massive pannus or mons pubis, with or without underlying phimosis, has had several severe necrotizing infections in our experience.

Nonspecific signs of Fournier gangrene include tenderness, swelling, erythema, and pain. Unfortunately, these signs mimic non-life-threatening infections such as cellulitis and erysipelas. In our experience and in the literature [3, 4], the most common distinguishing feature is severe pain and tenderness in the genitals. This pain is out of proportion to the exam findings. As the infection advances, this pain progresses to paresthesias and numbness, indicating destruction of the cutaneous nerves. Similarly, with advanced infection, the skin changes appearance from red, hot, and swollen with ill-defined borders to pale, mottled, blistered, and gangrenous with sharp lines of demarcation. Hemorrhagic bullae are a late finding, but suggestive of the disease. The odds ratio (OR) of bullae for necrotizing fasciitis compared to a cellulitis was found to be 3.5 with a 95% confidence interval (CI) of 1.0–11.9 [6].

Subcutaneous emphysema is an often-sought finding of necrotizing fasciitis and Fournier gangrene. However, the diagnosis must not be excluded if there is no crepitus on exam or air on radiograph. The majority of cases of Fournier gangrene we have treated have not had subcutaneous emphysema. This finding is only seen when gas-forming organisms are present.

The role that imaging such as X-ray, computed tomography (Fig. 43.2), and magnetic resonance imaging plays in the diagnosis of Fournier gangrene is debatable. They should only be considered as an adjunct to the clinical exam in doubtful cases and should not be used to determine the extent of surgical debridement. In addition, performing these studies prolongs the time to treatment. If imaging studies are performed, it is important to reiterate that the clinical exam should supersede image finding. Gas seen on scans is usually an indication for operative inter-

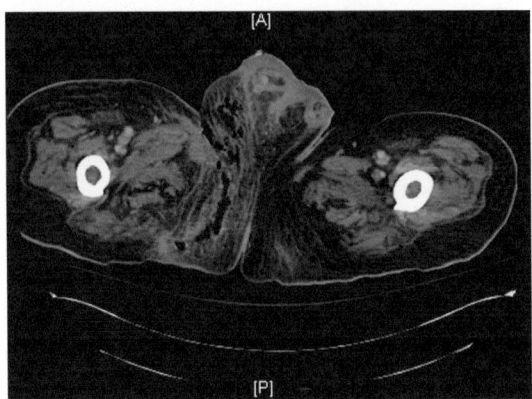

Fig. 43.2 Chronic stage IV right ischial pressure sore that progressed to Fournier gangrene. The patient had radical debridement of his right scrotum, right orchiectomy, and lower right anterior abdominal wall

vention; however, in patients with chronic pressure sores, gas can be seen in the absence of Fournier gangrene.

Ultrasonography has also been used in Fournier gangrene, mainly to assess blood flow to the testes. However, in our experience, it is very difficult to perform this test, as patients cannot tolerate the pain from direct pressure on the involved tissue.

If a frozen biopsy is needed to assist in the diagnosis, the pathognomonic findings of Fournier gangrene are (1) inflammation and necrosis of the fascia, (2) fibrinoid coagulation of the nutrient arterioles and veins, (3) polymorphonuclear cell infiltration, and (4) microorganisms within the deep tissue. The skin is often minimally involved in the disease process until very late.

43.4 Treatment

Fournier gangrene requires both emergent medical and surgical treatment. Patients with Fournier gangrene should receive immediate, empiric antibiotic therapy and emergent surgical debridement of the involved tissue. Aggressive measures should be taken to ensure normal end-organ perfusion. It is critical that these three measures be taken before pursuing unnecessary diagnostic maneuvers:

1. Resuscitation.
2. Parenteral broad-spectrum antibiotics.
3. Surgical debridement.

A multispecialty approach is mandatory, with the involvement of surgeons, infectious disease experts, and intensivists. The hospital course is often prolonged, and nosocomial complications are frequent. Urinary or rectal diversion may be necessary and, if so, should be done early.

The current antibiotic regimen of choice varies by region and hospital. The antibiotic spectrum should cover *Streptococcus*, *Staphylococcus*, the Enterobacteriaceae family, and anaerobes. Common first-line antibiotics for suspected polymicrobial Fournier gangrene are:

1. Ampicillin-sulbactam or piperacillin-tazobactam plus clindamycin plus ciprofloxacin.
2. Imipenem/cilastatin or meropenem.
3. Cefotaxime plus metronidazole or clindamycin.

It is essential that anaerobes be covered.

Clindamycin merits special mention in the antibiotic treatment of Fournier gangrene. It works by inhibiting bacterial protein synthesis, specifically decreasing the production of such proteins as SpeB [7]. Furthermore, its mechanism of action makes it not subject to the inoculum effect that occurs when large numbers of bacteria become slow growing and decrease expression of penicillin-binding proteins [7]. In animal models, clindamycin has been shown to be much more effective in the treatment of necrotizing streptococcal infections compared to penicillin and erythromycin, even when the treatment is delayed [8].

Ultimately, antibacterial coverage is tailored to culture results. With the initial debridement, blood cultures, a gram stain, KOH stain, and tissue cultures should be sent. If the patient defervesces and the clinical picture improves, the results from these tests can then be used to narrow antibiotic coverage. Most consider Fournier gangrene a deep infection and treat it with antibiotics for 4–6 weeks [9].

Antifungal agents are not used empirically in Fournier gangrene, as many are nephrotoxic. However, if the initial KOH stain shows fungi, amphotericin B or caspofungin should be instituted.

Many adjuvant medical therapies have been explored for the treatment of Fournier gangrene. Two of the more commonly discussed are intravenous immunoglobulin (IVIG) and hyperbaric oxygen (HBO). IVIG is postulated to work by neutralizing streptococcal toxins, mitigating the exaggerated cytokine response from them. Several authors have advocated for its use based on their experience in small series [10, 11]. HBO has also been advocated based on the results from small series [12, 13]. It is important to note that HBO is not without risk and has been reported to cause reversible myopia, barotraumas, pneumothorax, and cramps. Also, it should never take precedence over proper surgical debridement. Better studies are needed before IVIG, and HBO can be fully endorsed in the treatment of Fournier gangrene.

The unique role of medical comorbidities in Fournier gangrene merits special discussion. As mentioned previously, conditions such as diabetes, alcoholism, and immunosuppression are often predisposing diseases in Fournier gangrene. Strict glucose control and nutritional supplementation are two of the more vital adjuvant interventions.

While the medical management is important, ultimately the most critical part of treating Fournier gangrene remains surgical debridement. It must be swift and decisive. Any delay in surgery will increase mortality. As soon as Fournier gangrene is suspected, the patient must be brought emergently to the operating room for an aggressive and extensive debridement. Signs suggestive of Fournier gangrene are necrosis of the superficial fascia and fat, thrombosis of superficial vessels, and foul-smelling drainage. In early Fournier gangrene, the fascia appears edematous, while later in the disease, it becomes more gray and dusky.

With Fournier gangrene, tissue should be resected beyond the involved borders to healthy, bleeding edges. If the tissue edge is not bleeding, the vessels are likely thrombosed due to the inflammatory, necrotic process. It is our experience that with Fournier gangrene there is easy separation of the subcutaneous tissue from the fascia by blunt dissection. The margin of resection must extend beyond this easily separated plane. The deep fascia and muscle are spared in true Fournier gangrene; however, it may be involved due to the inciting event, such as a rectal fistula or anogenital trauma. If necrotic, it must also be aggressively resected to healthy muscle. Similarly, the testicles are often not involved in the necrotizing process. If they are exposed, though, they should be buried in a subcutaneous pocket or placed in a moist dressing to prevent desiccation. If necrotic, one should not hesitate to do an orchiectomy.

Reconstructive concerns are secondary as this is a life-threatening condition. Before leaving the operating room at the initial debridement, the wound should be reinspected for any remaining signs of gangrene. A dilute Betadine- or Dakin-soaked dressing is often used to cover the initial wound at this stage.

"Second-look" surgeries are often necessary within 12–24 h of the initial debridement (Fig. 43.3). Less urgency is often placed on these "second-look" surgeries. However, it must be remembered that this is the same rapid, aggressive, disease process, and it merits the same expediency as the initial presentation. Multiple "second-look" procedures may be necessary. Based on our experience, we make every effort to resect all actively infected and necrotic tissue from the start. We do not plan on "second looks" and have found that many times with an aggressive, proper debridement, the infection can be contained in the initial operating room visit. Our ideal treatment regimen is one thorough debridement followed by the placement of a vacuum-assisted closure (VAC) device. In general, healthy granulation tissue on the first VAC change is an excellent sign that adequate debridement has occurred.

Finally, if perineal involvement is extensive, the surgeon can consider diverting the fecal stream to prevent fecal contamination of the wounds. Modern rectal devices often avoid the

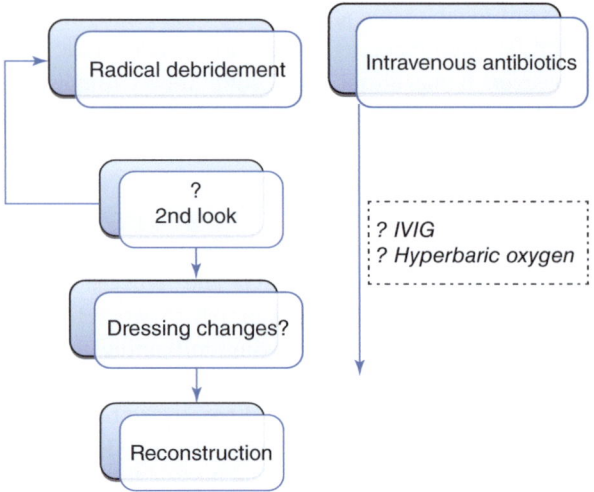

Fig. 43.3 Basic treatment algorithm of Fournier gangrene

need for colostomy. Urinary diversion can usually be accomplished with a urethral or suprapubic catheter.

43.5 Reconstruction

The reconstructive process begins with the preparation of the wound bed. To maximize success, the systemic condition must be addressed. Hemodynamic stability must be achieved, and severe anemia corrected. Like patients with large burns, nutritional support is mandatory from the first day of admission. A tremendous amount of protein and fluid is lost from these large, inflamed wounds, and it is easy for the patient to spiral into a catabolic state. Enteral feeding tubes may be necessary.

While the patient is being systemically optimized, dressing changes to the involved area are being done. The surgeon should not be rigid about one type of dressing, but rather flexible in dressing choices depending on the wound status. A typical regimen is to begin with dilute Betadine dressings for several days. Once the infection is clearly resolved, this is transitioned to a wet-to-dry saline-soaked dressing with or without topical antibiotics. The wound should be kept moist to avoid desiccation while preventing maceration. Subsequently, a hydrogel dressing may be employed to promote granulation. Another alternative is negative-pressure wound therapy (NPWT) devices, also commonly referred to as vacuum-assisted closure (VAC) devices. NPWT devices reduce the days of hospitalization, decrease patient discomfort and pain medication use, and allow for more prompt reconstructive surgery in patients with Fournier gangrene [14]. The NPWT devices have become very popular in the management of these large wounds, and we tend to employ it in all of our patients once the infectious process is under control. When a clean and well-vascularized wound bed is achieved, surgical closure can then be considered.

The workhouse of Fournier gangrene reconstruction is the split-thickness skin graft. Cadaver allografts can be considered if the surgeon is uncertain about the cleanliness of the recipient site. If these grafts take, the sites can easily be grafted with autografts in 1–2 weeks. While primary closure, local tissue rearrangement, and local flaps (such as the medial thigh myocutaneous flap [3]) may be employed for some wounds, most patients with Fournier gangrene receive a skin graft. Prior to any of these operations, the surgical bed is further prepared in the operating room. Any remaining necrotic tissue is removed, and microbial colonization is reduced with debridement and irrigation. Areas of hypergranulation are also debrided. The wound edges are excised to remove fibrotic tissue and obtain a uniform, level edge.

Split-thickness skin grafts are meshed to allow better contouring to the wound and expansion of the skin. We mesh at 1:1.5 or 1:2 for most wounds. The skin graft is secured with staples or absorbable sutures. Some surgeons use fibrin glue to assist with immobilization. A bolster dressing or NPWT device is placed over the graft. Those wounds where infection remains a significant concern can be moistly dressed with 5% mafenide acetate solution, dilute Betadine, or ¼ strength Dakin solution. If a bolster or NPWT device is placed, it is removed at 4–7 days or earlier if indicated.

Postoperatively, the patient must be rehabilitated from a demanding hospital course. The patients are usually extremely debilitated and benefit from physical and occupational therapy as well as nutritional replacement. They frequently develop lower extremity edema and may benefit from compression garment therapy. The debilitated patient may also require recovery in an inpatient rehabilitation facility. Long-term deficits should not be ignored. One study found that nearly 50% of men who had penile involvement had pain upon arousal, related to scarring and limited mobility of the genitalia [15]. Consultation with a psychiatrist is often important as well to assist in managing the altered self-image.

43.6 Conclusion

Fournier gangrene is a rare but serious infection that has a high mortality rate. Early diagnosis is critical. Patients presenting with pain out of proportion to the exam, spreading erythema, systemic laboratory abnormalities, and clinical deterioration should raise significant suspicion. Once suspected, the treatment must be prompt and definitive. Broad-spectrum antibiotic therapy should be administered and the patient brought immediately to the operating room. The surgical debridement should be aggressive until healthy, bleeding tissue is encountered. Reconstruction concerns are secondary, and the surgical intent should be to rid the necrotizing infection definitively, rather than plan on needing "second looks." Dressing care can transition to a VAC device, which assists in creating an ideal wound bed for skin graft, primary closure, or local tissue rearrangement. Much remains to be discovered in the pathogenesis of Fournier gangrene; however, unique virulence factors and abnormal interactions with the immune system have been recognized. It is hoped that one day, these insights will contribute to a reduction in the mortality rate of this aggressive disease.

References

1. Corman ML. Classic articles in colonic and rectal surgery. Jean-Alfred Fournier. Dis Colon Rectum. 1988;31:984–8.
2. Burch DM, Barreiro TJ, Vanek VW. Fournier's gangrene: be alert for this medical emergency. JAAPA. 2007;20:44–7.
3. Paty R, Smith AD. Gangrene and Fournier's gangrene. Urol Clin North Am. 1992;19:149–62.
4. Jiménez-Pacheco A, Arrabal-Polo MÁ, Arias-Santiago S, Arrabal-Martín M, Nogueras-Ocaña M, Zuluaga-Gómez A. Fournier gangrene: description of 37 cases and analysis of associated health care costs. Actas Dermosifiliogr. 2012;103:29–35.
5. Meleney FL. Hemolytic Streptococcus gangrene. Arch Surg. 1924;9:317–21.
6. Frazee BW, Fee C, Lynn J, et al. Community-acquired necrotizing soft tissue infections: a review of 122 cases presenting to a single emergency department over 12 years. J Emerg Med. 2008;34:139–46.
7. Bisno AL, Stevens DL. Streptococcal infections of skin and soft tissues. N Engl J Med. 1996;334:240–5.
8. Stevens DL, Gibbons AE, Bergstrom R, Winn V. The Eagle effect revisited: efficacy of clindamycin, erythromycin, and penicillin in the treatment of streptococcal myositis. J Infect Dis. 1988;158:23–8.
9. Shimizu T, Tokuda Y. Necrotizing fasciitis. Intern Med. 2010;49:1051–7.
10. Barry W, Hudgins L, Donta ST, Pesanti EL. Intravenous immunoglobulin therapy for toxic shock syndrome. JAMA. 1992;267:3315–6.
11. Lamothe F, D'Amico P, Ghosn P, Tremblay C, Braidy J, Patenaude JV. Clinical usefulness of intravenous human immunoglobulins in invasive group A Streptococcal infections: case report and review. Clin Infect Dis. 1995;21:1469–70.
12. Korhonen K, Hirn M, Niinikoski J. Hyperbaric oxygen in the treatment of Fournier's gangrene. Eur J Surg. 1998;164:251–5.
13. Hollabaugh RS Jr, Dmochowski RR, Hickerson WL, Cox CE. Fournier's gangrene: therapeutic impact of hyperbaric oxygen. Plast Reconstr Surg. 1998;101:94–100.
14. Assenza M, Cozza V, Sacco E, et al. VAC (vacuum assisted closure) treatment in Fournier's gangrene: personal experience and literature review. Clin Ter. 2011;162:e1–5.
15. Hejase MJ, Simonin JE, Bihrle R, Coogan CL. Genital Fournier's gangrene: experience with 38 patients. Urology. 1996;47:734–9.

Open Access This chapter is licensed under the terms of the Creative Commons Attribution-NonCommercial-NoDerivatives 4.0 International License (http://creativecommons.org/licenses/by-nc-nd/4.0/), which permits any non-commercial use, sharing, distribution and reproduction in any medium or format, as long as you give appropriate credit to the original author(s) and the source, provide a link to the Creative Commons license and indicate if you modified the licensed material. You do not have permission under this license to share adapted material derived from this chapter or parts of it.

The images or other third party material in this chapter are included in the chapter's Creative Commons license, unless indicated otherwise in a credit line to the material. If material is not included in the chapter's Creative Commons license and your intended use is not permitted by statutory regulation or exceeds the permitted use, you will need to obtain permission directly from the copyright holder.

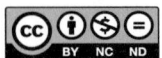

Infection Context: Necrotizing Fasciitis

Sadanori Akita

44.1 Introduction

The deep skin and soft tissue infections (SSTIs) primarily caused by group A *Streptococcus* (GAS) consist of necrotizing fasciitis and muscle necrosis. Necrotizing fasciitis is an infection of the subcutaneous tissue that rapidly destroys fat and fascia. It can be either monomicrobial (type II), where GAS alone or in combination with *Staphylococcus aureus* is the most common cause, or polymicrobial (type I), in which a mixture of Gram-positive and Gram-negative aerobes and anaerobes is present. Monomicrobial necrotizing fasciitis is more frequently seen in community-acquired or idiopathic cases, while polymicrobial causes are more typical after head and neck or genitourinary tract surgeries, such as Fournier's gangrene. The risk factors for invasive GAS SSTIs are numerous, including minor injuries, recent varicella zoster virus infection (which can lead to superinfected lesions), diabetes, and use of nonsteroidal anti-inflammatory drugs. These infections can occur even in healthy individuals [1]. Necrotizing fasciitis caused by group A *Streptococcus* was once considered rare, but population-based studies estimate there to be as many as 1500–3000 cases per year [2]. The high incidence, rapid clinical manifestations, and high morbidity and mortality rates of necrotizing fasciitis have been a focus of study in pathogenesis. Despite extensive research, the essential questions about the pathogenesis of GAS in necrotizing fasciitis remain unanswered [3].

44.2 Epidemiology

The US Centers for Disease Control and Prevention (CDC) reported that more than 500–1000 cases of necrotizing fasciitis (NF) are diagnosed in the USA each year. However, it is difficult to confirm an accurate estimate due to the use of various synonyms for these conditions. The annual rate of NF has been estimated at 0.4 cases per 100,000 populations, and it is increasing at an exponential rate [4]. NF is caused by an infection with a predisposing factor such as drugs, hypersensitivity, cardiovascular diseases, burns, insect bites, or trauma. NF can lead to severe sepsis, particularly among patients who are immunocompromised, are diabetic, have cancer, abuse drugs, or have chronic kidney disease. NF is more common in the winter, with the exception of necrotizing fasciitis caused by *Vibrio vulnificus*, which is more common in the summer and in males [4] and can occur at any age group. Approximately 50% of patients with NF

S. Akita (✉)
Department of Plastic Surgery, Tamaki-Aozora Hospital, Tokushima, Japan

Fukushima Medical University, Fukushima, Japan
e-mail: akitas@hf.rim.or.jp

have a history of skin injury, 25% have experienced blunt trauma, and 70% have at least one chronic disease. Half of all cases of necrotizing fasciitis occur in one lower limb and 30% in one upper limb.

44.3 Symptom

The early stage of necrotizing fasciitis (NF) is difficult to diagnose due to its nonspecific signs, such as swelling, erythema, and pain in the affected site, which can resemble non-severe soft tissue infections like cellulitis and erysipelas. However, magnetic resonance imaging (MR) may help differentiate necrotizing fasciitis from non-necrotizing infections by measuring the thickness and detecting the presence of low signal intensity in the deep fascia on fat-suppressed T2-weighted images, as well as the presence of non-enhancing areas in the deep fascia or involvement of three or more compartments in one limb [5]. NF is often accompanied by severe pain at onset, proportional to the physical findings [4].

44.4 Clinical Course and Features of Necrotizing Fasciitis

NF is a rapidly progressive and destructive bacterial infection affecting superficial and deep soft tissues, including the skin, subcutaneous tissue, fascia, and muscle. Within hours to days, the infection can progress from a seemingly benign skin lesion to a highly mortal condition (Fig. 44.1). Many clinical studies have reported that rapid and deep enough surgical debridement of infected tissue within 12–24 h from the onset of the original clinical manifestation is crucial for saving lives [4]. The bacterial infection spreads along the fascial and peri-ligamental planes, and excision of adjacent muscles or deep tissue is required. The fascia, with its loose fibrous connective tissue and neurovascular structures, provides a little anatomic barrier against the dissemination of pathogens. GAS proliferates in sterile sites and rapidly attacks acute inflammatory cells, resulting in severe tissue damage, which is compounded by potent proteases and degenerative virulent factors expressed by invading GAS and host-released polymorphonuclear (PMN) leukocytes (Fig. 44.2).

44 Infection Context: Necrotizing Fasciitis

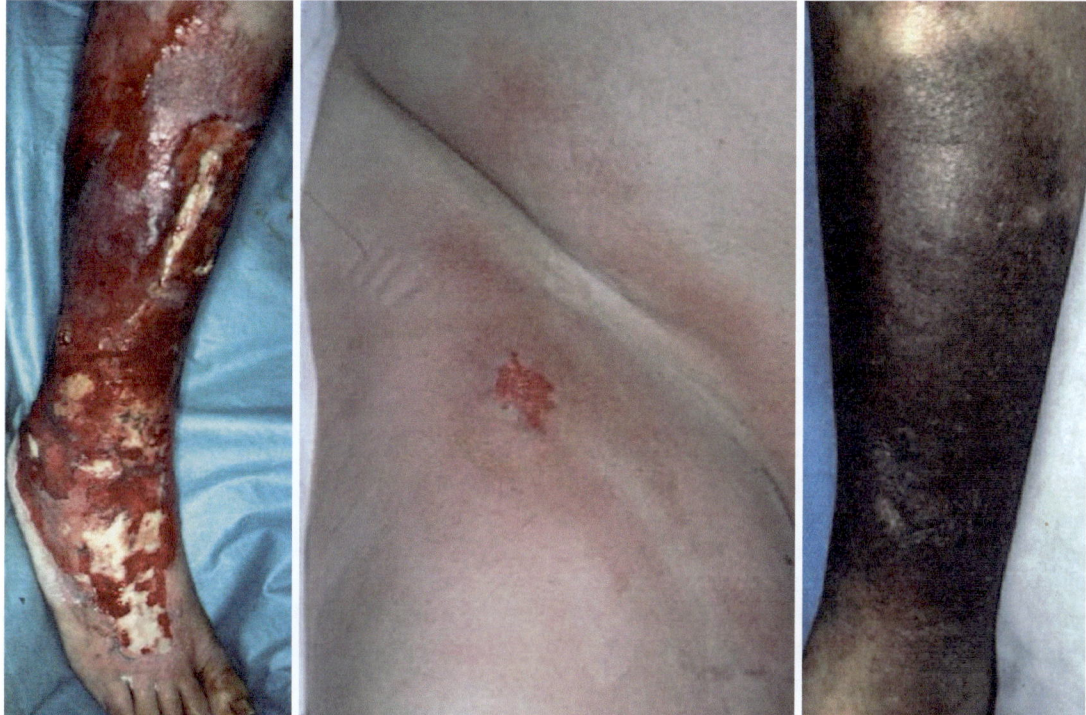

Fig. 44.1 A 66-year-old female, over years of medication of oral steroid (15 mg prednisolone) due to idiopathic thrombocytopenic purpura (ITP). Sudden onset of group A streptococcal necrotizing fasciitis in her right calf (*right*), ipsilateral thigh and inguinal lymph node inflammation (*middle*), and contralateral calf pigmentation largely due to ITP and continued hemorrhage (*right*)

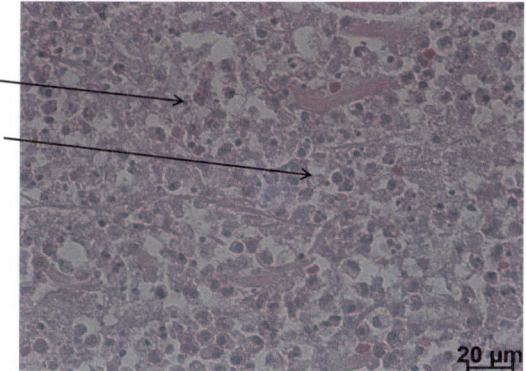

Fig. 44.2 Severe tissue damage deep to the fascia by invading group A streptococci and host-releasing polymorphonuclear (PMN) leukocytes (*arrows*)

44.5 Diagnosis and Tests

44.5.1 Physical Diagnosis

The odds ratios (ORs) between necrotizing fasciitis and non-severe soft tissue infections for fever, tachycardia, and hypotension are 3.4 (1.6–7.4), 4.5 (1.7–11.8), and 2.6 (1.1–6.0), respectively [6]. The likelihood of the presence of bullae in NF compared to non-severe soft tissue infections is 3.5 (1.0–11.9). Six percent of NF cases have skin necrosis, while only 2% of non-severe soft tissue infections have it. Initially, NF presents with erythematous and ecchymotic skin lesions, which quickly evolve into bleeding bullae, indicating that deep blood vessels in the fascia or muscle compartments have become occluded. The presence of bullae is therefore crucial for the clinical diagnosis of NF. Ludwig's angina (in the submandibular space) and Fournier's gangrene (in the scrotum, penis, or vulva) are variants of NF and often exhibit an explosive and aggressive clinical course.

44.5.2 Laboratory Tests

The Laboratory Risk Indicator for Necrotizing Fasciitis (LRINEC) score was developed to provide diagnostic clues for NF. A retrospective study suggests that a score of 6 or higher is highly indicative of NF, with a 92% positive predictive value and a 96% negative predictive value [7]. The LRINEC score is useful for categorizing patients into risk groups for NF.

44.6 Treatment

44.6.1 Medical Therapy

The broad-spectrum antibiotics should be empirically and immediately administered to suspected NF patients, as they may cover common suspected pathogens. The first-line antimicrobial agents for necrotizing fasciitis are listed in Table 44.1. In type I (polymicrobial) infections, the selection of an antimicrobial should be based on the patient's medical history, Gram staining, and culture results. Coverage against anaerobes is important in type I infections, and metronidazole, clindamycin, beta-lactams with a beta-lactamase inhibitor, or carbapenems are typically chosen. For patients who have been exposed to antibiotics previously, initial empirical therapy should take into account broader coverage against Gram-negative pathogens. Ampicillin-sulbactam, piperacillin-tazobactam, ticarcillin-clavulanate, newer cephalosporins, or carbapenems are potential options. In type II (monomicrobial) infections, the most common causative pathogen is group A *Streptococcus*, but sometimes methicillin-susceptible *Staphylococcus aureus* (MSSA) or methicillin-resistant *Staphylococcus aureus* (MRSA) can also be present. The use of tetracyclines and third-generation cephalosporins is crucial in managing *Vibrio* infections. The systemic antibiotic therapy for NF may continue for 4–6 weeks, as the deep-seated infection is established. Intravenous immunoglobulin (IVIG) is a desirable option for neutralizing streptococcal toxins.

Table 44.1 Treatment of necrotizing fasciitis, first-line antimicrobial agent

Mixed infection	*Streptococcus* infection
Ampicillin-sulbactam	Penicillin
or	plus
Piperacillin-tazobactam	Clindamycin
plus	*S. aureus* infection
Clindamycin	Cefazolin
plus	Vancomycin (for resistant strains)
Ciprofloxacin	Clindamycin
Imipenem/cilastatin	*Clostridium* infection
Meropenem	Clindamycin
Cefotaxime	Penicillin
plus	
Metronidazole	
or	
Clindamycin	

44.6.2 Surgical Therapy

Early and wide and deep enough surgical debridement is the mainstay treatment for NF and leads to better mortality compared to those who underwent surgery with a delay of a few hours [8]. When NF is suspected, the patient should be brought to the operating room for extensive surgical debridement. All infected tissue should be completely removed until there is no further evidence of infection. If further debridement is required, the patient should be returned to the operating room immediately. In this context, the use of artificial dermis after debridement is useful because it does not result in the loss of the patient's own tissue and makes it easier for "second-look" surgery or secondary reconstruction [9] (Fig. 44.3).

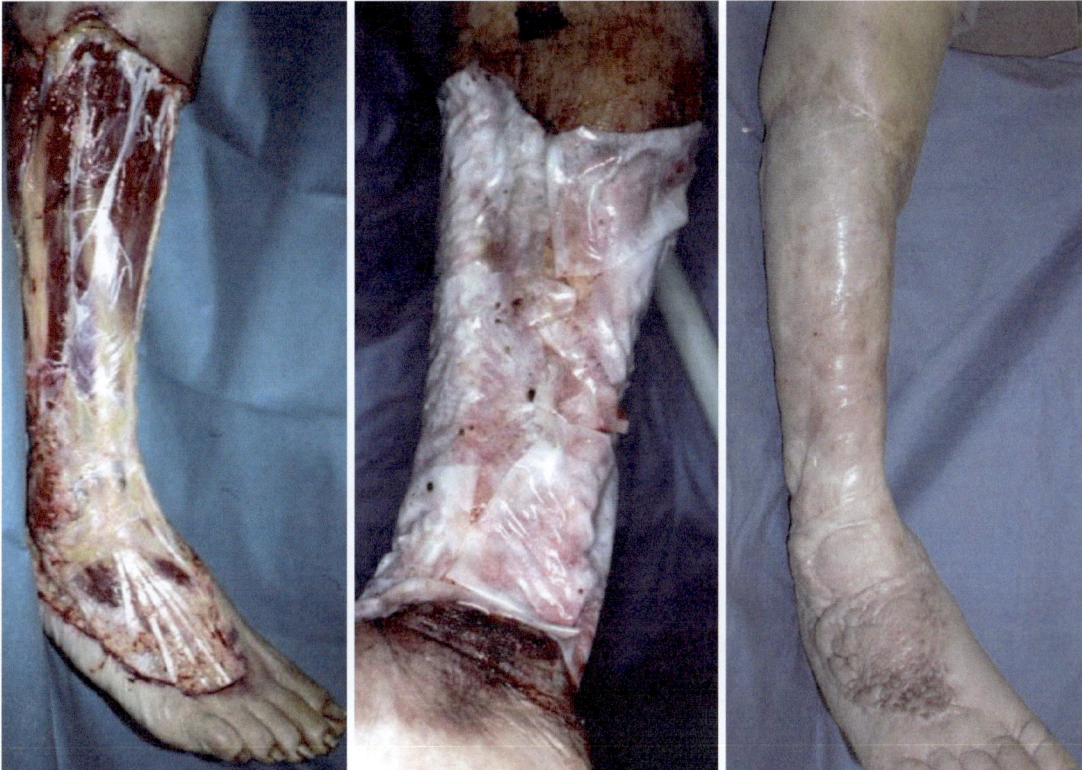

Fig. 44.3 Immediate (within 2 h from the onset) thorough debridement up to the fascia (*left*), temporal coverage with artificial dermis (*middle*), and 6 years after secondary split-thickness skin grafting (*right*)

References

1. Davies HD, McGeer A, Schwartz B, Green K, Cann D, Simor AE, Low DE. Invasive group A streptococcal infections in Ontario, Canada. Ontario group A streptococcal study group. N Engl J Med. 1996;335:547–54.
2. Carapetis JR, Steer AC, Mulholland EK, Weber M. The global burden of group A streptococcal soft-tissue diseases. Lancet Infect Dis. 2005;5:685–94.
3. Olsen RJ, Musser JM. Molecular pathogenesis of necrotizing fasciitis. Annu Rev Pathol. 2010;5:1–31. https://doi.org/10.1146/annurev-pathol-121808-102135.
4. Kaul R, McGeer A, Low DE, Green K, Schwartz B. Population-based surveillance for group A streptococcal necrotizing fasciitis: clinical features, prognostic indicators, and microbiologic analysis of seventy-seven cases. Ontario Group A streptococcal study. Am J Med. 1997;103:18–24.
5. Vinh DC, Embil JM. Rapidly progressive soft tissue infections. Lancet Infect Dis. 2005;5:501–13.
6. Frazee BW, Fee C, Lynn J, Wang R, Bostrom A, Hargis C, Moore P. Community-acquired necrotizing soft tissue infections: a review of 122 cases presenting to a single emergency department over 12 years. J Emerg Med. 2008;34:139–46.
7. Wong C, Wang Y. The diagnosis of necrotizing fasciitis. Curr Opin Infect Dis. 2005;18:101–6.
8. McHenry CR, Piotrowski JJ, Petrinic D, Malagoni MA. Determinants of mortality for necrotizing soft-tissue infections. Ann Surg. 1995;221:558–63.
9. Akita S, Tanaka K, Hirano A. Lower extremity reconstruction after necrotizing fasciitis and necrotic skin lesions using a porcine-derived skin substitute. J Plast Reconstr Aesthet Surg. 2006;59:759–63.

Open Access This chapter is licensed under the terms of the Creative Commons Attribution-NonCommercial-NoDerivatives 4.0 International License (http://creativecommons.org/licenses/by-nc-nd/4.0/), which permits any non-commercial use, sharing, distribution and reproduction in any medium or format, as long as you give appropriate credit to the original author(s) and the source, provide a link to the Creative Commons license and indicate if you modified the licensed material. You do not have permission under this license to share adapted material derived from this chapter or parts of it.

The images or other third party material in this chapter are included in the chapter's Creative Commons license, unless indicated otherwise in a credit line to the material. If material is not included in the chapter's Creative Commons license and your intended use is not permitted by statutory regulation or exceeds the permitted use, you will need to obtain permission directly from the copyright holder.

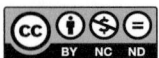

Part VI

Surgical Context of Skin Necrosis

Introduction to Skin Necrosis in Surgical Context

Luc Téot

Skin necrosis creates a local situation potentially leading to a spreading infection with vital consequences. Surgical debridement remains an issue as most of the surgeons may have concerns to introduce a septic patient in an OR which is not devoted to septic situations.

However, surgeons wiling to interfere more with skin necrosis may adopt recommendations concerning the post-debridement sequence leading to coverage and final closure.

Some wound situations need a surgeon involvement, particularly when a small orifice is hiding a large cavity or when there is a prolonged undermining or an apparent fistula with no skin exit (Figs. 45.1, 45.2, and 45.3).

Surgeons should understand the risk of spreading infection and the need for an adapted intervention depending on the local wound geomorphometrics but also on the general status of the patient and particularly on the vascular status.

In vascular leg ulcers, the degree of arteriopathy should be recognized with clinical signs (absence of pedal pulses), evaluated by ABPI (normal between 0.8 and 1.2), Doppler, and toe pressure and sent to a revascularization procedure by a vascular surgeon when needed.

In diabetic foot ulcers, some situations of skin necrosis are more frequently encountered:

– A distal necrosis involving a digit which does not cause huge difficulties.
– A part of the forefoot or a medial or lateral part of the foot where a collaboration between the avascular surgeon and the plastic/orthopedic surgeon is needed.
– A large infected cavity may develop with a limited entry usually located in a distal interdigital web. This situation requires inserting an instrument in the cavity to check how long the cavities are and in which direction (dorsal, plantar, lateral aspect of the foot). A counterincision is recommended by some authors, allowing to drain efficiently in a Seton mode (one entry, one exit) using wires or thin drainages. The drainage may limit the inner pressure and spreading infection, a factor of progressing tissue destruction.

The chapters presented in this part give an overview of the proposed surgical procedures concerning the different surgical strategies (Fig. 45.1) or exposing hidden pockets or draining subcutaneous cavities (Figs. 45.2 and 45.3).

L. Téot (✉)
Department of Plastic Surgery, Burns and Wound Healing, Montpellier University Hospital, Hôpital La Colombière, CICAT Occitanie, Montpellier Cedex 5, France
e-mail: l-teot@chu-montpellier.fr

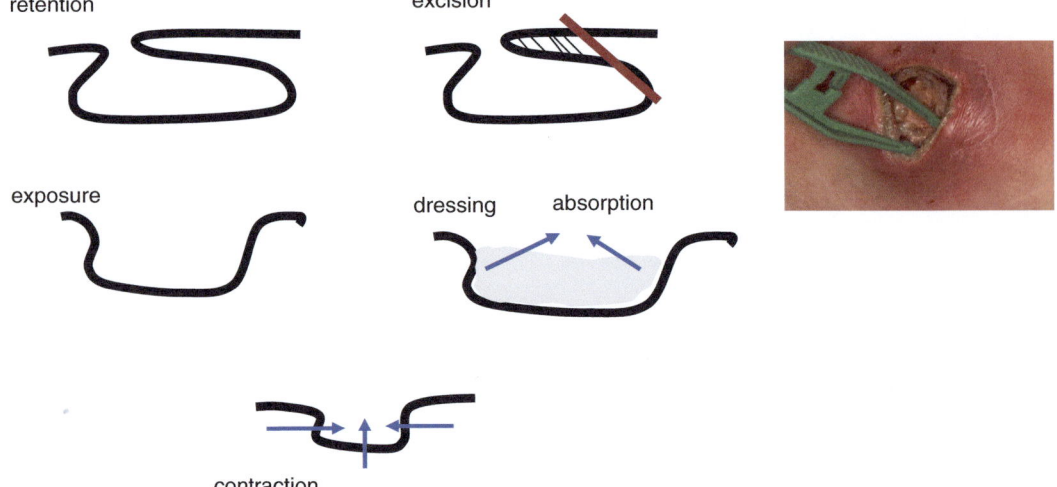

Fig. 45.1 The "deroofing" procedure consists in removing the cover of a poorly drained cavity prior to apply any type of dressing. This procedure allows to guarantee a full contact between the dressing and the edges of the wound, a prerequisite to start the granulation tissue formation and the contraction of the wound

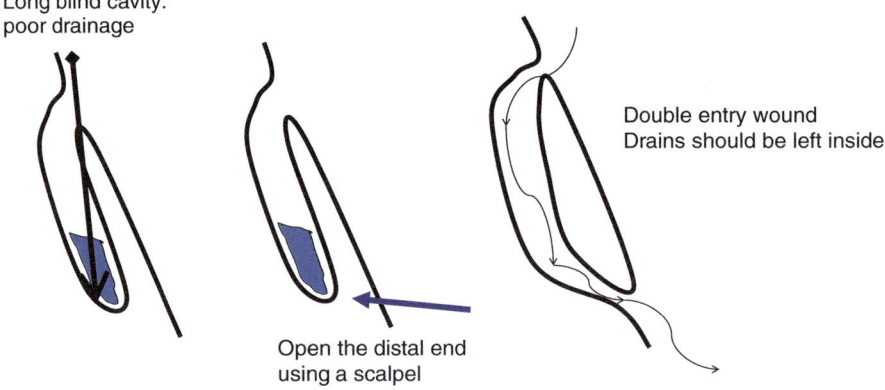

Fig. 45.2 Cavity wounds: drainage strategies

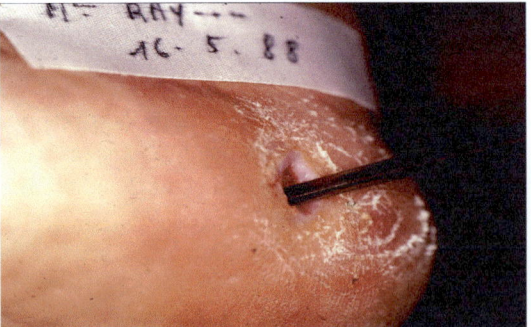

Fig. 45.3 emergency drainage in infected DFU reduces the purulent liquid pressure inside the wound and limits tissular damages

Open Access This chapter is licensed under the terms of the Creative Commons Attribution-NonCommercial-NoDerivatives 4.0 International License (http://creativecommons.org/licenses/by-nc-nd/4.0/), which permits any noncommercial use, sharing, distribution and reproduction in any medium or format, as long as you give appropriate credit to the original author(s) and the source, provide a link to the Creative Commons license and indicate if you modified the licensed material. You do not have permission under this license to share adapted material derived from this chapter or parts of it.

The images or other third party material in this chapter are included in the chapter's Creative Commons license, unless indicated otherwise in a credit line to the material. If material is not included in the chapter's Creative Commons license and your intended use is not permitted by statutory regulation or exceeds the permitted use, you will need to obtain permission directly from the copyright holder.

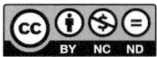

Skin Necrosis Over Osteosynthetic Material

Camille Rodaix

46.1 Introduction

Skin necrosis is a frequent complication in the management of traumatized extremity, particularly in the case of open fracture.

The treatment of open fracture is not the purpose of this chapter and will not be discussed here.

A prolonged period of hardware exposure ultimately leads to contamination, and then the goal of treatment is to prevent infection of hardware and underlying bone.

The traditional management of soft tissue defects and exposed hardware includes irrigation and debridement, intravenous antibiotics, and likely removal of the hardware. Obviously, preservation of the hardware would be the optimal goal to maintain stability and optimal reduction [1].

Skin necrosis covering osteosynthetic material can be divided into two groups: on the one hand that which happened early after the surgery because of soft tissue injury (contused or crushed) or too tensile strength in stitched and on the other hand that when a deep infection induces skin necrosis, early or later after the surgery.

In all cases, skin necrosis had to be removed, and bone and hardware had to be covered with soft tissue.

C. Rodaix (✉)

Department of Surgery, Montpellier Regional University Hospital, Montpellier, France

Orthopedic surgery, Polyclinique st Roch, Montpellier, France

46.2 Postoperative Skin Necrosis

In this case, skin necrosis is initially a soft tissue complication but can lead to a bone infection.

This is often seen in lower limb trauma with open or closed fracture. Skin necrosis appears because of a combination of soft tissue injuries (direct contusion, soft tissue degloving, displaced fracture fragments, articular dislocation, compartment syndrome), vascular injuries (hematoma, ischemia), early infection, and surgery (strength stitches, skin undermining, surgical approach).

46.2.1 Debridement

Those wounds require aggressive irrigation and debridement. This involves excision of all necrotic, devitalized, and contaminated tissue and bone as well as incisions for additional exposure and drainage [2] and had to be repeated every 24–48 h to ensure that all necrotic and devitalized tissue had been removed.

The aim of debridement is to prevent the risk of bacterial proliferation and to remove debris and necrotic tissue.

Many different techniques are available. Mechanical methods include water-jet dissection (Versajet hydrosurgery system [3]) or coblation technology (ArthroCare). Consensus on irrigation technique and additives (bacitracin, antiseptics, surfactants, or non-sterile soap) still remains to be determined. Other additions to wound care including the use of silver dressings [4] and negative-pressure wound therapy (NPWT) have proven successful in helping reduce infection rates. The use of NPWT has decreased the need for further debridements to every 48–72 h.

46.2.2 NPWTi

A modification of the NPWT system that adds automated intermittent wound irrigations was introduced nearly a decade ago. Instillation with normal saline can speed up wound fill with higher quality granulation tissue composed of increased collagen compared with traditional NPWT [5]. The instillation of an antimicrobial solution (antiseptic or antibiotic) into an infected wound can help decrease the bioburden and create a more favorable environment for wound healing [6]. In addition, analgesics may be mixed with some solutions to treat the pain that may be associated with NPWT therapy [7].

NPWT with instillation is particularly indicated to manage patients with infected orthopedic wounds (open fractures, osteomyelitis). Debridement of the infected and devitalized tissue and bone is important prior to the initiation of the NPWTi, especially for chronic infections where the presence of a biofilm may make penetration of antibiotics into tissues and bones and treatment of chronic infection more difficult.

The types of wound commonly treated from NPWTi are listed in Table 46.1.

46.2.3 Hardware Removal

In their review, Viol et al. [1] identified six parameters with prognosis relevance for the management of exposed hardware before soft tissue coverage and proposed an algorithm for treatment management (Fig. 46.1): location of the hardware, infection, type of bacteria, duration of infection, duration of exposure of hardware, and hardware loosening.

Absolute indications for hardware removal are the presence of hardware loosening, exposure of hardware for more than 2 weeks, and infection of hardware proved by positive cultures.

Table 46.1 Indications for NPWT with instillation

Wounds with persistent infection, especially after a trial of traditional negative-pressure wound therapy (NPWT)
Infected wounds with a foreign body in place (orthopedic hardware and total joint arthroplasty)
Exposed biologic or monofilament polypropylene mesh
Stalled wounds
Painful wounds
Wounds with significant biofilm present
Patients whose wounds are at a high risk of resulting in a major amputation due to the advanced nature of the wound and associated patient comorbidities
Wounds with a viscous exudate
Necrotizing fasciitis
Complex sternotomy wounds
Acute osteomyelitis
Chronic osteomyelitis after adequate debridement

Hardware removal is recommended in case of clinical signs of deep infection (the presence of purulent fluid and exposed hardware) and at the lower extremity when axial stability can be maintained with an external fixator device.

Osteosynthetic material for fractures or arthrodesis may be left in place for longer periods despite infection because the goal is bony consolidation, although the healing time may be prolonged. This is especially true for the spinal column, where the removal of hardware is only possible if stability is maintained.

Superficial infection without exposure of hardware can be treated without removal of the hardware but may nevertheless require additional soft tissue reconstruction [1].

46.2.4 Soft Tissue Reconstruction

In the case of exposed hardware as in open fracture, the concept of early coverage is important [8]. Patzakis et al. [9] have shown that only 18% of infections after open fractures are caused by an organism initially cultured from the traumatic wound, suggesting that many of the infections after open fractures are nosocomially acquired. For this reason, early coverage should be protective against infection.

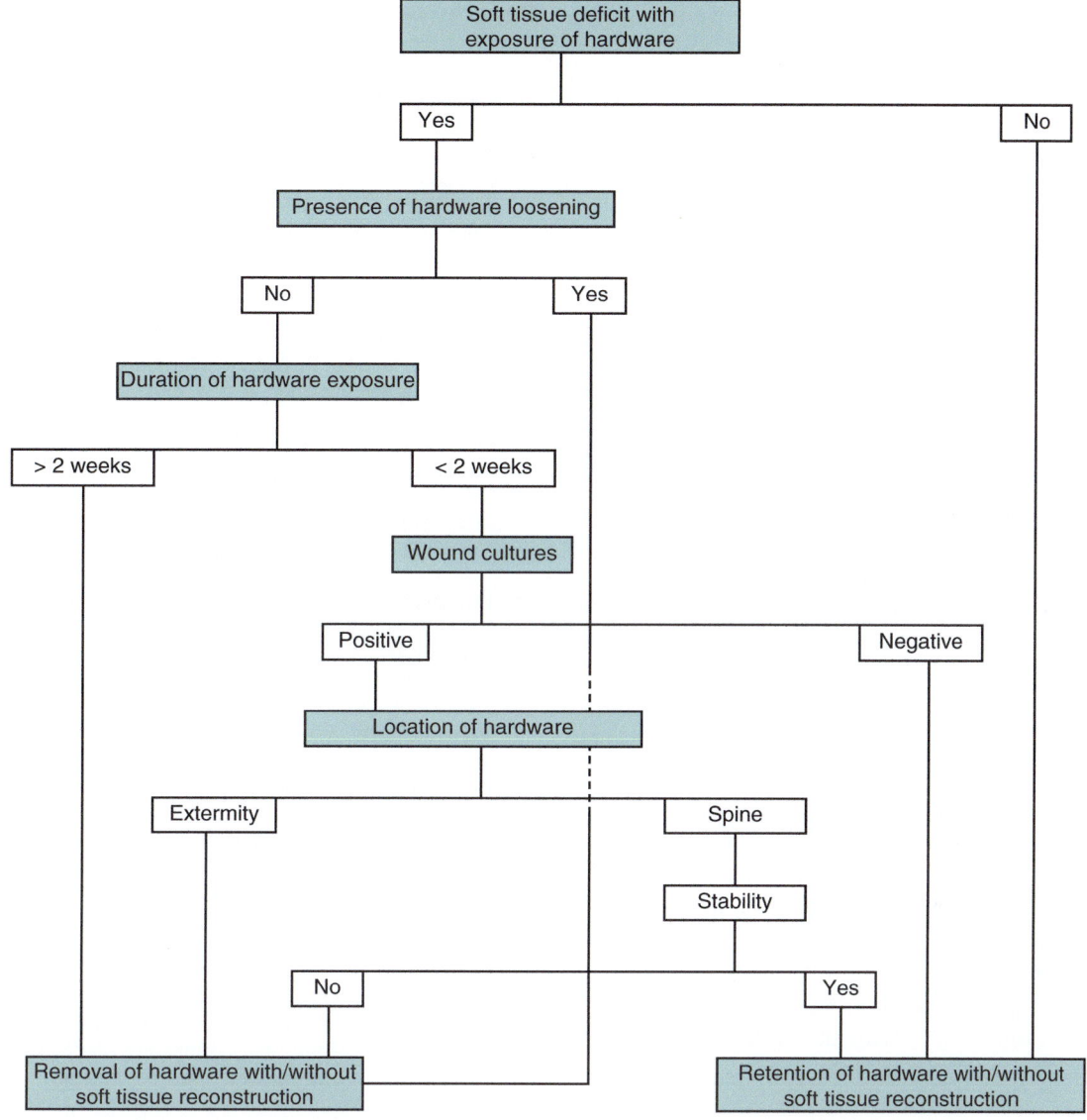

Fig. 46.1 Algorithm for management of soft tissue defects and exposed hardware according to the literature

Godina [10] found that early flap cover in primary trauma with a soft tissue defect was associated with a lower rate of failure of the flap, a lower rate of postoperative infection, a shorter time to bone healing, and a shorter mean length of hospital stay.

The local wound environment is usually ischemic and contaminated, with a soft tissue defect, and the use of free muscle flaps conveys a considerable advantage in such conditions because of their rich vascular supply and superior resistance to infection.

The ideal timing for free-flap reconstruction of these injuries has been controversial.

In the case of open fracture, free flaps transferred after 7 days had a significantly increased rate of infection and venous thrombosis [11]. Rates of flap take-back and osteomyelitis were significantly higher in patients who had metalware exposed for greater than 7 days compared to those who underwent free-flap coverage within 1 day of skeletal fixation.

Nowadays, local flaps decrease the need for free flaps in the reconstruction of the lower leg, and they are less expensive and time-consuming.

46.2.5 Alternatives to Flap Cover

Acellular skin substitutes (or artificial dermis), initially developed for acute burns, came to be used in the treatment of chronic wounds.

Because of the risk of infection and often poorly vascularized tissue, care must be taken in indications, and NPWT is often required to improve local environment.

Of course, skin substitutes as skin grafts must be used after removal of the hardware.

46.3 Delayed Skin Necrosis

Deep infection as osteitis, particularly in the case of internal fixation or arthroplasty, can lead to superficial wound and skin necrosis.

The definition of deep infection requires clinical signs and positive cultures. Radiographic signs of hardware loosening or bony infection seem to be not reliable enough to make decisions regarding the removal of hardware.

Management of infected prosthesis is quite the same with or without soft tissue defects, and early coverage is the rule.

46.4 Conclusion

Skin necrosis over osteosynthetic materiel requires debridement to avoid deep infection.

Deep infection, hardware loosening, and exposure of hardware for more than 2 weeks are indications for hardware removal if stability is achieved or can otherwise be maintained.

References

1. Viol A, Pradka SP, Baumeister SP, Wang D, Moyer KE, Zura RD, Olson SA, Zenn MR, Levin SL, Erdmann D. Soft-tissue defects and exposed hardware: a review of indications for soft-tissue reconstruction and hardware preservation. Plast Reconstr Surg. 2009;123(4):1256–63.
2. Baumeister S, Levin LS, Erdmann D. Literature and own strategies concerning soft-tissue reconstruction and exposed osteosynthetic hardware. Chirurg. 2006;77(7):616–21.
3. Klein MB, Hunter S, Heimbach DM, Engrav LH, Honari S, Gallery E, Kiriluk DM, Gibran NS. The Versajet water dissector: a new tool for tangential excision. J Burn Care Rehabil. 2005;26(6):483–7.
4. Dowsett C. The use of silver-based dressings in wound care. Nurs Stand. 2004;19(7):56–60.
5. Leung B, LaBarbera L, Carroll C, Diwi A, McNulty A. The effects of normal saline instillation in conjunction with negative pressure wound therapy on wound healing in a porcine model. Wounds. 2010;22:179–87.
6. Timmers M, Graafland N, Bernards A, et al. Negative pressure wound treatment with polyvinyl alcohol foam and polyhexanide antiseptic solution instillation in posttraumatic osteomyelitis. Wound Repair Regen. 2009;17:278–86.
7. Fleischmann W, Willy C. Vacuum instillation therapy. In: Willy C, editor. The theory and practice of vacuum therapy, Scientific bases, indication for use, case reports, practical advice. Ulm: Lindqvist Book-Publishing; 2006. p. 33–40.
8. Dedmond BT, Kortesis B, Punger K, Simpson J, Argenta J, Kulp B, Morykwas M, Webb LX. The use of negative-pressure wound therapy (NPWT) in the temporary treatment of soft-tissue injuries associated with high-energy open tibial shaft fractures. J Orthop Trauma. 2007;21(1):11–7.
9. Patzakis MJ, Bains RS, Lee J, et al. Prospective, randomized, double-blind study comparing single-agent antibiotic therapy, ciprofloxacin, to combination antibiotic therapy in open fracture wounds. J Orthop Trauma. 2000;14:529–33.
10. Godina M. Early microsurgical reconstruction of complex trauma of the extremities. Plast Reconstr Surg. 1986;78:285–92.
11. Shi Hao Liu D, Sofiadellis F, Ashton M, MacGill K, Webb A. Early soft tissue coverage and negative pressure wound therapy optimises patient outcomes in lower limb trauma. Injury. 2012;43:772–8.

Open Access This chapter is licensed under the terms of the Creative Commons Attribution-NonCommercial-NoDerivatives 4.0 International License (http://creativecommons.org/licenses/by-nc-nd/4.0/), which permits any non-commercial use, sharing, distribution and reproduction in any medium or format, as long as you give appropriate credit to the original author(s) and the source, provide a link to the Creative Commons license and indicate if you modified the licensed material. You do not have permission under this license to share adapted material derived from this chapter or parts of it.

The images or other third party material in this chapter are included in the chapter's Creative Commons license, unless indicated otherwise in a credit line to the material. If material is not included in the chapter's Creative Commons license and your intended use is not permitted by statutory regulation or exceeds the permitted use, you will need to obtain permission directly from the copyright holder.

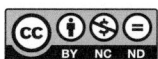

Necrotic Complications After Skin Grafts

47

Xavier Santos and Israel Iglesias

47.1 Introduction

Skin grafts are used in a variety of clinical situations. The essential indication for the application of a skin graft is wound closure. Skin grafts are usually the initial treatment of choice for many open wounds that cannot be closed primarily. Skin grafts are generally avoided in the management of more complex wounds. Anfractuous wounds; exposed bones, tendons, nerves, or vessels; and deep pressure ulcers normally require the use of flaps for stable wound coverage. Skin grafts have limited success in wounds with a compromised blood supply, such as irradiated wounds or ischemic ulcers.

Skin grafts can include either a portion of dermis (split-thickness graft) or the entire dermis (full-thickness graft). Split-thickness grafts can tolerate less vascularization of the recipient site but have a greater amount of contraction. The donor site generally heals spontaneously, through epithelialization from cells of hair follicles and sweat glands. Large areas of split-thickness grafts can be taken to cover big defects such as in large-surface-area burns. Full-thickness grafts require a better vascular bed for survival but undergo less contracture. Thus, if the recipient site is not well vascularized, full-thickness grafts have a greater chance to become necrotic. Full-thickness graft donor sites must be closed primarily. Thus, full-thickness grafts are only used to close small wounds, especially in the face because of better color matching and less contraction.

A skin graft is essentially a skin transplantation. The graft is completely severed from its blood supply, drainage system, and sensory innervation. The graft is placed onto a vascular bed so that it will become vascularized and sensate. So the survival of the graft completely depends on the recipient site. A skin graft becomes partial or totally necrotic when it fails to be vascularized from the recipient site. Necrosis of the transplanted skin is a complication of the procedure and can be related to the grafting technique, to the conditions of the recipient site, or to both of them.

47.2 Graft Survival

The process of graft survival has not been completely understood although it is accepted that it includes two phases: serum imbibition and revascularization.

Serum imbibition describes a well-understood series of events. After a graft is harvested, the graft vessels go into spasm, evacuating any old blood and serum. Once laid onto the recipient site, the graft passively absorbs the underlying serum. The graft becomes edematous and can increase in mass by as much as 30%. Metabolism in the graft

---

X. Santos (✉) · I. Iglesias
Department of Plastic Surgery, University Hospital Montepríncipe, Madrid, Spain
e-mail: unknown_user_562589@meteor.springer.com

converts to anaerobic metabolism, and the pH in the graft falls to 6.8. Metabolism waste products from anaerobic metabolism may stimulate the revascularization process. The graft remains edematous and in anaerobic metabolism for approximately 48 h until revascularization occurs, and the graft is able to unload its waste products.

Throughout the phase of serum imbibition, endothelial ingrowth from the host into the graft is occurring. Thus, vascular flow through the graft can be established as quickly as possible. Serum imbibition phase and revascularization phase can be thought of as overlapping rather than as mutually exclusive.

The phenomena occurring during the *revascularization phase* have been a matter of research for more than one century. In 1874, Thiersch proposed the theory of inosculation. This theory states that the cut vessels from the host bed line up with the cut ends of the vessels of the graft and form anastomoses. The process begins immediately, and vascular connections have been demonstrated as early as 22 h after grafting. At the beginning of the twentieth century, some authors proposed another theory. These works indicated that the original vasculature in the skin graft degenerates. Endothelial cells and capillary buds from the host invade the graft, restoring blood flow. Again, the process begins immediately, and as early as 9 h after grafting, inflammatory cells can be seen invading the graft. By the fourth postoperative day, flow through the graft has been reestablished. More recently, a third theory, first proposed by Henry, has evolved to describe skin graft revascularization. This theory states that the original vasculature of the graft does indeed degenerate. However, the acellular basal lamina persists, providing a conduit for the ingrowth of the new vascular tree from the host bed. Histologic studies have identified acellular patent vascular channels in the skin graft 48 h after grafting, which later become endothelialized from the invading host capillary buds.

There is strong evidence supporting all three of the proposed theories, and it is possible that graft revascularization involves all three processes. Inosculation may be responsible for early graft revascularization, allowing the graft to unload metabolic waste from the phase of serum imbibition. Concomitantly, the capillary buds and vascular endothelium developing in the bed invade the graft in both a random pattern and through patent vascular channels.

It is widely believed that a split-thickness graft can survive longer without revascularization than a full-thickness graft can. Split-thickness grafts contain fewer cellular elements than full-thickness grafts do. Also, a thick dermis acts as a barrier to diffusion of serum during the phase of serum imbibition. A thin split-thickness graft can survive longer during serum imbibition because there are fewer cellular elements to nourish, and there is a shorter distance of diffusion through the dermis. Thus, in managing a wound with marginal vascular bed, a thin graft is more likely to survive than a thick graft.

47.3 Graft Failure and Necrosis

Any development that disrupts the process of serum imbibition or revascularization will result in failure of the skin graft and necrosis of the transplanted skin. This failure of graft taking can be related to recipient site circumstances, intraoperative or postoperative complications, or technical errors. If a skin graft fails to be revascularized, the transplanted tissue will develop total or partial necrosis. It is important to make a correct indication for skin grafting with respect to the wound bed, graft thickness selection, meticulous technique, and adequate postoperative care.

47.3.1 Recipient Site

The process of skin graft take depends on a healthy and vascularized bed. One of the most common causes of skin graft failure is an inadequate bed. Exposed tendon, bone, and cartilage will not support a skin graft and can be considered a contraindication to skin graft application. Fat, peritenon, perichondrium, and periosteum are poorly vascularized, but they will support split-thickness skin graft. However, conservative treatment with dressings and/or negative pressure therapy can stimulate development of granulation

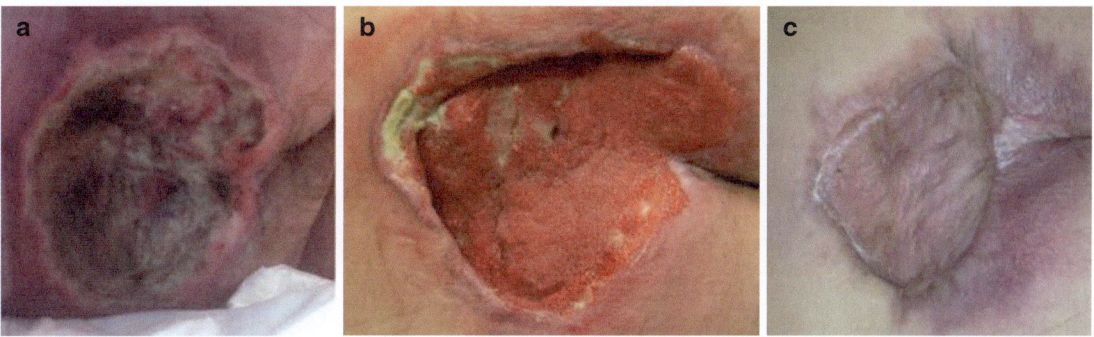

Fig. 47.1 Sacral pressure ulcer with necrotic tissues and exposed bone (**a**). Vascularized bed with granulation tissue developed after surgical debridement and negative-pressure therapy (**b**). Closure with split-thickness graft (**c**)

tissue, creating a vascularized bed, which improves the chances of skin graft take. In those cases in which a well-vascularized bed cannot be achieved (arterial ulcers, radiated bed), skin grafting will drive to necrosis of the transplant. In such situations, a well-vascularized flap must be the election.

The presence of necrotic tissues is an absolute contraindication for skin grafting. Necrotic tissue must be surgically removed and the wound treated in an adequate way to allow development of healthy granulation tissue. Once a well-vascularized bed is present, a split-thickness graft can be used to close the wound (Fig. 47.1).

47.3.2 Barriers Between Bed and Graft

Any barrier between the graft and the recipient bed can prevent revascularization of the graft. The most common barriers are blood, serum, and purulent material. Hematoma, seroma, and infection can lead to either partial or complete skin graft necrosis.

To prevent blood depots between the graft and the bed, careful hemostasis must be performed in the wound bed before the graft is placed. A useful preventive maneuver is to make small cuts in the graft to allow blood drainage (Fig. 47.2).

If in the postoperative period fluid collections develop under a skin graft, they can also be evacuated through small cuts in the graft, often saving a portion of the skin graft. It is better to cut a small hole in the graft over a hematoma than to

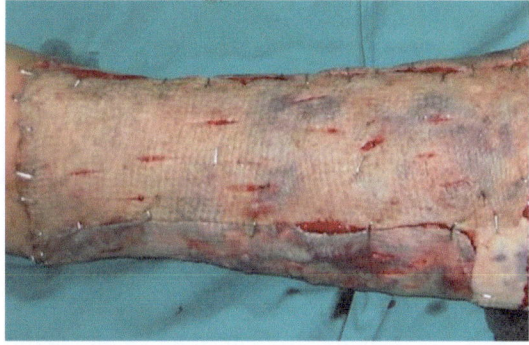

Fig. 47.2 Small cuts in a graft to allow drainage of blood

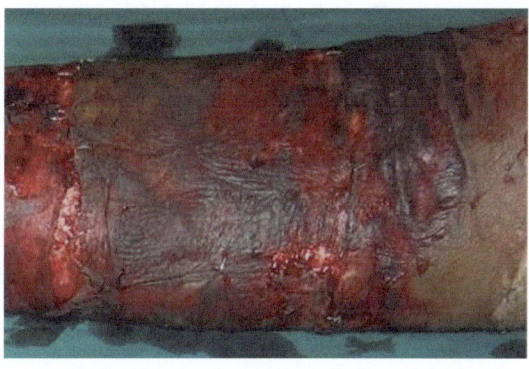

Fig. 47.3 Blood collection under a split-thickness graft that leads to necrosis of the graft

dislodge surrounding adherent graft to express the fluid through the graft periphery. If eschar is present, it should be debrided because eschar offers an excellent medium for bacteria. If large collections of blood accumulate between the graft and the bed, the more probable outcome will be the necrosis of the graft (Fig. 47.3).

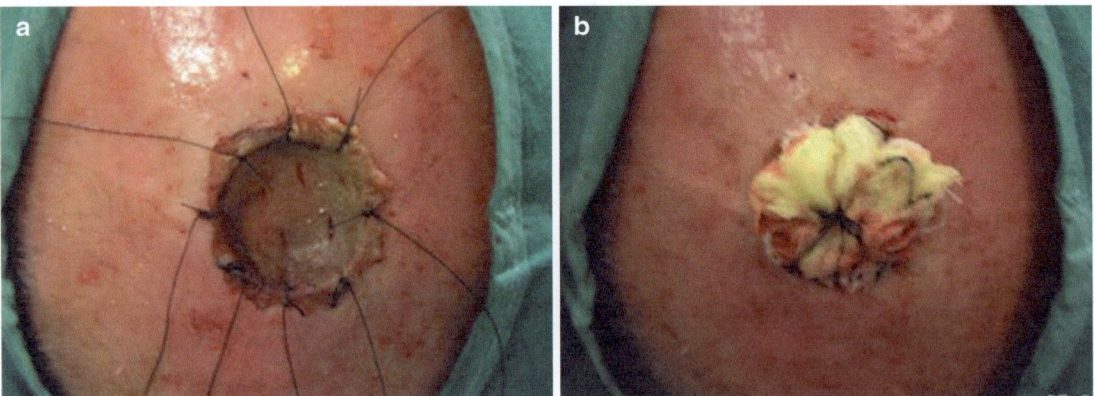

Fig. 47.4 Split-thickness skin graft to close the defect after excision of a basocellular carcinoma in the scalp (**a**). Bolus dressing to keep the graft in place (**b**)

To prevent fluid collection under the graft, it is recommended to apply a compressive dressing. Pressure should help to stop bleeding and seroma formation. In small grafts, it is very useful to apply a bolus or tie-over dressing to keep the contact between the graft and the bed and prevent fluid collections. To use a bolus dressing, the graft must be fixated with a permanent suture which is intentionally cut long. This leaves strands of suture that will be used to hold the dressing on. Once the sutures are placed, petrolatum gauze, Vaseline gauze, or Mepitel® is applied on top of the graft. Fluffed gauze or cotton balls are gently pressed onto the graft. The suture strands are then tied together so that they hold the dressing firmly onto the graft (Fig. 47.4). Apart from minimizing the risk of fluid collections under the graft, the bolus dressing prevents shearing forces from disrupting the graft.

In larger grafts, the dressing should apply gentle pressure on the graft to promote graft adherence without causing pressure necrosis. Cotton balls or fluffed gauze is pressed onto the wound to conform to the underlying bed. On an extremity, a circumferential wrap can be applied snugly across the wound to ensure contact between the graft and the host bed.

47.3.3 Graft Shearing

One of the most common causes of graft failure is shearing of the graft. The small capillaries that invade the graft are fragile and can be disrupted with a minimum force. Grafts can be devascularized during a dressing change or during movement in the early postoperative period. Consequently, grafts to the extremities are usually immobilized, and all dressing changes are performed with utmost care for the underlying graft. A nonadherent dressing must be applied over the graft. The silicone mesh dressings like Mepitel® have proved to adhere only to intact skin but not to the wound or the graft itself. The nonadherent properties of these types of dressings prevent the skin graft from being debrided off the wound at the time of the first dressing change.

If a portion of the graft appears to be sheared at the time of dressing change, it should be replaced and newly immobilized. In some cases, these displaced parts of the graft will take. If not, they should be removed with scissors, and if the defect is small, it will be re-epithelialized from the edges of the remaining graft.

47.3.4 Infection

Infection can cause destruction and necrosis of the graft without the formation of purulent drainage. It is generally accepted that a wound with more than 10^5 organisms per gram of tissue will not accept a skin graft. Some organisms, *Pseudomonas* being the most common, can destroy a skin graft with little or no purulence (Fig. 47.5). The infection does not have to be limited to the wound. In fact, some authors recom-

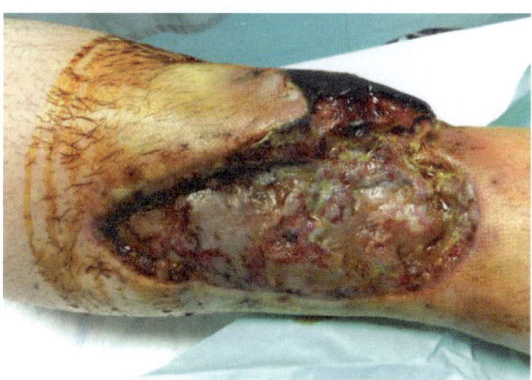

Fig. 47.5 Total destruction of a skin graft by *Pseudomonas* infection

mended that a patient be completely free of infection before skin grafting. Systemic infection can lead to poor wound healing and ultimately partial or total graft failure.

To prevent infection, apart from systemic antibiotics, local antiseptics should be used in the dressing. Nitrofurazone cream or povidone-iodine gel can be used on top of the graft before the compression dressing is placed.

Once an infection has destroyed a skin graft, the wound must be managed with extensive debridement, local and systemic antimicrobial treatment, and prevention of new grafting until the wound is clinical and microbiologically free of infection.

47.3.5 Poor Systemic Conditions

Unfavorable systemic conditions can lead to poor graft take and necrosis of the transplanted skin. Malnutrition, diabetes, vasculitis, malignant disease, steroids, and chemotherapeutic medications have all been shown to impair wound healing and to impair graft take. Radiation injury impairs the recipient bed and can lead to total or partial skin graft failure.

47.3.6 Technical Errors

Technical errors during grafting are a relatively uncommon cause of graft failure today. Grafts can be applied upside-down or they can be handled roughly, leading to total or partial necrosis. Dermatomes can be too hot after sterilization and burn the graft during the preparation phase.

First dressing change should be done at postoperative fifth day. If it is done earlier, there is a significant chance of shearing and disruption of the small capillaries penetrating the graft.

47.4 Graft Rescue

When there is a partial graft failure not caused by infection, there are some chances to rescue the already taken graft. The necrotic portion of the graft should be removed with scalpel or scissors. If the defect is not too large, it will be re-epithelialized from the edges of the defect. Adequate nonadherent dressing should be applied to allow this process. If the defect is large, it should be regrafted.

When the cause of graft failure is infection, the more probable outcome will be the total loss of the graft. In such cases, the wound should be managed as an infected one and when sterile regrafted.

Open Access This chapter is licensed under the terms of the Creative Commons Attribution-NonCommercial-NoDerivatives 4.0 International License (http://creativecommons.org/licenses/by-nc-nd/4.0/), which permits any non-commercial use, sharing, distribution and reproduction in any medium or format, as long as you give appropriate credit to the original author(s) and the source, provide a link to the Creative Commons license and indicate if you modified the licensed material. You do not have permission under this license to share adapted material derived from this chapter or parts of it.

The images or other third party material in this chapter are included in the chapter's Creative Commons license, unless indicated otherwise in a credit line to the material. If material is not included in the chapter's Creative Commons license and your intended use is not permitted by statutory regulation or exceeds the permitted use, you will need to obtain permission directly from the copyright holder.

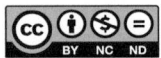

Arterial Leg Ulcers

48

Josef Aschwanden, Jurg Hafner, Vincenzo Jacomella, and Severin Läuchli

48.1 Introduction

Leg ulcers are not a diagnosis but a symptom of many different diseases. In this chapter, we will describe leg ulcers caused by arterial disease. However, many other causes should be considered in refractory ulceration on the lower extremity such as venous disease, neuropathy, and miscellaneous causes like vasculitis, malignancy, and autoimmune disease and even rare causes like pyoderma gangrenosum [1], thromboangiitis obliterans, or arterial-venous malformation. Martorell hypertensive ischemic leg ulcers [2] as part of the arterial causes are not discussed here as they are described in another chapter. Very often, the ulcers of the lower leg result from a combination of factors [3]. Therefore, it is important to rule out arterial insufficiency even when other causes or clinical signs are present. For example, about 15% of all leg ulcers are of a mixed arterial-venous origin [4–6]. We postulate that every patient with ulceration on the lower leg should receive an arterial workup, not only because a concomitant arterial disease may delay healing but also because of the underlying systemic process (arteriosclerosis) for which the patient might profit from an appropriate systemic therapy [7, 8].

48.2 Epidemiology and Classification

Chronic ulceration of the lower leg can result from several underlying factors as mentioned above. The most common cause is venous insufficiency in about 75%, followed by ulcers of mixed venous and arterial (15%) and those of primarily arterial (4%) origin [4, 5]. Arterial leg ulcers are caused by an oxygen deficit in the tissue resulting from reduced tissue blood perfusion due to occlusion of the arterial lumen. The most common cause for this occlusion is peripheral arterial occlusive disease (PAOD) due to an arteriosclerotic process. Generalized arteriosclerosis is therefore the most common cause not only of cardiovascular and cerebrovascular disease but also of peripheral vascular disease. The prevalence of PAOD in the general population varies between 7% and 21% [9]. It is related to age, gender, and definition of PAOD (by the cutoff value of the ankle-brachial index (ABI) and/or the presence of symptoms). The Fontaine stages classify the clinical appearance of PAOD (Table 48.1). Before progressing to a clinically symptomatic stage such as intermittent claudication or even critical limb ischemia, PAOD is typically asymptomatic for several years. Approximately 23% of all patients are asymptomatic, and this is proba-

J. Aschwanden · J. Hafner · S. Läuchli (✉)
Department of Dermatology, University Hospital Zürich, Zurich, Switzerland
e-mail: Severin.laeuchli@usz.ch

V. Jacomella
Department of Angiology, University Hospital Zürich, Zurich, Switzerland

Table 48.1 Fontaine classification for PAOD

Stage I	Asymptomatic
Stage II	Intermittent claudication
	Walking distance:
IIA	>200 m, with no disablement
IIB	<200 m with disablement
Stage III	Resting pain
Stage IV	Peripheral necrosis/gangrene

bly one reason that PAOD stage I seems to be underestimated [8]. Sometimes, symptoms can also be masked by reduced walking distance due to other reasons or by polyneuropathy secondary to diabetes. In stage II with intermittent claudication as the main symptom, rest pain is normally missing. Stage III ischemic rest pain is typically a nocturnal pain. Approximately 15–20% of patients with intermittent claudication will progress to critical ischemia. The distinction between arterial insufficiency and critical ischemia is not clearly outlined in the literature, and critical limb ischemia occurs only in a minority of patients with PAOD [10]. In 1996, *the Second European Consensus* [11] outlined criteria for the diagnosis of chronic critical limb ischemia: recalcitrant rest pain or distal necrosis of more than 2 weeks' duration in the presence of (A) a systolic ankle pressure (AP) 50 mmHg or less, (B) a systolic toe pressure of 30 mmHg or less, or (C) a transcutaneous oxygen pressure ($tcPO_2$) of 10 mmHg or less. In the last few years, the threshold for critical ischemia has been raised several times. Necrotic ulceration occurs in stage IV, usually on the toes or the back of the feet, but can also occur in stage II after trauma or in combination with chronic venous disease and is then generally considered a "complicated" stage IIB. In fact, the majority of arterial ulcers occur in "complicated" stage IIB on the lateral lower leg and do not match the criteria for critical ischemia. The angiosome concept is one possible explanation for the occurrence of nonhealing ulcers above the threshold of critical ischemia. It was first described by reconstructive plastic surgeons in 1987 [12]. They divided the tissue into specific three-dimensional sectors of the body supplied by specific arteries and veins, named angiosomes. Each angiosome therefore consists of a topographically specific arteriosome and corresponding venosome supply, which build block systems of perfusion. Neighboring angiosomes are linked by numerous communicating vessels, so-called choke vessels. In ischemic conditions, these interconnections between adjacent angiosomes create a very effective compensatory system in non-atherosclerotic and nondiabetic limbs [13]. In atherosclerotic or other changes of the large collateral vessels, such as those typically accompanying diabetic arterial disease below the knee and end-stage renal disease (ESRD), this natural "rescue system" between adjacent angiosomes may be jeopardized.

48.3 Clinical Findings

The typical localization for arterial leg ulcers is the lateral malleolar region for PAOD stage IIB (Fig. 48.1), whereas distal arterial necrosis (PAOD stage IV) is usually localized in the foot and toe region (Fig. 48.2). Arterial leg ulcers often have irregular edges and/or a "punched-out" appearance. The ulcer base is usually poorly developed with a grayish granulation tissue. Signs of chronic venous disease are missing except in mixed ulcers. Painful and necrotic areas are the typical appearance for all ischemic ulcers.

48 Arterial Leg Ulcers

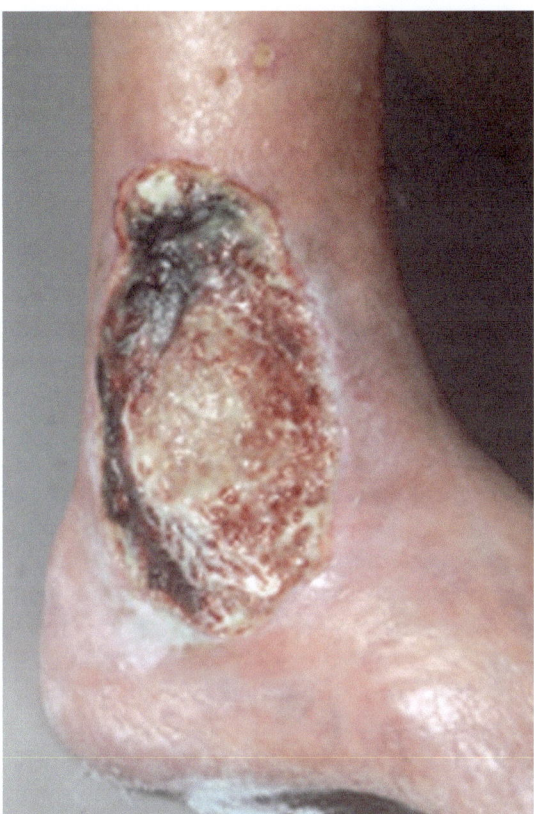

Fig. 48.1 Typical arterial leg ulcer on the lateral malleolar aspect of the lower leg (PAOD complicated stage IIB)

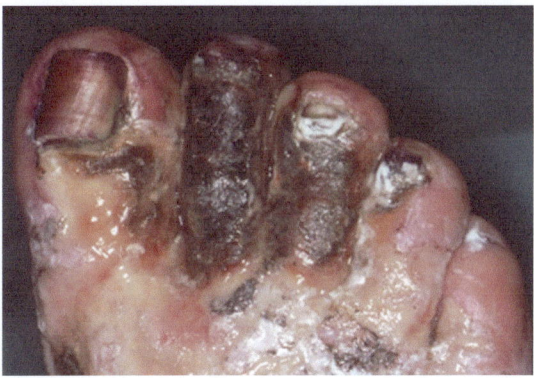

Fig. 48.2 Distal arterial necrosis due to PAOD stage IV

48.4 Diagnosis

The first test to rule out arterial insufficiency should be the palpation of the pedal pulses. It should be mentioned that the dorsalis pedis pulse

Table 48.2 Doppler ankle-brachial ratio [15]

0.91–1.4	Normal, if under exercise no ABI loss
0.5–0.85	PAOD, claudication (mild to moderate disease); a wound can heal
<0.5	Severe PAOD, threat of tissue and limb loss
>1.4	May be due to diabetes, Mönckeberg disease, renal disease

is missing in about 10% of individuals and the palpation of the posterior tibial pulse may be difficult due to swelling or presence of ulceration caused by a concomitant chronic venous insufficiency. If a pulse is palpable, we can assume that the ankle pressure is >100 mmHg [14] and wound healing should be possible. If no pulses can be detected, noninvasive vascular testing should always be performed.

As a fast and simple test, the ankle-brachial index (ABI) can be measured very easily with a cheap and simple continuous-wave (CW) Doppler probe (8–10 mMHz). The ABI is defined as the systolic ankle pressure divided by the systolic arm pressure and is considered an accurate and reliable marker of symptomatic and asymptomatic PAOD (Table 48.2). Significant arteriopathy is normally defined as an ABI <0.91 and an ABI <0.5 as severe arterial insufficiency [16]. The ABI measurement can therefore identify patients at risk of any systemic atherothrombotic events even in an asymptomatic stage. Identification of asymptomatic PAOD also leads to intensified targeted prophylactic anti-atherothrombotic treatment that can reduce morbidity and mortality as mentioned above [8].

To recognize critical ischemia, the measurement of ankle systolic pressure is the most accurate test. If the pressure is below the level of critical limb ischemia as defined with an ankle systolic pressure <50 mmHg [11], leg ulcers will only heal in 20% of cases, and aggressive revascularization therapy should be performed [17]. In contrast, a systolic pressure over 70 mmHg can nearly exclude arterial insufficiency as a cause for the ulcers. If the arteries are not compressible, i.e., the ABI is higher than 1.4 or the difference of the measured pressure between ankle and arm exceeds 75 mmHg, calcification of the arteries should be considered. In these cases, a toe sys-

Table 48.3 Use of noninvasive vascular tests to predict the presence of underlying severe arteriopathy [18]

Noninvasive avascular testing	Findings	Severe arteriopathy
Pedal pulses	Present	Unlikely
	Absent	Possible[a]
Ankle systolic pressure	>70 mmHg	Unlikely
With ulcer	<50–70 mmHg	Possible[a]
Without ulcer, with rest pain	<30–50	Likely
Toe systolic pressure	>50 mmHg	Unlikely
	<50 mmHg	Likely
tcPO$_2$	>30 mmHg	Unlikely
	<30 mmHg	Likely

[a]Proceed with further, noninvasive vascular tests to confirm or rule out severe arteriopathy especially if clinical evolution is poor

Table 48.4 Risk factors for arteriosclerosis and PAOD

Hypertension
Diabetes
Elevated cholesterol, especially low-density lipoprotein
Smoking

tolic pressure or a tcPO$_2$ measurement should be performed. In cases of Mönckeberg mediacalcinosis, the pole test technique can also give further information concerning the critical ischemia of the lower limbs. A toe systolic pressure lower than 50 mmHg or a tcPO$_2$ lower than 30 mmHg is diagnostic for critical ischemia (Table 48.3). If the tcPO$_2$ is over 30 mmHG, a wound can heal. Ultrasonic duplex scanning or arteriography can localize the arterial lesion but cannot make any statement about the severity of the arterial disease. In contrast, it is a very good surveillance tool after an invasive intervention or as first-step screening in order to evaluate an invasive procedure. The gold standard to investigate PAOD is still angiography, especially when an intervention is planned. Recently, magnetic resonance angiography has emerged as a noninvasive imaging modality without the risks associated with conventional angiography (e.g., arterial puncture, plaque embolization, and contrast-induced nephropathy).

48.5 Treatment

The arteriosclerotic process as a systemic problem needs an interdisciplinary approach. The common arteriosclerotic risk factors should be treated aggressively (Table 48.4). Whenever possible, revascularization should be attempted by angioplasty or vascular surgery. This is the only effective therapeutic option to allow wound healing when ischemic necrosis is present. Furthermore, it often provides the most efficient pain relief. If revascularization by interventional or surgical means is not possible, intravenous application of iloprost can ameliorate the situation, but this is often limited by side effects (e.g., hypotension, headaches). Exercise also plays an important role in improving the maximal walking distance and thus increasing the blood perfusion. Adjuvant medical treatment with antithrombotic or rheological agents can improve the outcome [19].

For the local therapy, the common principles of modern wound care should be applied. Sharp surgical debridement is of foremost importance to remove the bioburden, which can delay wound healing. However, as arterial ulcers often reach to deeper structures, it should be performed by surgeons or wound care experts with adequate training. Enzymatic debridement and biosurgery with maggots can be viable alternatives. Local wound infection can be treated with wound antiseptics or silver dressings; if signs of systemic infection are present, systemic antibiotics have to be utilized.

The choice of wound dressing must take into consideration the amount of exudation and necrosis and the phase of wound healing. Generally, occlusive dressings should be avoided, as their main mode of action, a local increase of CO_2 tension, is not desirable for ischemic ulcers and the detection of wound infection could be delayed. Semiocclusive dressings can be utilized with caution, if granulation tissue exceeds necrotic areas and there are no signs of wound infection. The type of wound dressing does not significantly influence healing times [20, 21]. Therefore, the choice of wound dressing should be guided by patient-centered concerns such as exudate management and pain control [22]. Wound pain is one of the main concerns of patients [23].

Dressings that avoid desiccation of the wound and which do not traumatize the wound when the dressing is changed are therefore ideal.

Arterial leg ulcers can show a very protracted healing time, especially if surgical or interventional revascularization is not possible. In these cases, advanced methods often have to be utilized, such as acellular matrices, keratinocyte cultures, or growth factors. In many instances, split-thickness skin grafts can improve the wound pain immediately and accelerate healing, even if the wound bed does not show sufficient granulation for a full graft take.

References

1. Pannier F, Rabe E. Differential diagnosis of leg ulcers. Phlebology. 2013;28(Suppl. 1):55–60.
2. Hafner J, Nobbe S, Partsch H, Lauchli S, Mayer D, Amann-Vesti B, et al. Martorell hypertensive ischemic leg ulcer: a model of ischemic subcutaneous arteriolosclerosis. Arch Dermatol. 2010;146:961–8.
3. Fukaya E, Margolis DJ. Approach to diagnosing lower extremity ulcers. Dermatol Ther. 2013;26:181–6.
4. Koerber A, Schadendorf D, Dissemond J. Genese des Ulcus cruris. Hautarzt. 2009;60:483–8.
5. Läuchli S, Bayard I, Hafner J, Hunziker T, Mayer D, French L. Unterschiedliche Abheilungsdauer und Häufigkeit der Hospitalisation bei Ulcus cruris verschiedener Ursachen. Hautarzt. 2013;64(12):917–22.
6. Ghauri AS, Nyamekye I, Grabs AJ, Farndon JR, Poskitt KR. The diagnosis and management of mixed arterial/venous leg ulcers in community-based clinics. Eur J Vasc Endovasc Surg. 1998;16:350–5.
7. van Kuijk JP, Flu WJ, Poldermans D. Risk factors and peripheral arterial disease; a plea for objective measurements. Atherosclerosis. 2011;214:37–8.
8. Hayoz D, Bounameaux H, Canova CR. Swiss Atherothrombosis Survey: a field report on the occurrence of symptomatic and asymptomatic peripheral arterial disease. J Intern Med. 2005;258:238–43.
9. Alzamora MT, Fores R, Baena-Diez JM, Pera G, Toran P, Sorribes M, et al. The peripheral arterial disease study (PERART/ARTPER): prevalence and risk factors in the general population. BMC Public Health. 2010;10:38.
10. Hafner J, Schaad I, Schneider E, Seifert B, Burg G, Cassina PC. Leg ulcers in peripheral arterial disease (arterial leg ulcers): impaired wound healing above the threshold of chronic critical limb ischemia. J Am Acad Dermatol. 2000;43:1001–8.
11. Anon. Second European Consensus Document on chronic critical leg ischemia. Circulation. 1991;84:IV1–26.
12. Taylor GI, Palmer JH. The vascular territories (angiosomes) of the body: experimental study and clinical applications. Br J Plast Surg. 1987;40:113–41.
13. Attinger CE, Evans KK, Bulan E, Blume P, Cooper P. Angiosomes of the foot and ankle and clinical implications for limb salvage: reconstruction, incisions, and revascularization. Plast Reconstr Surg. 2006;117:261S–93S.
14. Christensen JH, Freundlich M, Jacobsen BA, Falstie-Jensen N. Clinical relevance of pedal pulse palpation in patients suspected of peripheral arterial insufficiency. J Intern Med. 1989;226:95–9.
15. Ray SA, Buckenham TM, Belli AM, Taylor RS, Dormandy JA. The nature and importance of changes in toe-brachial pressure indices following percutaneous transluminal angioplasty for leg ischaemia. Eur J Vasc Endovasc Surg. 1997;14:125–33.
16. Norgren L, Hiatt WR, Dormandy JA, Nehler MR, Harris KA, Fowkes FG. Inter-society consensus for the management of peripheral arterial disease (TASC II). J Vasc Surg. 2007;45(1):S5–67.
17. Wütschert R, Bounameaux H. Quantification de l'insuffisance artérielle des membres inférieurs: méthodes et applications. Med Hyg. 1998;56:137–40.
18. Hafner J, Ramelet AA, Schmeller W, Brunner UV. Management of leg ulcers. Curr Probl Dermatol. 1999;27:4–7.
19. Coccheri S, Palareti G, Fortunato G. Antithrombotic drugs in peripheral obliterative arterial diseases. Haemostasis. 1994;24:118–27.
20. Chaby G, Senet P, Vaneau M, Martel P, Guillaume JC, Meaume S, et al. Dressings for acute and chronic wounds: a systematic review. Arch Dermatol. 2007;143:1297–304.
21. Nelson EA, Bradley MD. Dressings and topical agents for arterial leg ulcers. Cochrane Database Syst Rev. 2007;(1):CD001836.
22. Gottrup F, Apelqvist J, Price P. Outcomes in controlled and comparative studies on non-healing wounds: recommendations to improve the quality of evidence in wound management. J Wound Care. 2010;19:237–68.
23. Woo KY, Sibbald RG. The improvement of wound-associated pain and healing trajectory with a comprehensive foot and leg ulcer care model. J Wound Ostomy Continence Nurs. 2009;36:184–91. quiz 92–3

Open Access This chapter is licensed under the terms of the Creative Commons Attribution-NonCommercial-NoDerivatives 4.0 International License (http://creativecommons.org/licenses/by-nc-nd/4.0/), which permits any non-commercial use, sharing, distribution and reproduction in any medium or format, as long as you give appropriate credit to the original author(s) and the source, provide a link to the Creative Commons license and indicate if you modified the licensed material. You do not have permission under this license to share adapted material derived from this chapter or parts of it.

The images or other third party material in this chapter are included in the chapter's Creative Commons license, unless indicated otherwise in a credit line to the material. If material is not included in the chapter's Creative Commons license and your intended use is not permitted by statutory regulation or exceeds the permitted use, you will need to obtain permission directly from the copyright holder.

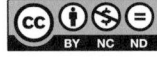

Prevention of Skin Necrosis in Cosmetic Medicine

49

Hugues Cartier, Leonie Schelke, and Peter Velthuis

49.1 Introduction

Aesthetic medicine is a constantly evolving field, which includes minimally invasive treatments, i.e., considered as nonsurgical.

Nevertheless, the current evolution makes some procedures more intrusive.

Most of the patients treated are healthy people looking for an aesthetic improvement, so the treatments performed must be as safe as possible.

This treatment cannot be done without a medical diagnosis, a precise history, informed information, and a choice of treatment options to be weighed against a benefit-risk ratio.

49.1.1 Aesthetic Procedures

49.1.2 Filling Products

Filling products play a significant role in aesthetic medicine. The rheology of the products has not stopped evolving over the last 20 years. Fortunately, nonabsorbable products such as silicone, Gore-Tex, and acrylamides have been banned in Europe.

At present, four types of products that integrate well into the cutaneous and subcutaneous tissue and that are slowly resorbable can be identified: hyaluronic acid, calcium hydroxyapatite, polycaprolactone, and polylactic acid, which is in the form of powder to be diluted in sterile water.

Of these four filling or collagen stimulation products, only hyaluronic acid can be dissolved rapidly with hyaluronidase in case of complications (such as bad placement, accumulation of product, associated infection, sterile inflammatory reaction, or vascular occlusion).

The major complication is vascular occlusion or compression. At best, they cause cutaneous and subcutaneous suffering that is resolved thanks to the contiguous arterial network. At worst, they cause extensive and deep necrosis in the vascularized area. Cases of occlusion of the central retinal artery with loss of ocular function due to migration of the product in the bloodstream are fortunately rare compared to the number of injections performed every day in the world but nevertheless regularly reported and published.

Vascular complication can occur at any time, especially since needles or fine cannulas are used that can easily perforate an artery. The reason for this is simple: even though all doctors who perform injections of filling products must know the facial anatomy, injections are done blindly. We do have the blood aspiration test technique, but it

H. Cartier (✉)
Saint-Jean Dermatologic Center, Arras, France

L. Schelke · P. Velthuis
Dermatology Department, Erasmus University Medical Center, Rotterdam, Netherlands
e-mail: leonie.schelke@cutaneous.org; p.velthuis@erasmusmc.nl

is far from reliable. To date, only ultrasound imaging, a dynamic, noninvasive examination to be used prior to injection, can supply an answer, but it requires training, a certain amount of dexterity, and adequate equipment. The world of aesthetics is discovering this technique, which cannot guarantee to ban this complication but contributes to reducing this risk [1].

Venous embolisms rarely cause skin suffering at first because they are diluted in the general vascular system. However, there have been reports of cavernous sinus thrombosis in facial injections and pulmonary embolism in genital or gluteal injections with massive quantities of filler.

The cutaneous signs of arterial vascular complications are with important variations:

– Immediate pain like a cramp
– Immediate or delayed blanching extending as a livedoid pattern
– Progressive cyanosis of the skin that may look like bruises but may not be declining but ascending
– Pustules, inflammation that may resemble the false vesicular eruptions of herpes or shingles
– Cyanotic suffering with extensive tissue necrosis depending on the vascular territory

49.1.3 Lifting Effect or Collagen Stimulation by Threads

A distinction is made between absorbable and nonabsorbable threads. In themselves, the threads only cause a confined inflammation around them. Depending on their characteristics, the threads can also pull the skin to give this tensor effect.

Intrinsically, they do not cause skin necrosis, but a cutaneous or subcutaneous injury. This tearing of the tissues during their introduction under the skin by needles of varying lengths induces microtrauma, even more so since they are armed with small spines allowing for better fixation and maintenance over time. Avoid combination with radiofrequency to stimulate neocollagenesis because it induces more exaggerated inflammatory responses such as development of nodular panniculitis and adipocyte necrosis [2].

Moreover, the number of threads accumulated under the skin can cause vascular breaches and poor tissue integration. We have seen cutaneous suffering and even necrosis, particularly on the nose.

49.1.4 Laser and EBD

In general, the effect of lasers and EBD treatment is mediated by controlled damage to tissue. After this, regeneration occurs that should lead to an improved appearance [3].

49.1.4.1 Ablative Lasers

Ablative lasers are represented by the CO2 laser and the erbium-YAG laser.

They cause vaporization of the epidermis and middle dermis in resurfacing mode. In fractionated mode, ablative lasers cause micro-wells that perforate the skin to a depth of up to 3.5 mm. This is a focused necrosis that forms just around the well due to the brutal heating of the skin tissue. This is normally a controlled burn if the energy delivered and the density of the points that are juxtaposed are not too high. The higher these two parameters are, the greater the thermal trauma. The burn is then uncontrollable, leading to skin necrosis and consequently to vicious, flanged, and hypochromic scars.

The skin structure plays a key role because the tissue regeneration is induced by this skin vaporization and the thermal effect. Thus, the healing process is very variable depending on the type of the skin, its age, and density in pilosebaceous appendages and in vascular network that contributes to it. Outside the face, the risk of burning is increased since densities of these structures are much less.

49.1.4.2 Non-ablative Thermal Lasers

Non-ablative lasers induce a thermal effect that is supposed to regenerate the dermis. There are numerous devices, fractionated or not. If too much heat is accumulated, the effect of the laser radiation can cause skin suffering up to the point of skin necrosis. This is nevertheless rare and related to a bad use or an error of parameterization.

49.1.4.3 Vascular Lasers

We distinguish the KTP laser, the pulsed dye laser, the vascular diode, the yellow laser, the pulsed lights with vascular filter, and the long-pulse Nd-YAG laser.

Vascular lasers are characterized by wavelengths that are preferentially absorbed by the redness of the skin. It is important to distinguish skin redness from inflammation, which is rarely a good indication for vascular lasers.

In fact, all vascular lasers cause inflammation that should not be added to an already existing inflammation.

This inflammation causes an edema that will vary according to the type of laser and its photon energy setting, the size of the vascular target to be destroyed, and the intrinsic drainage of the skin in each case or according to the site treated.

In addition, depending on the type of laser and the adjustment of emission time and energy, a purpura can be seen in the presence of purple spots that will fade in 5–10 days.

The burn is the consequence of an excessive accumulation of energy with a dispersion of the heat that is not well done. We can therefore have a surface epidermolysis, which is to say a blow-out or a real cutaneous necrosis which will leave a hypochromic scar.

On tanned or self-tanning skin or for a phototype above III on the Fitzpatrick scale, there is an increased risk of burning and reactive hyperpigmentation.

Special mention should be made of the long-pulse Nd-YAG laser, which delivers very high light energy and should be used with caution, as it induces the most dermal necrosis with systematic scarring.

49.1.4.4 Pigment Lasers

A distinction is made between hair removal lasers and those used to erase sunspots or tattoos. The wavelengths are identical, but it is the emission time of the laser beam that will change.

For tattoos, we can only use picosecond or nanosecond lasers. The energy delivered must be high enough to burst the tattoo pigment and dissolve it progressively. Other pigment lasers deliver their photonic energy in milliseconds. If these are used for tattoos, they will systematically cause skin necrosis by deep burning. Indeed, the instantaneous accumulation of dermal pigment in tattoos is so important and brutal that the skin does not have time to disperse the heat.

For laser hair removal, the laser radiation follows the hair like an electric current follows a conducting wire. The heat accumulation causes its destruction, but if the skin is tanned, covered with self-tanner or on phototype beyond IV on the Fitzpatrick scale, then the photons will also be absorbed by the skin surface which by itself becomes a target and causes a surface burn, from epidermolysis to dermolysis. And thus, at best a hypochromia and at worst a burn will occur which will be deep enough to leave definitive hypochromic scars. In these cases, Nd-YAG long-pulse lasers or hair removal diodes are recommended, unlike alexandrite and pulsed light lasers.

For sunspots, all these lasers can be used, and it is only a question of setting and wavelength. The spots will turn into small superficial scabs that will disintegrate in a few days without leaving any trace. A deeper burn is in most cases secondary to a bad use of the device.

49.1.4.5 Radiofrequency

Radiofrequency is an electric current that disperses heat according to its operating mode. Contact with a handpiece that is swept over the skin surface accumulates local heat and causes tissue remodeling. Fractional radiofrequency aims to place contact microelectrodes on the surface of the skin to induce dermal-epidermal micro-bulges and finally radiofrequency with microneedles. The microneedles penetrate the skin up to 4 mm deep; they are protected up to the tip or not, depending on the device.

The electrical effect causes skin coagulation, tissue, and vascular damage, which is supposed to regenerate the skin. Too long an emission time, too much energy, and repetition of passages can cause tissue damage. From the spike scar to the loss of skin substance by dermal-epidermal burn, everything is possible but rare.

49.1.5 EBD

49.1.5.1 LEDs

The diodes juxtaposed on a panel are athermal. The mode of operation therefore does not cause skin necrosis unless they are used to activate a photosensitizing substance. In this case, they contribute to cause it. LEDs emit in the visible spectrum and therefore do not contain UV radiation.

49.1.5.2 High-Intensity Focused Ultrasound (HIFU)

Focused ultrasound concentrates its energy on a focal point at 1.5 mm, 3 mm, 4.5 mm, 6 mm, or more. The sudden rise in temperature causes coagulation and punctual necrosis in the form of aligned micro-points. Paresis due to nerve damage has been seen.

Used to obtain a firming and tensing effect on the oval of the face, it is necessary to multiply the lines of points to obtain a result. The closer the lines of stitches are to each other, the more skin suffering is induced.

Skin burns are rare unless the handpiece is not applied correctly to the skin.

49.1.5.3 Cryolipolysis

Cryolipolysis is based on the freezing of a volume of skin and fat caught in a vacuum chamber. The combination of cold, up to $-12\ °C$, and suction to fix the volume to be melted by destroying the adipocytes has proved its medical interest with numerous publications to support it. Nevertheless, many devices have appeared on the world market of aesthetic medicine and aesthetic centers of nondoctors. Medical ability is necessary to avoid complications such as thermal burns caused by the cold. Cases of surface burns and even skin necrosis of the bedsore type have even been reported. They are much more frequent when the temperature descent is not progressive, when the skin contact interface has been forgotten or is not confirmed for this use, or when the duration of the cold and the suction force is not adapted to the volume of the fat mass.

49.1.6 Peelings

49.1.6.1 Epidermal Peel

The leader in epidermal peels is glycolic acid. All its exfoliating agents can give epidermolysis, rarely deeper burns.

49.1.6.2 Medium and Deep Dermal Peels

They are essentially represented by trichloroacetic acid and phenol associated with croton oil. These peels are of varying concentrations and pH. They aim at provoking a dermal-epidermal regeneration. Incorrect use, i.e., too many applications and too high a concentration, can cause serious burns with permanent scarring. Learning to use them is essential to set limits to their use.

It should be remembered that healthy skin serves as a natural protection, if one causes skin breaches.

49.1.7 Other Injectable Active Ingredients

Mesotherapy with unsuitable products can cause skin necrosis at the injection site, as can deoxycholate, a chemical agent designed to destroy localized fatty areas.

49.2 Complications

Complications are multiple but essentially inflammatory, scarring, and infectious.

49.2.1 Inflammation and Pigmentation

The inflammation caused by all the techniques mentioned above is a normal phenomenon that is the consequence of any trauma. This normal process is gradually reduced, but if it persists, it can cause a resurgence of pigment on the surface, hypersensitivity, or sensitive skin. It is mainly embarrassing but does not lead to tissue destruction but can give way to fibrosis.

49.2.2 Scars

All types of scars can be observed: depressed scars due to loss of substance following dermal necrosis or dermal collapse, retractile scars, or hypertrophic scars due to the effect of tension, always related to damage to the middle/deep dermis, and of course keloids if the genetic profile is suitable, as in the case of black skins.

Any incident on the middle and especially deep dermis exposes the patient to these risks. In order to avoid them, it is necessary to know and master the healing process.

49.2.3 Infectious

Fortunately rare, they are often secondary to *Staphylococcus aureus* but also to commensal germs or those carried by lack of hygiene. Herpetic infections, on the other hand, can cause irrevocable and sometimes extensive scarring on skin that is still healing after an essentially abrasive technique that involves the dermis. They cause dermal necrosis, which can only be avoided by recommending a preventive and systematic antiviral treatment.

49.3 Conclusion

Each aesthetic technical procedure can be a source of complications. Necrosis affecting the dermis will inevitably leave a visible structural scar with fibrosis or colorimetric scarring with permanent hypochromia. An evaluation and knowledge of the procedure are the basis of a benefit-risk ratio in favor of the patient.

References

1. Habib SM, Schelke LW, Velthuis PJ. Management of dermal filler (vascular) complications using duplex ultrasound. Dermatol Ther. 2020;33(4):e13461.
2. Li K, Zhang X, Guo W, Wang L, Wang G, Gao L. Polydioxanone thread insertion in combination with radio frequency treatment does not exhibit synergistic efficacy: animal study with pigs. J Cosmet Dermatol. 2022;21(8):3479–85.
3. Cartier H, Dahan S, Pusel B. Les lasers en dermatologie—4e édition Doin ISBN 978-2-7040-1532-0

Open Access This chapter is licensed under the terms of the Creative Commons Attribution-NonCommercial-NoDerivatives 4.0 International License (http://creativecommons.org/licenses/by-nc-nd/4.0/), which permits any non-commercial use, sharing, distribution and reproduction in any medium or format, as long as you give appropriate credit to the original author(s) and the source, provide a link to the Creative Commons license and indicate if you modified the licensed material. You do not have permission under this license to share adapted material derived from this chapter or parts of it.

The images or other third party material in this chapter are included in the chapter's Creative Commons license, unless indicated otherwise in a credit line to the material. If material is not included in the chapter's Creative Commons license and your intended use is not permitted by statutory regulation or exceeds the permitted use, you will need to obtain permission directly from the copyright holder.

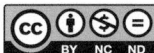

50

Leeches in Prevention of Skin Necrosis in Flap Surgery

Luc Téot

50.1 Introduction

Historically, the use of leeches started in ancient Egypt. Mainly used in the middle of the nineteenth century, leeches were forgotten for more than a century until microsurgery could become a standardized procedure with its possible venous congestion. Salvage of microvascular free tissue using leeches became popular since 1981 [1] and is still recognized as useful in saving compromised situations.

Leeches reappeared in reconstructive microsurgery during the last 15 years, as a potential option in compromised flap vascularization after having realized microsutures. Leeches are more indicated in venous congestion but have also been proposed for enhancing the arterial blood flow. Local blood flow may be impaired by several local factors (see Horch chapter).

Leeches have been used by reconstructive surgeons to facilitate replanted digits, ears, lips, and nasal tips [2].

Peer-reviewed evidence suggests that the survival of compromised, venous-congested tissues is improved by early application of a leech. Other clinical indications could anecdotally be described.

L. Téot (✉)
Department of Plastic Surgery, Burns and Wound Healing, Montpellier University Hospital, Hôpital La Colombière, CICAT Occitanie, Montpellier Cedex 5, France
e-mail: l-teot@chu-montpellier.fr

50.2 Mode of Action

Leeches possess capacities to treat venous-compromised tissue thanks to different secretions. Once they are fixed on a perforated skin or a suture edge, their saliva will provide an anticoagulant and a histamine-like vasodilator. A local bleeding is then promoted, which should be quantified and compensated if considered in excess [3].

Leeches also secrete different factors like a local anesthetic and an enzyme, the hyaluronidase [4]. The suction effect is activated by a peristaltic movement. Once completely fed, the leech may fall apart or remain attached to the skin. A leech can ingest 1 milliliter per minute of blood, and the area of attachment can bleed from 10 h to 7 days.

50.3 Conservation and Use

In microsurgical centers, leeches are stored either in the pharmacy or in a refrigerated area and used on demand.

After having collected the patient authorization and providing an adapted information, the application starts with a scalpel puncture of the compromised skin. Optimal frequency of application ranges from 2 to 8 h, while average overall duration ranges from 4 to 10 days. The number of leeches to be applied can be determined depending on the volume of the flap. In 50% of the cases reported in the literature, the patients required transfusion. Antibiotic prophylaxis against *Aeromonas* is highly advisable, as post-leech infection could be observed (ciprofloxacin and trimethoprim-sulfamethoxazole combination currently appears as the most relevant prophylactic antibiotherapy). Hemoglobin should also be regularly checked in order to prevent experimental anemia.

The leeches have to remain visible to the nurse during the whole period of application. The nurse will regularly check the proper suction effect on the leech movements and change the leech when necessary. The patient should be informed that the leech may fall apart and circulate on the dressing, a psychological condition which should be anticipated. An adapted information should detail before the microsurgical procedure the possibility of using these living animals considered as repulsive.

50.4 Clinical Indications

Treatment of venous insufficiency in pedicled or free flaps after revision surgery had failed to improve flap vascularization in cases where flap revision was not appropriate. However, the leech does not attach and/or initiate the suction effect in case of completely necrosed skin.

A systematic review of leech therapy for flap salvage between 1960 and 2015, analyzing 121 articles and subsequently taking into consideration 41 studies [5], indicated that the success rate of leech therapy ranged from 65% to 85% according to the situations encountered.

50.5 Conclusion

Hirudotherapy is a reliable treatment in cases of patent venous insufficiency of pedicled or free flaps (or when revision surgery is not recommended). Even though the relevant literature is highly heterogeneous, we have attempted to put forward a specific protocol bringing together dosage, delivery route, frequency of administration, and appropriate prophylactic antibiotherapy. An algorithm for the treatment and management of venous congestion and a practical information sheet have been placed at the disposal of plastic surgery teams.

References

1. Whitaker IS, Rao J, Izadi D, et al. Historical article: hirudo medicinalis: ancient origins of, and trends in the use of medicinal leeches throughout history. Br J Oral Maxillofac Surg. 2004;42:133–7.
2. Hackenberger PN, Janis JE. A comprehensive review of medicinal leeches in plastic and reconstructive surgery. Plast Reconstr Surg Glob Open. 2019;7(12):e2555. https://doi.org/10.1097/GOX.0000000000002555.
3. Kraemer BA, Korber KE, Aquino TI, Engleman A. Use of leeches in plastic and reconstructive surgery: a review. J Reconstr Microsurg. 1988;4(5):381–6. https://doi.org/10.1055/s-2007-1006947.
4. Conforti ML, Connor NP, Heisey DM, Hartig GK. Evaluation of performance characteristics of the medicinal leech (Hirudo medicinalis) for the treatment of venous congestion. Plast Reconstr Surg. 2002;109(1):228–35.
5. Herlin C, Bertheuil N, Bekara F, Boissiere F, Sinna R, Chaput B. Leech therapy in flap salvage: systematic review and practical recommendations. Ann Chir Plast Esthet. 2017;62(2):e1–e13. https://doi.org/10.1016/j.anplas.2016.06.004.

Open Access This chapter is licensed under the terms of the Creative Commons Attribution-NonCommercial-NoDerivatives 4.0 International License (http://creativecommons.org/licenses/by-nc-nd/4.0/), which permits any non-commercial use, sharing, distribution and reproduction in any medium or format, as long as you give appropriate credit to the original author(s) and the source, provide a link to the Creative Commons license and indicate if you modified the licensed material. You do not have permission under this license to share adapted material derived from this chapter or parts of it.

The images or other third party material in this chapter are included in the chapter's Creative Commons license, unless indicated otherwise in a credit line to the material. If material is not included in the chapter's Creative Commons license and your intended use is not permitted by statutory regulation or exceeds the permitted use, you will need to obtain permission directly from the copyright holder.

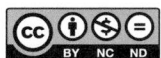

Revascularization Techniques to Prevent Limb Amputation Presenting Distal Necrosis

51

Francis Pesteil, Romain Chauvet, Lucie Chastaingt, Rami El Hage, Maxime Gourgue, Raphaël Van Damme, Loïc Prales, and Philippe Lacroix

In 2010, the prevalence of peripheral arterial disease was 202 million patients globally, an increase of 23.5% compared to 2000 [1]. In its most severe forms, peripheral arterial disease presents as chronic limb-threatening ischemia (CLTI). It is an advanced stage of disease with ischemic rest pain and/or presenting ischemic ulcer or gangrene for at least 2 weeks and severe alteration of lower limb perfusion characterized by ankle-brachial index inferior to 0.4, ankle pressure inferior to 50 mmHg, toe pressure inferior to 30 mmHg, and transcutaneous partial pressure of oxygen ($tcPO_2$) inferior to 30 mmHg [2]. It is associated with a high risk of amputation and death. The prevalence increases dramatically with age, from 6.5% in men aged 60–69 years to 29.4% in men over 80 years [3]. Without revascularization, 31.6% died and 23% required major amputation within 2 years [4]. In a Danish registry, a reduction of major amputation rate was observed from 41.67 for 100,000 subjects per year to 32.53 between two periods: 1997–2002 and 2009–2014. This was coupled with an increase in vascular surgeon referrals from 25.7% to 31.3% from 1997 to 2014 [5].

Compared to rest pain, wounds are associated with a higher risk of amputation (OR = 4.93, 95% CI 4.18–5.81, and OR = 2. 48, 95% CI 1.29–4.76) and death (OR = 1.42, 95% CI 1.16–1.74, and OR = 1.50, 95% CI 0.91–2.47) in the setting of CLTI [6, 7].

These multiple factors led to the creation of the WIfI classification, which incorporates three key elements: wound, ischemia, and foot infection (Tables 51.1, 51.2, and 51.3) [8]. The WIfI score is correlated with amputation risk, limb salvage, and wound healing (Tables 51.4 and 51.5) [9]. This classification highlights the importance for wound care and infection treatment in addition to revascularization.

Some studies highlighted the interest of direct revascularization (DR) for patients affected by CTLI and wounds. The angiosome concept is based on the segmental vascularization of vasculature in the foot. Improving perfusion of the vessel responsible for the segment with tissue loss could be helpful to improve wound healing, prevent major amputation, and improve survival [10].

F. Pesteil (✉) · R. Chauvet · L. Chastaingt · R. El Hage
M. Gourgue · R. Van Damme · L. Prales · P. Lacroix
Vascular Medicine and Surgery Department,
Dupuytren University Hospital, Limoges, France
e-mail: romain.chauvet@chu-limoges.fr;
lucie.chastaingt@chu-limoges.fr;
rami.elhage@chu-limoges.fr;
maxime.gourgue@chu-limoges.fr;
philippe.lacroix@unilim.fr

Table 51.1 Classification for ischemia in WIFI score

Grade	ABI	Ankle systolic pressure	TP, $TcPO_2$
0	≥0.80	>100 mmHg	≥60 mmHg
1	0.6–0.79	70–100 mmHg	40–59 mmHg
2	0.4–0.59	50–70 mmHg	30–39 mmHg
3	≤0.39	<50 mmHg	<30 mm

© The Author(s) 2024
L. Téot et al. (eds.), *Skin Necrosis*, https://doi.org/10.1007/978-3-031-60954-1_51

Table 51.2 Wound evaluation for WIfI score

Grade	Ulcer	Gangrene
0	None	None
1	Small, no exposed bone (excludes digits)	None
2	Deeper, exposed bone, joint, tendon (excludes calcaneal involvement)	Limited to digits
3	Extensive, bone, joint, and/or tendon involvement to mid/rearfoot	Extensive, involving forefoot and/or midfoot and/or rearfoot

Table 51.3 Infection evaluation for WIfI score

SVS	IDSA infection severity	Clinical manifestation
0	Uninfected	No symptoms or signs
1	Mild	Local infection confined to skin and sub Q. No systemic SOI
2	Moderate	Local infection within deeper tissues, periwound erythema >2 cm. Includes bone and joint. No SIRS
3	Severe	Local infection with SIRS (2 or more: temp, HR, RR, WBC)

Table 51.4 WIfI classification

Risk of amputation	Proposed clinical stages	WIfI spectrum score (W, I, fI)
Very low	Stage 1	000, 001, 010, 011, 100, 101, 110
Low	Stage 2	002, 011, 020, 021, 030, 102, 111, 120, 200, 201
Moderate	Stage 3	003, 021, 022, 031, 032, 103, 112, 121, 130, 131, 202, 210, 211, 220, 300, 301
High	Stage 4	013, 023, 033, 113, 122, 123, 132, 133, 203, 212, 213, 221, 222, 223, 230, 231, 232, 233, 302, 303, 310, 320, 330, 321, 323, 331, 332, 333

Table 51.5 One-year amputation rate

Author	Year	Limb (n)	One-year amputation rate stage 1	One-year amputation rate stage 2	One-year amputation rate stage 3	One-year amputation rate stage 4
Cull	2014	151	3	10	23	40
Zhan	2015	201	0	0	8	37
Darling	2015	551	0	10	11	24
Causey	2016	160	0	25	21	31
Beropoulis	2016	126	13	19	19	38
Ward	2017	98	0	14	21	34
Darling	2017	992	0	4	4	21
Mean		2279	**0**	**10**	**19**	**34**

In a study on diabetic patients suffering from CLTI with ischemic wounds treated by femoropopliteal bypasses, complete wound healing was obtained in 56 ± 18 days after DR and 112 ± 45 days after indirect revascularization (IR) ($p = 0.01$). Amputation-free survival rates were 91%, 65%, and 58% at 1, 3, and 5 years after DR and 66%, 24%, and 18% after IR ($p = 0.03$). There was no difference in mortality and primary patency: 80%, 55%, and 36% after DR versus 83%, 68%, and 36% after IR [11]. In two meta-analyses, wound healing and limb salvage were improved after DR when compared to IR. Amputation-free survival after DR was 86.2% and 84.9% at 1 and 2 years, respectively, after DR and 77.8% and 70.1% after IR [12, 13]. However, these results have not been observed in a study of 177 patients treated by femorotibial bypasses. Median time to complete wound healing was 5.4 months for DR and 8.7 for IR ($p = 0.28$). 72%

and 85% of patients in the DR arm achieved complete wound healing after 6 and 12 months, respectively, versus 69% and 79% after IR ($p = 0.48$). There were also no significant differences in major amputations and mortality rates: The amputation rate was 28.5% after IR and 17.3% after DR ($p = 0.071$), and the mortality rate was 41.3% after IR and 36.8% after DR ($p = 0.088$). These results can be explained by the quality of the perimalleolar collateral vasculature and the plantar arch quality [14]. In addition to these two factors, the conflicting results are also explained by the heterogeneity in the types of revascularizations [15–19].

Patients suffering from CLTI usually present multiple comorbidities and have a higher risk of perioperative morbidity and mortality with a poor mid- and long-term outcome. Coronary disease, end-stage renal disease, malnutrition, poor functional status, and frailty have to be evaluated. The surgeon has to take this into account before elaborating his strategy based on **p**atient, **l**imb, and **an**atomy (**PLAN**) [5]. A risk stratification has to be taken into account to choose the best modalities for anesthesia and surgical techniques. Older and frail patients will be preferentially treated under local anesthesia with endovascular techniques. Before proposing a treatment plan, the WIfI score needs to be calculated to estimate the risk of amputation after 1 year, a risk that should be clearly communicated to the patient.

The pressures measured for the WIfI score will also help the physician decide if a revascularization is needed:

- No revascularization if the ABI is higher than 0.6, ankle systolic pressure higher than 70 mmHg, and toe pressure and $TcPO_2$ higher than 50 mmHg
- Revascularization if the ABI is lower than 0.4, ankle systolic pressure lower than 50 mmHg, and toe pressure and $TcPO_2$ lower than 30 mmHg

For the patients who do not fill the above criteria, 2-week trial of medical treatment should be proposed and then surgery if the wound worsens or does not get better.

Next, the arterial lesions need to be evaluated by examining the level of disease (aortoiliac, femoropopliteal and/or tibial and pedal), extent of disease, and degree of disease (stenosis or occlusion). This will help develop an operative strategy that will answer the four following questions:

1. From? Where is the percutaneous access site, or what is the bypass donor site?
2. To? The target artery that the surgeon wants to revascularize
3. How? Endovascular therapy, open surgery (anatomical or extra-anatomical bypass), or hybrid surgery
4. Using? Endarterectomy, autologous vein conduit, prosthesis, balloon angioplasty, drug-coated balloon, bare metal stent (BMS), drug-eluting stent (DES), covered stent (CS), or a combination of all the above

Many classifications have been proposed to help the surgeon choose the best treatment plan. First, the Trans-Atlantic Society Consensus (TASC) classification was used to stratify the lesions as aortoiliac, femoropopliteal, and infrapopliteal. However, in patients affected by CLTI, all levels are interested by atherosclerosis and have to be treated. If technically feasible (and if there is no risk of worsening the patient's condition), a direct pulsatile in-line flow to the foot is needed to achieve a fast and complete wound healing. TASC was initially helpful to choose between endovascular surgery for short and segmental lesions and endarterectomy or bypass for complex and extensive lesions. Nowadays, endovascular tools and techniques have evolved and are used to successfully treat long stenosis and occlusions previously thought to be not amenable to endovascular treatment by the classification.

The Global Limb Anatomic Staging System (GLASS) was proposed next. The physician needs to determine a target artery pathway (TAP) that will restore a pulsatile flow to the ankle. The TAP is then graded from I to III, which correlates with low-, intermediate-, or high-complexity lesions and also with immediate success and 1-year permeability for endovascular treatment [5].

Bypass surgery requires adequate inflow and outflow and also a suitable conduit, ideally autologous GSV more than 3 mm in diameter for an infra-inguinal bypass (Fig. 51.1). PTFE or Dacron grafts are used for aortoiliac revascularizations (Fig. 51.2) and can also be used for infra-inguinal bypasses with acceptable results for above-knee revascularizations. Although acceptable, these remain inferior to GSV in above-knee revascularizations. Patency is significantly better with GSV for below-knee bypasses. If no vein is available, reinforced vascular grafts should be used to avoid plication (Fig. 51.3). GSV can be used reversed or in situ after devalvulation for infra-inguinal bypass. No statistically significant differences in patency were found between the two techniques [20]. Vessels need to be clamped to control blood flow before arteriotomy. This can be challenging in case of extensive arterial calcifications. In some cases, an extensive ulcer is a contraindication for a distal bypass especially if the target vessel is a distal posterior tibial artery or a pedal artery. General, spinal, epidural, or locoregional anesthesia is mandatory for open surgery. Patients with severe comorbidities can be at high risk for open surgery, and endovascular-first approach appears to be safer for limb salvage. Local anesthesia and sedation are usually sufficient for endovascular treatments, and general, spinal, or epidural anesthesia is not necessary except for long and complex interventions.

In contrast, successful endovascular treatment depends essentially on the extent or length of occlusions and the severity of calcifications. Improved wires, low-profile and dedicated catheters, and long and low-profile balloons are available to treat occlusions (Fig. 51.4) and complex and distal lesions (Fig. 51.5). The access site generally used is the femoral artery, but brachial or radial arteries can also be used. Ultrasound guidance is helpful to choose the best site for arterial puncture and avoid complications and is helpful for retrograde access (Fig. 51.6). Renal insufficiency is not a contraindication for endovascular treatment in case of CLTI. Injection through a long sheath or catheter and dilution of the iodine contrast are helpful techniques to limit iodine contrast use during procedures. Stenting is indicated after angioplasty in case of residual stenosis, dissection, severe calcified lesions, or treatment for occlusion. Self-expandable nitinol stents are generally used for infra-inguinal lesions and balloon expandable steel, chrome-cobalt, or covered stents for iliac lesions. Drug-coated balloons and stents are used to prevent restenosis after angioplasty.

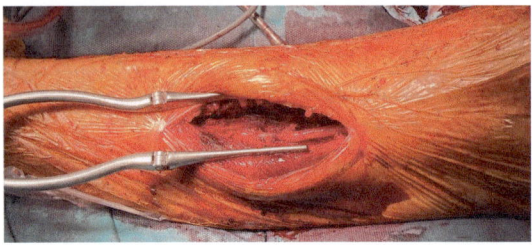

Fig. 51.1 Femorotibial bypass with *GSV* distal anastomosis

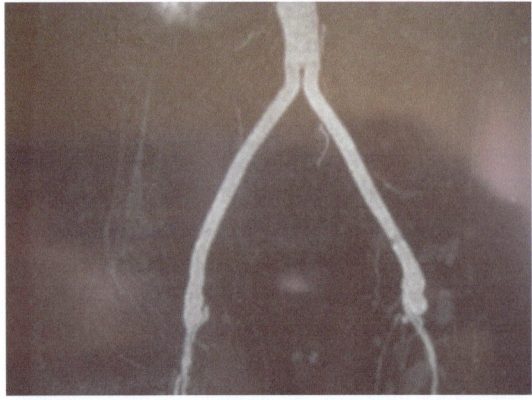

Fig. 51.2 Aorto-bifemoral bypass to treat aorto-bi-iliac extensive occlusion

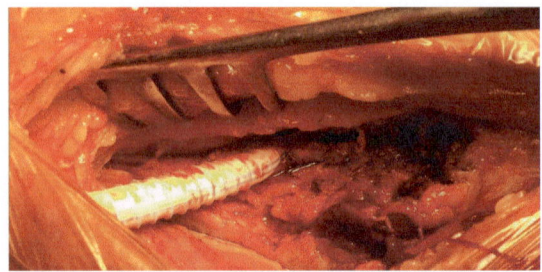

Fig. 51.3 Femoropopliteal bypass below the knee with a PTFE-strengthened prosthesis

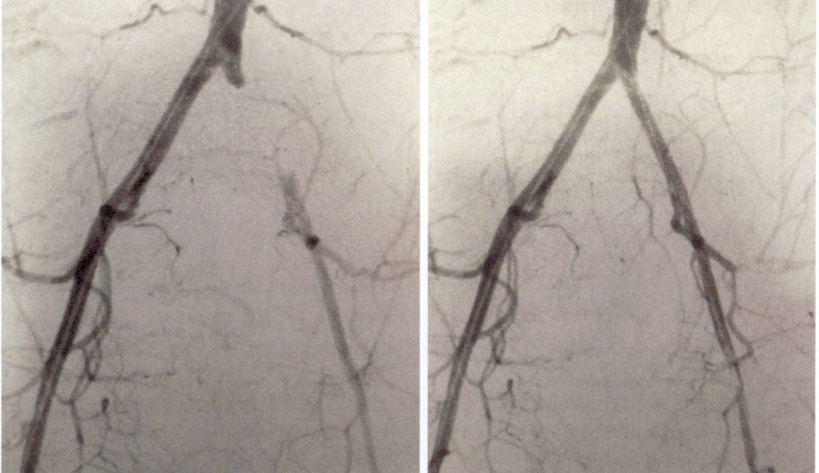

Fig. 51.4 Common left iliac artery recanalization

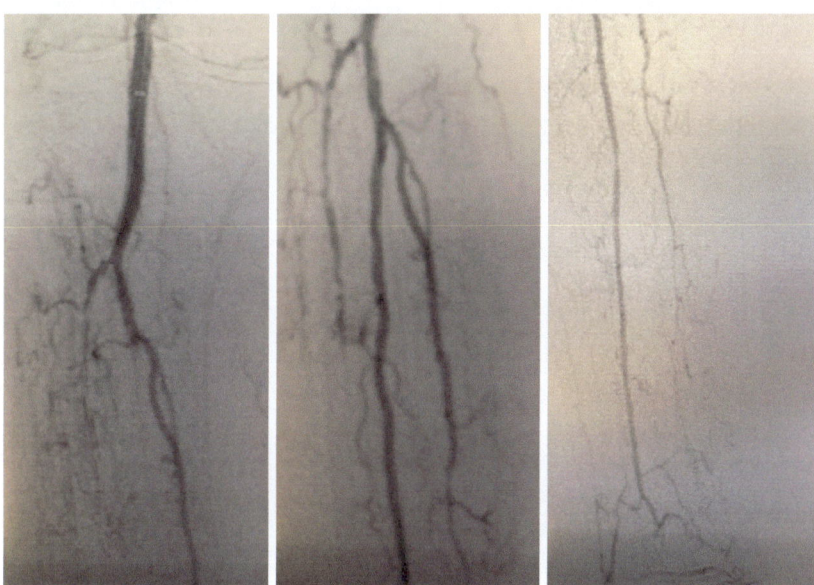

Fig. 51.5 Peroneal artery recanalization

Multilevel and extensive lesions are challenging, and all open and endovascular techniques can be associated to propose the best treatment for each patient. These hybrid procedures are helpful to treat these challenging lesions.

Perioperative mortality, morbidity, limb salvage, and patency for bypasses are summarized in Tables 51.6, 51.7, 51.8, and 51.9. 8602 patients suffering from CLTI treated by infra-inguinal revascularization were reviewed. Subjects with infra-popliteal disease treated by GSV graft had higher patency rates at 1 and 2 years (primary: 87%, 78%; secondary: 94%, 87%) compared to all other types of interventions. Prosthetic bypass outcomes were significantly worse in terms of amputation and patency rates, especially for bellow-knee revascularizations. Survival, major amputation, and amputation-free survival (AFS) at 2 years were similar between endovascular interventions and vein bypasses, with prosthetic bypasses having higher rates of limb loss [21].

Another randomized trial (**BASIL** study) evaluated **b**ypass versus **a**ngioplasty in **s**evere **i**schemia of the **l**eg. Technical success was better in the bypass group: 97.4% versus 80.0% ($p = 0.01$). However, there was no statistical dif-

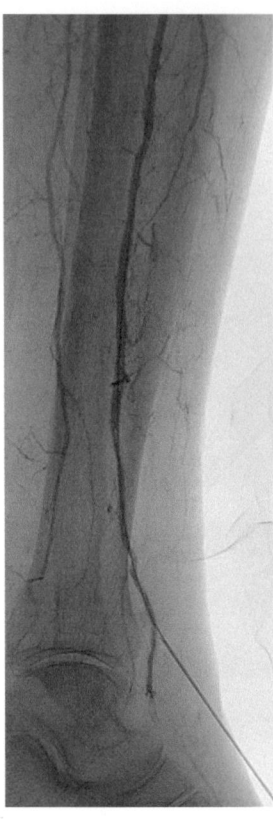

Fig. 51.6 Anterior tibial artery recanalization by retrograde approach

ference for survival and AFS 2 years after surgery. After 2 years, survival and AFS were improved in the bypass group [22].

A meta-analysis compared endovascular treatment and bypass for CLTI (20,903 patients). Endovascular treatment was associated with lower perioperative mortality (OR = 0.69, 95% IC 0.51–0.95), lower major cardiovascular events (OR = 0.42, 95% IC 0.29–0.61), and less surgical site infection (OR = 0.31, 95% IC 0.19–0.51). Primary permeability (HR = 1.31, 95% IC 1.08–1.58) and limb salvage (HR = 1.41, 95% IC 1.02–1.94) were improved in the bypass group [23].

In a single-center prospective monocentric randomized controlled trial, venous bypasses and angioplasty with nitinol stenting were compared for patients affected by long femoropopliteal lesions (53% suffering from CLTI). Technical success was 88% in the stent group. During a 4-year follow-up, primary patency, freedom from target lesion revascularization, limb salvage, survival, and complications showed no significant differences between the groups. 48 months' secondary permeability was 73% for the bypass group and 50% in the stent group ($p = 0.021$). Clinical improvement was significantly superior in the bypass group with 52% versus 19% reaching Rutherford 0 category ($p < 0.001$) [24].

In a retrospective study, 153 patients had a revascularization of both femoropopliteal and infra-popliteal vessels (48 by bypass and 105 by an endovascular treatment). There was no significant difference in technical success rates (98.0% in the bypass group and 95.2% in the endovascular group), perioperative mortality (8.3% and 7.7% [$p = 0.25$], 3-year survival: 73.4% and 61.3% [$p = 0.25$]), or 3-year limb salvage (53.3% and 59.7% [$p = 0.24$]) [25].

A meta-analysis of 17,118 patients compared CLTI treatment results in octogenarians and non-octogenarians. One-year mortality was greater in octogenarians: 32% (95% CI, 27–37) versus 17% (95% CI, 11–22) (OR = 2.52, 95% CI, 1.93–3.29). No significant difference was observed in major amputations between the two groups (15% for non-octogenarians [95% CI, 11–18] and 12% for octogenarians [95% CI, 7–14]). One-year AFS was lower for octogenarians (OR 1.55, 95% CI, 1.03–2.43), 64% (95% CI, 54–74), and 69% for non-octogenarians (95% CI, 58–81). No difference was observed in amputation rate between endovascular and open surgical treatment. A higher mortality was observed with conservative treatment compared to amputation or revascularization (OR 1.76, 95% CI, 1.19–2.60) [26].

Recovery after open surgery and endovascular treatment for CLTI was studied in octogenarians. There was no statistical difference in perioperative mortality (respectively, 4% and 2% [$p = 0.697$]), morbidity (13.7% vs. 10.3% [$p = 0.716$]), primary patency (76%, 59%, and 50% and 82%, 75%, and 32%, respectively, at 1, 2, and 4 years [$p = 0.467$]), and limb salvage (91%, 90%, and 89% and 94%, 87%, and 86% [$p = 0.939$] at 1, 2, and 4 years). Complete recovery was observed in 34.3% and 35.7% of patients after 1 and 6 months in the open surgery group

Table 51.6 Perioperative mortality after bypasses

Revascularization	Author	Publication year	Patients (N)	Revascularizations (N)	Perioperative mortality
Popliteal and distal heparin-bonded ePTFE prosthetic bypasses	Daenens	2009	240	240	0.41%
ePTFE distal bypasses	Scandinavian Miller Collar Study	2010	77	77	**10%**
ePTFE distal bypasses with cuff	Scandinavian Miller Collar Study	2010	69	69	5%
Infra-malleolar venous bypasses (in situ 60.6%)	Brochado Neto	2010	116	122	13%
Pedal branch venous bypasses	Brochado-Neto	2012	25	25	8%
ePTFE heparin-bonded distal bypasses and venous cuff	Neville	2012	62	62	0%
GSV distal bypasses	Neville	2012	50	50	0%
Perigenicular vessel bypasses	De Latour	2007	57	59	3.5%
GSV, arm veins, PTFE distal bypasses	Slim	2011	164	179	2.20%
GSV, arm veins, PTFE pedal bypasses	Slim	2011	45	51	**0%**
PTFE reinforced prosthetic distal bypasses with venous cuff	Neville	2012	252	270	0.5%
Contralateral GSV, SSV, arm veins bypasses	Nierlich	2020	–	644	1.9%

Table 51.7 Perioperative morbidity after bypasses

Revascularization	Author	Publication year	Morbidity
Popliteal and distal heparin-bonded ePTFE prosthetic bypasses	Bosiers	2006	**0%**
Supra-popliteal PTFE with cuff bypasses	Rückert	2009	**29%**
Popliteal and distal venous bypasses	Daenens	2009	0%
Popliteal and infra-popliteal heparin-bonded ePTFE bypasses	Daenens	2009	0.83%
ePTFE distal bypasses	Scandinavian Miller Collar Study	2010	10%
ePTFE distal bypasses with cuff	Scandinavian Miller Collar Study	2010	6%
Infra-malleolar venous bypasses (in situ 60.6%)	Brochado Neto	2010	2.4%
Pedal branch venous bypasses	Brochado-Neto	2012	24%
ePTFE heparin-bonded distal bypasses and venous cuff	Neville	2012	1.6%
GSV distal bypasses	Neville	2012	4%
Composite autologous and umbilical vein distal bypasses	Neufang	2007	26%
Perigenicular vessel bypasses	De Latour	2007	9.1%
Cryopreserved venous infra-popliteal bypasses	Randon	2010	11.1%
Infra-malleolar venous bypasses	Saarinen	2016	5.0%

Table 51.8 Limb salvage after bypasses

Revascularization	Author	Publication year	Limb salvage rate	Limb salvage rate evaluation time
Popliteal and distal heparin-bonded ePTFE prosthetic bypasses	Bosiers	2006	87%	1 year
Popliteal and distal venous bypasses	Daenens	2009	100% above the knee, 91% below the knee, **96% tibial arteries**	2 years
Popliteal and distal ePTFE heparin-bonded bypasses	Daenens	2009	92% above the knee, 98% below the knee, 87% tibial arteries	2 years
ePTFE distal bypasses	Scandinavian Miller Collar Study	2010	**44%**	3 years
ePTFE distal bypasses with cuff	Scandinavian Miller Collar Study	2010	59%	3 years
Popliteal pedal venous bypasses (in situ 78.5%)	Good	2011	81.8%, 81.8%, 81.8%	1, 3, and 5 years
Infra-malleolar venous bypasses (in situ 60.6%)	Brochado Neto	2010	70.0%, 50.4%	3 and 5 years
Popliteal distal venous bypasses (meta-analysis)	Albers	2006	77.7 ± 4%	5 years
Pedal branch venous bypasses	Brochado-Neto	2012	81.7%, 69%	1 and 3 years
ePTFE heparin-bonded distal bypasses and venous cuff	Neville	2012	80%	1 year
GSV distal bypasses	Neville	2012	80%	1 year
Composite autologous and umbilical vein distal bypasses	Neufang	2007	87%	5 years
Perigenicular vessel bypasses	De Luccia	2011	73.5 ± 7%	3 years
Perigenicular vessel bypasses	De Latour	2007	90.0 ± 4%	3 years
Cryopreserved venous infra-popliteal bypasses	Randon	2010	84.91%, 77.1%, 62%, 58%	1, 2, 3, and 5 years
GSV, arm veins, PTFE distal bypasses	Slim	2011	92%	1 year
GSV, arm veins, PTFE pedal bypasses	Slim	2011	96%	1 year
Reinforced ePTFE distal bypasses with venous cuff	Neville	2012	80.6%, 78.0%, 75.7%, 67.5%	1, 2, 3, and 4 years
Infra-malleolar venous bypasses	Saarinen	2016	78.6%, 72.0%, 67.2%	1, 5, and 10 years
Contro-lateral GSV, SSV, arm veins bypasses	Nierlich	2020	73%, 79%, 74%	5 years

and 48.2% and 59.6% in the endovascular treatment group ($p = 0.01$ at 6 months) [27]. Elderly patients are more likely to undergo endovascular treatment with 1-year amputation rates greater than younger patients. Furthermore, perioperative and 1-year mortality increase with age [28]. However, elderly patients are perhaps referred more for palliative care, which might explain sometimes the better results observed for limb salvage in this population.

The BEST-CLI group in its recent international randomized trial enrolling 1830 patients with infra-inguinal peripheral artery disease suffering from CLTI showed lower incidence of major adverse limb event or death in the surgical group in case of adequate great saphenous vein (42.6%) compared to endovascular group (57.4%) (HR 0.68; 95% CI: 0.59–0.79; $p < 0.001$) and less major amputations (10.4% versus 14.9%) (HR 0.73; 95% CI, 0.54–0.98) but no difference in case of an alternative bypass conduit: major adverse limb event or death in the surgical group: 42.8% and 47.7% in the endovascular

Table 51.9 Permeability for bypasses

Revascularization	Author	Publication year	Primary permeability	Time to evaluation (years)	Secondary permeability	Secondary permeability assessment time
Popliteal and distal venous bypasses	Daenens	2009	91%, 80% sus-art, 72%, 72% popliteal, 69%, 64% distal	1 and 2	?	?
Popliteal and distal ePTFE heparin-bonded prosthetic bypasses	Daenens	2009	92%, 83% sus-art, 92%, 83% sous-art, 79%, 69% jambiers	1 and 2	?	?
ePTFE distal bypasses	Scandinavian Miller Collar Study	2010	17%	3	**20%**	3 years
ePTFE distal bypasses with cuff	Scandinavian Miller Collar Study	2010	20%	3	22%	3 years
Popliteal pedal venous bypasses (in situ 78.5%)	Good	2011	63.3%, 63.3%, 63.3%	1, 3, and 5	74.6%, 74.6%, 74.6%	1, 3, and 5 years
Infra-malleolar venous bypasses (in situ 60.6%)	Brochado Neto	2010	51.4%, 46.7%	3 and 5	58.2%, 53.4%	3 and 5 years
Popliteal distal venous bypasses (meta-analysis)	Albers	2006	63.1% ± 4.3%	5	70.7% ± 4.6%	5 years
ePTFE heparin-bonded distal bypasses and venous cuff	Neville	2012	75.4%	1	?	?
GSV distal bypasses	Neville	2012	86%	1	?	?
Composite autologous and umbilical vein distal bypasses	Neufang	2007	35%	5	42%	5 years
Perigenicular vessel bypasses	De Luccia	2011	74.7 ± 7%	3	83.4 ± 8%	3 years
Perigenicular vessel bypasses	De Latour	2007	65 ± 7%	3	70 ± 7%	3 years
Cryopreserved allograft venous infra-popliteal bypasses	Randon	2010	56%, 32%, 17%	1, 3, and 5	73%, 60%, 38.5%	1, 3, and 5 years
GSV, arm veins, PTFE distal bypasses	Slim	2011	61.7%	1	87.4%	1 years
GSV, arm veins, PTFE pedal bypasses	Slim	2011	61.9%	1	87.4%	1 year
Reinforced ePTFE distal bypasses with venous cuff	Neville	2012	79.8%, 75.6%, 65.9%, 51.2%	1, 2, 3, and 4	?	?
Infra-malleolar venous bypasses	Saarinen	2016	71.2%, 59.7%, 49.0%	1, 5, and 10	81.0%, 70.7%, 68.4%	1, 5, and 10 years
Contralateral GSV, SSV, arm vein bypasses	Nierlich	2020	59%, 66%, 63% and 48%, 50%, 39%	1 and 5	?	?

group (HR 0.79; 95% CI, 0.58–1.06; $p = 0.12$) [29].

Endovascular treatment encompasses different modalities: angioplasty, Bare Metal Stent (BMS), drug-coated balloons, Drug Eluting Stent (DES), and Covered Stent (CS). They were reviewed for the treatment of supra-popliteal lesions (23 randomized controlled trials, 3314 patients affected by claudication: 85% or CLTI: 15%). Fifteen studies failed to show a benefit for stenting when compared to angioplasty alone. There was no clinical benefit, but a lower target lesion revascularization was observed in four studies with coated balloons. Four trials failed to show a clinical benefit for DES compared to BMS. However, there is a lack of data concerning the best strategy for patients suffering from CLTI [30]. For infra-popliteal lesions, 12 trials were reviewed (1145 patients, 90% affected by CLTI). BMS and DES do not improve clinical results after angioplasty. Another trial compared plain old balloon angioplasty (POBA) and drug-coated balloon angioplasty. Drug-coated balloon use was associated with improved wound healing (RR: 1.28; 95% CI: 1.05–1.56; $p = 0.01$), improved Rutherford stage (RR: 1.32; 95% CI: 1.08–1.60; $p = 0.008$), lower target lesion revascularization (RR: 0.41; 95% CI: 0.23–0.74; $p = 0.002$), and a lower rate of restenosis (RR: 0.36; 95% CI: 0.24–0.54; $p < 0.0001$) among diabetic patients at 12 months. No differences were observed between DES and BMS [31].

IN.PACT SFA Randomized Trial compared drug-coated angioplasty and POBA for femoropopliteal lesions (220 patients in the first group and 111 in the second, Rutherford 4: 5.0% and 5.4%, Rutherford 5: 0.0% and 0.9%, respectively). Technical success was comparable between groups: 99.5% and 98.2%; primary patency was, respectively, 82.2 and 52.4% ($p < 0.001$); target lesion revascularization at 12 months was lower in drug-coated angioplasty group: 2.4% versus 20.6% ($p < 0.001$); and clinical improvement was more frequent in the drug-coated balloon group: 85.2% versus 68.9% ($p < 0.001$). Walking distance improvement was comparable: 72.7 ± 31.4% and 73.6 ± 29.5% ($p = 0.59$). One-year life quality was comparable. No procedure-related mortality was observed. No patient needed major amputation at 1 year. Targeted lesion occlusion after 1 year was observed in 1.4% and 3.7%, respectively ($p = 0.10$) [32].

DES demonstrated improved patency over BMS in infra-popliteal arteries (primary patency: 73% versus 50% at 1 year) and was at least comparable to balloon angioplasty (66% primary patency) [21]. BMS, DES, and CS were compared in a retrospective cohort study for SFA lesions. The unadjusted primary patency at 12, 24, and 48 months were 57%, 47%, and 44% for BMS; 81%, 66%, and 53% for DES; and 62%, 49%, and 42% for CS (log-rank $p = 0.044$). Compared to CS, DES was associated with improved primary-assisted patency (HR for patency loss: 0.35, $p = 0.008$) and secondary patency (HR: 0.32, $p = 0.011$). Across the entire follow-up period, stent occlusions occurred in 40% BMS, 57% CS, and 19% DES ($p < 0.001$). Among them, ALI occurred in 5% BMS, 33% CS, and 9% DES ($p = 0.01$). The relative risk of presenting with acute limb ischemia as opposed to claudication was 27 times greater among patients re-presenting with occluded CS compared to BMS ($p = 0.02$). There was no significant difference in AFS or all-cause mortality across the three cohorts [33].

Revascularization is a key factor to prevent major amputation during CLTI. Endovascular treatments and bypasses show similar results during the first 2 years. Endovascular treatment can be proposed as the first-line strategy especially for elderly and frail patients. When life expectancy is superior to 2 years, open surgery seems to offer better results than endovascular treatment. GSV is the best conduit for infra-popliteal bypasses. Angioplasty and selective stenting represent the reference for endovascular treatments, but drug-coated balloons, drug-eluting stents, and covered stents are helpful to prevent restenosis and improve target lesion revascularization.

References

1. Aboyans V, Sevestre MA, Désormais I, Lacroix P, Fowkes G, Criqui M. Epidémiologie de l'artériopathie des membres inférieurs. Presse Med. 2018;47(1):38–46.
2. Conte MS, Bradbury AW, Kohl P, White JV, Dick F, Fitridge R, Mills JL, Ricco JB, Suresh KR, Hassanmurad M, Aboyans V, Aksoy M, Alexandrescu VA, Armstrong D, Azuma N, Belch J, Bergoeing M, Bjorck M, Chakfé N, Cheng S, Dawson J, Debus ES, Dueck A, Duval S, Eckstein HH, Ferraresi R, Gambhir R, Garguilo RM, Geraghty P, Goode S, Gray B, Guo W, Gupta PC, Hinchliffe R, Jetty P, Komori K, Lavery L, Liang W, Lookstein R, Menard M, Misra S, Miyata T, Moneta G, Munoa Prado JA, Munoz A, Paolini JE, Patel M, Pomposelli F, Powell R, Robless P, Rogers L, Schanzer A, Schneider P, Taylor S, De Ceniga MV, Veller M, Vermassen F, Wang J, Wang S, GVG Writing Group for the Joint Guidelines of the Society for vascular Surgery (SVS), European Society for Vascular Surgery (ESVS), World Federation of Vascular Societies (WFVS). Global vascular guidelines on the management of chronic limb-threatening ischemia. Eur J Vasc Endovasc Surg. 2019;58:S1–S109.
3. Hirsch AT, Allison MA, Gomes AS, Corriere MA, Duval S, Ershow AG, et al. A call to action: women and peripheral artery disease: a scientific statement from the American Heart Association. Circulation. 2012;125:1449–72.
4. Marston WA, Davies SW, Armstrong B, Farber MA, Mendes RC, Fulton JJ, et al. Natural history of limbs with arterial insufficiency and chronic ulceration treated without revascularization. J Vasc Surg. 2006;44:108–14.
5. Londero L, Hoegh A, Houlind K, Lindholt J. Major amputation rates in patients with peripheral arterial disease aged 50 years and over in Denmark during the period 1997–2014 and their relationship with demographics, risk factors, and vascular services. Eur J Vasc Endovasc Surg. 2019;58:729–37.
6. Brahmandam A, Gholitabar N, Cardella J, Nassiri N, Dardik A, Georgi M, Chaar CI. Discrepancy in outcomes after revascularization for chronic limb-threatening ischemia warrants separate reporting of rest pain and tissue loss. Ann Vasc Surg. 2021;70:237–43.
7. Tsay C, Luo J, Zhang Y, Attaran R, Dardik A, Chaar CI. Perioperative outcomes of lower extremity revascularization for rest pain and tissue loss. Ann Vasc Surg. 2020;66:493–501.
8. Mills JL, Conte MS, Armstrong DG, Pomposelli FB, Schanzer A, Sidawy AN, Andros G, on behalf of the Society for Vascular Surgery lower Extremity Guidelines Committee. The society for vascular surgery lower limb extremity threatened limb classification system: risk stratification based on wound, ischemia, and foot infection (WIFI). J Vasc Surg. 2014;59(1):220–34.
9. Mills JL. The application of the Society for Vascular Surgery Wound, Ischaemia, and foot Infection (WIFI) classification to stratify amputation risk. J Vasc Surg. 2017;65(3):591–3.
10. Taylor GI, Palmer JH. The vascular territories (angiosomes) of the body: experimental study and clinical applications. Br J Plast Surg. 1987;40:113–41.
11. Lejay A, Georges Y, Tartaglia E, Gaertner S, Geny B, Thaveau F, Chakfe N. Long-term outcomes of direct and indirect below-the-knee open revascularization based on the angiosome concept in diabetic patients with critical limb ischemia. Ann Vasc Surg. 2014;28(4):983–9.
12. Bosanquet DC, Glasbey JCD, Williams IM, Twine CP. Systematic review and meta-analysis of direct versus indirect angiosomal revascularisation of infrapopliteal arteries. Eur J Vasc Endovasc Surg. 2014;48(1):88–97.
13. Biancari F, Juvonen T. Angiosome-targeted lower limb revascularization for ischemic foot wounds: systematic review and meta-analysis. Eur J Vasc Endovasc Surg. 2014;47(5):518–22.
14. Harth C, Randon C, Vermassen F. Impact of angiosome targeted femorodistal bypass surgery on healing rate and outcome in chronic limb threatening ischaemia. Eur J Vasc Endovasc Surg. 2020;60:68–75.
15. Sumpio BE, Forsythe RO, Ziegler KR, Van Baal JG, Lepantolo MJ, Hinchliffe RJ. Clinical implications of the angiosome model in peripheral vascular disease. J Vasc Surg. 2013;58:814–26.
16. Chae KJ, Shin JY. Is angiosome-targeted angioplasty effective for limb salvage and wound healing in diabetic foot? A meta-analysis. PLoS One. 2016;11:e0159523.
17. Jongsma H, Bekken JA, Akkersdijk GP, Hoeks SE, Verhagen HJ, Fioole B. Angiosome-directed revascularization in patients with critical limb ischemia. J Vasc Surg. 2017;65(4):1208–19.
18. Azuma N, Uchida H, Kokubo T, Koya A, Akasaka N, Sasajima T. Factors influencing wound healing of critical ischaemic foot after bypass surgery: is the angiosome important in selecting bypass target artery? Eur J Vasc Endovasc Surg. 2012;43:322–8.
19. Rashid H, Slim H, Zayed H, Huang DY, Wilkins CJ, Evans DR, et al. The impact of arterial pedal arch quality and the angiosome revascularization on foot tissue loss healing and infrapopliteal bypass outcome. J Vasc Surg. 2013;57:1219–26.
20. Chang H, Veith FJ, Rockman CB, Maldonado TS, Jacobowitz GR, Cayne NS, Garg K. Comparative analysis of patients undergoing lower extremity bypass using in-situ and reversed great saphenous vein graft techniques. Vascular. 2022;31(5):931–40. https://doi.org/10.1177/17085381221088082.
21. Almasri J, Adusumalli J, Asi N, Lakis S, Alsawas M, Prokop LJ, Bradbury A, Kohl P, Conte MS, Murad MH. A systematic review and meta-analysis of revascularization outcomes of infra-inguinal chronic limb-threatening ischemia. Eur J Vasc Endovasc Surg. 2019;58:S110–9.

22. Bradbury AW, Adam DJ, Bell J, Forbes JF, Fowkes FG, Gillespie I, et al. Bypass versus angioplasty in severe ischemia of the leg (BASIL) trial: analysis of amputation free and overall survival by treatment received. J Vasc Surg. 2010;51(5):18S–31S.

23. Wang J, Shu C, Zhao J, Huang B, Huang D, Yang Y, Bian H, He Y, Wang Z. Percutaneous vascular interventions versus bypass surgery in patients with critical limb ischemia: a comprehensive meta-analysis. Ann Surg. 2017; https://doi.org/10.1097/SLA.0000000000000344.

24. Enzmann FK, Nierlich P, Hölzenbein T, Aspalter M, Kluckner M, Hitzl W, Popperer M, Linni K. Vein bypass versus nitinol stent in long femoropopliteal lesions: 4-year results of a randomized controlled trial. Ann Surg. 2022; https://doi.org/10.1097/SLA.0000000000005413.

25. Benaduce Casella I, Holanda Sartori C, Brito Faustino C, Vieira Mariz MP, Presti C, Puech-Leao P, De Luccia N. Endovascular therapy provides similar results of bypass graft surgery in the treatment of infrainguinal multilevel arterial disease in patients with chronic limb-threatening ischemia in all GLASS stages. Ann Vasc Surg. 2020;68:400–8.

26. Wübbeke LF, Naves CCLM, Daemen JWHC, Jacobs MJ, Mees BME. Mortality and major amputation after revascularisation in octogenarians versus non-octogenarians with chronic limb threatening ischemia: a systematic review and meta-analysis. Eur J Vasc Endovasc Surg. 2020;60:231–41.

27. Lejay A, Thaveau F, Georges Y, Bajcz C, Kreitz JG, Chakfe N. Autonomy following revascularisation in 80-year-old patients with critical limb ischemia. Eur J Vasc Endovasc Surg. 2012;44(6):562–7.

28. Kim TI, Aboian E, Fischer U, Zhang Y, Guzman RJ, Chaar CI. Lower extremity revascularization for chronic limb threatening ischemia among patients at the extremes of age. Ann Vasc Surg. 2021;72:517–28.

29. Farber A, Menard MT, Conte MS, Kaufman JA, Powell RJ, Choudhry NK, Hamza TH, Assmann SF, Creager MA, Cziraky MJ, Dake MD, Jaff MR, for the BEST-CLI Investigators. Surgery or endovascular therapy for chronic limb-threatening ischemia. N Engl J Med. 2022; https://doi.org/10.1056/NEJMoa2207899.

30. Jens S, Conijn AP, Koelemay MJW, Bipat S, Reekers JA. Randomized trials for endovascular treatment of infrainguinal arterial disease: systematic review and meta-analysis (part 1: above the knee). Eur J Vasc Endovasc Surg. 2014;47(5):524–35.

31. Jens S, Conijn AP, Koelemay MJW, Bipat S, Reekers JA. Randomized trials for endovascular treatment of infrainguinal arterial disease: systematic review and meta-analysis (part 2: below the knee). Eur J Vasc Endovasc Surg. 2014;47(5):536–44.

32. Tepe G, Laird J, Schneider P, Brodmann M, Krishnan P, Micari A, Metzger C, Scheinert D, Zeller T, Cohen DJ, Snead DB, for the IN PACT SFA Trial Investigators. Drug-coated balloon versus standard percutaneous transluminal angioplasty for the treatment of superficial femoral and popliteal peripheral artery disease 12-month results from the IN.PACT SFA randomized trial. Circulation. 2015:495–502.

33. Zamani N, Sharath SE, Browder RC, Barshes NR, Braun JD, Mills JL, Kougias P, Younes HK. Outcomes after endovascular stent placement for long-segment superficial femoral artery lesions. Ann Vasc Surg. 2021;71:298–307.

Open Access This chapter is licensed under the terms of the Creative Commons Attribution-NonCommercial-NoDerivatives 4.0 International License (http://creativecommons.org/licenses/by-nc-nd/4.0/), which permits any non-commercial use, sharing, distribution and reproduction in any medium or format, as long as you give appropriate credit to the original author(s) and the source, provide a link to the Creative Commons license and indicate if you modified the licensed material. You do not have permission under this license to share adapted material derived from this chapter or parts of it.

The images or other third party material in this chapter are included in the chapter's Creative Commons license, unless indicated otherwise in a credit line to the material. If material is not included in the chapter's Creative Commons license and your intended use is not permitted by statutory regulation or exceeds the permitted use, you will need to obtain permission directly from the copyright holder.

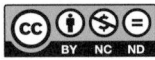

Skin Reconstruction Using Dermal Substitutes After Skin Necrosis

Franco Bassetto and Carlotta Scarpa

52.1 Introduction

Even if due to different etiopathogeneses (for example, trauma, burns, post-oncological excision), skin necrosis is still a challenge for plastic surgeons who must personalize the treatment on different kinds of patients.

Indeed, after the removal of necrotic tissue and a good debridement, which can be performed both with blade and devices, as for example negative-pressure therapy with or without instillation or hydrodebridement, the surgeon has to analyze not only the residual loss of substance but also the features of the involved area (for example, if it is a leg or a thoracic region or a scalp) and the features of the interested patient (for example, if he/she is young or old, if there are comorbidities as diabetic or vascular impairments) in order to choose the correct closure procedure.

Nowadays, many procedures are available such as skin grafts, local/perforating/free flaps, and physical therapies (as for example the acoustic waves or the fluorescent light energy), but since their introduction in the 1950s, dermal substitutes have become one of the most popular treatments in order to obtain a good skin reconstruction, especially when old and/or very compromised patients have to be treated.

Also known as acellular matrices, these products have the capability of modulating scar tissue formation avoiding its hypertrophy and/or retraction; they can come from different animals like pigs, fishes, or cows; they can be composed of different elements like collagen with or without elastin; and they can be covered by a silicone layer which permits to protect the dermal matrix in case we need a new and functional dermal layer before final closure.

These features combined with different surface density, porosity, and time of degradation have given rise to a huge heterogeneity of different matrices, each with different indications and time of scaffold's reabsorption [1, 2].

For these reasons in these last years, it has been proposed to differentiate the matrices into two main classes: (1) in the first class, we can recognize acellular matrices whose scaffold remains after the intake period of 14–21 days; (2) in the second class, the scaffold can be reabsorbed immediately after 7 days stimulating the growth of a "good-quality" granulation tissue.

In this chapter, we will generally talk about the most popular acellular dermal matrices used in European countries for skin reconstruction.

F. Bassetto · C. Scarpa (✉)
Plastic Surgery Unit, University of Padova, Padova, Italy
e-mail: franco.bassetto@unipd.it; carlotta.scarpa@unipd.it

52.2 The Different Acellular Matrices

As said earlier, different acellular dermal matrices have different indications depending on different areas and different kinds of loss of substance.

Dermal regeneration template [3–7]: derived from cows, it is featured by the presence of collagen and other components as chondroitin-6-sulfate but it is without elastin. Nowadays, the dermal regeneration template has been widely used to obtain (1) full-thickness reconstruction, (2) healing stabilization, and (3) low rate of recurrence. These features have made it a valuable treatment for skin necrosis after burns, diabetic lesions, post-traumatic necrosis, and acute and chronic ulcers of the leg due to vascular impairment and also for post-oncological excision when radicality is demonstrated.

This template can be immediately covered by a skin graft, or it can present a removable silicone layer to prepare a new and efficient derma before final closure with skin graft after 14–21 days; interestingly, the scaffold remains present after the intake period.

Even if this dermal substitute has been widely considered and used since its introduction, in our experience, it is preferable to avoid it if there is a high risk of infection or when noble structures are exposed (Fig. 52.1).

Bilayered three-dimensional porous matrix [3, 8, 9]: featured by a stabilized bovine origin type I collagen, this matrix seems to improve the colonization as fibroblasts recognize collagen fibers. As others, it can be immediately covered by a skin graft or, in a dual-step procedure, can be used for the treatment of losses of substances after burns, post-oncological excisions, trauma, and/or acute or chronic ulcers. Also in this case, we prefer to avoid it in high risk of infection areas or patients (Fig. 52.2).

Acellular dermal matrix with elastin [10, 11]: made of purified, freeze-dried bovine collagen mixed with 3% elastin hydrolysate, this matrix is widely used when treated areas require pliability and there is need of tissue sliding, for example on tendon areas. Differently from the previous one, this dermal matrix does not present silicon layer

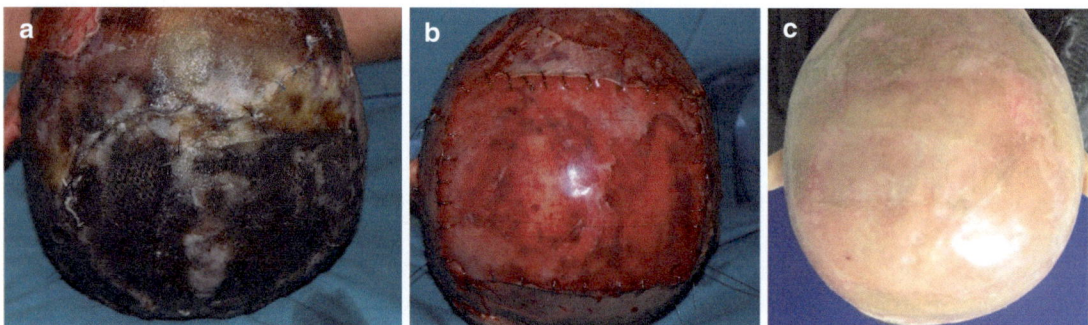

Fig. 52.1 Post-traumatic necrosis of the scalp: (**a**) pre-op after skin necrosis; (**b**) autologous skin graft plus dermal matrix; (**c**) after 1 month of final closure with skin grafts

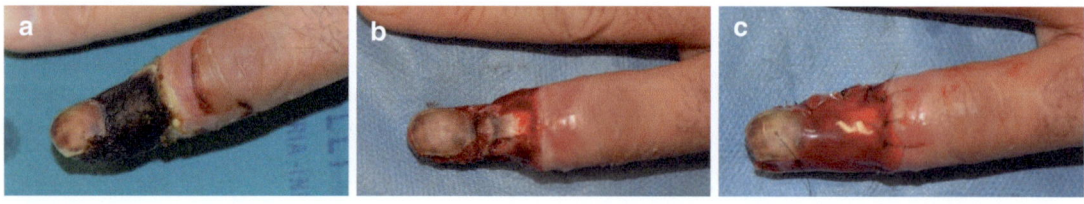

Fig. 52.2 Post-traumatic necrosis on right hand-II finger: (**a**) pre-op; (**b**) post-necrosis removal; (**c**) bilayer three-dimensional porous matrix

on its top, but it can equally be used in multistep procedures; indeed, even if it is more frequently immediately covered by a skin graft, it is possible to use a thicker dermal matrix (2 mm) and cover it after 14 days from the first procedure. Also in this case, in our experience, it is preferable to avoid it if there is high risk of infection (Fig. 52.3).

Porcine origin matrix [12, 13]: composed by atelocollagen derived by porcine tendon, this matrix is available both with and without silicone layer and in fenestrated type, so it can be used both in one- and dual-step procedures also in very exudating lesions. Indicated for skin loss that is partial thickness to deep dermis, in our experience, this matrix is highly recommended in areas/patients at high risk of infections, as for example in post-traumatic lesions or diabetic patients (Fig. 52.4).

Fish-derived acellular matrix [14–16]: featured by intact decellularized fish skin derived from cod, this matrix is very rich in omega-3. It seems that these features could both induce a "good-quality" granulation tissue and reduce pain before, during, and after the dressing. As other matrices, this product can be immediately covered by a skin graft, but it is also possible to delay the final closure to obtain a better granulation tissue. In this case, the matrix can be reabsorbed after 7 days, and some new application can be required to reach both the desired granulation tissue and the required thickness of the dermal layer. In our experience, this matrix can be used in cases in which pliability can be required as, for example, in joints as heel or knee (Fig. 52.5).

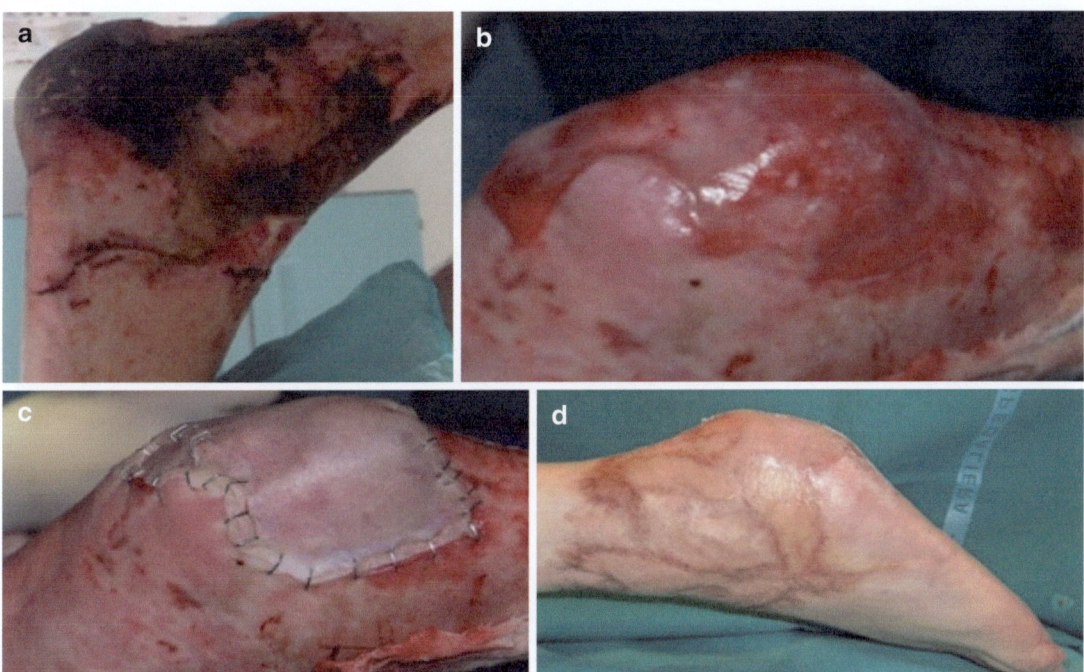

Fig. 52.3 Post-traumatic necrosis of the foot: (**a**) preoperative; (**b**) after necrosis removal, we used the dermal matrix, (**c**) immediate skin graft; (**d**) 3-month follow-up

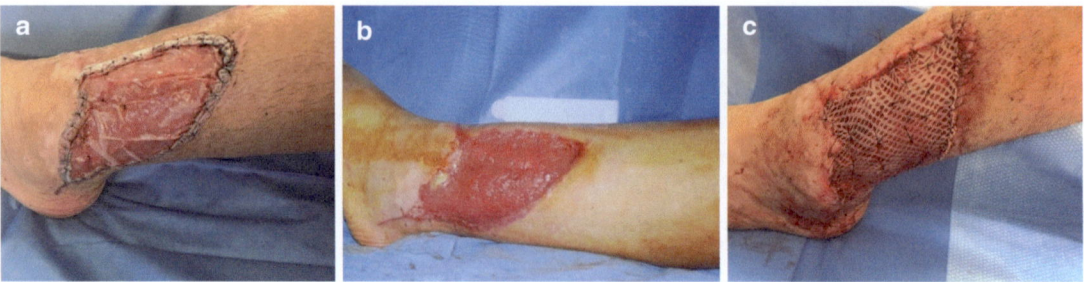

Fig. 52.4 Post-traumatic lesion in obese and diabetic patient—high risk of infection: (**a**) post-necrosis removal, we applied fenestrated one; (**b**) after 14 days; (**c**) post-final closure with skin graft

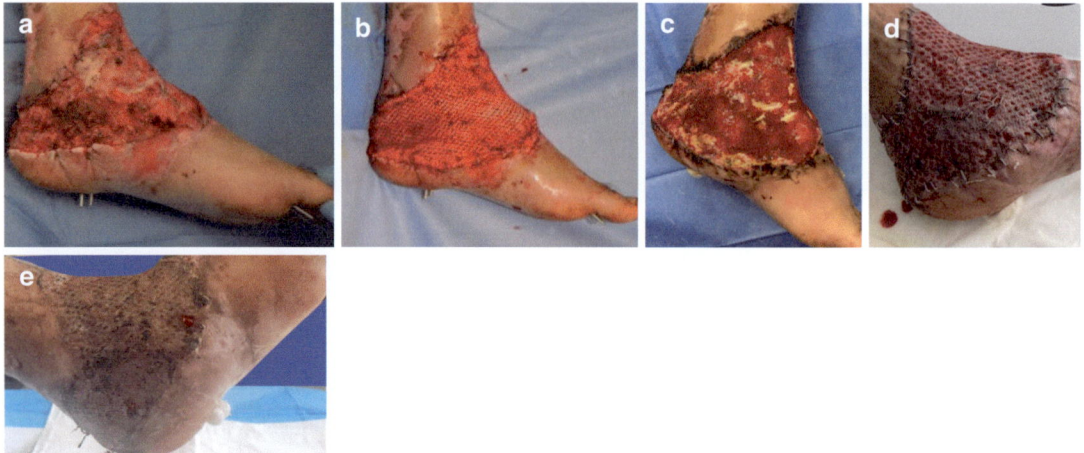

Fig. 52.5 Post-traumatic skin necrosis of the heel and dorsal foot: (**a**) post-necrosis removal; (**b**) fish-derived matrix positioning; (**c**) after 2 weeks and a new dressing with fish skin; (**d**) 1 week post-skin graft; (**e**) 1-month follow-up

52.3 Conclusion and Take-Home Messages

As briefly described, many are the available opportunities to perform skin reconstruction after skin necrosis, but most of all, many are the possibilities to choose the right dermal matrix in order to customize the treatment matching the right matrix to a specific patient and the specific features of the skin.

References

1. Dai C, Shih S, Khachemoune A. Skin substitutes for acute and chronic wound healing: an updated review. Dermatol Treat. 2020;31(6):639–64.
2. Piaggesi A, Låuchli S, Bassetto F, Biedermann T, Marques A, Najafi B, Palla I, Scarpa C, Seimetz D, Triulzi I, Turchetti G, Vaggelas A. Advanced therapies in wound management: cell and tissue based therapies, physical and bio-physical therapies smart and IT based technologies. J Wound Care. 2018;27(Suppl. 6a):S1–S137. https://doi.org/10.12968/jowc.2018.27.Sup6a.S1.
3. Giovannini UM, Teot L. Long-term follow-up comparison of two different bi-layer dermal substitutes in tissue regeneration: clinical outcomes and histological findings. Int Wound J. 2020;17(5):1545–7. https://doi.org/10.1111/iwj.13381.
4. Dalla Paola L, Cimaglia P, Carone A, Boscarino G, Scavone G. Use of integra dermal regeneration template for limb salvage in diabetic patients with no-option critical limb ischemia. Int J Low Extrem Wounds. 2021;20(2):128–34. https://doi.org/10.1177/1534734620905741.
5. Choughri H, Weigert R, Heron A, Dahmam A, Abi-Chahla ML, Delgove A. Indications and functional outcome of the use of integra® dermal regeneration template for the management of traumatic soft tissue defects on dorsal hand, fingers and thumb. Arch

Orthop Trauma Surg. 2020;140(12):2115–27. https://doi.org/10.1007/s00402-020-03615-z.
6. Gonzalez SR, Wolter KG, Yuen JC. Infectious complications associated with the use of integra: a systematic review of the literature. Plast Reconstr Surg Glob Open. 2020;8(7):e2869. https://doi.org/10.1097/GOX.0000000000002869.
7. Lv Z, Yu L, Wang Q, Jia R, Ding W, Shen Y. The use of dermal regeneration template for treatment of complex wound with bone/tendon exposed at the forearm and hand, a prospective cohort study. Medicine (Baltimore). 2019;98(44):e17726.
8. Yiğitbaş H, Yavuz E, Beken Özdemir E, Onen O, Pençe HH, Meriç S, Çelik A, Çelebi F, Yasti AC, Sapmaz T, Zilan A, Turan M. Our experience with dermal substitute Nevelia® in the treatment of severely burned patients. Ulus Travma Acil Cerrahi Derg. 2019;25(5):520–6. https://doi.org/10.14744/tjtes.2019.24358.
9. De Angelis B, Orlandi F, Morais D'Autilio MFL, Di Segni C, Scioli MG, Orlandi A, Cervelli V, Gentile P. Vasculogenic chronic ulcer: tissue regeneration with an innovative dermal substitute. J Clin Med. 2019;8(4):525. https://doi.org/10.3390/jcm8040525.
10. Bloemen MC, van Leeuwen MC, van Vucht NE, van Zuijlen PP, Middelkoop E. Dermal substitution in acute burns and reconstructive surgery: a 12-year follow-up. Plast Reconstr Surg. 2010;125:1450–9.
11. Maitz J, Wang Y, Fathi A, Ximena Escobar F, Parungao R, van Zuijlen P, Maitz P, Li Z. The effects of cross-linking a collagen-elastin dermal template on scaffold bio-stability and degradation. J Tissue Eng Regen Med. 2020;14(9):1189–200. https://doi.org/10.1002/term.3082.
12. Lisa AVE, Galtelli L, Vinci V, Veronesi A, Cozzaglio L, Cananzi FCM, Sicoli F, Klinger M. Adoption of a newly introduced dermal matrix: preliminary experience and future directions. Biomed Res Int. 2020;2020:3261318.
13. Lv Z, Wang Q, Jia R, Ding W, Shen Y. Pelnac® Artificial dermis assisted by VSD for treatment of complex wound with bone/tendon exposed at the foot and ankle, a prospective study. J Invest Surg. 2020;33(7):636–41. https://doi.org/10.1080/08941939.2018.1536177.
14. Kotronoulas A, Jónasdóttir HS, Sigurðardóttir RS, Halldórsson S, Haraldsson GG, Rolfsson Ó. Wound healing grafts: Omega-3 fatty acid lipid content differentiates the lipid profiles of acellular Atlantic cod skin from traditional dermal substitutes. J Tissue Eng Regen Med. 2020;14(3):441–51. https://doi.org/10.1002/term.3005.
15. Alam K, Jeffery SLA. Acellular fish skin grafts for management of split thickness donor sites and partial thickness burns: a case series. Mil Med. 2019;184(Suppl. 1):16–20. https://doi.org/10.1093/milmed/usy280.
16. Michael S, Winters C, Khan M. Acellular fish skin graft use for diabetic lower extremity wound healing: a retrospective study of 58 ulcerations and a literature review. Wounds. 2019;31(10):262–8.

Open Access This chapter is licensed under the terms of the Creative Commons Attribution-NonCommercial-NoDerivatives 4.0 International License (http://creativecommons.org/licenses/by-nc-nd/4.0/), which permits any non-commercial use, sharing, distribution and reproduction in any medium or format, as long as you give appropriate credit to the original author(s) and the source, provide a link to the Creative Commons license and indicate if you modified the licensed material. You do not have permission under this license to share adapted material derived from this chapter or parts of it.

The images or other third party material in this chapter are included in the chapter's Creative Commons license, unless indicated otherwise in a credit line to the material. If material is not included in the chapter's Creative Commons license and your intended use is not permitted by statutory regulation or exceeds the permitted use, you will need to obtain permission directly from the copyright holder.

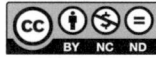

Skin Necrosis of the Diabetic Foot and Its Management

53

J. Karim Ead, Miranda Goransson, and David G. Armstrong

53.1 Introduction

The global prevalence of diabetes mellitus has risen by 16% in the last 2 years (DM) and is expected to continue this trajectory. Indeed, it is estimated to affect 537 million people in 2021, with this figure expected to rise to 643 million by 2030 and 783 million by 2045 [1]. Diabetes is primarily caused by the body's inability to produce or respond to insulin, resulting in carbohydrate metabolic dysfunction [1]. Chronic insulin resistance can raise blood and urine glucose levels [1]. Diabetes patients are more likely to develop other systemic pathologies that can affect the feet, eyes, skin, kidneys, and cardiovascular systems. Because of the harmful nature of this disease process, it is a major risk factor for atherosclerotic disease. Peripheral artery disease (PAD) is a type of occlusive disease that typically affects the lower extremities. PAD is now thought to affect approximately 12 million people in the United States. Patients with PAD are more likely to have lower extremity amputations, and it can be an early warning sign of other harmful cardiovascular pathologies. Most of these amputations begin with diabetic foot ulcers [2]. A patient with a diabetic foot ulcer has a 2.5 times higher risk of death at 5 years than a patient with diabetes who does not have a foot ulcer. Infection occurs in more than half of diabetic ulcers. Approximately 20% of moderate or severe diabetic foot infections result in amputation. Peripheral artery disease raises the risk of nonhealing ulcers, infection, and amputation on its own [3].

Hyperglycemia is derived from the Greek word hyper (high [4]) + glykys (sweet/sugar) + haima (blood). Hyperglycemia is the physiologic state of blood glucose greater than 125 mg/dL while fasting and greater than 180 mg/dL 2 h postprandial [4]. A patient has impaired glucose tolerance, or considered "prediabetes," with a fasting plasma glucose of 100–125 mg/dL. Hyperglycemia has the potential to cause several systemic life-threatening complications that include damage to the eye, kidneys, nerves, heart, and peripheral vascular system [4]. Hence, it is vital for patients with diabetes to manage hyperglycemia effectively and efficiently to prevent complications of the disease and improve patient outcomes.

J. K. Ead (✉)
Podiatric Medicine & Surgery, CHRISTUS Health, Alexandria, LA, USA

M. Goransson
Podiatric Medicine & Surgery, HCA Florida: Westside Hospital, Plantation, FL, USA

D. G. Armstrong
Keck School of Medicine, Los Angeles, CA, USA

53.2 The Biochemical Consequences of Hyperglycemia

Between 30% and 70% of patients with diabetes mellitus, both type 1 and type 2, will present with a cutaneous complication of diabetes mellitus at some point during their lifetime. Hyperglycemia is an inflammatory condition that causes sensory and motor nerve defects, which blunt the perception of adverse stimuli and produce an altered gait. Peripheral neuropathy, vascular disease, and metabolic dysfunction all play a key role in diabetic tissue necrosis (Fig. 53.1). Altered lower extremity biomechanics can increase the likelihood of developing foot ulcers and other osseous malformations. DM causes a pathogenic environment, which induces abnormal cellular responses to infection, immunological and microvascular dysfunction, and peripheral neuropathy. These dynamic processes are implicated in the pathogenesis of the wound healing impairment and the diabetic foot ulcer. The skin houses a dense network of sensory nerve afferents and nerve-derived modulators, which communicate with epidermal keratinocytes and dermal fibroblasts bidirectionally to effect normal wound healing after trauma. Damage to autonomic nerve fibers causes a reduction in tissue hydration (sweat), which may leave skin in the lower extremity dehydrated and prone to fissures and secondary infection [5]. As the disease progresses, hyperglycemia injures target cells through multiple pathways, including the effects of aldose reductase, advanced glycation end products, polyol accumulation, oxidative stress, protein kinase C isoforms, growth factors, and atherosclerosis.

Hyperglycemia causes tissue damage and oxidative stress through four major mechanisms (Fig. 53.2):

- Increased flux of glucose and other sugars through the polyol pathway [6]:
  - Aldose reductase affinity for glucose to also increase
  - Leads to the increased production of sorbitol

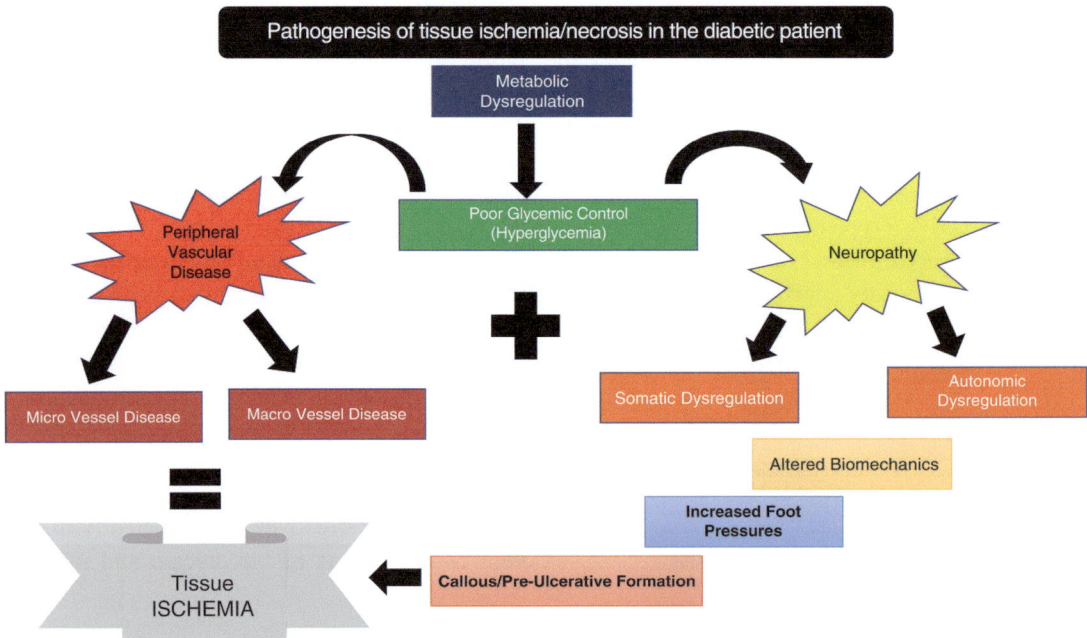

Fig. 53.1 Pathogenesis of diabetic foot related complications as it pertains to ischemia leading to tissue necrosis

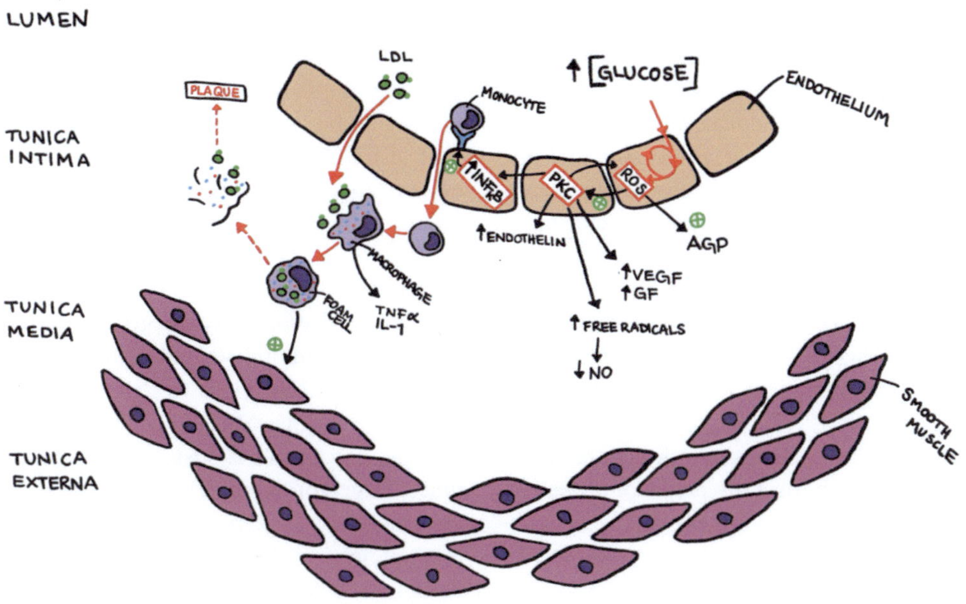

Fig. 53.2 The biochemical response to a hyperglycemic state

- Accumulation of sorbitol reduces the activity of Na+K+-ATPase:
    Reduces the physiological reserve of nerve cells and leads to commensurate reduction of nerve conduction velocity
- Increased intracellular formation of advanced glycation end products (AGEs) [6]:
  - AGEs increase cellular apoptosis
  - Decrease the proliferation of fibroblasts
  - Reduce the activity of growth factors such as fibroblast growth factor
- Activation of protein kinase C (PKC) isoforms [6]:
  - Increases deleterious free radicals:
      Inhibiting the activity of nitric oxide (NO)
      - Leading to damage of the endothelial function
- Overactivity of the hexosamine pathway [6]:
  - Instigates macrophage dysfunction increases and prolongs inflammation

These four pathways cause a biochemical imbalance by increasing the production of inflammatory mediators, pericyte degeneration, thickening basement membrane, endothelial hyperplasia, NO reduction, and impaired vasodilation. The proinflammatory biomarkers include IL-6, TNF-α, D-dimer, and PAI-1 [7]. All of these are in one way or another involved in the development of diabetic microangiopathy [8]. Previous studies have revealed that the cytokines and proteins associated with inflammation (interleukins IL-6 and IL-8; tumor necrosis factor alpha, TNF-α [7]; C-reactive protein; fibrinogen) were significantly elevated in the diabetic patients at baseline [7]. Hyaluronan (HA) plays an important role in the integumentary physiology. HA is a key glycosaminoglycan that facilitates the reepithelialization process [9]. HA is an integral part of the extracellular matrix of basal keratinocytes, which are major constituents of the epidermis which foster keratinocyte proliferation and migration. Hyperglycemia primes the degradation of HA in the glycocalyx of endothelial cells, consequently increasing leukocyte recruitment and creating a proinflammatory microenvironment [10]. Therefore, the thickness of the glycocalyx on blood vessel endothelia is significantly reduced, leading to the loss of protective functions and other deleterious changes [10]. This leads to an imbalance of free radicals and antioxidants in the body, which results in the overproduction of reactive oxygen species (ROS) [6, 11]. Excess ROS can lead to cell and tissue damage and delayed wound healing. Therefore, decreasing ROS levels through antioxidative systems may reduce oxidative stress-induced damage to improve healing [6, 11].

Endothelial cell damage secondary to hyperglycemia induces vascular impairment, consequently decreasing the delivery of oxygen and vital nutrients to organ systems. Additionally, the alteration of the capillary or arteriolar vessel structure also hinders activated white blood cells to specific tissues, increasing the susceptibility, and accelerates the occurrence and progression of diabetic ulcers and infectious/gangrenous processes [6, 11]. A hyperglycemic state causes a decrease in the oxygen, nutrient supply, and vascular impairment resulting in hair alterations like hair thinning, hair fragility, sparseness of hair, or decreased hair growth speed. Some studies have found that lower leg hair loss could be an early predictor of diabetic foot through vascular impairment [12].

53.3 Wound Wars: The Limb Preservation Team Strikes Back!

The development of diabetic foot infections is attributed to several comorbidities that include peripheral neuropathy, PAD, and/or structural deformities of the lower extremity. Additionally, diabetic patients are four times more likely to develop chronic limb-threatening ischemia (CLTI) than patients without diabetes mellitus. Clinicians should consider the possibility of infection occurring in any foot wound in a patient with diabetes. High-risk patients should be assessed for the degree of potential ischemia, but also on the extent and depth of the wound and the presence and severity of infection [13].

Factors that increase the risk for DFI include [13]:

- A wound for which the probe-to-bone (PTB) test is positive
- Ulceration present for >30 days
- A history of recurrent foot ulcers
- A traumatic foot wound
- Presence of peripheral vascular disease in the affected limb
- Previous lower extremity amputation
- Loss of protective sensation
- Presence of renal insufficiency
- Poor glycemic management

The Society of Vascular Surgery (SVS) opined that the current classification systems of diabetic foot ulcers/infection have two major problems: "(1) the validity and natural history of the concept of CLTI and (2) the failure of most existing systems to assess and grade the major factors that influence both risk of limb loss and clinical management" [13]. The proposed SVS Lower Extremity Threatened Limb Classification System is based simply on grading each of the three major factors (wound, ischemia, and foot infection [WIfI]) [13]. Uncontrolled diabetes typically presents with several deleterious factors of which ischemia is just one component of a much larger problem. They devised a dynamic classification system that integrates a global methodology in the stratification of these disease pathologies: wound extent, ischemia, and foot infection [13] (Fig. 53.3). This resulted in a paradigm shift in evaluating the risks of amputation and the potential benefits of vascular intervention [13]. The target population of the WIfI system incorporates patients across a broad spectrum of lower extremity vascular disease etiologies [13]. The main idea behind this new classification system was to help patients categorize their condition in a similar fashion to the TNM (tumor, nodes, metastasis) system commonly utilized in malignancies [9, 13]. Clinicians should then document and classify the severity of the infection based on its extent and depth and the presence of any systemic findings of infection. Grades are

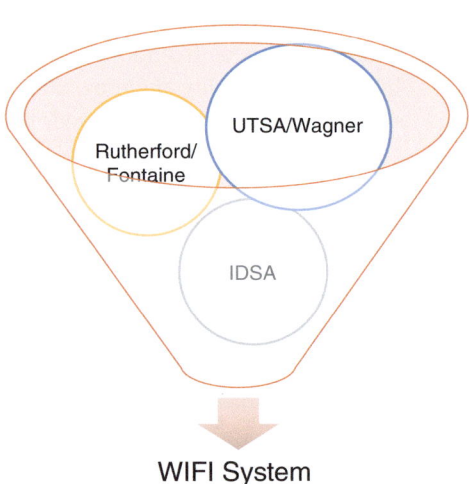

Fig. 53.3 WIFI system

calculated separately by measuring the wound depth; ischemia based on TBI, ABI, and $TcPO_2$; and systemic to local infection from the IDSA guideline [13]. Once the grades are combined and calculated, a risk of amputation is generated [13]. For infected wounds, we recommend that clinicians send appropriately obtained specimens for culture prior to starting empiric antibiotic therapy, if possible [13].

Liu et al. devised the medial arterial calcification (MAC) score, which is a simple metric that describes the potential effects of lower extremity arterial calcification using plain foot radiographs. These scores were conducted by a single-blinded reviewer using two-view minimum plain foot radiographs [14].

Study parameters [14]:

- Each patient was assigned a score from 0 to 5:
  - 1 point given for calcification in each of the following arterial segments:
  - >2 cm in the dorsalis pedis, plantar, and metatarsal arteries
  - >1 cm in the hallux and lesser digital arteries
- A random sampling of plain radiographs from 10% of the cohort was scored by an additional blinded reviewer to assess for interobserver variability.
- The limbs were stratified using the SVS WIfI staging system.

These investigators found that a higher MAC score was significantly associated with the risk of major amputation [14]. These findings have provided evidence for the clinical significance of pedal arterial calcifications, an incidental finding frequently observed when foot radiographs are obtained to evaluate the severity of wounds and infection in patients with CLTI [14]. The ability to prognosticate the risk of limb loss is paramount in the care of patient with CLTI, because it guides the decision-making process for patient counseling and potential immediate and future interventions [14].

In order to effectively treat the assortment of complications that pertains to the diabetic foot, a transdisciplinary approach is critical in order to optimize patient outcomes. Limb preservation programs consist of interdisciplinary teams that work synergistically to exchange information, discuss assessment, and create joint plans to achieve the goal of limb salvage in an integrated model. This model often incorporates podiatric and vascular surgeons ("toe and flow" model) as the core of an interdisciplinary team but which may include other medical specialties as well.

A holistic limb preservation program needs four key elements:

- Hot foot line:
  - In the acute setting, diabetic foot complications presenting to the emergency room or on the inpatient wards should be reported to a single "hot foot line."
  - Once initiated, the limb preservation team will promptly assess the patient and internally triage the patient.
- Access to a wound-healing clinic:
  - The primary focus of the clinic is to determine the etiology of the lower extremity wound and implement evidence-based modalities to accelerate wound closure, moving patients into remission.
- Remission clinic:
  - Studies have demonstrated that recurrence rates of foot ulcerations are noted to be 40% at 1 year, nearly 66% at 2 years, and 75% at 5 years, focus on stopping severe recurrence should replace a focus on preventing every recurrence [1]. Maximizing ulcer-free, hospital-free, and activity-rich days in remission is a primary goal. Individualized patient self-care and monitoring education are a vital function of the remission clinic, along with home-based monitoring program coordination, as they have shown to reduce ulcer recurrence [1].
- Screening clinic:
  - Patients with diabets should be screened according to the updated ADA (American Diabetes Association) Diabetic Foot Risk Assessment guideline protocol. This would include a detailed examination of the lower extremity in regard to the cardiovascular, neurological, dermatological, and musculoskeletal systems.

References

1. Armstrong DG, Boulton AJM, Bus SA. Diabetic foot ulcers and their recurrence. N Engl J Med. 2017;376(24):2367–75. https://doi.org/10.1056/NEJMra1615439.
2. Khan TH, Farooqui FA, Niazi K. Critical review of the anklebrachialindex.CurrCardiolRev.2008;4(2):101–6. https://doi.org/10.2174/157340308784245810.
3. Edmonds M, Manu C, Vas P. The current burden of diabetic foot disease. J Clin Orthop Trauma. 2021;17:88–93. https://doi.org/10.1016/j.jcot.2021.01.017.
4. Mouri M, Badireddy M. Hyperglycemia. In: StatPearls. Treasure Island (FL): StatPearls Publishing; 2021. Available from: https://www.ncbi.nlm.nih.gov/pubmed/28613650.
5. Rosen J, Yosipovitch G. Skin manifestations of diabetes mellitus. In: Feingold KR, Anawalt B, Boyce A, Chrousos G, de Herder WW, Dhatariya K, et al., editors. Endotext. South Dartmouth (MA): MDText.com, Inc.; 2018. Available from: https://www.ncbi.nlm.nih.gov/pubmed/29465926.
6. Azevedo RA, Carvalho HF, de Brito-Gitirana L. Hyaluronan in the epidermal and the dermal extracellular matrix: its role in cutaneous hydric balance and integrity of anuran integument. Micron. 2007;38(6):607–10. https://doi.org/10.1016/j.micron.2006.09.008.
7. Shakya S, Wang Y, Mack JA, Maytin EV. Hyperglycemia-induced changes in hyaluronan contribute to impaired skin wound healing in diabetes: review and perspective. Int J Cell Biol. 2015;2015:701738. https://doi.org/10.1155/2015/701738.
8. Deng L, Du C, Song P, Chen T, Rui S, Armstrong DG, et al. The role of oxidative stress and antioxidants in diabetic wound healing. Oxid Med Cell Longev. 2021;2021:8852759. https://doi.org/10.1155/2021/8852759.
9. Cano Sanchez M, Lancel S, Boulanger E, Neviere R. Targeting oxidative stress and mitochondrial dysfunction in the treatment of impaired wound healing: a systematic review. Antioxidants (Basel). 2018;7(8) https://doi.org/10.3390/antiox7080098.
10. Miranda JJ, Taype-Rondan A, Tapia JC, Gastanadui-Gonzalez MG, Roman-Carpio R. Hair follicle characteristics as early marker of type 2 diabetes. Med Hypotheses. 2016;95:39–44. https://doi.org/10.1016/j.mehy.2016.08.009.
11. Nowak NC, Menichella DM, Miller R, Paller AS. Cutaneous innervation in impaired diabetic wound healing. Transl Res. 2021;236:87–108. https://doi.org/10.1016/j.trsl.2021.05.003.
12. Mills JL Sr, Conte MS, Armstrong DG, Pomposelli FB, Schanzer A, Sidawy AN, et al. The society for vascular surgery lower extremity threatened limb classification system: risk stratification based on wound, ischemia, and foot infection (WIfI). 50 Landmark Papers Every Vascular and Endovascular Surgeon Should Know. 2020, p. 43. Available from: https://books.google.com/books?hl=en&lr=&id=bp3yDwAAQBAJ&oi=fnd&pg=PT217&dq=Mills+JL+Sr+Conte+MS+Armstrong+DG+The+Society+for+Vascular+Surgery+Lower+Extremity+Threatened+Limb+Classification+System+risk+stratification+based+on+Wound+Ischemia+and+foot+Infection+(WIfI)+J+Vasc+Surg+2014+59+220-34+e1&ots=fxB6NPl2b-&sig=R2vVFxdLszZTYJCAMlD93polKxY.
13. Lipsky BA, Berendt AR, Cornia PB, Pile JC, Peters EJG, Armstrong DG, et al. 2012 Infectious Diseases Society of America clinical practice guideline for the diagnosis and treatment of diabetic foot infections. Clin Infect Dis. 2012;54(12):e132–73. https://doi.org/10.1093/cid/cis346.
14. Khan T, Shin L, Woelfel S, Rowe V, Wilson BL, Armstrong DG. Building a scalable diabetic limb preservation program: four steps to success. Diabet Foot Ankle. 2018;9(1):1452513. https://doi.org/10.1080/2000625X.2018.1452513.

Open Access This chapter is licensed under the terms of the Creative Commons Attribution-NonCommercial-NoDerivatives 4.0 International License (http://creativecommons.org/licenses/by-nc-nd/4.0/), which permits any non-commercial use, sharing, distribution and reproduction in any medium or format, as long as you give appropriate credit to the original author(s) and the source, provide a link to the Creative Commons license and indicate if you modified the licensed material. You do not have permission under this license to share adapted material derived from this chapter or parts of it.

The images or other third party material in this chapter are included in the chapter's Creative Commons license, unless indicated otherwise in a credit line to the material. If material is not included in the chapter's Creative Commons license and your intended use is not permitted by statutory regulation or exceeds the permitted use, you will need to obtain permission directly from the copyright holder.

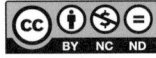

Skin Necrosis of Diabetic Foot and Its Management

Joon Pio Hong

54.1 Introduction

The chapter describes the statistics related to diabetic foot ulceration, pathology of necrosis formation, types of necrosis, and current surgical management of diabetic foot skin necrosis.

According to the statistics given in the USA, approximately 3–4% of individuals with diabetes currently have foot ulcers or deep infections and 25% will develop foot ulcers sometime during their life [1, 2]. Their risk of lower leg amputation increases by a factor of 8 once an ulcer develops. It is estimated that the age-adjusted rate of lower extremity amputation in diabetic patients is 15-fold that of nondiabetics [3]. Intractable diabetic foot ulcers can bring not only decreased physical, emotional, and social functions but also huge economic impact to the patient [4–6]. Furthermore, the 5-year mortality after major amputations may range from 39% to as high as 80% [1, 7]. The necrosis is often seen in the late stages of the diabetic foot. The presence of skin necrosis is a serious implication leading to the loss of limb. Their respective indications vary depending essentially on criteria like the hardness of the black cover, the extent of necrosis in depth, and the extent of necrotic tissue over the skin.

J. P. Hong (✉)
Department of Plastic Surgery, Asan Medical Center, Univeristy of Ulsan, Seoul, South Korea
e-mail: joonphong@amc.seoul.kr

In neuropathic foot, infection is usually the cause, whereas it can be solely due to ischemia alone with slow onset of mummification like dry necrosis.

54.2 Risk Factors for Diabetic Foot Skin Necrosis

Risk factors involved for ulceration are peripheral neuropathy, vascular disease, limited joint mobility, foot deformities, abnormal foot pressures, minor trauma, history of ulceration or amputation, and impaired visual acuity [8]. Superimposed infection in neuropathic or neuroischemic types will lead to wet necrosis, whereas occlusion of arteries will lead to dry necrosis. The dry necrosis frequently coincides with the angiosome territory of the macrovascular supply [9].

54.3 Clinical Presentation

54.3.1 Detecting Early Change

Early signs of necrosis may begin with sudden change in color of the skin. Previously pink skin may change to a blue or purple color when hit by infection. Skin turning from pink to pale white may be from lack of circulation. Sudden change of ulcer character may also imply potential change to dry or wet ischemia. A close fol-

54.3.2 Wet Necrosis

Wet necrosis is due to severe infection and ulceration. This is the most frequently seen necrosis of the diabetic foot. Untreated infections and recent traumatic wounds may lead to necrosis. One must stay alert during the follow-up for patients especially being treated with immunosuppressive drugs after kidney transplants. Clinical characteristics suggesting serious infection may be ulcers penetrating to subcutaneous tissues, involvement of deep tissues, extensive cellulitis expanding more than 2 cm from ulceration, and local signs such as severe inflammation, crepitus, bullae, swelling, discoloration, and necrosis [10]. Deep tissue specimens should be sent to identify pathogen. Patients should be hospitalized for possible surgical intervention, fluid resuscitation, treatment with antibiotics, and control of diabetes (Fig. 54.1).

54.3.3 Dry Necrosis

Dry necrosis is a black, hard, mummified tissue often with clear demarcation from the surrounding tissue. It may have infection but usually is from severe ischemia resulting from vasculopathy. In cases where peripheral artery disease progresses slowly among ischemic-neuropathic diabetic foot patients, it gradually develops vascular compromise of the skin, and thus perception of ischemic pain is reduced [11]. The result is that the prevalence of claudication in the diabetic population with PAD is lower than the prevalence of critical limb ischemia (CLI) in this population. Thus, eye inspection becomes a very important tool to diagnose the dry necrotic change among this group.

In diabetic patients with acute ischemia, sudden onset of pain is noted with pallor and coldness of the foot followed by mottling of the skin and shiny appearance of the texture.

Regardless of the duration of the peripheral artery disease, intervention of the artery is required to reperfuse the ischemic skin. Failure to reperfuse the foot will end in dry necrosis and loss of the tissue. Intervention angioplasty or bypass surgery should be applied accordingly to ensure better outcome after removal of dry necrotic skin [12]. Otherwise, further complication and increase in necrosis may occur in resection without vascular intervention. One must also be aware of the reperfusion injury after intervention. Once reperfused, inflammation will ensue and the wound around the dry necrosis will turn wet and increase the risk for infection. Debridement must follow reperfusion (Fig. 54.2).

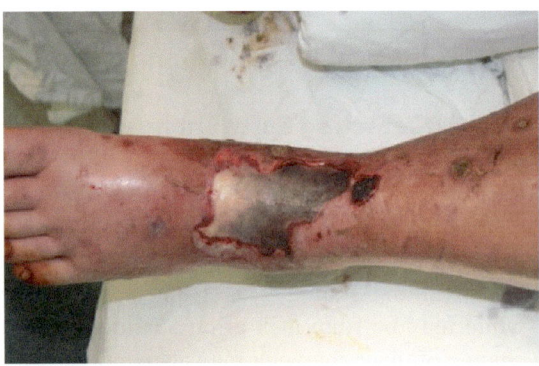 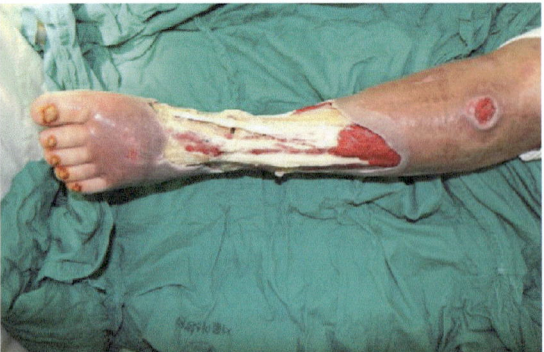

Fig. 54.1 Patient with wet necrosis extending to the deep fascia tissue, and debridement was performed. Note the extent of necrosis after the debridement of all necrotic tissue

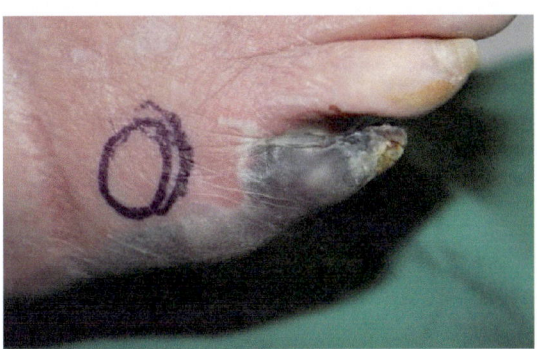

Fig. 54.2 Dry necrosis with relatively well-demarcated wound

54.4 Treatment and Reconstruction

When considering the diabetic foot for reconstruction, there are multiple issues to be addressed. These issues can be effectively approached though a multidisciplinary approach [13]. The first step is to control the systemic aspect of diabetes. Then malnutrition, chronic renal disease, and hypertension have to be addressed properly and treatment schedules made before and after surgery especially hemodialysis and perioperative blood sugar control. While the systemic condition of the patient is being optimized, specific attention can be directed to the foot ulcer. Depending upon the general condition; peripheral vascular status; bone pathology; wound depth, location, and duration; involvement of chronic osteomyelitis; and patient motivation, wounds can be treated with debridement and other related surgical procedures. Another important issue concerns the vascular pathology of the patient. The vascular surgery consultation is warranted when the patient is symptomatic with ischemic pain or a nonhealing ulcer. Neuropathic ulcers require debridement of nonviable or infected tissue, combined with local wound care and off-loading. If the diabetic wound is not improved by such procedures or aggressive wound care, foot salvage procedures can be considered. A robust predictor of healing is 53% change in the wound area of diabetic foot ulcers [14]. In our center, we monitor the change in wound size and depth, and when wound healing is stalled despite good standard of care such as off-loading, infection control, edema control, and advanced dressings, then additional treatment with hyperbaric oxygen, cell therapy, growth factor treatment, and negative-pressure wound therapy is considered. But depending on the complexity of the wound, some of these secondary modalities are used primarily as well. Again, wound healing progress is closely monitored, and stalled healing despite these multimodal therapies may become one of the indicators for reconstruction. Figure 54.3 shows the spectrum of care for diabetic foot ulcers from general care to reconstruction or amputation.

54.4.1 Debridement

The first step of treatment for diabetic foot wound is to evaluate, debride, and treat infection [9]. Missing timely management will lead to amputations and longer hospital days [15]. If symptoms and signs of infection are clinically suspected, proper treatment must be provided without delay. If superficial infection is suspected without systemic infection, antibiotic treatment along with non-weight-bearing of the foot should be ensued. Optimal management of diabetic foot infection can potentially reduce incidence of major limb amputations and other related morbidities. All nonviable and infected soft tissue and bone should be excised during debridement. Milking along the proximal tendon can be helpful to identify and limit ascending infection. Tissue culture should be sent. Sufficient irrigation should follow after debridement to reduce bacterial count [16]. Recent advance in technology introduced a hydrosurgery system that allows to debride while preserving viable tissues and irrigate simultaneously, allowing reduced surgical time [17, 18]. Biodebridement such as maggot therapy has also been useful in clearing the necrotic tissue [19]. Application of negative-pressure wound therapy has also played a role in reconstruction as they are used as an indicator and a wound preparation method of achieving clean wound with reasonable vascularity.

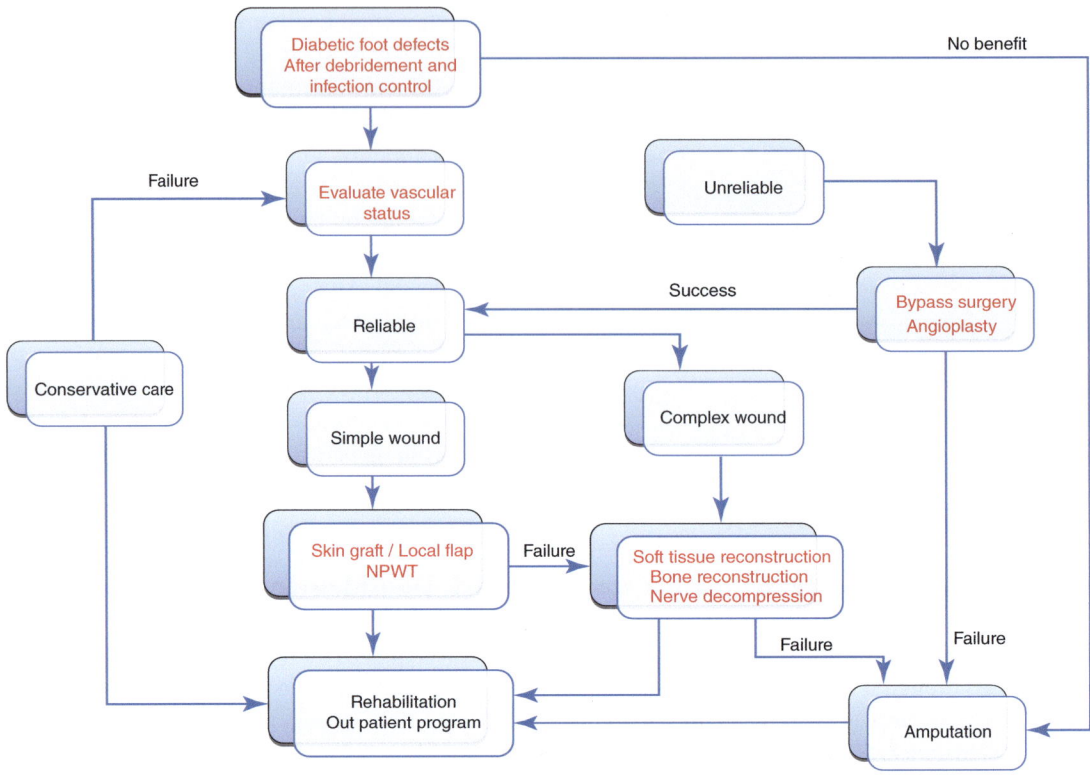

Fig. 54.3 Algorithm for diabetic foot reconstruction after debridement of necrotic diabetic wound

The understanding of vascular distribution of the foot, angiosome, helps to plan not only reconstruction but also debridement [20]. When planning for reconstruction, one can avoid violating the angiosome territory when designing a local flap that may lead to flap breakdown [21]. Also by performing debridement according to the angiosome territory, one may enhance flap survival by increasing the chance for marginal vascularization from healthy surrounding angiosome territory.

Repetitive debridement should be performed as part of wound preparation for reconstruction while monitoring C-reactive protein for possible hidden infections and using it as an index for possible infection after reconstruction.

54.4.2 Vascular Intervention

In our surgical algorithm, all patients considered for microsurgical reconstruction undergo a non-invasive CT angiogram to evaluate the vascular status. The CT angiogram provides information regarding general vascular anatomy of the lower extremity and shows atherosclerotic change of vessels, which is useful information when choosing recipient vessels. The overview is important as collateral vessels may be the main trunk to the distal limb. Without this information, one may elevate the flap harvesting the main arterial source to the distal limb and cause limb ischemia. If vascular status is in doubt, then revascularization by angioplasty or bypass surgery is referred. Although preoperative angiograms may indicate intact anatomy of the artery to the foot, actual findings upon surgery can be different. In order to confirm the distal vascular flow, we use ultrasound duplex scans. A study by Kim et al. showed correlation of peak blood flow velocity over 40 cm/s to flap survival [22]. However, in an ongoing study at our center, we hypothesized that the preoperative measurement of flow will not influence the survival of the flap, but the perioperative flow will play a more important factor. For now, ultrasound duplex scan provides information in the selection of recipient vessels or can be used to refer for vascular intervention when no recipient vessels can be identified. The transcutaneous oxygen measurement (TcPO2) also plays a role in our protocol. Measurement over 30 mmHg in normobaric oxygen is a relative predictive factor for successful healing, whereas pressure less than that of 30 mmHg is likely to follow an unfavorable course [23, 24]. The wound, if measured under this level after vascular intervention, was treated with hyperbaric oxygen. If peri-wound $TcPO_2$ measurements were over 30 mmHg, then further treatment including reconstructive procedures was planned; otherwise, amputations at according levels were performed. The ankle-brachial index (ABI) is not used as it is not reliable in diabetic patients due to the high incidence of calcified vessels causing falsely elevated values [25].

In diabetic patients, the most significant atherosclerosis occurs in the crural arteries often sparing the arteries of the foot [26]. Bypass to the dorsalis pedis or posterior tibial artery of the foot or angioplasty with or without stent placement procedures results in high success to restore perfusion pressure to the distal circulation of the foot reestablishing palpable pulse. The timing of when to perform reconstruction after vascular intervention is not clear. Reports have shown successful free flap transfer with simultaneous vascular reconstruction to salvage the limb [27]. But early bypass failures within 30 days are reported to be high [28, 29]. In our experience, partial flap loss or total loss was suddenly noted after 2–3 weeks in the cases combined with simultaneous or reconstruction following few days after vascular interventions. This may suggest that there should be a sufficient stabilization period after vascular intervention.

Reperfusion is most essential prior to microsurgery reconstruction. If vascular intervention fails and wound progresses, amputation is warranted.

54.4.3 Reconstruction Using Free Flaps

Once an adequate debridement and reasonable vascular perfusion are achieved, in extensive and complex diabetic foot defects, reconstruction should be considered. In my experience, local flaps such as reverse sural, medial plantar, or lateral supramalleolar for large defects have not been as successful as free flap reconstruction. Especially when reconstructing diabetic foot with reduced vascular flow, the utilization of local flaps may breach the distal flow of the small collateral vessels. One must consider current vascular status as well as future flow where small collateral vessels may play an important role for distal circulation. In this sense, my choice for moderate and large defects is the reconstructive microsurgery to transfer free flaps. Inclusion criteria from a meta-analysis of free tissue transfer in 528 diabetic patients in 18 studies suggest (1) lower limb defect which has not displayed any signs of granulation or healing despite adequate debridement or necrotic tissue and conservative treatment, (2) no significant renal function impairment, (3) no significant systemic illness likely to be exacerbated by multiple operations and prolonged rehabilitation, (4) previously ambulatory with the aim to restore a functional limb, (5) likely to engage with the significant physiotherapy required for return to normal living, and (6) peak flow velocity of >40 cm/s in the recipient artery. We generally agree with the suggested inclusion criteria except for the significant renal disease. In our experience, we have not found an increased risk for failure despite the fact that uremia may cause a decrease in cell-mediated immunity and impair wound healing [30–32]. But we did report a significant risk of 4.857 times higher odds for flap failure in patients using immunosuppressive agents after renal transplant ($p < 0.041$) [31]. Another progress we have made recently was introducing the concept of supermicrosurgery to diabetic foot reconstruction [33–36]. This is especially useful in reconstructing diabetic foot with poor perfusion. This concept utilized small vessels as recipients for flaps where the blood supply is from the newly formed collateral vessels instead of major axial arteries, which are frequently calcified with lack of flow [13, 37]. This approach salvages even in the ischemic diabetic foot with dry eschar.

I would rather prefer to present the contraindication rather than the indications for flap reconstruction as microsurgery technique evolves using small recipient vessels rather than major vessels for reconstruction [38]. The most important factor may be the perfusion of the recipient vessel. If any small vessel is seen with good pulsatile flow, it would be indicated for microsurgery. Thus, an absolute contraindication would be no flow to the foot without any sign of perfusion from any distal small vessels [31]. This supermicrosurgery and freestyle reconstruction approach, however, will require a refined skill along with a paradigm shift for reconstruction (Figs. 54.4, 54.5, 54.6, 54.7, and 54.8).

It is important to take into consideration the long-term follow-up for patients who undergo reconstruction. One of the biggest challenges is seen when reconstructing the plantar surface. However, one must remember the actual cause of the necrosis itself, which often starts with an imbalance in the mechanics of the musculoskel-

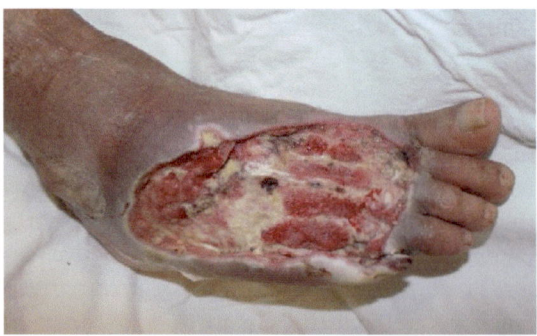

Fig. 54.5 Complete debridement with respect to angiosome territory. The patient then underwent NPWT (CuraVAC®, Daewoong Pharmaceuticals, Seoul, Korea) for 10 days to prepare the wound for microsurgical reconstruction

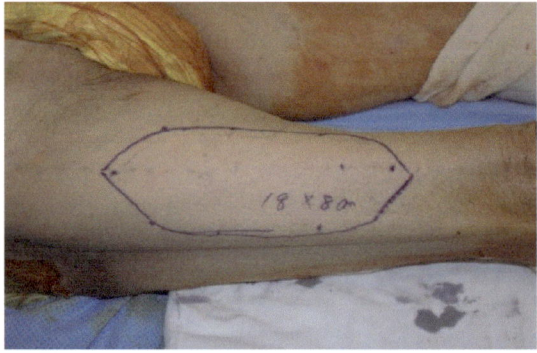

Fig. 54.6 Anterolateral thigh flap was used to reconstruct the feet

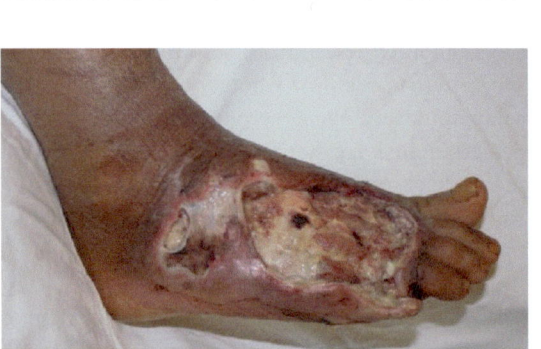

Fig. 54.4 Necrotic diabetic foot with neuroischemic wound. Poor vascular supply of the anterior tibial artery was noted. Endovascular intervention was performed successfully increasing the flow to the feet

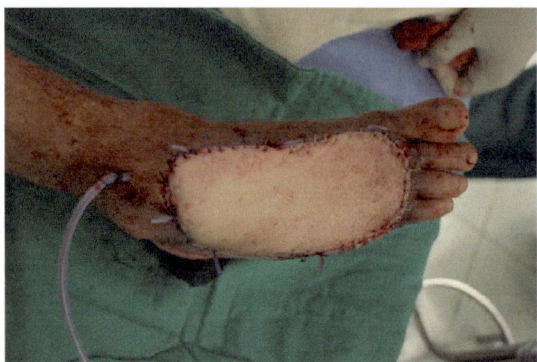

Fig. 54.7 The anterolateral thigh flap artery was anastomosed to the dorsalis pedis end-to-side fashion

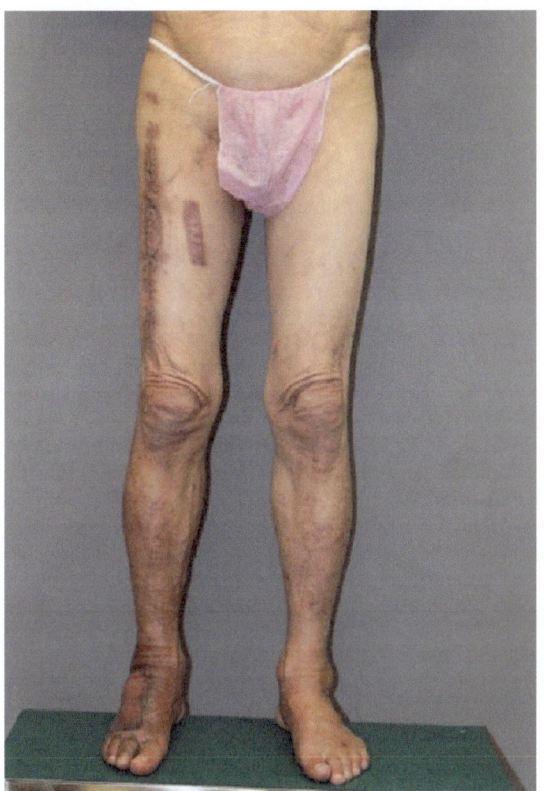

Fig. 54.8 The patient at a 2-year follow-up shows good contour and function of the foot without signs of recurrence

etal structure of the foot. Without addressing the issue for mechanical imbalance, the newly reconstructed soft tissue will not last long and will break down. Thus, one must approach reconstruction with the idea of orthoplastic approach. When reconstruction is done properly, the long-term soft tissue change will actually show better perfusion as the flap settles in the ischemic foot and generally provides long-lasting resurfacing of the foot [39].

References

1. Reiber GE. The epidemiology of diabetic foot problems. Diabet Med. 1996;13(Suppl 1):S6–11.
2. Singh N, Armstrong DG, et al. Preventing foot ulcers in patients with diabetes. JAMA. 2005;293(2):217–28.
3. Most RS, Sinnock P. The epidemiology of lower extremity amputations in diabetic individuals. Diabetes Care. 1983;6(1):87–91.
4. Apelqvist J, Ragnarson-Tennvall G, et al. Long-term costs for foot ulcers in diabetic patients in a multidisciplinary setting. Foot Ankle Int. 1995;16(7):388–94.
5. Reiber GE, Lipsky BA, et al. The burden of diabetic foot ulcers. Am J Surg. 1998;176(2A Suppl):5S–10.
6. Saar WE, Lee TH, et al. The economic burden of diabetic foot and ankle disorders. Foot Ankle Int. 2005;26(1):27–31.
7. Moulik PK, Mtonga R, et al. Amputation and mortality in new-onset diabetic foot ulcers stratified by etiology. Diabetes Care. 2003;26(2):491–4.
8. Frykberg RG, Zgonis T, et al. Diabetic foot disorders. A clinical practice guideline (2006 revision). J Foot Ankle Surg. 2006;45(5 Suppl):S1–66.
9. Attinger CE, Bulan EJ. Debridement. The key initial first step in wound healing. Foot Ankle Clin. 2001;6(4):627–60.
10. Lipsky BA. A report from the international consensus on diagnosing and treating the infected diabetic foot. Diabetes Metab Res Rev. 2004;20(Suppl 1):S68–77.
11. Faglia E. Characteristics of peripheral arterial disease and its relevance to the diabetic population. Int J Low Extrem Wounds. 2011;10(3):152–66.
12. Conte MS. Diabetic revascularization: endovascular versus open bypass—do we have the answer? Semin Vasc Surg. 2012;25(2):108–14.
13. Suh HP, Park CJ, Hong JP. Special considerations for diabetic foot reconstruction. J Reconstr Microsurg. 2021;37(1):12–6.
14. Sheehan P, Jones P, et al. Percent change in wound area of diabetic foot ulcers over a 4-week period is a robust predictor of complete healing in a 12-week prospective trial. Plast Reconstr Surg. 2006;117(7 Suppl):239S–44.
15. Reiber GE, Vileikyte L, et al. Causal pathways for incident lower-extremity ulcers in patients with diabetes from two settings. Diabetes Care. 1999;22(1):157–62.
16. Badia JM, Torres JM, et al. Saline wound irrigation reduces the postoperative infection rate in Guinea pigs. J Surg Res. 1996;63(2):457–9.
17. Granick M, Boykin J, et al. Toward a common language: surgical wound bed preparation and debridement. Wound Repair Regen. 2006;14(Suppl 1):S1–10.
18. Granick MS, Posnett J, et al. Efficacy and cost-effectiveness of a high-powered parallel water-jet for wound debridement. Wound Repair Regen. 2006;14(4):394–7.
19. Edwards J, Stapley S. Debridement of diabetic foot ulcers. Cochrane Database Syst Rev. 2010;1:CD003556.
20. Clemens MW, Attinger CE. Angiosomes and wound care in the diabetic foot. Foot Ankle Clin. 2010;15(3):439–64.
21. Attinger C, Cooper P, et al. The safest surgical incisions and amputations applying the angiosome principles and using the Doppler to assess the arterial-arterial connections of the foot and ankle. Foot Ankle Clin. 2001;6(4):745–99.

22. Kim JY, Lee YJ. A study of the survival factors of free flap in older diabetic patients. J Reconstr Microsurg. 2007;23(7):373–80.
23. Christensen KS, Klarke M. Transcutaneous oxygen measurement in peripheral occlusive disease. An indicator of wound healing in leg amputation. J Bone Joint Surg Br. 1986;68(3):423–6.
24. Got I. Transcutaneous oxygen pressure (TcPO2): advantages and limitations. Diabetes Metab. 1998;24(4):379–84.
25. Goss DE, de Trafford J, et al. Raised ankle/brachial pressure index in insulin-treated diabetic patients. Diabet Med. 1989;6(7):576–8.
26. Strandness DE Jr, Priest RE, et al. Combined clinical and pathologic study of diabetic and nondiabetic peripheral arterial disease. Diabetes. 1964;13:366–72.
27. Randon C, Jacobs B, et al. A 15-year experience with combined vascular reconstruction and free flap transfer for limb-salvage. Eur J Vasc Endovasc Surg. 2009;38(3):338–45.
28. Bush HL Jr, Nabseth DC, et al. In situ saphenous vein bypass grafts for limb salvage. A current fad or a viable alternative to reversed vein bypass grafts? Am J Surg. 1985;149(4):477–80.
29. Shenaq SM, Dinh TA. Foot salvage in arteriolosclerotic and diabetic patients by free flaps after vascular bypass: report of two cases. Microsurgery. 1989;10(4):310–4.
30. Berman SJ. Infections in patients with end-stage renal disease. An overview. Infect Dis Clin N Am. 2001;15(3):709–20. vii
31. Oh TS, Lee HS, et al. Diabetic foot reconstruction using free flaps increases 5-year-survival rate. J Plast Reconstr Aesthet Surg. 2013;66(2):243–50.
32. Yue DK, McLennan S, et al. Effects of experimental diabetes, uremia, and malnutrition on wound healing. Diabetes. 1987;36(3):295–9.
33. Suh HS, Oh TS, Hong JP. Innovations in diabetic foot reconstruction using supermicrosurgery. Diabetes Metab Res Rev. 2016;32(Suppl 1):275–80.
34. Suh HS, Oh TS, Lee HS, Lee SH, Cho YP, Park JR, et al. A new approach for reconstruction of diabetic foot wounds using the Angiosome and Supermicrosurgery concept. Plast Reconstr Surg. 2016;138(4):702e–9e.
35. Hong JP, Pak CJ, Suh HP. Supermicrosurgery in lower extremity reconstruction. Clin Plast Surg. 2021;48(2):299–306.
36. Hong JPJ, Song S, Suh HSP. Supermicrosurgery: principles and applications. J Surg Oncol. 2018;118(5):832–9.
37. Suh HP, Kim Y, Suh Y, Hong J. Multidetector computed tomography (CT) analysis of 168 cases in diabetic patients with Total superficial femoral artery occlusion: is it safe to use an anterolateral thigh flap without CT angiography in diabetic patients? J Reconstr Microsurg. 2018;34(1):65–70.
38. Hong JP. The use of supermicrosurgery in lower extremity reconstruction: the next step in evolution. Plast Reconstr Surg. 2009;123(1):230–5.
39. Kwon JG, Cho MJ, Pak CJ, Suh HP, Hong JP. A retrospective case series on free flap reconstruction for ischemic diabetic foot: the nutrient flap further explained. Plast Reconstr Surg. 2022;149(6):1452–61.

Open Access This chapter is licensed under the terms of the Creative Commons Attribution-NonCommercial-NoDerivatives 4.0 International License (http://creativecommons.org/licenses/by-nc-nd/4.0/), which permits any non-commercial use, sharing, distribution and reproduction in any medium or format, as long as you give appropriate credit to the original author(s) and the source, provide a link to the Creative Commons license and indicate if you modified the licensed material. You do not have permission under this license to share adapted material derived from this chapter or parts of it.

The images or other third party material in this chapter are included in the chapter's Creative Commons license, unless indicated otherwise in a credit line to the material. If material is not included in the chapter's Creative Commons license and your intended use is not permitted by statutory regulation or exceeds the permitted use, you will need to obtain permission directly from the copyright holder.

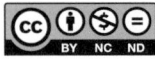

Exposed Necrotic Tendons

55

Luc Téot

55.1 Introduction

Tendon necrosis may be observed in several types of wounds, traumas, or chronic wounds like pressure ulcers, diabetic foot ulcers, or arterial leg ulcers, as a consequence of skin necrosis. The subcutaneous anatomical position of the tendons makes them directly exposed when the skin necroses. The origin of tendon necrosis is multifactorial, exposure to air, desiccation of poorly vascularized structures, and infection being most frequently observed. An appropriate debridement is possible when the deep parts of the tendons remain vascularized enough. A partial loss of depth of the tendon does not severely impact its mechanical resistance and function. Wound bed preparation using negative pressure wound therapy is necessary to enhance the tendon embedding into granulation tissue. Coverage can be done using dermal substitutes followed by split thickness skin grafts, a guarantee for tendon gliding recovery. Flaps are sometimes preferred but more invasive and needing secondary procedures. Direct skin grafting being not recommended as leading to secondary tendinous adherences. Immobilization of the tendon is the key element to prevent infection to spread along the tendon sheets and develop tunnels. Tendon necrosis should be considered as an emergency in order to preserve the functional results. The introduction of microsurgery and NPWT has drastically modified the capacity to conserve exposed tendinous structures and prevent loss of function.

55.2 Clinical Features: Staging the Living Tendinous Tissue

Three different stages of severity can be observed (Fig. 55.1a–c). The tendon may be simply exposed, and the paratenon becomes necrotic on its exposed aspect, or partially necrotic, or completely destroyed.

Stage 1: The paratenon is exposed and looks inert, dry, more or less hard. A few opening may be observed, giving access to the tendon itself. When properly managed, the paratenon may recover, be revascularized by the surrounding living structures.

Stage 2: The paratenon is lost, and the tendon is directly exposed, some areas presenting a dead fleshy aspect, tendon fibers being easily dissociated. It is not easy to differentiate the still living areas from the dead parts, but the mechanical resistance to dissociation and the tendon fibers consistency and hardness differ (Fig. 55.2). Risks of complete loss of the tendon are important as infection of the exposed tendon may extend under the tendon sheets up and down and develop a large infected pocket. Modern management including negative pressure therapy after a surgi-

L. Téot (✉)
Department of Plastic Surgery, Burns and Wound Healing, Montpellier University Hospital, Hôpital La Colombière, CICAT Occitanie, Montpellier, France
e-mail: l-teot@chu-montpellier.fr

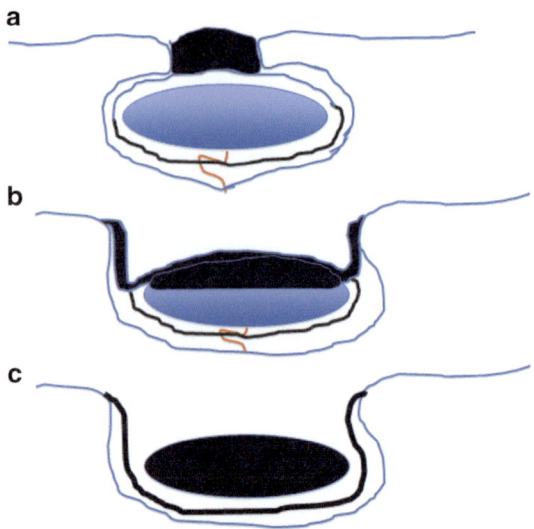

Fig. 55.1 (**a**) The tendon is intact under a necrotic cover. The vascularisation is intact. NPWT may obtain a full coverage by granulation tissue formation. (**b**) The tendon is partially destroyed but the vascularisation is conserved. Excision of the necrotic part, plus NPWT may end to a salvage of the tendon functionality. (**c**) The tendon is completely necrosed, the vascularisation is destroyed. A complete excision is needed

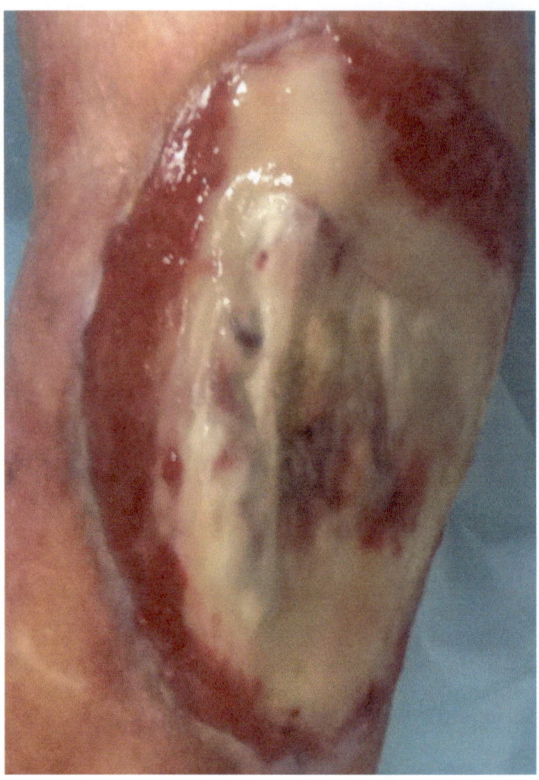

Fig. 55.2 Sloughy tendon. A partial excision is needed, and NPWT Instill may complete the debridement and embed the tendon granulation tissue

cal adapted debridement will enhance the progression of the granulation tissue coming from the edges and the deep part of the wound. The tendon will progressively be incorporated into this granulation tissue, and a coverage technique using either dermal substitute or flap will allow tendon salvage.

Stage 3: Clinically the tendon looks dry, hard, and having lost suppleness. No more connexion with the underlying structures is observed, the tendon lying inert over the wound (Figs. 55.3 and 55.4). Tunnels on each extremity are long, and pus may be present. The tendon should be removed on the whole exposed area including tunnels.

When not managed properly, complications of tendon exposure are multiple, the necrotic extension to the surrounding structure being often observed, infection may progress along the tendon sheath, issuing to secondary at distance infected wounds and complete destruction of the tendon and paratenon.

55 Exposed Necrotic Tendons

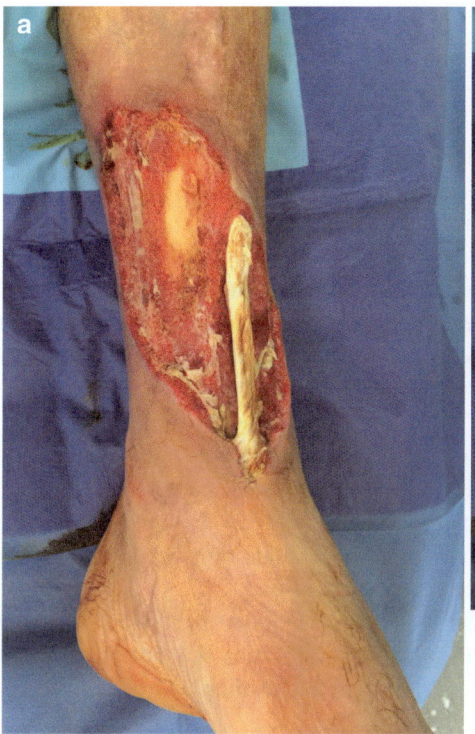
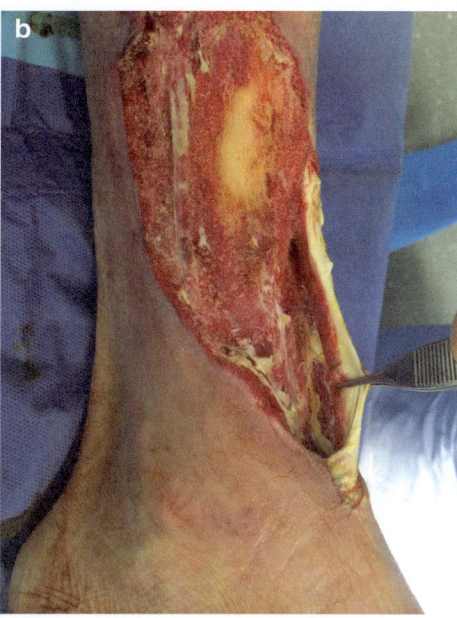

Fig. 55.3 (**a**) The tendon can be detached from the bed. (**b**) The vascularisation remains intact. This tendon is candidate to NPWT in order to embed it into granulation tissue

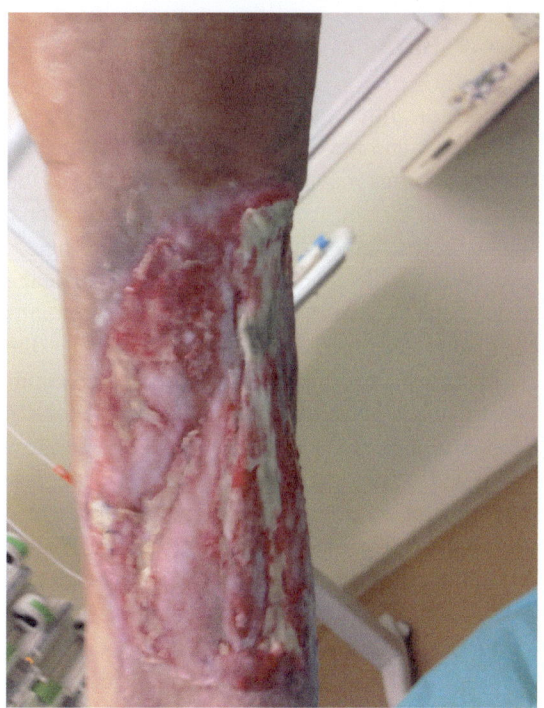

Fig. 55.4 Spontaneous healing of an exposed tendon, with zones of epidermisation and areas ot the tendon destroyed by local infection

55.3 Mode of Treatment

55.3.1 Immobilization

Immobilization is a technique adapted to the involved segment of limb. Tendons being less rigid than bones, a strict tight immobilization is not required. On the other hand, the course of a tendon of the foot being comprised between 2 and 4 cm, it is easy to understand that infection will tend to move with tendon along the sheets and induce secondary infected zones involving the subcutaneous areas and the skin itself. In some situations, most often discovered lately, infection may run along the tendons or aponeurosis of the muscles and emerges as a secondary infection at the other extremity of a segment (seen in ischiatic pressure ulcers with a distal emergence of infection at the level of the knee).

55.3.2 Negative Pressure Wound Therapy

NPWT became a key factor to enhance tendon revascularization and salvage. This technique represents a good alternative to flaps with less morbidity and more chances to save function, as the negative pressure acts as a booster for granulation tissue formation. The tendon is progressively embedded into the granulation tissue, providing a neovascularization and preventing spreading of local infection. In an initial series of 16 patients, Lee et al. [1, 2] reported that NPWT facilitates the rapid formation of healthy granulation tissue on open wounds in the foot and ankle region, and thus, to shorten healing time and minimize secondary soft tissue defect coverage procedures, reducing the need for a free flap to one single case. NPWT was also effective on infected patellar tendon salvage. Hong et al. [3] proposed an algorithm of decisions in soft tissue defects including NPWT.

55.3.3 Artificial Dermis

Several authors recently published clinical results concerning the use of artificial dermis in tendon coverage and more largely in soft tissue defects in upper and lower extremities.

Attinger et al. [4] resume these possibilities as a step by step management of complex wounds with debridement, negative pressure wound therapy, and coverage using dermal substitutes. These techniques are utilized in chronic wounds, acute trauma wounds, and burns [5, 6] with good results. Products used may be double layer dermis, mainly used in USA, covered with a silicone film secondarily skin grafted, contrarily to one stage immediately covered single layers proposed in Europe [7, 8] and Asia [9]. Other dermal substitutes have recently emerged on the market, aiming to the same objective which is to bring suppleness and prevent adherences of skin grafting to the underlying structures.

Dermal substitutes may also be used in upper limbs [10] with good results in terms of mechanical possibilities of recovering skin capacities.

55.3.4 Flaps

Flaps remain adapted to cover a tendon. This technique leads to few adherences, a soft covering allowing tendon to glide underneath with some potential complications, like excess of fat tissue or wrinkling observed when the transferred flap is too deep. Local flaps or regional sural flaps like distally based neurosural flaps [11] can be used, and free flaps being used in large defects or in acute wounds for young patients with adapted vascularization [12].

Flaps are more available in upper arm where many possibilities of local or regional skin flaps are used and available directly or in reverse.

55.4 Causes and Specific Management

55.4.1 Burns

Tendons are often exposed in third-degree burns. Both upper and lower extremities can be touched. Electrical burns may be terribly devastating at the wrist level, issuing to an exposure of all tendons, with a destruction of the paratenons and a progressive lysis of the tendinous structures. Coverage using flaps [12] may be proposed but it remains difficult to diagnose clinically tendon necrosis, the flap possibly covering already necrosed anatomical structures. Negative pressure therapy is usually proposed prior reconstructive or covering surgery, combined to tendon immobilization. A progressive separation between dead and living tissue appears, the remaining living tendon being slowly incorporated into a granulation bed after excision of the dead part. Coverage may then be obtained using a dermal substitute secondarily grafted using a partial thickness skin graft. Tendon repair may be planned some months after, ideally more than 1 year in order to prevent recurrence of inflammation source of secondary adherences.

55.4.2 Trauma

Traumatic skin avulsion in upper or lower limbs issues to a direct exposure of the tendon. If properly debrided and immobilized, tendons will preferably be covered using skin flaps in young patients presenting no comorbidities. Microsurgery is often proposed [3].

Chronic wounds like pressure ulcer, DFU, and LU may expose infected tendons. The tendon vascularization is difficult to assess if the tendon is still attached to the depth by the paratenon of not. In DFU series of cases using NPWT to enhance the granulation tissue, then covered using dermal substitutes plus split thickness skin grafts to cover exposed tendons were reported [13, 14].

55.4.3 Miscellaneous

Infected post corticosteroid injection sites may lead to tendon exposure and necrosis. This situation obliges to treat and debride the necrosed structures, cover the wound, and plan after several months a reconstructive procedure for tendon repair.

Management of tendon exposure on the dorsum of the hand using a dermal matrix has also been described [15].

References

1. Lee HJ, Kim JW, Oh CW, Min WK, Shon OJ, Oh JK, Park BC, Ihn JC. Negative pressure wound therapy for soft tissue injuries around the foot and ankle. J Orthop Surg Res. 2009;4:14. https://doi.org/10.1186/1749-799X-4-14.
2. Lee SY, Niikura T, Miwa M, Sakai Y, Oe K, Fukazawa T, Kawakami Y, Kurosaka M. Negative pressure wound therapy for the treatment of infected wounds with exposed knee joint after patellar fracture. Orthopedics. 2011;34(6):211. https://doi.org/10.3928/01477447-20110427-27.
3. Hong JP, Oh TS. An algorithm for limb salvage for diabetic foot ulcers. Chir Plast Surg. 2012;39(3):341–52. https://doi.org/10.1016/j.cps.2012.05.004. Epub 2012 May 30.
4. Iorio ML, Shuck J, Attinger CE. Wound healing in the upper and lower extremities: a systematic review on the use of acellular dermal matrices. Plast Reconstr Surg. 2012;130(5 Suppl 2):232S–41S. https://doi.org/10.1097/PRS.0b013e3182615703.
5. Yeong EK, Yu YC, Chan ZH, Roan TL. Is artificial dermis an effective tool in the treatment of tendon-exposed wounds? J Burn Care Res. 2013;34(1):161–7. https://doi.org/10.1097/BCR.0b013e3182685f0a.
6. Shores JT, Hiersche M, Gabriel A, Gupta S. Tendon coverage using an artificial skin substitute. J Plast Reconstr Aesthet Surg. 2012;65(11):1544–50. https://doi.org/10.1016/j.bjps.2012.05.021. Epub 2012 Jun 20.
7. Heckmann A, Radtke C, Rennekampff HO, Jokuszies A, Weyand B, Vogt PM. [One-stage defect closure of deperiosted bone and exposed tendons with MATRIDERM® and skin transplantation. Possibilities and limitations]. Unfallchirurg. 2012;115(12):1092–8.
8. Hamuy R, Kinoshita N, Yoshimoto H, Hayashida K, Houbara S, Nakashima M, Suzuki K, Mitsutake N, Mussazhanova Z, Kashiyama K, Hirano A, Akita S. One-stage, simultaneous skin grafting with artificial dermis and basic fibroblast growth factor successfully improves elasticity with maturation of scar formation. Wound Repair Regen. 2013;21(1):141–54.
9. Wollina U, Meseg A, Weber A. Use of a collagen-elastin matrix for hard to treat soft tissue defects. Int Wound J. 2011;8(3):291–6. https://doi.org/10.1111/j.1742-481X.2011.00785.x. Epub 2011 Mar 30.
10. Weigert R, Choughri H, Casoli V. Management of severe hand wounds with Integra® dermal regeneration template. J Hand Surg Eur Vol. 2011;36(3):185–93. https://doi.org/10.1177/1753193410387329. Epub 2010 Nov 15.
11. Peng F, Wu H, Yu G. Distally-based sural neurocutaneous flap for repair of a defect in the ankle tissue. J Plast Surg Hand Surg. 2011;45(2):77–82. https://doi.org/10.3109/2000656X.2011.558732.
12. Oni G, Saint-Cyr M, Mojallal A. Free tissue transfer in acute burns. J Reconstr Microsurg. 2012;28(2):77–84. https://doi.org/10.1055/s-0031-1284239. Epub 2011 Aug 2.
13. Alagaratnam S, Choong A, Loh A. Dermal substitute template use in diabetic foot ulcers: case reports. Int J Low Extrem Wounds. 2012;11(3):161–4. Epub 2012 Jun 3.
14. Clerici G, Caminiti M, Curci V, Quarantiello A, Faglia E. The use of a dermal substitute (integra) to preserve maximal foot length in a diabetic foot wound with bone and tendon exposure following urgent surgical debridement for an acute infection. Int J Low Extrem Wounds. 2009;8(4):209–12. https://doi.org/10.1177/1534734609350553.
15. Melamed E, Melone CP Jr. Coverage of hand defects with exposed tendons: the use of dermal regeneration template. Am J Orthop (Belle Mead NJ). 2018;47(5). https://doi.org/10.12788/ajo.2018.0030.

Open Access This chapter is licensed under the terms of the Creative Commons Attribution-NonCommercial-NoDerivatives 4.0 International License (http://creativecommons.org/licenses/by-nc-nd/4.0/), which permits any non-commercial use, sharing, distribution and reproduction in any medium or format, as long as you give appropriate credit to the original author(s) and the source, provide a link to the Creative Commons license and indicate if you modified the licensed material. You do not have permission under this license to share adapted material derived from this chapter or parts of it.

The images or other third party material in this chapter are included in the chapter's Creative Commons license, unless indicated otherwise in a credit line to the material. If material is not included in the chapter's Creative Commons license and your intended use is not permitted by statutory regulation or exceeds the permitted use, you will need to obtain permission directly from the copyright holder.

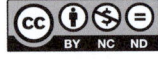

Dissecting Haematomas in Patients Submitted to Anticoagulation

Sergiu Fluieraru

56.1 Introduction

Large haematomas of the lower limbs are more frequently observed in patients submitted to anticoagulants [1]. Skin necrosis is limited in size, but the blood collection largely extends below the apparent lesion, inducing a vast dissecting collected space with clinical consequences comparable to compartment syndrome, with muscular and tendinous consequences.

56.2 Clinical Signs

After a mild trauma linked to a fall, or a consequence of compression bandaging, the apparent skin lesions are usually reported by the patient. Pain is moderate to intense, the local colour darkening progressively. The skin lesions are not extending over the skin surface during the next days, with a limited clinical symptomatology. This creeping lesion may induce extensive devascularisation of tendons and muscles located in the leg compartment involved, issuing to devastative loss of substances.

The leg volume slightly increases when the haematoma extends. However, the patients are usually aged and the symptoms are not always recognised, the clinical exam being rarely conclusive, a reason why the diagnosis is often delayed.

56.3 Anatomical Lesions on the Skin Spreading to the Depth

Skin apparent lesions are relatively limited, usually located over the anterior part of the tibia and sometimes over the medial aspect of the knee joint or the calf muscles. Low impact traumas are most of the time reported by the patients who are submitted to anticoagulants.

Lesions are linked to the dissecting hyperpressure of blood in a non-expandable zone, inducing self-ischaemia of soft tissues like tendons and muscles. This progressive necrosis is often underestimated as the skin itself is not extensively destroyed. It looks like a limited consequence of a localised trauma with a mild haematoma.

Lately inflammation is present, issuing to exudation from the opened necrotic skin, contemporarily with coagulated blood extruding from the wound. Infection is quickly spread, depending on the size of the collection, inducing a potential risk for septicaemia [2].

This life-threatening complication may induce spreading of infection to other tissues like the cardiac valves. The situation may lead to death.

S. Fluieraru (✉)
Wound Healing Unit, Montpellier University Hospital, Montpellier, France
e-mail: s-fluieraru@chu-montpellier.fr

56.4 Complementary Exams

Ultrasonography is mandatory to assess the presence of blood still below the normal skin located around the visible necrotic skin. This collection may be still under liquid form, accessible to syringe aspiration, or under coagulated form, observed after some days. This collection is highly susceptible of becoming infected.

Magnetic resonance imaging (MRI) is sometimes needed to assess the soft tissues involvement, muscles being destroyed partially or completely.

56.5 Surgical Management

Extensive surgical debridement is needed to eliminate the whole infected pocket when the skin is opened. Ultrasonography will define the anatomical limits, and the surgeon will excise the necrotised skin and the surrounding cover. This surgical decapitation is needed to promote granulation tissue formation over a clean wound, without persistent undermining. Negative pressure therapy will rapidly induce a healthy granulation tissue within 2 weeks and allow a surgical coverage using skin grating (Figs. 56.1, 56.2, and 56.3).

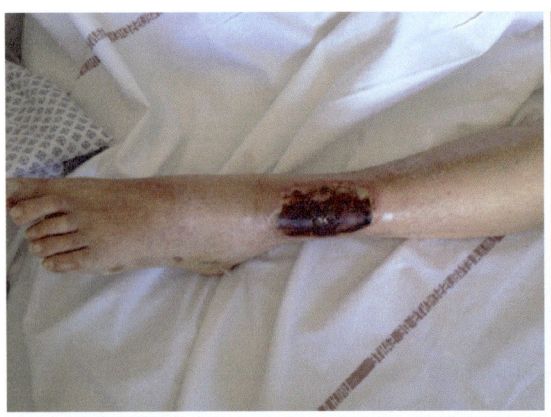
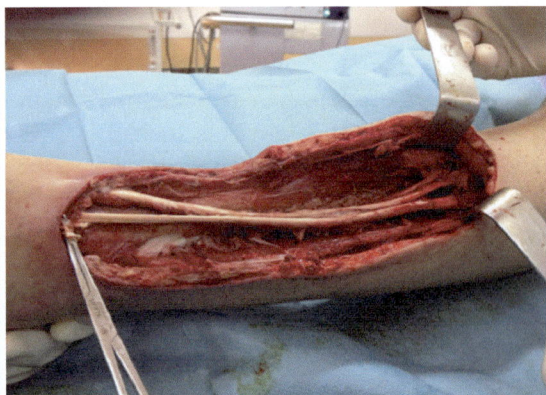
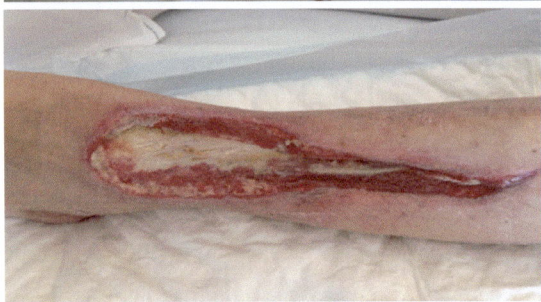

Figs. 56.1, 56.2, and 56.3 Extensive necrosis of the anterior compartment of the leg (compartment syndrome), inducing a septicaemia with cardiac valve destruction and thrombosis of the ipsilateral femoral artery. In spite of several attempts of debridement and promotion of granulation tissue, below knee (*BK*) amputation was needed.

References

1. Aliano K, Gulati S, Stavrides S, Davenport T, Hines G. Low-impact trauma causing acute compartment syndrome of the lower extremities. Am J Emerg Med. 2013;31(5):890.e3–4. https://doi.org/10.1016/j.ajem.2013.01.004. Epub 2013 Mar 6.

2. Daggett JR, Chung S, Smith PD. Bilateral spontaneous, simultaneous lower extremity hematomas in a patient on dalteparin. Int J Surg Case Rep. 2013;4(12):1080–3. https://doi.org/10.1016/j.ijscr.2013.07.036. Epub 2013 Sep 9.

Open Access This chapter is licensed under the terms of the Creative Commons Attribution-NonCommercial-NoDerivatives 4.0 International License (http://creativecommons.org/licenses/by-nc-nd/4.0/), which permits any non-commercial use, sharing, distribution and reproduction in any medium or format, as long as you give appropriate credit to the original author(s) and the source, provide a link to the Creative Commons license and indicate if you modified the licensed material. You do not have permission under this license to share adapted material derived from this chapter or parts of it.

The images or other third party material in this chapter are included in the chapter's Creative Commons license, unless indicated otherwise in a credit line to the material. If material is not included in the chapter's Creative Commons license and your intended use is not permitted by statutory regulation or exceeds the permitted use, you will need to obtain permission directly from the copyright holder.

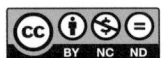

Management of the Patient After Flap Failure

57

Raymund E. Horch, Justus Osterloh, Christian Taeger, Oliver Bleiziffer, Ulrich Kneser, Andreas Arkudas, and Justus P. Beier

57.1 Introduction

The loss of a free flap is always a catastrophe in reconstructive surgery. This chapter describes possible approaches and algorithms how to manage the patient after the loss of a free, microsurgically transferred flap.

First, the possible pathophysiologic causes that may lead to malperfusion or stop of perfusion and to a subsequent partial or complete flap loss will be discussed. Reasons for flap failure are then analyzed dependent on their origin. They may be either patient inherent and irreversible or can be due to outer circumstances which can in principle be reversible and correctable.

We presented an algorithm on the management of a patient after failure of free tissue transfer. The appropriate decision-making depends on a large variety of factors. These include the persistence and differently pronounced urgency of reconstructive needs of the patient, the underlying cause of flap failure and its potential reversibility, the altered geometry and size of the defect, presence of sufficient recipient vessels, as well as the remaining selection of donor sites.

R. E. Horch (✉) · J. Osterloh · C. Taeger · O. Bleiziffer · U. Kneser · A. Arkudas · J. P. Beier
Department of Plastic and Hand Surgery, University Hospital Erlangen, Friedrich Alexander University Erlangen-Nuernberg, Erlangen, Germany
e-mail: raymund.horch@uk-erlangen.de; justus.osterloh@uk-erlangen.de; Ulrich.Kneser@bgu-ludwigshafen.de

57.2 Etiology and Pathogenesis

Over the past decades, free tissue transfer has become one of the mainstays in the reconstructive plastic surgeon's armamentarium to solve complex reconstructive problems in the whole body arising from tumor resection, trauma, congenital defects, or malformations [1]. Success rates of free flap transfer have reached an average of 95% in specialized centers, making this kind of procedure a very safe one in recent years [2].

All the more, it is a devastating event for the patient but also for the reconstructive microsurgeon if the rare event occurs and the free flap fails [3, 4].

In principle, early flap failure must be differentiated form late or even long-term flap failure. Flap necrosis is caused either by a lack of blood flow and oxygen to the tissue or by a venous congestion. Vascular compromise of free flaps most commonly occurs in the immediate postoperative period, in association with failure of the microvascular anastomosis. Conversely, rarely do flaps fail in the late postoperative period.

It is of crucial importance to determine the underlying cause of flap failure as soon as possible because it will affect the future reconstructive strategy and whether to consider a repeat free flap or not to a significant extent.

However, the pathomechanisms of the final steps leading to eventual flap failure are the same in every single case and have their background in the normal physiology of blood flow within the

© The Author(s) 2024
L. Téot et al. (eds.), *Skin Necrosis*, https://doi.org/10.1007/978-3-031-60954-1_57

vessels [5]. Regarding blood flow velocity within recipient or flap vessels, knowledge of the optimal perfusion pressures and flow values have still been scarce. Latest investigations into the various blood flow patterns and flow pressure values as well as flow transit times are ongoing and could be relevant to shed more light into the intraoperative aspects of intravascular blood flow. Matching the optimal relations of blood flow between flaps vessel capacity and recipient vessel blood flow dynamics could help to prevent flow mismatch and flap failure [6].

In addition, exact determination of the blood flow transit time utilizing indocyanine green near infrared fluorescence angiography after completing the microvascular anastomosis can also add significant information to either correct an anastomosis or prevent vascular flow mismatch and to detect any microcirculatory problem within the flap at the earliest possible time point [6].

When vascular injury occurs at the site of the microvascular anastomosis, the natural reaction is adherence of blood platelets at the site of injury which acts in a thrombogenic way due to denudation of the endothelium. The growing thrombus created by platelets following the thrombogenic stimulus is counteracted by the shear stress caused by the blood flowing physiologically through the vessel at the site of anastomosis. At the moment when a balance between these two processes is reached, a fibrin clot will be generated at the site of platelet accumulation and will stabilize and prevent further prothrombotic platelet adherence. Within a week, the endothelial surface will be restored making thrombotic occlusion of the vessel wall and subsequent flap failure a very unlikely event.

If the described balance is not preserved, the growing accumulation of platelets will eventually lead to occlusion of the vessel at the anastomosis leading to subsequent flap failure [7].

The introduction of intraoperative indocyanine green near infrared fluorescence angiography has dramatically added safety to determine the optimally perfused zones of a flap intraoperatively. By trimming and customizing any flap to the zones that are safely perfused, partial flap necrosis and postoperative fat necrosis can widely be avoided [8–11].

57.3 Causes of Flap Failure

Causes of flap failure will be discussed as far as they directly relate or impact decision-making for the subsequent steps in patient management. This applies particularly when a second free flap is considered to achieve the reconstructive goal (Table 57.1).

57.3.1 Reversible Causes Due to Outer Circumstances

57.3.1.1 Microsurgical Technique and Intraoperative Flap Handling

The initial thought after failure of a free flap procedure will generally lead a self-critical microsurgeon to investigate whether technical reasons are directly responsible for the flap loss [13]. Indeed, many flap losses are attributable to inadequate surgical technique and planning [14, 15]. It is also well known that around 90% of anasto-

Table 57.1 Causes of flap failure

Reversible	Irreversible
Technical problems	Vascular disease
Microsurgical techniques	Atherosclerosis
Reduced blood flow	Radiation injury
Postoperative management/anticoagulation	Malformations
Patient positioning	Hypercoagulability
Delay in diagnosis	Systemic disease
Delay in salvage	

Modified after Neligan and Wei [12]

motic thromboses occur in the venous part and that therefore it has to be considered as the most frequent cause of anastomotic failure [16]. Therefore, immediate revision is mandatory when there is the slightest suspicion of thrombosis formation postoperatively [17, 18].

Using coupler systems for venous anastomosis has been shown to lower the complication rate on the venous side [19, 20]. Coupler systems safe hypoxia time and by the nature of the system align intima to intima without any suture material at the inner lumen. Implantable ultrasonic devices to readily detect anastomotic problems postoperatively have been propagated but suffer from not yet sufficient reliability [21].

Risk of vessel injury and increased endothelial lesion followed by excessive platelet adhesion can be minimized by meticulous technique [22].

This includes avoiding to grasp the intima unduly with sharp instruments, avoiding tension at the anastomosis site, or undue clamping of vessels resulting in inner intimal lesions, not directly visible from the outside. It is advisable that if in doubt, vascular interpositional grafts should be used. Size match of flap vessel and recipient vessel should be ensured to avoid blood flow disturbances. At flap inset, tension on and kinking of the pedicle should be avoided [23]. In our own clinical practice, we found it helpful to protect the microanastomosis from kinking and from direct compression from the outside (such as by hematoma or seroma formation) and hence pressure on the pedicle in the postoperative period by covering the anastomotic site with fibrin sealant [2, 24]. Others have confounded this technical tool and reported on several hundreds of successful applications with free flap anastomotic "fibrin sheltering" [2, 24].

57.3.1.2 Postoperative Management

Careful positioning of the patient to prevent compression of the pedicle or the flap itself is crucial for successful outcome of free flap transfers, e.g., in the lower extremity or in the perineal or sacral region.

If in free muscle flaps skin pedicles are used, one has to make sure that the monitor island is sufficiently perfused and reflects the perfusion status of the muscles itself to rule out a false decision-making [25].

The use of systemic anticoagulation varies widely, but routine use is not uniformly agreed upon by all microsurgeons [26, 27]. Dextran, aspirin, heparin, and low-molecular weight heparins have been used as the most commonly used pharmacologic agents. However, dextran which influences hemodilution has been withdrawn from the market in some countries because of systemic side effects. Recent studies showed that it did not demonstrate better outcomes in terms of flap survival. Because it can cause serious systemic complications, it is better not to administer it routinely [28]. Aspirin has similarly not been shown to be effective enough to be recommended. Particular indications such as bypass free flaps—especially in the lower extremity— have been the subject of a more aggressive anticoagulative regimen. Given that evidence-based recommendations are not available thus far, the German-Speaking Society for Microsurgery has published its attempts to formulate potential guidelines for anticoagulation regimen after microsurgical free flap transfer [29].

When a second microvascular free flap is going to be performed to achieve a reconstructive goal following flap failure, systemic anticoagulation is often applied if risk factors persist as unfavorable conditions that are not correctable such as radiation tissue injury or radionecrosis [30]. This holds also true for complex microsurgical procedures including arterial bypasses or arteriovenous loops between flap and recipient site. In such interdisciplinary cases in our institution, we apply oral medication for systemic anticoagulation for half a year.

Through technical advances, it has become possible to perform microvascular anastomosis even when the intima is extremely fragile and usually not suitable for microanastomosis. By suturing the intima with a few stitches to the adventitia in extremely calcified arteries, a delicate second anastomosis can solve the problem when flap ischemia time is still within the range and prevent flap loss [31].

57.3.1.3 Patient-Inherent Irreversible Causes

These issues need to be considered in particular when evaluating the reconstructive options after free flap loss since they cannot be altered and may pose a limiting factor to secondary free flap reconstruction that has not been considered thoroughly enough at initial evaluation.

57.3.1.4 Vascular Disease

Atherosclerosis is one major threat to successful microsurgical free flap reconstruction. In particular, recipient vessels in the head and neck and in the lower extremity may often be of poor quality, increasing the risk of anastomosis-related complications, embolism, or thrombosis formation. When there is peripheral vascular disease of the lower extremity, free flap surgery itself may threaten survival of an already hypoperfused limb, necessitating the use of combined approaches using a bypass or vessel loop to provide both sufficient recipient vessels and secure perfusion of the compromised lower extremity [32, 33].

A history of diabetes and radiation injury may also severely compromise the quality of flap or recipient site vessels [34], the latter being of particular importance and frequently encountered in autologous breast reconstruction and sarcoma patients. When free flaps are buried, PET scanning may be helpful to determine the necessary measures [35] when Doppler or duplex sonography is not sufficient.

It can be important to avoid severing a vascular pedicle of a free flap even after several years of flap patency, since secondary flap losses have been described during secondary revisional operations. However, the questions of long-term flap autonomization have been studied recently [36, 37].

57.3.1.5 Systemic Disease

Especially in multimorbid patients and complex reconstructions, a failed free flap may worsen the patient's general condition, giving the patient an even greater risk when secondary free flap reconstruction is considered [38]. In such cases, stabilization of the patient's overall condition is advisable before a second free flap is attempted.

Clotting disorders including factor V Leiden, protein C and S deficiencies, and other conditions are not common, but an important cause to consider and identify before further efforts are undertaken to start another reconstructive effort using microsurgery [39, 40].

Myocardial infarction, stroke, respiratory failure, and morbid obesity and malnutrition are other severe conditions possibly precluding microsurgical reconstruction. When such conditions can be managed and the patient is recovered, another attempt of free flap transplantation may be warranted.

In each single case, the reconstructive goals must be reevaluated and potential new factors included in the analysis of patients after free flap failure.

57.4 Reevaluation of Reconstructive Goals

After a thorough assessment of the clinical course has been carried out and the cause for failure of the free flap procedure has been identified, a careful reevaluation of the status quo and the reconstructive goals is warranted.

The following factors must now be considered before the next step toward a secondary reconstruction is being made, in particular if a second attempt for free flap microsurgical reconstruction is considered: first, the possible limitation of donor sites; second, the new defect that may be potentially larger than the first defect; and third, previously available recipient vessels that may no longer be available. Taking all these factors together, a second free flap may be more technically challenging, increasing the risk for another free flap failure in the same patient. The need and urgency to reach a reconstructive goal by the use of a free flap may vary considerably, reaching from indications mainly for restoration of aesthetic appearance (breast reconstruction, reanimation of the paralyzed face), functional reconstruction (reanimation of the paralyzed face), and limb salvage (lower leg reconstruction) to the essential coverage of vital structures such as major blood vessels [33] (Fig. 57.1).

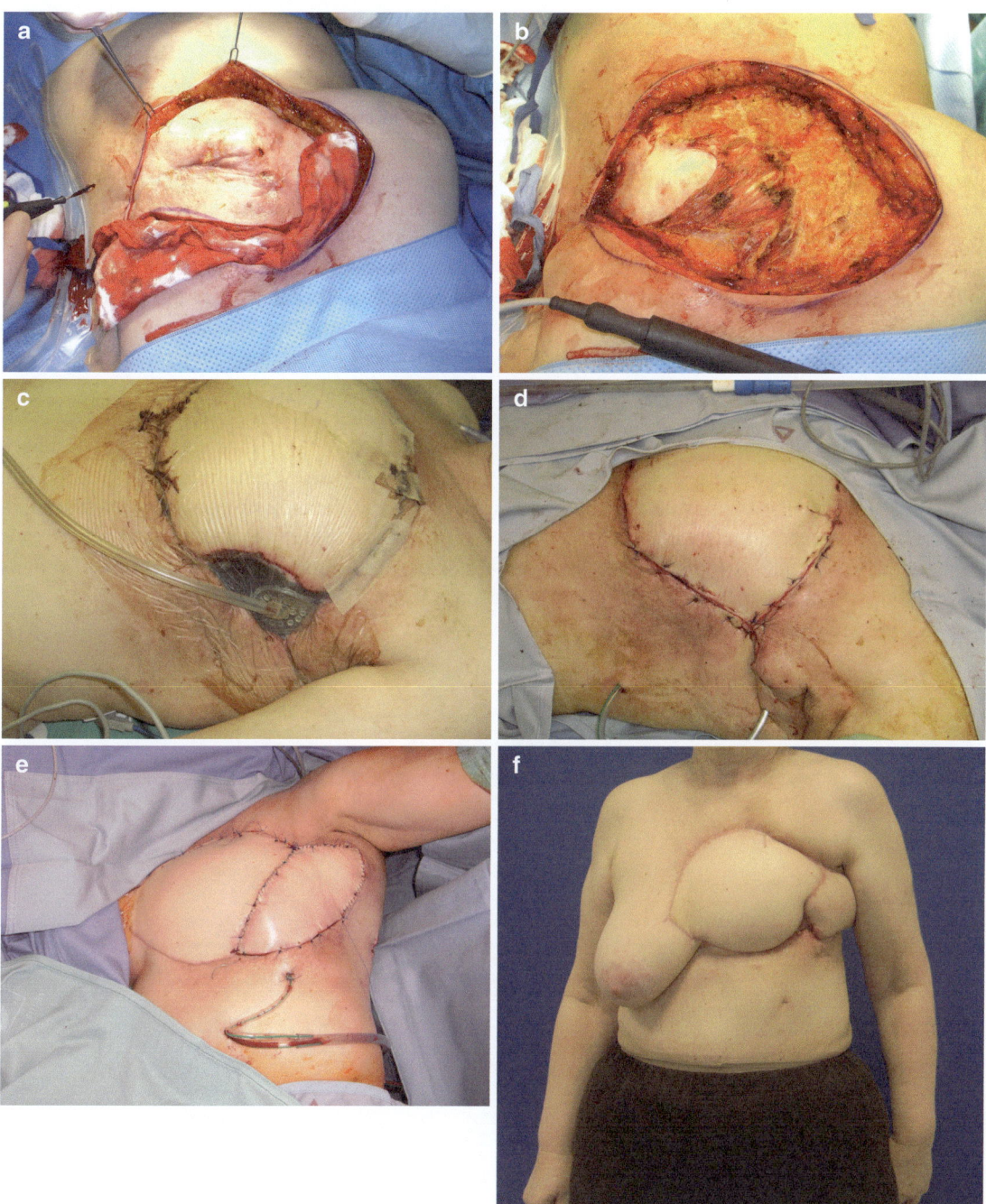

Fig. 57.1 (a) Palliative resection in fistulating inflammatory breast cancer after mastectomy and repeated irradiation (first cycle due to breast conserving therapy and second radiotherapy after mastectomy). (b) 43 cm × 27 cm large defect after palliative resection of fistulating inflammatory breast cancer. (c) After inset of extended DIEP flap to cover the large area, partial necrosis in zone IV occurred, necessitating debridement of the tip of the flap. We attempted wound conditioning with topical negative pressure therapy (TNP). (d) Secondary closure in the heavily irradiated field was attempted after wound conditioning with TNP. (e) Following wound breakdown after the secondary closure, a pedicled latissimus dorsi myocutaneous flap was necessary to achieve stable cover of the large wound area in the irradiated field. Note the fibrotic tissue changes and skin alteration below the latissimus dorsi flap in the upper abdominal wall soft tissue where the drain is placed through the skin. (f) Finally the wound was closed with conservative treatment of minor secondary healing in the lower wound margin between the latissimus dorsi and the DIEP flap within the irradiated area in this palliative situation rendering improved quality of life. The patient deceased 1 year later from pulmonary metastasis

57.4.1 Repeat Free Flap Procedure

Typical indications for where a repeat free flap procedure is recommended include the coverage of major vessels or vital structures, limb-threatening wounds in the extremity, and timely wound healing for potentially life-saving radiation. In such cases, it may be advisable to not risk another free flap but instead solve the problem with a pedicled flap to cover vital structures if possible [41–43].

Contraindications include deteriorating general conditions and severe uncontrollable local wound infection.

Typical flap choices will usually be the contralateral side of the initial donor site, "easy to perform" safe and standard flaps that the surgeon is experienced and comfortable with, and flaps with sufficiently long and strong-caliber pedicles (Fig. 57.2).

57.4.2 Non-microsurgical Therapy

Several factors may lead to the conclusion that another attempt to microsurgical free flap transplantation may not be the best reconstructive option for a particular option. When the patient's general condition deteriorates or when there is severe uncontrollable infection, alternative strategies of problem-solving must be implemented. These include local flap coverage, skin transplantation, and healing by secondary intention.

Treatment of free large flaps other than small skin flaps with the use of leeches is not advisable. It leads to anemia necessitating blood transfusions and does not alter the underlying condition. This is different when fingers are replanted, where the application of leeches due to the often immanent problem of lacking venous vessels may help to overcome the initial period of venous congestion in replanted digits [44].

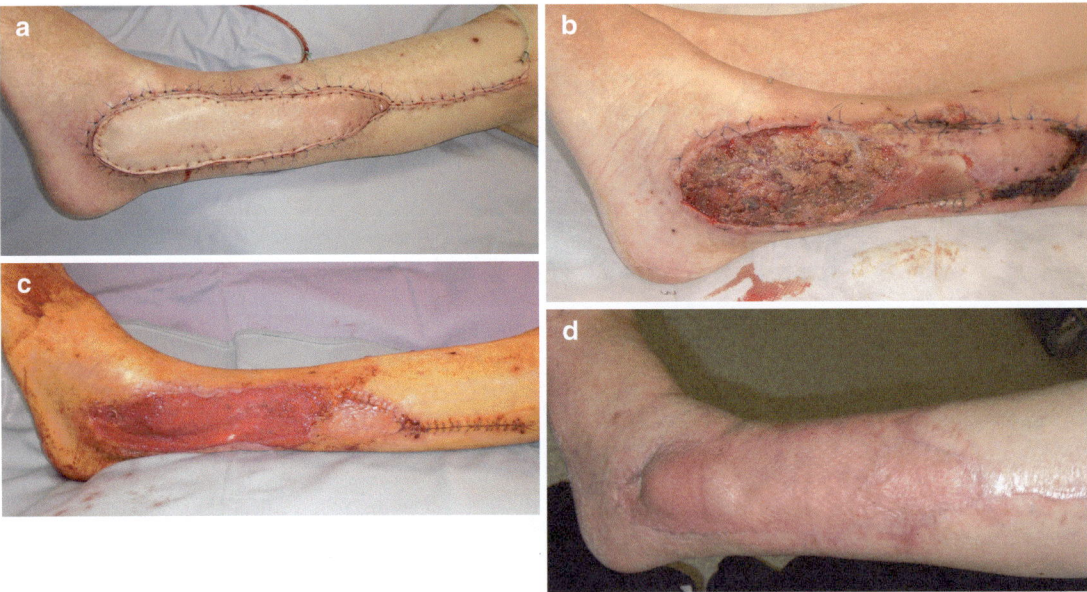

Fig. 57.2 (**a**) The patient initially suffered from a combined pilon tibiale and fibula fracture. After initially successful osteosynthesis, further clinical course was complicated by an unstable scar followed by soft tissue breakdown. After radical surgical debridement and removal of the exposed hardware, a propeller flap based on a perforator from the fibular artery was performed for defect coverage. (**b**) In the postoperative course, malperfusion occurred, mainly in the distal part of the flap. After debridement, the remaining defect was covered with a free gracilis flap which again became necrotic in its distal part. The remaining defect then was covered after a partial debridement of the gracilis flap with a peroneus brevis flap. (**c**) After wound conditioning using negative pressure therapy, a healthy well-perfused wound bed was visible. (**d**) The wound bed was then amenable to split-thickness skin grafting. The further course was uneventful, and the patient had long-term stable soft tissue coverage

57 Management of the Patient After Flap Failure

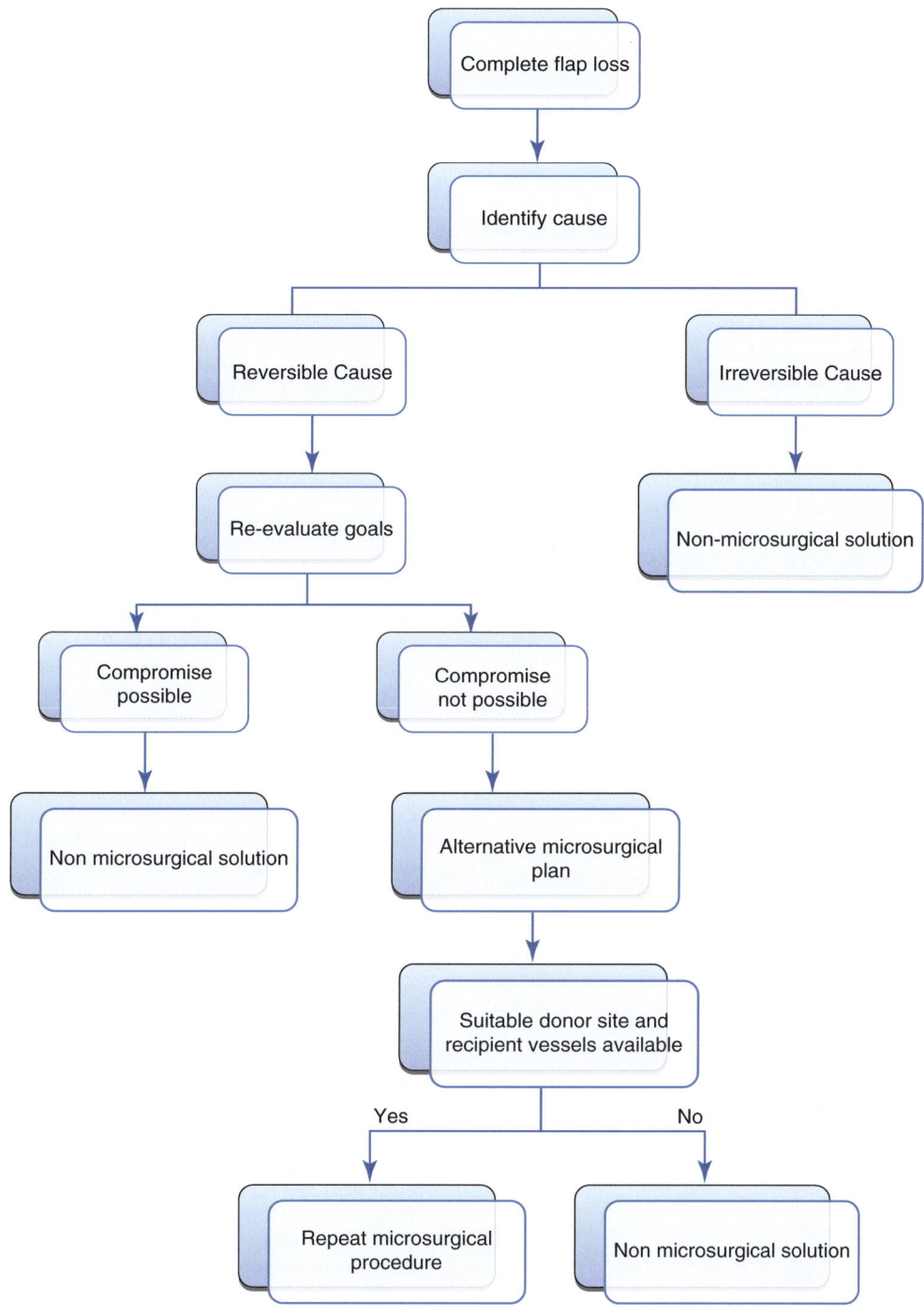

Flow sheet—Surgical decision-making after complete flap loss

References

1. Horch RE, Stark GB. The rectus abdominis free flap as an emergency procedure in extensive upper extremity soft-tissue defects. Plast Reconstr Surg. 1999;103(5):1421–7.
2. Langer S, et al. Development of a surgical algorithm and optimized management of complications—based on a review of 706 abdominal free flaps for breast reconstruction. Med Sci Monit. 2010;16(11):Cr518–22.
3. Wei F, Mardini S. Flaps and reconstructive surgery. Saunders-Elsevier; 2010.
4. Godina M. Preferential use of end-to-side arterial anastomoses in free flap transfers. Plast Reconstr Surg. 1979;64(5):673–82.
5. Atchabahian A, Masquelet AC. Experimental prevention of free flap thrombosis. I: a model of free flap failure. Microsurgery. 1996;17(12):710–3.
6. Geierlehner A, et al. Intraoperative blood flow analysis of DIEP vs. ms-TRAM flap breast reconstruction combining transit-time flowmetry and microvascular indocyanine green angiography. J Pers Med. 2022;12(3).
7. Lidman D, Daniel RK. Evaluation of clinical microvascular anastomoses—reasons for failure. Ann Plast Surg. 1981;6(3):215–23.
8. Müller-Seubert W, et al. Intra- and early postoperative evaluation of malperfused areas in an irradiated random pattern skin flap model using Indocyanine green angiography and near-infrared reflectance-based imaging and infrared thermography. J Pers Med. 2022;12(2).
9. Geierlehner A, et al. A Myocutaneous latissimus Dorsi propeller flap based on a single dorsal intercostal perforator. Plast Reconstr Surg Glob Open. 2021;9(11):e3881.
10. Ludolph I, et al. Leaving the perfusion zones? Individualized flap design in 100 free DIEP and ms-TRAM flaps for autologous breast reconstruction using indocyanine green angiography. J Plast Reconstr Aesthet Surg. 2022;75(1):52–60.
11. Müller-Seubert W, et al. Novel imaging methods reveal positive impact of topical negative pressure application on tissue perfusion in an in vivo skin model. Int Wound J. 2021;18(6):932–9.
12. Neligan P, Wei F. Microsurgical reconstruction of the head and neck. St. Louis: QMP; 2007.
13. Skrbić S, Stanec Z. Early rupture of the arterial anastomoses with free flap survival. Injury. 1995;26(7):494–6.
14. Daigeler A, et al. Microsurgical training—report on the consensus workshop of the 31st annual meeting of the German-language group for microsurgery of the peripheral nerves and vessels 2009 in Erlangen. Handchir Mikrochir Plast Chir. 2010;42(4):273–6.
15. McKee NH. Operative complications and the management of intraoperative flow failure. Microsurgery. 1993;14(3):158–61.
16. Murray DJ, et al. Free tissue transfer and deep vein thrombosis. J Plast Reconstr Aesthet Surg. 2008;61(6):687–92.
17. Hidalgo DA, Jones CS. The role of emergent exploration in free-tissue transfer: a review of 150 consecutive cases. Plast Reconstr Surg. 1990;86(3):492–8; discussion 99–501.
18. Beckingham IJ, et al. Free flap failure due to venous occlusion secondary to previous intravenous cannulation: a case report. Microsurgery. 1992;13(6):348–9.
19. Steiner D, et al. Interdisciplinary treatment of breast cancer after mastectomy with autologous breast reconstruction using abdominal free flaps in a university teaching hospital-a standardized and safe procedure. Front Oncol. 2020;10:177.
20. Ahn CY, et al. Clinical experience with the 3M microvascular coupling anastomotic device in 100 free-tissue transfers. Plast Reconstr Surg. 1994;93(7):1481–4.
21. Kind GM, et al. The effect of an implantable Doppler probe on the salvage of microvascular tissue transplants. Plast Reconstr Surg. 1998;101(5):1268–73; discussion 74–5.
22. Horch RE. The development of plastic surgery: retrospective view of 80 years of "Der Chirurg" (the surgeon). Chirurg. 2009;80(12):1132–9.
23. Selvaggi G, Anicic S, Formaggia L. Mathematical explanation of the buckling of the vessels after twisting of the microanastomosis. Microsurgery. 2006;26(7):524–8.
24. Andree C, et al. Improved safety of autologous breast reconstruction surgery by stabilisation of microsurgical vessel anastomoses using fibrin sealant in 349 free DIEP or fascia-muscle-sparing (fms)-TRAM flaps: a two-centre study. Breast. 2008;17(5):492–8.
25. Beier JP, et al. Perforator-based monitoring skin islands in free muscle flaps: teaching old dogs new tricks. Plast Reconstr Surg. 2012;129(3):586e–7e.
26. Lecoq JP, et al. Thromboprophylaxis in microsurgery. Acta Chir Belg. 2006;106(2):158–64.
27. Brands MT, et al. Prevention of thrombosis after microvascular tissue transfer in the head and neck. A review of the literature and the state of affairs in Dutch Head and Neck Cancer Centers. Int J Oral Maxillofac Surg. 2010;39(2):101–6.
28. Filipan D, et al. The effects of dextran on postoperative thrombosis and hemodilution in microvascular head and neck reconstruction. Ann Plast Surg. 2020;85(1):38–42.
29. Schmitz M, et al. [Perioperative coagulation management in microsurgery: report of the consensus workshops in the course of the 31st and 32nd annual meeting of the German-language Working Group for microsurgery of the peripheral nerves and vessels (DAM) November 2009 in Erlangen and November 2010 in Basel]. Handchir Mikrochir Plast Chir. 2011;43(6):376–83.
30. Holm C, et al. The intrinsic transit time of free microvascular flaps: clinical and prognostic implications. Microsurgery. 2010;30(2):91–6.

31. Cai A, Horch RE, Arkudas A. The impossible anastomosis: intima-to-adventitia suture technique for microanastomosis of severely calcified arteries. Plast Reconstr Surg Glob Open. 2021;9(10):e3866.
32. Lang W, Horch RE. [Distal extremity reconstruction for limb salvage in diabetic foot ulcers with pedal bypass, flap plasty and vacuum therapy]. Zentralbl Chir. 2006;131(Suppl 1):S146–50.
33. Horch RE, Horbach T, Lang W. The nutrient omentum free flap: revascularization with vein bypasses and greater omentum flap in severe arterial ulcers. J Vasc Surg. 2007;45(4):837–40.
34. Salama AR, et al. Free-flap failures and complications in an American oral and maxillofacial surgery unit. Int J Oral Maxillofac Surg. 2009;38(10):1048–51.
35. Dragu A, et al. Interesting image. Tc-99m sestamibi SPECT/CT as a new tool for monitoring perfusion and viability of buried perforator based free flaps in breast reconstruction after breast cancer. Clin Nucl Med. 2010;35(1):36–7.
36. Rother U, et al. Wound closure by means of free flap and arteriovenous loop: development of flap autonomy in the long-term follow-up. Int Wound J. 2020;17(1):107–16.
37. Ludolph I, et al. Indocyanine green angiography and the old question of vascular autonomy—long term changes of microcirculation in microsurgically transplanted free flaps. Clin Hemorheol Microcirc. 2019;72(4):421–30.
38. Wang TY, et al. A review of 32 free flaps in patients with collagen vascular disorders. Plast Reconstr Surg. 2012;129(3):421e–7e.
39. Dragu A, et al. Acute and diffuse postoperative bleeding after free latissimus dorsi flap—factor XIII deficiency: a case report and review of the literature. Med Sci Monit. 2009;15(1):Cs1–4.
40. Schleich AR, Oswald TM, Lineaweaver WC. Complete salvage of impending free flap failure in heparin induced thrombocytopenia by emergent institution of therapy with argatroban. J Plast Reconstr Aesthet Surg. 2008;61(10):1263–4.
41. Horch R, Stark GB. Prosthetic vascular graft infection—defect covering with delayed vertical rectus abdominis muscular flap (VRAM) and rectus femoris flap. Vasa. 1994;23(1):52–6.
42. Kneser U, et al. Comparison between distally based peroneus brevis and sural flaps for reconstruction of foot, ankle and distal lower leg: an analysis of donor-site morbidity and clinical outcome. J Plast Reconstr Aesthet Surg. 2011;64(5):656–62.
43. Loos B, et al. Post-malignancy irradiation ulcers with exposed alloplastic materials can be salvaged with topical negative pressure therapy (TNP). Eur J Surg Oncol. 2007;33(7):920–5.
44. Beier JP, Horch RE, Kneser U. Chemical leeches for successful two-finger re-plantation in a 71-year-old patient. J Plast Reconstr Aesthet Surg. 2010;63(1):e107–8.

Open Access This chapter is licensed under the terms of the Creative Commons Attribution-NonCommercial-NoDerivatives 4.0 International License (http://creativecommons.org/licenses/by-nc-nd/4.0/), which permits any non-commercial use, sharing, distribution and reproduction in any medium or format, as long as you give appropriate credit to the original author(s) and the source, provide a link to the Creative Commons license and indicate if you modified the licensed material. You do not have permission under this license to share adapted material derived from this chapter or parts of it.

The images or other third party material in this chapter are included in the chapter's Creative Commons license, unless indicated otherwise in a credit line to the material. If material is not included in the chapter's Creative Commons license and your intended use is not permitted by statutory regulation or exceeds the permitted use, you will need to obtain permission directly from the copyright holder.

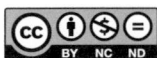

Part VII

Techniques Applicable to Skin Necrosis

Introduction to Techniques Applicable to Skin Necrosis

Luc Téot

Different strategies should be developed and proposed when facing a skin necrosis.

The knowledge of the anatomical region is crucial, as the underlying structure may be fat and subcutaneous tissues, or a muscular aponeurosis, a tendon or a bone. So the initial assessment of a skin necrosis should be the location on the body surface.

Before choosing the technique the, nature and origin of the skin necrosis should be determined. A medical expertise has to be completed prior to any management proposal.

The causes of skin necrosis may be multiple, as developed in this book. A good knowledge of the main pathologies is required, and experts in dermatology, infectious diseases, traumatology, geriatrics, diabetology, systemic collagen diseases, and vascular specialists should be contacted in order to accurately determine the medical context when needed.

Debridement has always been considered as the most efficient strategy to remove undesired tissues, and even if evidence-based medicine is still considered as not having fully demonstrated its efficiency, debridement is recommended by a majority of experts.

Techniques for removing necrotic tissues may vary, from non-invasive adsorbing dressings like alginates or hyperabsorbent dressings, to curette or scalpel removing gradually necrotic tissues or to negative pressure wound therapy plus instillation combined with perforated foams. In deep infection like in diabetic foot ulcer, the carcinologic excisions realized in the operative room should be referred to specialists, who will debride and redebride as required by the local evolution. Some authors considered that a complete debridement should be obtained before day 4, but algorithms considering the variability, the availability, and the skill needed for using appropriately the different technical options render this principle somehow difficult to apply.

A nurse at home has not the same capacities of complete debridement on a painful patient than a surgeon working under general anaesthesia in the OR. Here again, the clinical assessment of the risks/benefits ratio should work, in order to prevent infection but not imposing excessive difficulties to the nursing staff. However, a strong consensus exists concerning that the more the wound is infected the more repetitive debridement is needed.

L. Téot (✉)
Department of Plastic Surgery, Burns and Wound Healing, Montpellier University Hospital, Hôpital La Colombière, CICAT Occitanie, Montpellier, France
e-mail: l-teot@chu-montpellier.fr

Dressing types applicable in skin necrosis	Absorbant	Highly absorbant	Hyper absorbant	Permanent aspiration + edge effect	Antibacterial necrosis stabilization
Hydrocolloid	X				
Hydrofibers		X			
Alginate		X			
Polycarbonate			X		
NPWT Instill				X	
Flammacerium					X

Types of dressings proposed in skin necrosis

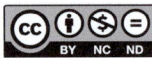

Open Access This chapter is licensed under the terms of the Creative Commons Attribution-NonCommercial-NoDerivatives 4.0 International License (http://creativecommons.org/licenses/by-nc-nd/4.0/), which permits any noncommercial use, sharing, distribution and reproduction in any medium or format, as long as you give appropriate credit to the original author(s) and the source, provide a link to the Creative Commons license and indicate if you modified the licensed material. You do not have permission under this license to share adapted material derived from this chapter or parts of it.

The images or other third party material in this chapter are included in the chapter's Creative Commons license, unless indicated otherwise in a credit line to the material. If material is not included in the chapter's Creative Commons license and your intended use is not permitted by statutory regulation or exceeds the permitted use, you will need to obtain permission directly from the copyright holder.

59

Dressings for Necrosed Skin

Christine Faure-Chazelles and Sylvie Meaume

59.1 Introduction

During the physiological process of healing, the initial stage of debridement and inflammation is realized spontaneously. Moist wound healing favors the activity of proteolytic enzymes and the macrophages phagocytosing dead cells, and it allows absorption of tissue debris. However, this slow natural process may lead to negative consequences for wound healing. The necrotic process stops the formulation of granulation tissue and creates a milieu that favors bacterial development. This necrosis may be black and dry or humid or fibrinous, the color depending on the accompanying bacterial colonization. The presence of a biofilm prolongs the inflammatory stage and exposes the wound to recurrent infectious episodes [1]. Modern dressings based on the concept of moist wound healing contribute to the acceleration of autolytic debridement [2].

This chapter presents the different dressings recognized to be effective during debridement and their mode of use. Depending on the type of necrosis—hard and dry or soft and humid—these recommended dressings are mostly absorbent or mixed hydrating/absorbent. These dressings may be gauzes, sheets, or gels [3, 4]. Some dressings with osmotic properties are also used for debridement and are briefly described below.

59.2 Dressings and Autolytic Debridement

59.2.1 Hydrating Dressings

59.2.1.1 Hydrogels

Hydrogels are mainly composed of water (around 80%) to which is added, depending on the adsorbing components (carboxymethyl cellulose [CMC], alginate, etc.), hydrating agents (gelatin, pectin, etc.), thickening agents (xanthan gum, guar gum), and bacteriostatic agents (propylene glycol, etc.). Gels are mostly used for debridement, but they also exist in the form of gauzes impregnated with gel and transparent sheets.

The physical properties of hydrogels should combine a relatively low viscosity favoring the maximal coverage of the wound and good adherence, preventing the gel from gliding over the wound. Because of their composition, they hydrate and soften the necrotic plaque to facilitate debridement of hard, dry necrosis or adherent fibrin (Fig. 59.1). Gels are presented differently depending on the manufacturer: classic tubes, accordion tubes, and syringes. Unexpected events may be observed, such as

C. Faure-Chazelles (✉)
Medical Device Pharmacy Department, Montpellier University Hospital, Montpellier, France
e-mail: c-faurechazelles@chu-montpellier.fr

S. Meaume
Geriatric and Wound Care Department, Rothschild University Hospital, Assistance Publique Hôpitaux de Paris, Sorbonne Université of Paris, Paris, France
e-mail: sylvie.meaume@aphp.fr

© The Author(s) 2024
L. Téot et al. (eds.), *Skin Necrosis*, https://doi.org/10.1007/978-3-031-60954-1_59

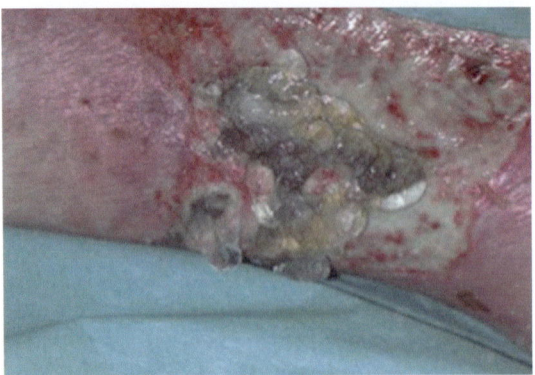

Fig. 59.1 Appearance of hydrogel applied on necrotic tissue: the gels stick to the wound, and the product layer should not be applied on the wound edges

maceration of the wound edges in the case of heavy exudation or when the gel is applied in excess. Good care should be taken to apply a uniformly thin layer of hydrogel over a previously cleaned and dried wound bed. The choice of the secondary dressing is crucial, as it will enhance the moisturizing effect of the gel. Any absorbing dressing should be avoided. Facility of use of the applicator is the main element of differentiation among the products currently on the market: a long nose for deep wounds, the sharpness of application, and the ease of use of the product as a whole.

59.2.1.2 Hydrogel-Like Devices

Over the last few years, the classic formulations of hydrogels have changed. Adding antiseptics was proposed, and of the products currently on the market, the following could be mentioned:

- A matrix of hydroxyethyl cellulose polymers, insoluble and hydrophilic, containing 85% water and octenidine dichlorhydrate, a cationic antibacterial belonging to the bipyridine family [5];
- A solution containing hydrogel, but also polyhexamethylene biguanide (PHMB) together with betaine. PHMB is an antimicrobial belonging to the biguanide family, whose property is to reduce the bacterial load by acting on the phospholipids of the bacterial membrane. Betaine is a tensioactive agent called a surfactant, whose action is to dissolve fibrinous material on the wound surface [6].

One of the main expected actions of these devices is to eliminate and prevent biofilm formation.

59.2.2 Mixed "Hydrating/Absorbent" Dressings

59.2.2.1 Irrigo-Absorbents

Irrigo-absorbent dressings are gaining popularity among debridement dressings, although only one dressing has been launched under TenderWet, now known as HydroClean Plus. It is a multilayer dressing presenting a shape of a cushion whose center is mainly composed of polyacrylate particles activated by an adequate volume of Ringer solution. The superabsorbent polyacrylate presents an increased attraction for wound exudate rich in proteins compared with the Ringer solution. The combined action of irrigation is due to the continuous delivery of Ringer and the drainage of exudates. Peri wound blanching may be observed when the dressing lies over the wound edges; a water paste or zinc oxide paste can be proposed. The Cleansite study [7] demonstrates the superiority of the product over normal hydrogel in long-term undebrided chronic leg ulcer.

59.2.2.2 Hydrocolloids

Considered to be active at all wound healing stages, hydrocolloids occupy a relatively modest position in the list of debriding agents. These older dressings have been progressively supplanted by more adaptive dressings. Composed mostly of sodium CMC, they jellify when in contact with fibrin or necrosis and provide an optimal level of moisture (Fig. 59.2a). The absorption of exudate occurs slowly and moderately, and their use is indicated in the presence of humid necrosis and mainly for superficial wounds owing to the speed of action.

They can be found as fairly thick sheets, opaque or transparent and with anatomical shapes (sacrum, heel, and elbow). All are adhesive and do not require secondary dressings. The dressing

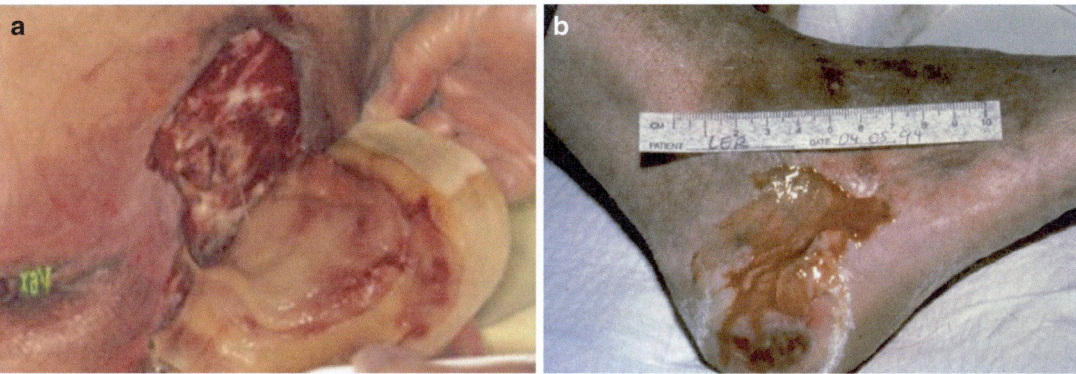

Fig. 59.2 (**a**) Aspect of hydrocolloid after 2 days. (**b**) Jellification smells and look like pus

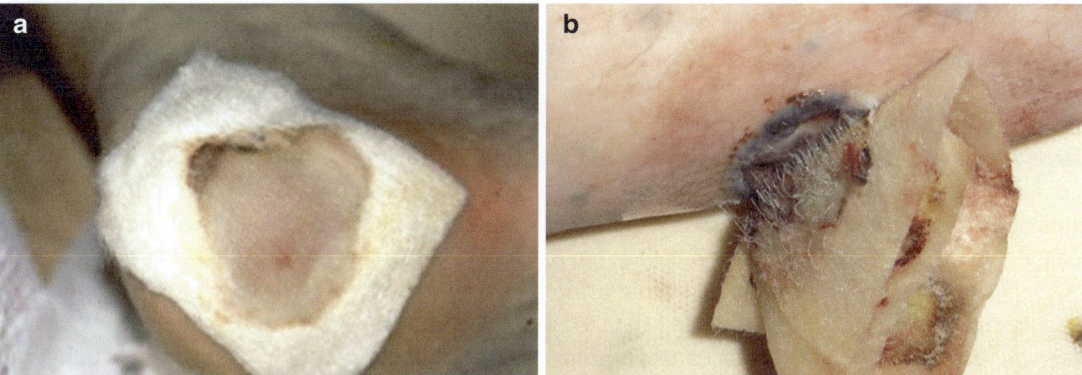

Fig. 59.3 (**a**) Highly exudating wound covered with an alginate will be changed when saturated. (**b**) Saline is applied over an alginate in order to facilitate the dressing removal

should lie at least 3 cm over the edges of the wound to obtain maximal adhesion (Fig. 59.2b). In some cases, an adhesive tape can be used to secure the edges of the dressing in place.

59.2.3 Absorbent Dressings

Absorbent dressings are composed of various materials such as alginate, CMC, polyacrylate, or others polymers. Their main characteristic is that they jellify when in contact with exudates without being destroyed. To be active during the debridement stage, the dressing should not dry out between two successive changes. They are available as gauzes or meshes.

59.2.3.1 Alginates

Alginates are polymers of alginic acid obtained from brown algae. They are differentiated from each other by their chemical composition and thus their physical properties. When guluronic acid is predominant compared with mannuronic acid, the dressing will be more rigid. Ca++ and Na+ concentrations and the presence or absence of CMC provide different levels of absorption and jellification. The jellification of alginate fibers is concomitant with the formation of Na alginate, which is soluble in water and highly hydrophilic, and/or with the presence of CMC (Fig. 59.3).

Maintaining the adapted level of moisture without occlusiveness allows better efficacy.

Their hemostatic capacity is also an interesting property [8]. In order to facilitate the removal of the dressing, saline or water may be used (Fig. 59.3). Alginates are contraindicated over dry wounds or during the epidermization stage. Sequential use of alginates during the debridement stage is recommended by numerous guidelines [9].

59.2.3.2 Fiber Dressings

Hydrofiber technology was introduced in 1999 when launching the first unwoven dressing composed of sodium CMC (Aquacel), a vertical and horizontal matrix containing regenerated cellulose. Other fiber dressings containing CMC are now available and even other polymer-like polyvinyl alcohol.

Those fiber dressings are characterized by their high degree of hydrophilia combined with a large capacity for absorption. Looking at their composition, when they contains CMC they are similar to hydrocolloids as they jellify when in contact with exudates (Fig. 59.4), but they have the capacity to retain moisture and bacteria inside the matrix (bacterial sequestration) [10]. The recently developed matrix enhances these properties; thus, it is possible to cover the dressing with a secondary dressing, allowing some moisture (hydrocolloid, foams). Removal of all type of those new fiber dressings is facilitated by hydration. Those dressings are suitable for rather exuding wound and allow painless dressing removal which is very comfortable for patients with acute or chronic fibrinous wounds.

59.2.3.3 Polyacrylate Fibers Dressing for Debridement and Combined with NOSF to Boost Wound Healing Process

There is one unique dressing in this category. It consists of a gauze composed of polyacrylate fibers and coated in a micro-adherent lipido-colloid layer (TLC-Contact). The mesh version does not contain lipido-colloid. Together with the hydro-debriding fibers, polyacrylate fibers jellify and adhere to fibrinous residues and microorganisms, absorb them and drain them in order to enhance their elimination: this mechanism favors autolytic debridement (Fig. 59.5b). Resistance to traction is also observed. The clinical study EARTH, whose publication is in process, has confirmed advantage of these dressings in highly exudative, chronic wounds with non-inferiority to hydrofibers with CMC [11] (Fig. 59.5a).

The recently developed Urgostart Plus dressing contains NOSF (Nano-Oligosaccharide Factor) in addition to TLC fibers which regulate metalloproteases which are in excess in chronic wounds and which have shown through several randomized controlled trials significant efficacy in wound healing only chronic wounds [12, 13], and which is recommended to be used first-line [14] in the local treatment of chronic wounds. Indeed, the NOSF acts as soon as the granulation tissue appears after the effect of the polyacrylate fibers which helps in debridement allowing the wounds to heal more quickly. This dressing can be used from debridement to epithelialization of chronic moist wounds.

59.2.3.4 Dressings and Osmotic Pressure

Dressings Containing Salts
Salts with 20% NaCl were added to the initial composition of hydrogels to form a hyperosmotic dressing. This formulation is more adapted to the necrotic plaques, which are black, hard, and dry. The periwound has to be specifically checked

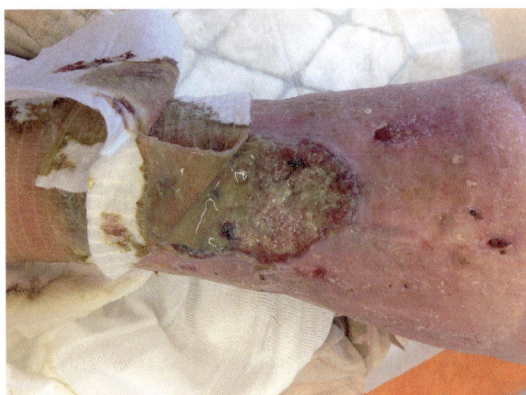

Fig. 59.4 Hydrofiber removal is easy thanks to the CMC gelification

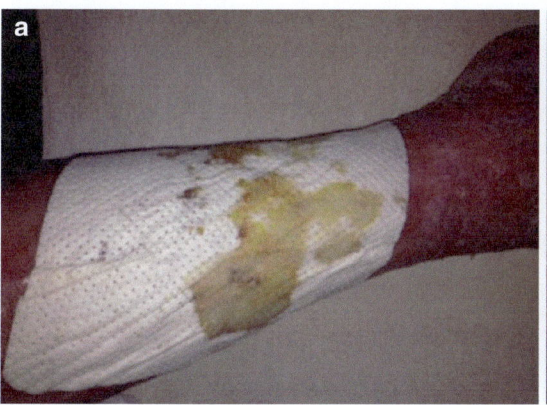 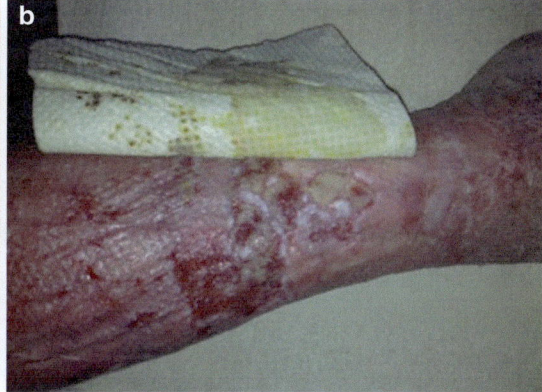

Fig. 59.5 (**a**) Polyacrylate fiber dressing is a fast remover of undesired tissues over a fibrinous leg ulcer. (**b**) When saturated the polyacrylate dressing is mechanically resistant enough to be removed as a whole, without leaving debris over the wound

when using these dressings with high risk of maceration and sometime uncomfort, that can prevent using protection with zinc paste.

Medical Honey Dressings

Sterile dressings are now available. They have physicochemical and microbiological properties that are comparable to the ancient description of honey when it was used empirically in ancient times [15]. Its high osmolarity favors wound exudation and mechanically induces the elimination of dead tissues and foreign bodies (including microorganisms). This mechanism induces a moist ambience that favors wound healing. This debridement is accompanied by an antibacterial effect on Gram-positive, Gram-negative, and Gram-resistant bacteria, whatever their presentation, whether planktonic or biofilm. Honey is either attached to the gauze or present as a paste.

59.3 How to Use These Dressings

Hygiene should be respected during the dressing change. Whichever dressing is used, the protocol is important. The wound should be cleaned carefully (with water and soap) and rinsed, and the periwound should be dried. The dressing should then be applied respecting the mode of use specified by the manufacturer, and the frequency of the dressing change is usually every 1 or 2 days at this phase. The use of these debriding dressings does not prevent an active mechanical debridement at each dressing change.

59.4 How to Choose the Dressing

This autolytic debridement is suitable for all types of wound, except for infected or heavily exudating wounds. It acts on the tissues in a selective manner. It is easy to use requiring no training before use, which makes them easily accessible to nurses. The cost is moderate compared with surgical debridement. Its main inconvenience is the slow process, but the absence of pain and bleeding, preventing microtrauma on the surface of the wound, is an advantage.

References

1. Winter GD. Effect of air drying and dressings on the surface of wounds. Nature. 1963;197:91–3.
2. James GA, Swogger E, Wolcott R, et al. Biofilms in chronic wounds. Wound Repair Regen. 2008;16(1):37–44.
3. Vaneau M, Chaby G, Guillot B, Martel P, Senet P, Téot L, Chosidow O. Consensus panel recommendations for chronic and acute dressings. Arch Dermatol. 2007;143(10):1291–4.
4. Chaby G, Senet P, Vaneau M, Martel P, Guillaume JC, Meaume S, Téot L, Debure C, Dompmartin A, Bachelet H, Carsin H, Matz V, Richard JL, Rochet

JM, Sales-Aussias N, Zagnoli A, Denis C, Guillot B, Chosidow O. Dressings for acute and chronic wounds: a systematic review. Arch Dermatol. 2007;143(10):1297–304.
5. Hämmerle G, Strohal R. Efficacy and cost-effectiveness of octenidine wound gel in the treatment of chronic venous leg ulcers in comparison to modern wound dressings. Int Wound J. 2014;13:182. https://doi.org/10.1111/iwj.12250.
6. Horrocks A. Prontosan wound irrigation and gel: management of chronic wounds. Br J Nurs. 2006;15(22):1222, 1224–8.
7. Humbert P, Faivre B, Véran Y, Debure C, Truchetet F, Bécherel PA, Plantin P, Kerihuel JC, Eming SA, Dissemond J, Weyandt G, Kaspar D, Smola H, Zöllner P, CLEANSITE study group. Protease-modulating polyacrylate-based hydrogel stimulates wound bed preparation in venous leg ulcers—a randomized controlled trial. J Eur Acad Dermatol Venereol. 2014;28(12):1742–50.
8. Sayag J, Meaume S, Bohbot S. Healing properties of calcium alginate dressings. J Wound Care. 1996;5(8):357–62.
9. Belmin J, Meaume S, Rabus MT, Bohbot S. Sequential treatment with calcium alginate dressings and hydrocolloid dressings accelerates pressure ulcer healing in older subjects: a multicenter randomized trial of sequential *versus* non sequential treatment with hydrocolloid dressing alone. J Am Geriatr Soc. 2002;5à(2):269–74.
10. Barnea Y, Amir A, Leshem D, Zaretski A, Weiss J, Shafir R, Gur E. Clinical comparative study of Aquacel and paraffin gauze dressing for split-skin donor site treatment. Ann Plast Surg. 2004;53(2):132–6.
11. Meaume S, Dissemond J, Addala A, Vanscheidt W, Stücker M, Goerge T, Perceau G, Chahim M, Wicks G, Perez J, Tacca O, Bohbot S. Evaluation of two fibrous wound dressings for the management of leg ulcers: results of a European randomised controlled trial (EARTH RCT). J Wound Care. 2014;23(3):105–16.
12. Meaume S, Truchetet F, Cambazard F, Lok C, Debure C, Dalac S, Lazareth I, Sigal ML, Sauvadet A, Bohbot S, Dompmartin A, CHALLENGE Study Group. A randomized, controlled, double-blind prospective trial with a Lipido-Colloid Technology-Nano-OligoSaccharide Factor wound dressing in the local management of venous leg ulcers. Wound Repair Regen. 2012;20(4):500–11.
13. Edmonds M, Lázaro-Martínez JL, Alfayate-García JM, Martini J, Petit JM, Rayman G, Lobmann R, Uccioli L, Sauvadet A, Bohbot S, Kerihuel JC, Piaggesi A. Sucrose octasulfate dressing versus control dressing in patients with neuroischaemic diabetic foot ulcers (explorer): an international, multicentre, double-blind, randomised, controlled trial. Lancet Diabetes Endocrinol. 2018;6(3):186–96.
14. Munter KC, Meaume S, Augustin M, Senet P, Kerihuel JC. The reality of routine practice: a pooled data analysis on chronic wounds treated with TLC-NOSF wound dressings. J Wound Care. 2017;26(suppl 2):4–15.
15. Vandamme L, Heyneman A, Hoeksema H, Verbelen J, Monstrey S. Honey in modern wound care: a systematic review. Burns. 2013;39(8):1514–25.

Open Access This chapter is licensed under the terms of the Creative Commons Attribution-NonCommercial-NoDerivatives 4.0 International License (http://creativecommons.org/licenses/by-nc-nd/4.0/), which permits any non-commercial use, sharing, distribution and reproduction in any medium or format, as long as you give appropriate credit to the original author(s) and the source, provide a link to the Creative Commons license and indicate if you modified the licensed material. You do not have permission under this license to share adapted material derived from this chapter or parts of it.

The images or other third party material in this chapter are included in the chapter's Creative Commons license, unless indicated otherwise in a credit line to the material. If material is not included in the chapter's Creative Commons license and your intended use is not permitted by statutory regulation or exceeds the permitted use, you will need to obtain permission directly from the copyright holder.

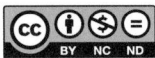

Surgical Debridement

Sadanori Akita

60.1 Introduction

Surgical debridement in acute and chronic wounds plays a crucial role in the wound healing process. Debridement is believed to accelerate wound healing and reduce the wound area by removing necrotic tissue, hyperkeratotic epidermis, necrotic dermis, foreign debris, and bacterial pathogens, which all have inhibitory effects on wound healing [1]. Microarray analysis has shown marked cytoplasmic reduction and localization of the epidermal growth factor receptor (EGFR) in the epidermis, indicating that non-healing keratinocytes have a diminished capacity to respond to EGF. Additionally, fibroblasts derived from non-healing wounds demonstrate decreased migration [2]. This molecular analysis suggests that proper surgical debridement may be an effective solution to overcome these challenges. However, the evidence and rationale for this technique should be further discussed for each specific pathologic condition, such as leg and diabetic foot ulcers.

Prior to surgical debridement, it is important to optimize the patient's nutrition. If these criteria are not met, it may be best to delay wound closure until conditions are more favorable for the surgeon, physician, and patient. Debridement can be beneficial for both acute and chronic wounds. If a wound is able to produce granulation tissue without bacterial overload, it is typically ready for subsequent skin grafting or flap coverage. For wounds that are unable to develop a granulation tissue bed, bioactive dressings or topical growth factors may be used.

60.2 Pathophysiology of the Underlying Diseases and Conditions in Surgical Debridement

60.2.1 Burns

In the case of deep burns (third-degree burns, which penetrate all skin layers), surgical debridement of dead, eschar, and necrotic tissues is nearly always necessary. In general, surgical debridement continues until fresh tissue and bleeding are observed. This procedure may be performed in a multiplane fashion. After complete and thorough surgical debridement, skin coverage with a skin graft, flap, or bioengineered material such as an artificial dermis is usually required. Skin grafting is the most commonly used method for skin coverage as it can cover larger post-surgical debrided wound beds and is easier to handle. Split-skin grafting is used for less vascular beds, as it has a lower metabolic demand compared to full-thickness grafts. These

S. Akita (✉)
Department of Plastic Surgery,
Tamaki-Aozora Hospital, Tokushima, Japan

Fukushima Medical University, Fukushima, Japan
e-mail: akitas@hf.rim.or.jp

areas with limited vascularity include the paratenon (tendon sheath), periosteum (bone envelope), and perineurium (neural envelope). Adequate debridement and skin coverage are particularly crucial in pediatric burn cases (Fig. 60.1).

In the case of deep dermal burns (second-degree burns, partial-thickness burns), surgical debridement is typically used in conjunction with skin grafting, but the debate continues. Some deep dermal burn wounds may heal within 2–3 weeks, and aggressive surgical debridement may not be necessary in such cases. However, the current standard techniques for determining burn depth and making treatment decisions are largely dependent on the subjective assessment of the clinician and can be inaccurate, even among experienced surgeons. A porcine contact deep dermal burn of 50 cm^2 in size, which takes more than 3 weeks to heal through re-epithelialization by proliferation and migration of keratinocytes from the skin appendages in the deep dermis, is a model that can best demonstrate the impact of surgical interventions on burn healing [3].

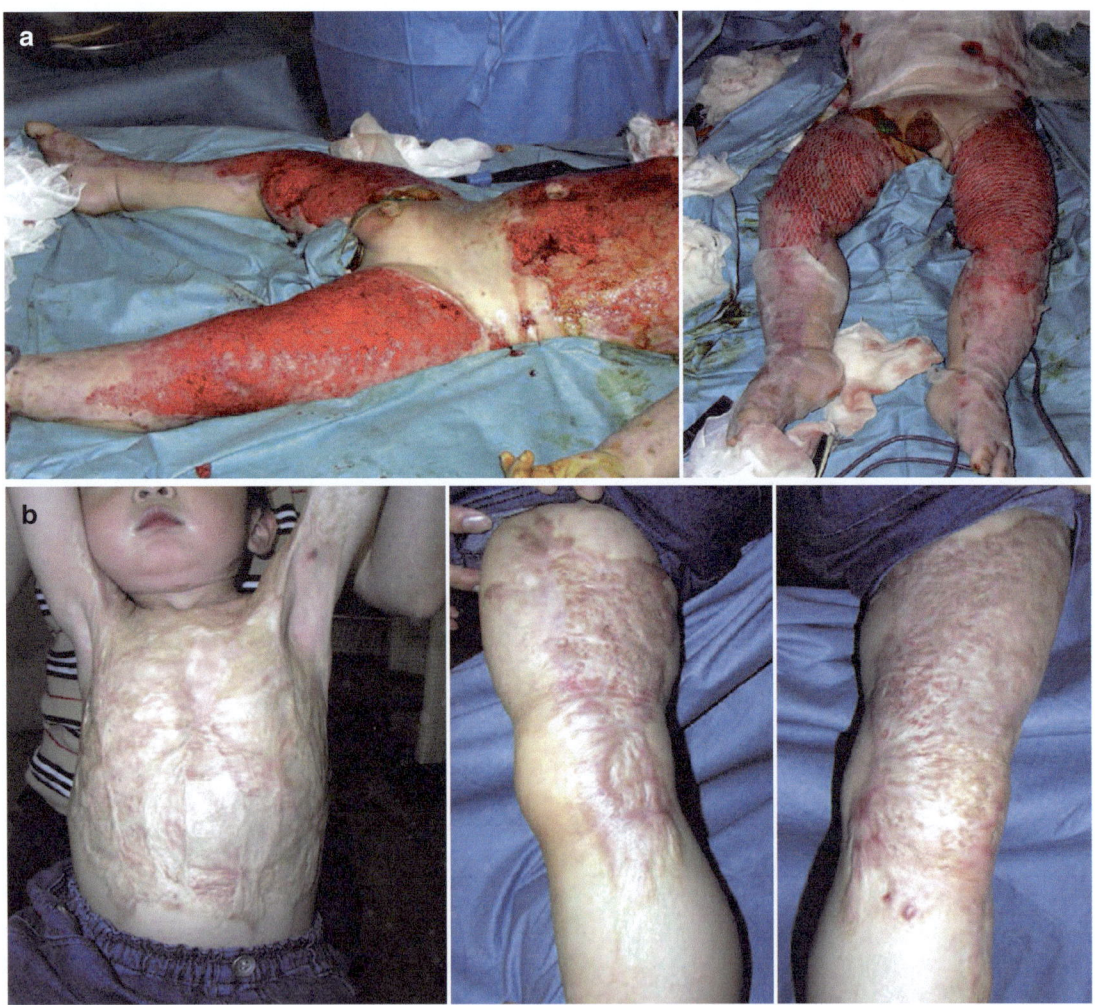

Fig. 60.1 (**a**) A 9-month-old boy, extensive scald burn, debridement, and mesh skin grafting. (**b**) A 1.5 years after surgery

60.2.2 High-Energy Trauma Wound

As is often observed in the orthopedic specialty, high-energy open fractures often result in deep infections due to extensive damage and the presence of necrotized tissue [4]. In a study comparing the use of negative pressure wound therapy (NPWT) and a control group, 5.4% of the NPWT group developed delayed deep infections, while 28% of the control group developed deep infections. High-energy wounds are prone to infection due to both acute and delayed insufficient blood supply and extensive tissue damage.

Traumatic wounds can be caused by both blunt and penetrating injuries. Blunt trauma typically results in a larger area of tissue damage and can include injuries such as crush, degloving, and avulsion. The extent of these wounds is not always clear and may change after aggressive debridement of non-vitalized tissue, bacterial control, and fluid maintenance. In these cases, temporary coverage with artificial dermis and further assessment may improve proper healing (Fig. 60.2).

60.2.3 Pressure Injury

Pressure ulcers are a reflection of a patient's systemic health, including physical, nutritional, social, and psychological status. The complex pathophysiology of pressure injuries requires several stages of evolution. Firstly, sustained pressure or shear force is applied to the soft tissue between the body mass, bony process, and surface. This reduces capillary vessel flow and oxygen and nutrient transfer, leading to occlusion of blood vessels and lymphatic vessels and capillary thrombosis. The tissues become ischemic, causing an increase in capillary permeability and fluid accumulation in the third space (extravascular space). Pressure-related intact discolored areas of the skin are described as non-blanching erythema or suspected deep tissue injury. The prevalence of

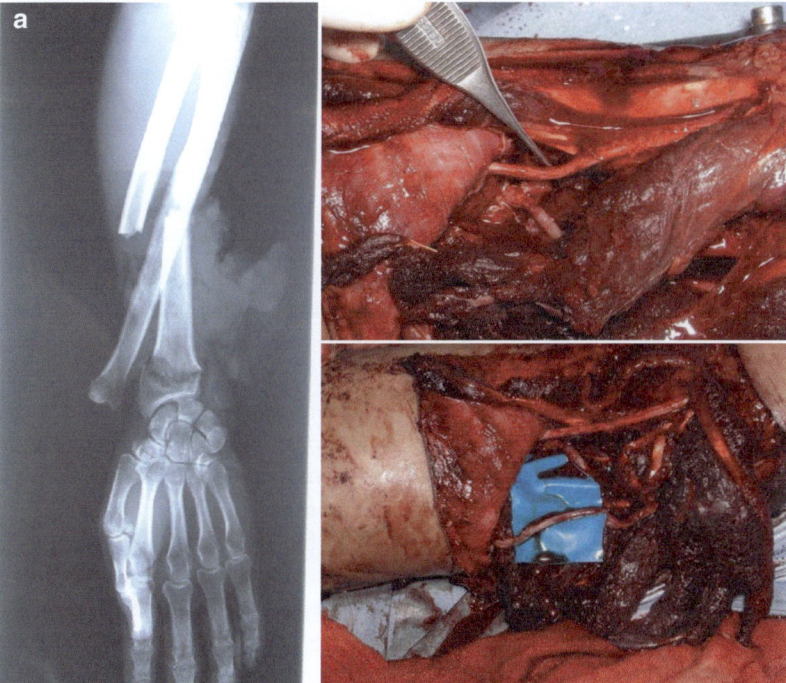

Fig. 60.2 (a) A 67-year-old man, high-energy injury, open fractures of the ulna and radius, externally intact but later found thrombus-formed radial artery (*right above*) and severed ulnar artery after microanastomosis. (b) External fixation with thorough debridement and artificial dermis (*top*), 10 days later, some tissues are still necrotic and further debridement and flap reconstruction (*middle*), 2 years after reconstruction (*bottom*)

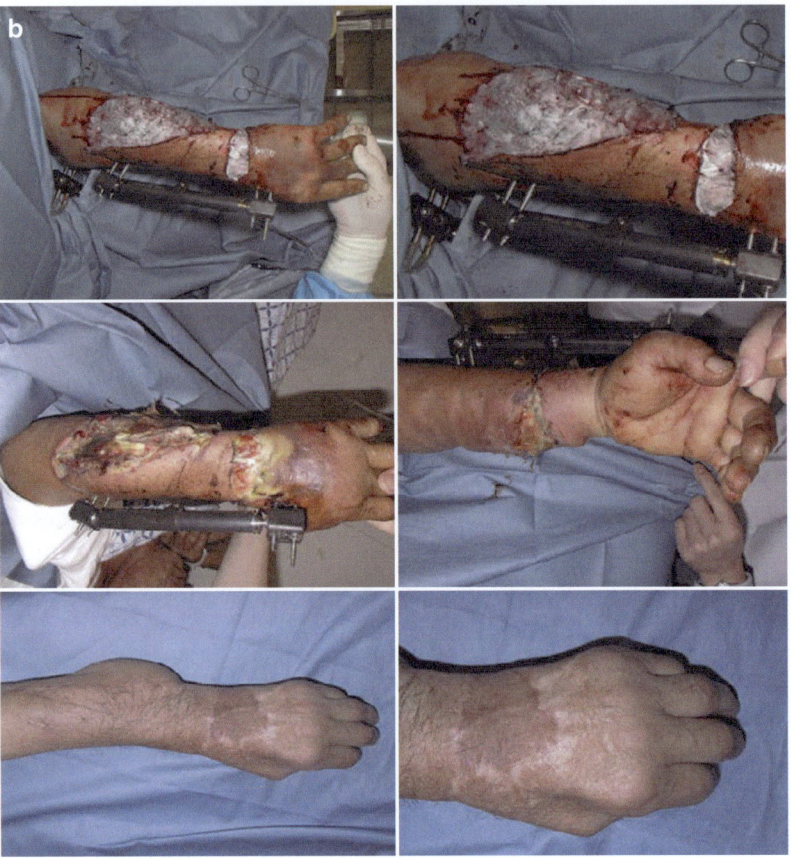

Fig. 60.2 (continued)

suspected deep tissue injury is more frequent than deeper pressure ulcers such as stage III or IV and has increased more recently than any other stages of pressure ulcers [5]. Edematous tissues may result in necrosis, which is irreversible. Precise debridement is considered when necrosis of tissue has occurred. The deep surgical intervention may start with evaluating the necrosis of the tissue and how to effectively remove it from the healthy surrounding tissue (Fig. 60.3).

60.2.4 Diabetic Foot Ulcer

The etiology of diabetic foot is a result of several combined factors, including peripheral vascular (arterial) disease, as well as sensory, motor, and autonomic neuropathy [6]. It is essential to evaluate the patient objectively for ischemia and underlying deep tissue issues, such as bone infections. Standard of care for the diabetic foot involves surgical debridement, proper wound dressings, and appropriate off-loading to promote moist wound healing. This can help to convert a chronic non-healing wound into an acute wound healing environment by removing senescent or non-vital cells, thereby improving the wound environment and enabling better local treatment response [7].

A biopsy of the edge of a non-healing chronic wound shows a hyperproliferative epidermis with hyper- and parakeratotic elements [2]. This is largely due to repetitive stress in the foot with sensory disturbances. Despite the activation of keratinocytes at the non-healing edge, wound healing is still impaired. Nuclear localization of β-catenin leads to downstream activation of c-Myc and the glucocorticoid pathway, resulting

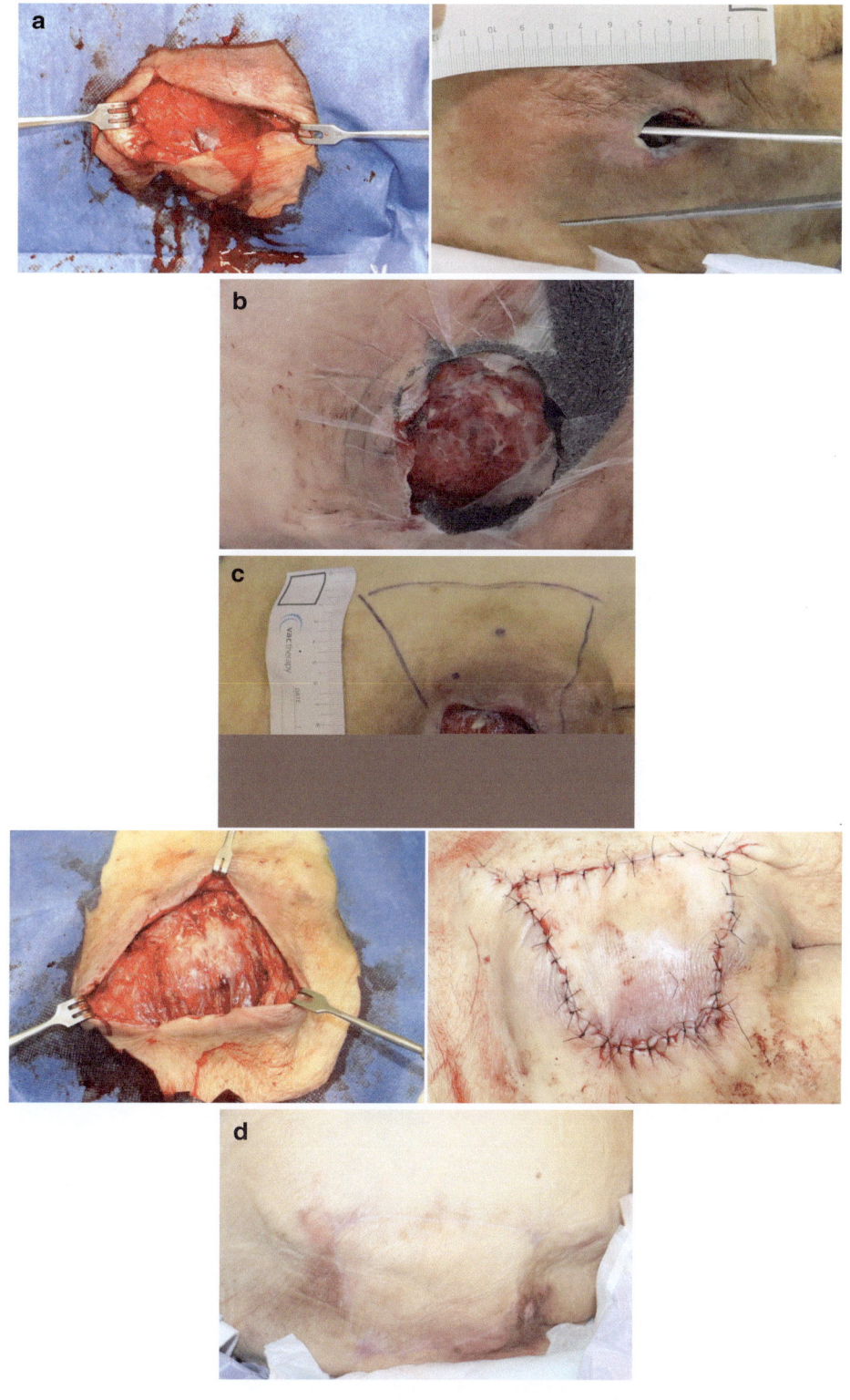

Fig. 60.3 A 92-year-old male, sacral pressure ulcer (**a**) Sacral pressure ulcer proved by a instrument. Wound opened fully. (**b**) 3-week negative pressure wound therapy provied an optimal wound bed with good granulation tissue (**c**) A perforator arterialized flap designed (**d**) Flap covered the defect and remained closed at 9 months post-operatively

in the inhibition of keratinocyte migration [8]. Microarray analysis of non-healing ulcers reveals a reduction and cytoplasmic localization of EGFR, which decreases responsiveness to EGF. The fibroblasts at the edges of non-healing wounds display a clear pathogenic phenotype and slower migration [2]. Diabetic foot ulcers with ischemic conditions are often seen in hemodialysis would develop a rapid progression of necrosis and may result in major amputation (Fig. 60.4).

60.2.5 Leg Ulcer

Although venous ulcers are always linked to venous hypertension during ambulation, the exact mechanism connecting the pathological hemodynamics in venous circulation to the formation of necrotic lesions in the skin remains unknown. It appears that the underlying causes are more complex than previously anticipated. Numerous experiments have shown that tissue injury in venous ulcer patients is caused by leukocytes. These cells become trapped in the microcirculation of the legs when they are in a dependent position. Subsequently, several authors have confirmed that this process is exacerbated in patients with chronic venous insufficiency (CVI). It is believed that the increased trapping of leukocytes in patients with CVI is due to an increase in the expression of adhesion molecules in the capillaries of the papillary dermis. In patients with CVI, leukocytes enter the microvascular regions affected by venous hypertension. As the distance between leukocyte adhesion molecules and endothelial adhesion molecules is less than 1 μm, the first step in the leukocyte–endothelial interaction is the displacement of leukocytes toward the endothelium by erythrocytes. This process occurs predominantly in postcapillary venules. When circulating leukocytes

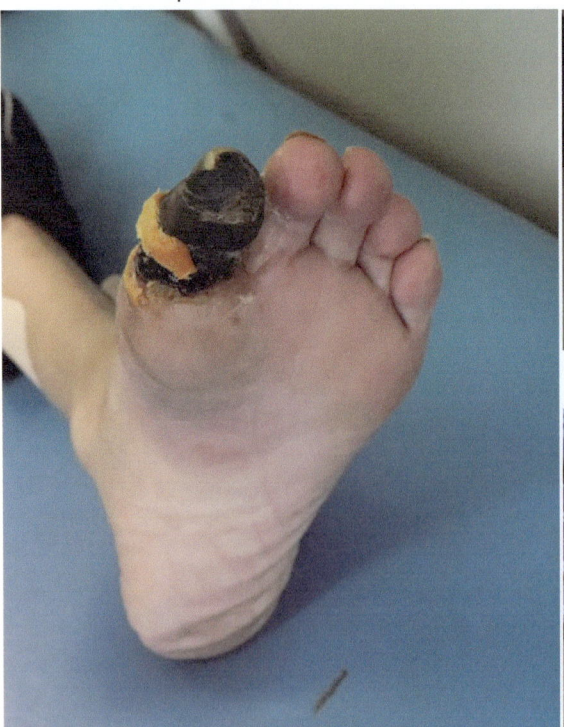

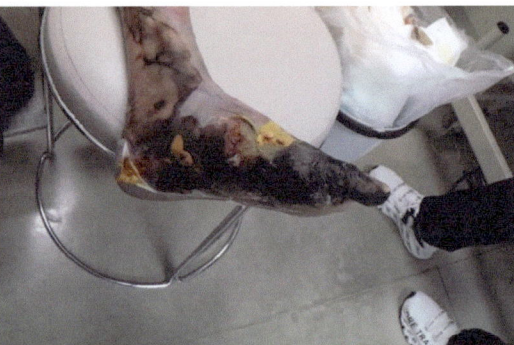

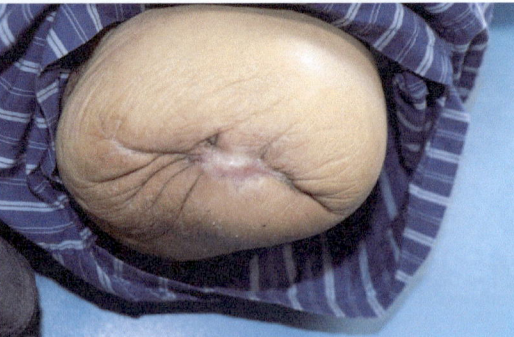

Fig. 60.4 A 73-year-old male, neuro-ischemic diabetic foot ulcer and necrosis resulted in a major amputation

encounter the endothelium, they may start to form weak, rolling adhesive interactions mediated by L-selectin and P-selectin glycoprotein ligand-1 (PSGL-1) on leukocytes and P-selectin and E-selectin on endothelial cells. Hypertension in postcapillary venules has been shown to increase leukocyte rolling and adhesion. Rolling leukocytes can then develop into stationary adhesion, which is dependent on the interaction between adhesion molecules CD11/CD18 on leukocytes and intercellular adhesion molecule-1 (ICAM-1) on endothelial cells. Once the leukocytes are firmly adhered to the vascular wall, they can migrate into the extravascular space, become activated, and trigger an inflammatory process in the skin and surrounding tissues. VCAM-1 is another adhesion molecule that plays a role in the process of leukocyte adhesion to the endothelium, and its expression is heightened in patients with CVI [9].

60.3 Choice of the Surgical Debridement

Wound bed preparation through sharp and mechanical debridement using surgical instruments is the most essential step in managing wound healing. This method effectively and selectively reduces the bio-burden of a wound. Elimination of necrotic tissue, which serves as a breeding ground for bacteria competing for the same nutrients and oxygen needed for wound healing, is crucial for promoting normal tissue healing. If the boundary between healthy and devitalized skin is not clear, consider tangential excision, starting from the center of the necrotic skin, until scattered bleeding is seen in the dermis. However, bleeding is not necessarily an indicator for debridement of subcutaneous tissue as fat tissue has less vascularity compared to skin. The debridement should continue until the shimmering yellowish fat tissue level is reached. Hemostasis can be achieved through clamping or compression, and scattered bleeding can be controlled through electrocautery. If bleeding from larger diameter vessels is observed, ligation should be attempted.

Fascia that is not vascularized should be removed with caution to avoid damaging the neurovascular bundles in the superficial area. Muscles, tendons, cartilage, and bones can be resected if there is no visible blood supply. In the case of deep tissue injury in pressure ulcers, sharp penetration to the muscle and deeper tissue level can be useful in determining the extent of the wound.

Surgical equipment includes scalpel blades, pickups, electrocautery, scissors, curettes, rongeurs, elevators, chisels, osteotomes, saws, rasps, burrs, the Harmonic scalpel, Cavitron ultrasonic surgical aspirator (CUSA®), water-jet (hydro-jet) system (Versajet II), radio-frequency energy system (Coblation® technology), low-frequency ultrasound debriding device (SonicVac), and more. Further information will be covered in Part VI.

References

1. Cardinal M, Eisenbud DE, Armstrong DG, Zelen C, Driver V, Attinger C, Phillip T, Harding K. Serial surgical debridement: a retrospective study on clinical outcomes in chronic lower extremity wounds. Wound Repair Regen. 2009;17:306–11.
2. Brem H, Stojadinovic O, Diergelmann RF, Entero H, Lee B, Pastar I, Golinko M, Rosenberg H, Tomic-Canic M. Molecular markers in patients with chronic wounds to guide surgical debridement. Mol Med. 2007;13:30–9.
3. Wang XQ, Kempf M, Liu PY, Cuttle L, Chang HE, Kravchuk O, Mill J, Phillips GE, Kimble RM. Conservative surgical debridement as a burn treatment: supporting evidence from a porcine model. Wound Repair Regen. 2008;16:774–83.
4. Stannard JP, Volgas DA, Stewart R, McGwin G Jr, Alonso JE. Negative pressure wound therapy after severe open fractures: a prospective randomized study. J Orthop Trauma. 2009;23:552–7.
5. VanGilder C, MacFarlene GD, Harrison P, Lachenbruch C, Meyer S. The demographics of suspected deep tissue injury in the United States: an analysis of the international pressure ulcer prevalence survey 2006–2009. Adv Skin Wound Care. 2010;23:254–61.
6. Edwards J, Stapley S. Debridement of diabetic foot ulcers. Cochrane Database Syst Rev. 2010;1:CD003556.
7. Everett E, Nestoras Mathioudakis N. Update on management of diabetic foot ulcers. Ann N Y Acad

8. Stojadinovic O, Brem H, Vouthounis C, Lee B, Fallon J, Stallcup M, Merchant A, Galiano RD, Tomic-Canic M. Molecular pathogenesis of chronic wounds: the role of beta-catenin and c-myc in the inhibition of epithelialization and wound healing. Am J Pathol. 2005;167:59–69.

9. Coleridge S. Deleterious effects of white cells in the course of skin damage in CVI. Int Angiol. 2002;21:26–32.

Open Access This chapter is licensed under the terms of the Creative Commons Attribution-NonCommercial-NoDerivatives 4.0 International License (http://creativecommons.org/licenses/by-nc-nd/4.0/), which permits any non-commercial use, sharing, distribution and reproduction in any medium or format, as long as you give appropriate credit to the original author(s) and the source, provide a link to the Creative Commons license and indicate if you modified the licensed material. You do not have permission under this license to share adapted material derived from this chapter or parts of it.

The images or other third party material in this chapter are included in the chapter's Creative Commons license, unless indicated otherwise in a credit line to the material. If material is not included in the chapter's Creative Commons license and your intended use is not permitted by statutory regulation or exceeds the permitted use, you will need to obtain permission directly from the copyright holder.

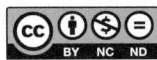

61

Stabilization of Necrotic Tissue Using Cerium Nitrate Silver Sulfadiazine

Chloé Geri

61.1 Introduction

The association in the form of a cream, silver sulfadiazine with cerium nitrate is a topical product conventionally used in the management of burns. Its antibacterial efficacy and its interest in stabilizing necrosis by the formation of a "scab" have made it an essential alternative to surgery in this indication.

Apart from burns, there are many wounds for which healing theoretically requires a rapid excision of the necrotic areas. Their management therefore begins with a careful assessment of the possibility or otherwise of debridement and the choice of the "surgical moment" [1, 2].

For example, a major vascular insufficiency will contraindicate debridement, the risk being a renecrosis of the edges; as a progressing cancer wound will represent a risk of dissemination when cleansing.

By extrapolation, the use of this effective, easy to use, topical antibacterial agent presenting few contraindications could therefore be an alternative to debridement, by stabilization of the crust due to a powerful antibacterial effect preventing the elimination fold to occur.

C. Geri (✉)
CICAT-Occitanie, Montpellier, France
e-mail: c-geri@chu-montpellier.fr

61.2 Burns Are the Classic Indication

Flammacerium has not been evaluated by the HAS working group which worked on the evaluation of dressings [3], but its current indication in France is the prevention and treatment of infections in extensive burns with deep lesions [4].

This antibacterial cream, effective against Staphylococcus aureus (85–93%) and Pseudomonas aeruginosa (83–98%) [5], is linked to an effect of combination of silver sulfadiazine and cerium nitrate. It helps preventing infection in severe burns [6]. In addition, it causes the formation of a protective crust on the burn. This crust promotes protection against bacterial colonization and could reduce water and calorie losses. Moreover, by maintaining this protection for a long time, it makes it possible to best choose the surgical moment.

A review of the literature in 2005 [7] established that this dressing reduced morbidity and mortality in the treatment of severe burns thanks to the mechanism of creating a "protection" on the burn as well as its capture of the lipid–protein complex released by the burned skin, responsible for profound local immunosuppression. It was also demonstrated that the application of Flammacérium® made it possible to delay, without short- or long-term consequences, the surgical treatment of serious burns [8]. A study published in 2007 on predictive markers of mortality in burn victims concluded that the use of Flammacerium® was a turning point in terms of morbidity and mortality [9], even if the great diversity of changes in the treatment of burns did not confirm that this treatment was the sole agent of these improvements.

61.3 Contraindications and Adverse Effects

There are currently no strict contraindications to its use.

However, it requires precautions for use in the event of allergy to sulfonamides, in patients with renal and hepatic impairment [10], and in pregnant or breastfeeding women (due to limited study data in these situations).

Rare adverse effects are reported in the studies: systemic passage of sulfonamides which may be responsible for adverse effects such as leukopenia (rarely observed) or methemoglobinemia [11–13] (in patients with very extensive burns) which normally disappear after discontinuation of treatment, a skin reaction such as dermatitis or eczema (due to an excipient: cetyl alcohol or propylene glycol) (less than 1% of cases) reversible on discontinuation of treatment [6], and granulomatous dermatitis (one case described in the literature [14]).

In addition to the direct antiseptic effects, cerium therefore helps to prevent sepsis and limit the systemic inflammatory response by fixing toxins. These beneficial effects have long been demonstrated in patients with severe burns [3, 15–19]; however, there is little or no literature regarding the use of this topical in other indications.

61.4 Clinical Indications Outside Burns

61.4.1 Arterial Leg Ulcer

When tissue necrosis is present on a wound, debridement may be necessary to remove necrotic tissue, reduce the risk of infection, accelerate wound healing, and prevent complications [20, 21]. However, it is not recommended to clean a wound on arterial ground, the risk being the extension of the necrosis. In the case of arterial ulcers, the recommendations state that debridement is contraindicated when vascular circulation is compromised at the level of the wound [22–24]. Indeed, guidelines specify that before performing any type of debridement of the extremities, in particular below the knee, the patient must be evaluated from an arterial point of view (level of evidence IV), by knowing the medical history, cardiovascular risk factors of the patient, palpation of the pulses and the measurement of the IPS/IPSO, and the realization of an arterial Doppler [25]. The guidelines also mention that debridement is contraindicated in the presence of dry gangrene or a dry ischemic wound until a complete vascular evaluation is carried out [22], and that while waiting for a revascularization procedure (or not), the necrosis must be preserved and mummified to protect against the risk of infection in the event of wet necrosis (Fig. 61.1).

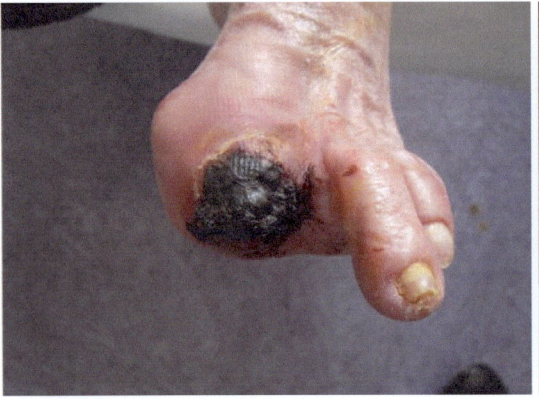 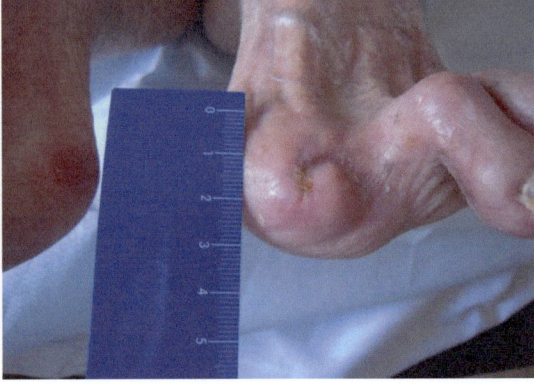

Fig. 61.1 Renecrosis after amputation in arteritic context

61.4.2 Heel Pressure Ulcer in the Elderly Patient

According to its 2006 recommendations, the HAS (French Ministry of Health) recommends systematic screening for PAD in patients at risk of pressure ulcers under the age of 65 and in all patients over the age of 65 [26].

A cohort survey conducted by S. Meaume in 2007 attempts to establish the link between PAD and heel pressure ulcers [27]. Strategies to relieve pressure on the heel seem to become insufficient to prevent pressure ulcers, probably due to the increase in PAD (often asymptomatic) in elderly patients.

And conversely, patients with heel ulcers may have associated risk factors such as peripheral vascular disease leading to delayed wound healing [27, 28]. Peripheral vascular disease should be assessed as a co-morbidity for lower extremity pressure ulcers [29, 30] by clinical assessment, including presence of pulse, capillary re-staining time, edema, or mobility. The purpose of carrying out a vascular diagnostic test by measuring the ABI >0.86 is to rule out arterial disease in a heel pressure sore, making it possible to help with the differential diagnosis and the classification of the severity of the disease arterial pathology [31]. Caution is advised to ensure the absence of PAD in these patients presenting with a heel sore [32]. A local lesion stabilization strategy is then proposed until the vascular assessment is completed in order to consider a revascularization procedure if this is possible. In a recent article, replacing the recommendations cited in the NPUAP, caution would lead to keeping necrotic tissue (mummification) as dry as possible to protect against infection and odor [33].

61.4.3 Diabetic Foot Ulcer

Similarly, diabetic foot wounds are often accompanied by distal arteriopathy, sometimes inaccessible to revascularization, with a high risk of necrosis and superinfection, placing this pathology at the forefront of causes of non-traumatic amputation [34–36]. Stabilization of wounds and necrotic tissues is also indicated until vascular assessment has been carried out (and revascularization if necessary) (Fig 61.2).

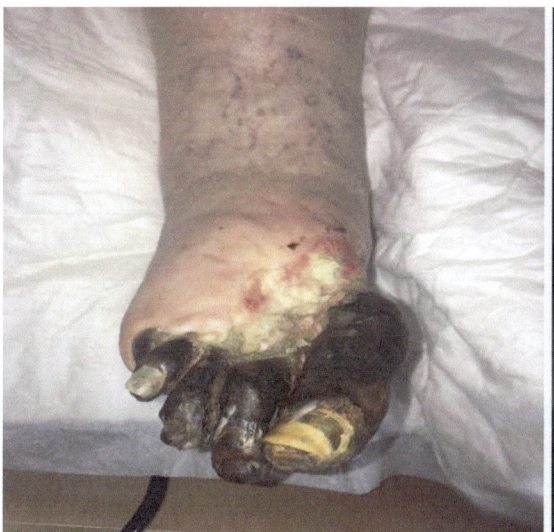
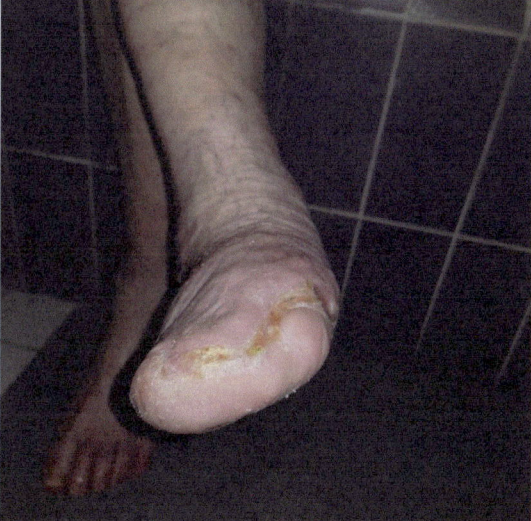

Fig. 61.2 Stabilization of distal necrosis then healing after spontaneous amputation in a demented ambulant patient with severe PAD

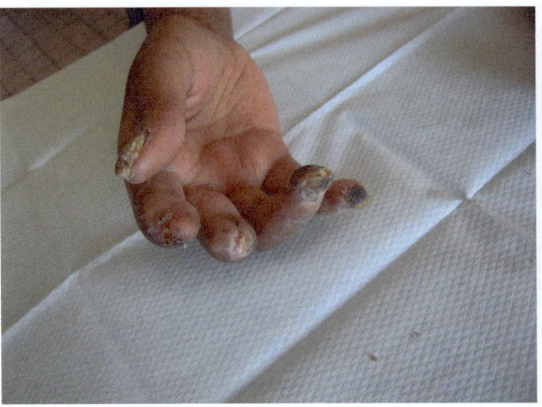 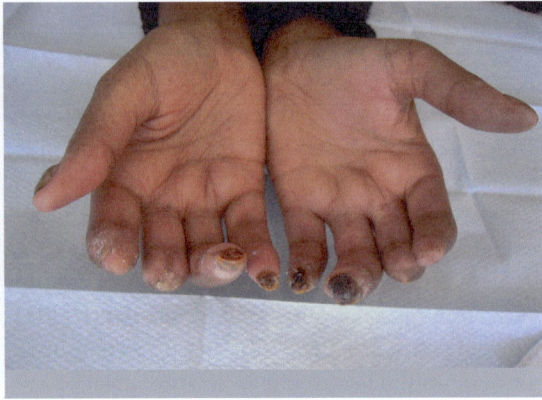

Fig. 61.3 Scleroderma

61.4.4 Cutaneous Lesions of Microvascular Etiology

In the forefront of which necrotizing angiodermatitis presents a contraindication to debridement linked on the one hand to the intensity of the pain but also because of the phenomenon of pathergy: each gesture of debridement causing worsening of the lesion with extension of the necrotic area.

For example, in Buerger's disease (thromboangiitis obliterans), cutaneous manifestations of vasculitis, or scleroderma, the microvascular pathology is partly responsible for necrosis and explains the effectiveness of treatment with ilomedin (Fig. 61.3).

61.5 Other Factors of Delayed Healing

61.5.1 Malignant Wound

The debridement of a tumor wound is a potentially hemorrhagic and painful act with a high risk of dissemination. Indeed, the bed of the tumoral wound and the necrosis which covers it or composes it, are constitutive of the tumor and the excision is impossible in many situations: the healing being only possible if the complete oncological excision is possible [37] (healthy wound edges and safety margins). The necrosis of these wounds is linked to the ischemia of the tumor mass. It is therefore the local consequence and not the cause of a local disease (primary cancer) or disseminated disease (cutaneous metastases), most often progressive. It is not always understood that necrosis can be left in place on a tumor wound, unlike the vast majority of other chronic wounds. However, the presence of necrotic tissue exposes the patient to a risk of infection, extension of the lesion, and numerous inconveniences such as significant exudate or nauseating odors generally linked to the presence of anaerobic germs [38]. The purpose of treatment is then not to move toward healing, but to make the wound cleaner, leading to a favorable evolution when the long-term treatment allows it (chemotherapy), or only to treat symptoms (odors, for example) in a palliative context [39, 40].

61.5.2 Radionecrosis

Radionecrosis is often a late complication of radiotherapy. When it escapes to standard treatment (anti-inflammatories, local care, etc.) [41], it requires surgical excision of all the damaged tissues with, most often, a reconstructive procedure (skin graft, flap, etc.). This excision is unfortunately not always possible.

Indeed, when the radionecrosis is complicated by osteoradionecrosis on areas such as the thorax or the skull, it is sometimes impossible to remove the bone and the underlying structures (pleura, meninges, etc.). After evaluation of the depth and extension of the necrosis by MRI imaging, a decision to stabilize the lesion can be considered as an alternative to a highly dilapi-

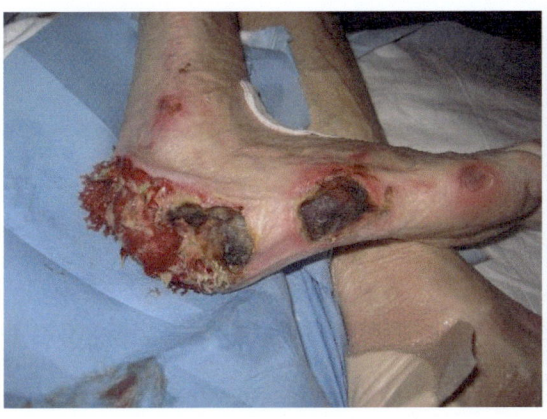 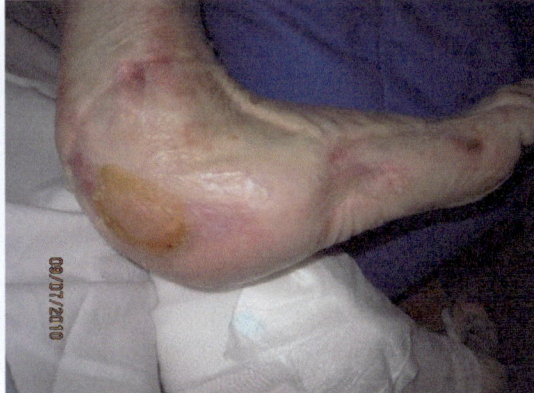

Fig. 61.4 Heel PU, malnutrition, arteriopathy

dated surgical procedure in patients who are sometimes fragile and elderly because the skin lesions can appear for many years even decades after radiotherapy.

61.5.3 Other Types of Wounds

Other situations, less classic, may present contraindications to cleansing, for example, wounds related to certain treatments (antimitotics, corticosteroids, etc.) or certain inflammatory pathologies with cutaneous manifestations. Only the suspension of the treatment in question or the treatment of the responsible pathology is likely to improve the healing prognosis. It should also be noted that, in certain situations, the treatment of the pathology in question can, itself, be deleterious for healing (corticosteroids, for example). Waiting solutions should be considered with the objective of "temporization" by stabilizing and protecting the wound, allowing a slow healing process out of germs, limiting painful symptoms and the risk of infection.

61.6 End of Life and/or Multiple Comorbidities

Although healing requires, whenever possible, the excision of necrotic tissue, clinical experience shows that the objective, when managing a complex wound, is not always healing. Indeed, severe malnutrition, extreme fragility, the association of multiple comorbidities, very old age, or the end of life sometimes orient management toward comfort care and contraindicate aggressive mechanical debridement. Dressing changes will be spaced out to avoid painful mobilizations, and exudates and odors must be managed with a view to dignity and to allow end-of-life support by those around them (Fig 61.4).

61.7 Discussion and Perspectives

A retrospective study was carried out in 2010 to determine the efficacy of Flammacerium® in stabilizing necrosis in chronic wounds [42]. It included 99 patients with wounds for which debridement was contraindicated (42 arterial ulcers, 30 bedsores, 5 cancerous wounds, 10 traumatic wounds, and 12 other types of wound). This study showed an improvement in pain, a decrease in exudates and bad odors, and a positive effect on quality of life, corresponding to an increase in patient comfort, participation in social activity and psychological well-being. In addition, by delineating the necrosis, the use of this topical gives practitioners more time to prepare for subsequent surgical treatment, including skin grafting.

In 2018, a study [43] on 50 patients completed this research and assessed the effectiveness of Flammacerium® on ischemic necrosis wounds of the lower limb as an alternative to amputation (50 patients, 25 in each group). Despite a non-significant difference, amputation-free survival was superior in the active treatment group compared to the standard group.

In addition to its role of stabilization by the formation of a protective "crust," Flammacerium® would then bring an element of comfort by its anti-inflammatory and analgesic properties, in particular on radionecrosis or in very painful pathologies such as angiodermatitis or necrosis digitalis related to scleroderma.

Following these initial elements, Flammacerium® was studied retrospectively more specifically on angiodermatitis [44] (out of 82 patients between 2013 and 2018: 25 benefited from a transplant, 23 from Flammacerium®, and 34 from two therapies). The treatment was compared versus the pellet graft, which is the usual treatment for an angiodermatitis flare-up. The results indicated that Flammacerium® could have a greater analgesic effect than skin grafting. In a second phase, a monocentric randomized pilot clinical trial in 2018 showed an analgesic benefit of Flammacerium® with an ability to restart the healing process at least as effective or even superior to skin grafting.

The anticancer potential of cerium compounds is being re-explored in an experimental setting, although the mechanistic basis remains to be elucidated [6].

61.8 Conclusion

Flammacerium® has long demonstrated its effectiveness in the prevention of sepsis in burn victims and its role in the inflammatory response. Its advantages include easy and painless application, limiting the necrotic area by the formation of a crust allowing good resistance to infection (Figs. 61.1, 61.2, 61.3, and 61.4).

But Flammacerium® seems to have a promising place in stabilizing necrosis in other chronic wounds for which debridement is contraindicated.

On all the wounds for which a vascular involvement is evoked, the stabilization of the necrotic zone could make it possible to limit and postpone the surgical excisions, and to be more conservative: the gesture of revascularization, if it is possible, can then be programmed under good conditions.

By extension, Flammacerium® can also be offered in all situations contraindicating debridement, whether related to pain, pathergy, or poor healing prognosis.

Finally, in a palliative situation, it can participate in the improvement of painful symptoms or stabilize the risk of infection.

Flammacerium® can then be considered as an interim solution, or even an alternative to surgery in much broader indications than burns.

References

1. Teot L. Debridement of wounds, review general. JPC. 1996;(3):7–12.
2. Téot L. [The "surgical moment" in the care of chronic wounds]. Soins. 2000;(642 Suppl):9–11.
3. Recommandations HAS. Evaluation des pansements primaires et secondaires. 2007.
4. French Edition. Recommendations Vidal. 2011.
5. Monafo WW, Tandon SN, Ayvazian VH, et al. Cerium nitrate: a new topical antiseptic for extensive burns. Surgery. 1976;80(4):465–73.
6. Jakupec MA, Unfried P, Keppler BK. Pharmacological properties of cerium compounds. Rev Physiol Biochem Pharmacol. 2005;153:101–11.
7. Garner JP, Heppell PSJ. Cerium nitrate in the management of burns. Burns. 2005;31(5):539–47.
8. Vehmeyer-Heeman M, Tondu T, Van den Kerckhove E, Boeckx W. Application of cerium nitrate-silver sulphadiazine allows for postponement of excision and grafting. Burns. 2006;32(1):60–3.
9. Vehmeyer-Heeman M, Van Holder C, Nieman F, Van den Kerckhove E, Boeckx W. Predictors of mortality: a comparison between two burn wound treatment policies. Burns. 2007;33(2):167–72.
10. Hirakawa K. [Determination of silver and cerium in the liver and the kidney from a severely burned infant treated with silver sulfadiazine and cerium nitrate]. Radioisotopes. 1983;32(2):59–65.
11. Attof R, Rachid A, Magnin C, et al. Methemoglobinemia by cerium nitrate poisoning. Burns. 2006;32(8):1060–1.
12. Poredos P, Gradisek P, Testen C, Derganc M. Severe methemoglobinaemia due to benzocaine-containing "burn cream": two case reports in an adult and in a child. Burns. 2011;37(7):e63–6.
13. Kath MA, Shupp JW, Matt SE, et al. Incidence of methemoglobinemia in patients receiving cerium nitrate and silver sulfadiazine for the treatment of burn wounds: a burn center's experience. Wound Repair Regen. 2011;19(2):201–4.

14. Boye T, Terrier J-P, Coillot C, et al. Cerium-induced granulomatous dermatitis. Ann Dermatol Venereol. 2006;133(1):50–2.
15. Hermans RP. Topical treatment of serious infections with special reference to the use of a mixture of silver sulphadiazine and cerium nitrate: two clinical studies. Burns Incl Therm Inj. 1984;11(1):59–62.
16. Boeckx W, Focquet M, Cornelissen M, Nuttin B. Bacteriological effect of cerium-flamazine cream in major burns. Burns Incl Therm Inj. 1985;11(5):337–42.
17. Scheidegger D, Sparkes BG, Lüscher N, Schoenenberger GA, Allgöwer M. Survival in major burn injuries treated by one bathing in cerium nitrate. Burns. 1992;18(4):296–300.
18. Ross DA, Phipps AJ, Clarke JA. The use of cerium nitrate-silver sulphadiazine as a topical burns dressing. Br J Plast Surg. 1993;46(7):582–4.
19. Koller J, Orsag M. Our experience with the use of cerium sulphadiazine in the treatment of extensive burns. Acta Chir Plast. 1998;40(3):73–5.
20. Bluestein D, Javaheri A. Pressure ulcers: prevention, evaluation, and management. Am Fam Physician. 2008;78(10):1186–94.
21. Langemo D, Thompson P, Hunter S, Hanson D, Anderson J. Heel pressure ulcers: stand guard. Adv Skin Wound Care. 2008;21(6):282–92; quiz 293–294.
22. National Guideline Clearinghouse. Chronic wounds of the lower extremity. 2007. http://www.guideline.gov/.
23. National Guideline Clearinghouse. Pressure ulcer prevention and treatment. Health care protocol. 2010. http://www.guideline.gov/.
24. National Guideline Clearinghouse. Guideline for prevention and management of pressure ulcers. 2010. http://www.guideline.gov/.
25. National Institute for Health and Clinical Excellence; Guidelines for the measurement of ankle brachial pressure index using doppler ultrasound. 2010. www.nice.org.uk/cg48.
26. Recommandation. Prise en charge de l'ulcère de jambe à prédominance veineuse hors pansement, HAS. 2006. http://www.has-sante.fr.
27. Meaume S, Faucher N. Heel pressure ulcers on the increase? Epidemiological change or ineffective prevention strategies? J Tissue Viability. 2008;17(1):30–3.
28. Graham J. Heel pressure ulcers and ankle brachial pressure index. Nurs Times. 2005;101(4):47–8.
29. Fowler E, Scott-Williams S, McGuire JB. Practice recommendations for preventing heel pressure ulcers. Ostomy Wound Manage. 2008;54(10):42–8, 50–52, 54–57.
30. Institute for Healthcare Improvement. Prevent pressure ulcers. 2007.
31. Rennert R, Golinko M, Yan A, et al. Developing and evaluating outcomes of an evidence-based protocol for the treatment of osteomyelitis in stage IV pressure ulcers: a literature and wound electronic medical record database review. Ostomy Wound Manage. 2009;55(3):42–53.
32. Ribal E, Lano J. Ankle-brachial index measurement: analysis of the consequences and implications for the debridement of heel pressure ulcers. J wound Technol. 2012;32–36(16).
33. St-Cyr D. [Decubitus ulcer of the heel: evidence concerning debridement]. Perspect Infirm. 2010;7(2):26–8.
34. Monteiro-Soares M, Boyko E, Ribeiro J, Ribeiro I, Dinis-Ribeiro M. Predictive factors for diabetic foot ulceration: a systematic review. Diabetes/metabolism research and reviews. 2012. http://www.ncbi.nlm.nih.gov/pubmed/22730196. Accessed 14 Sept 2012.
35. Chin JW, Teague L, McLaren A-M, Mahoney JL. Non traumatic lower extremity amputations in younger patients: an 11-year retrospective study. International wound journal. 2012. http://www.ncbi.nlm.nih.gov/pubmed/22329536. Accessed 14 Sept 2012.
36. Anon. Data Points Publication Series. Rockville, MD: Agency for Healthcare Research and Quality (US); 2011. http://www.ncbi.nlm.nih.gov/pubmed/22049561. Accessed 14 Sept 2012.
37. Fromantin I. [Debridement of cancerous wounds]. Soins. 2011;(752):53.
38. Lazelle-Ali C. Psychological and physical care of malodorous fungating wounds. Br J Nurs. 2007;16(15):S16–24.
39. Grocott P. The management of fungating wounds. J Wound Care. 1999;8(5):232–4.
40. Isabelle F, Kriegel I, Baffie A, Téot L. La place du Flammacerium® dans la prise en charge des plaies complexes en oncologie. J Plaies Cicatris. 2013;90(XVIII):25–8.
41. Delanian S, Lefaix J-L. Current management for late normal tissue injury: radiation-induced fibrosis and necrosis. Semin Radiat Oncol. 2007;17(2):99–107.
42. Signe-Picard C, Cerdan M-I, Naggara C, Téot L. Flammacérium in the formation and stabilisation of eschar in chronic wounds. J Wound Care. 2010;19(9):369–70, 372, 374 passim.
43. Vitse J, Tchero H, Meaume S, Dompmartin A, Malloizel-Delaunay J, Geri C, Faur C, Herlin C, Teot L. Silver sulfadiazine and cerium nitrate in ischemic skin necrosis of the leg and foot: results of a prospective randomized controlled study. Int J Low Extrem Wounds. 2018;17(3):151–60.
44. Toch S. Évaluation du Flammacérium versus greffe de peau pour la prise en charge de l'angiodermite nécrotique: étude pilote contrôlée randomisée, réalisée au Centre Hospitalier Universitaire de Montpellier Thèses d'exercice et mémoires - UFR de Médecine Montpellier-Nîmes.

Open Access This chapter is licensed under the terms of the Creative Commons Attribution-NonCommercial-NoDerivatives 4.0 International License (http://creativecommons.org/licenses/by-nc-nd/4.0/), which permits any non-commercial use, sharing, distribution and reproduction in any medium or format, as long as you give appropriate credit to the original author(s) and the source, provide a link to the Creative Commons license and indicate if you modified the licensed material. You do not have permission under this license to share adapted material derived from this chapter or parts of it.

The images or other third party material in this chapter are included in the chapter's Creative Commons license, unless indicated otherwise in a credit line to the material. If material is not included in the chapter's Creative Commons license and your intended use is not permitted by statutory regulation or exceeds the permitted use, you will need to obtain permission directly from the copyright holder.

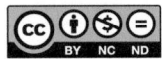

Honey Debridement

Vijay K. Shukla and Vivek Srivastava

62.1 Introduction

A wound is a disturbance in the normal structure and function of the epidermis, the first line of defence against infection. Wound healing is a complex process with many interdependent immunological and pathophysiological mediators to restore the cellular integrity of the damaged tissue. Four distinct and overlapping stages are involved: Hemostasis, inflammation, proliferation/regeneration and tissue re-modelling [1]. Presence of necrotic slough is a hindrance in the natural as well as assisted wound healing process and acts as a focus for infection. Additionally, it encourages the multiplication of anaerobic bacteria, which can cause wound malodour. Moreover, the TIME framework used in wound bed preparation also advocates removal of devitalized tissue in order to promote a reduction in the inflammatory response, encourage wound contraction and decrease in the bacterial burden of a wound. Debridement of slough and necrotic material is the key element associated with wound bed preparation and best practice guidelines [2, 3]. Among various methods of debridement, dressing with natural compounds like honey has been used with success in the last decade.

For thousands of years, honey has been used for medicinal applications. The beneficial effects of honey, particularly its antimicrobial activity, represent its useful option for management of various wounds [4]. Honey dressings contain major amounts of carbohydrates, lipids, amino acids, proteins, vitamin and minerals that have important roles in wound healing with advantage of minimum trauma during re-dressing. The mechanisms of action of honey in wound healing are majorly due to its hydrogen peroxide, high osmolality, acidity, non-peroxide factors, nitric oxide and phenols [5]. Honey promotes autolytic debridement, stimulates growth of wound tissues and anti-inflammatory activities and thus accelerates the wound healing processes [5–7].

62.2 Antibacterial Properties

Due to the high osmolarity of honey secondary to its high sugar content, microbial growth is greatly inhibited. Further, the sugar molecules within the honey hold onto the water molecules, and the bacteria are devoid of enough water to support their growth. This effect is lessened as the honey becomes more and more diluted by the wound exudates [6]. However, the antimicrobial properties are retained, even when the honey is diluted by exudate. This is due to the presence of hydrogen peroxide which is slowly released by action of the enzyme, glucose oxidase, which is added to the honey by the bees during production and becomes activated as the honey is diluted by exudate. This hydrogen peroxide which is released at

V. K. Shukla (✉) · V. Srivastava
Department of General Surgery, Institute of Medical Sciences, Banaras Hindu University, Varanasi, India

a concentration of 1000 times less than the traditional 3% solution of hydrogen peroxide is formerly used as a wound cleansing agent, thus negating the potential for cellular damage [6]. However, some honeys, particularly the Leptospermum or Manuka honeys, have been found to retain their bactericidal properties even without the presence of hydrogen peroxide and are effective against both antibiotic-sensitive and antibiotic resistant organisms [8] which are thought to be associated with an unidentified phytochemical component within the honey. It has been demonstrated that the antibacterial activity of honey persists in preventing Pseudomonas, Methicillin-resistant Staphylococcus aureus (MRSA) and Vancomycin-sensitive or resistant Enterococci, common pathogens found in chronic wounds and burns, even if the honey is diluted more than ten times by wound exudate [8].Therefore, Manuka honey is sold with a unique Manuka factor (UMF) rating (equivalent to the concentration of phenol which has the same activity against S. aureus), which rates the antimicrobial activity of its phytochemical component [6].

62.3 Debridement

Debridement is recognized to be an essential procedure for achieving wound healing in chronic wounds and wounds with devitalized tissue. Debridement needs to be done rapidly as slough is a potential substrate for bacterial growth. Debridement is also necessary to ascertain the extent of a wound, which will influence further management. As honey dressings provide a moist environment due to water retention, it provides an environment which can encourage autolytic debridement of sloughy and necrotic wounds. It has also been suggested that proteases within the tissues may be activated by the hydrogen peroxide present in honey, leading to the rapid debriding property of honey, along with the ability of honey to aid conversion of plasminogen to plasmin which facilitates breakdown of devitalized tissue within a wound. Successful outcomes in the reduction of slough and eschar of between 10 days to 10 weeks have been reported in patients with infected venous leg ulcers and burns [9]. In general, proteases are inactive in wound tissue and can be activated by oxidation. Proteases are also able to change the conformation of MMPs and make them active. It has been postulated that high protease activity in the wound may impair wound healing but such effect has never been proved. In fact, potent anti-inflammatory action of honey can prevent excessive proteolytic activity [10]. Plasmin digests the fibrin attached to the slough in wound surface, but does not digest the collagen matrix which is needed for tissue repair. Honey is able to inhibit production of the plasminogen activator inhibitor (PAI) by the macrophages. On the other hand, inflammation increases production of PAI, thus reduction in production of PAI by honey is a good reason for its anti-inflammatory activity.

Debridement is a basic necessity to induce the functional process of tissue repair. The standard procedure for the debridement of wounds is to surgically remove any dead tissue which may be a painful procedure and usually is performed under anaesthesia in operation room [10]. Aggressive and invasive debridement methods on the other hand may cause growth of infecting toxin producing bacteria which can destroy the surrounding tissues. Application of honey as wound dressing provides a moist environment that induces rapid debridement of wounds. The osmotic and water retaining property of honey owing to the high sugar content contributes to the painless lifting off of the slough and necrotic tissues.

Evidence to support the effectiveness of the various methods of debridement gained from randomized controlled trials is inadequate. Clinical evidence obtained before year 2000 was based on the use of generic honey and not on sterile, medical-grade honey [11] but in later years the effectiveness of medical-grade honey has been demonstrated with robust research designed specifically for wound management. There is now a growing body of evidence that supports the use of medical-grade honey as an effective autolytic debriding agent [7]. There have been several studies that highlight the effectiveness of honey as a debriding agent [12, 13].

A study done on 40 patients of non-responders of compression therapy venous ulcer patients showed a significant improvement in wound size and decrease in malodour and pain after application of Manuka honey with an average rate of reduction in wound area was 5.46% [14]. Similar results were seen in study by Gethin and Cowman [15] who compared honey to hydrogel in 108 patients with leg ulcers that had >50% slough and found honey to be a superior debriding agent. Biglari et al. [16] observed patients of category III and IV pressure ulcers following spinal trauma with Manuka honey application to support autolysis of necrotic and sloughy tissue. Encouraging results were found in form of negative swabs after a week of application and 18 out of 20 patients (90%) showed complete wound healing after a period of 4 weeks. Some interesting case reports of honey dressing for debridement and healing are also reported. A case study of an elderly patient with plantar aspect sloughy wound has been reported. Honey was used as a first-line antimicrobial dressing in a community hospital setup showing a positive outcome [17]. Within 2 weeks, there was a significant improvement in the wound and infection had improved significantly resulting in change of honey to hydro-fibre dressing. However, the following week, the wound deteriorated with friable granulation with increase in exudate volume. Honey dressings were reapplied, thus supporting the effectiveness of honey as a first-line antimicrobial agent.

A comparative study evaluating chemical and honey debridement method over a 15-day evaluation period in 20 patients was done. All patients were of diabetic foot sloughy ulcers in foot. Patients were divided into four groups including one for commercially available chemical debridement and others for different types of honey. The chemical group had daily dressing changes, as per manufacturer's directions, and the other three groups were changed every 3 days. The rate of debridement showed that the chemical agent was the slowest and 100% debridement was achieved with the honey which contained 100% pure medical-grade Manuka honey with no additives or preservatives [18].

Wounds in paediatric and neonatal group of patients need special and tender care. The skin tends to be very fragile and may have immature immune systems and impaired thermoregulation, putting them at higher risk of infection when necrotic or sloughy tissue is present. There may be a risk of percutaneous absorption of topical agents. In a study including 115 neonatal and paediatric, wounds needing debridement were treated with honey dressing. Successful debridement was achieved in 86.0% (104 wounds), and 77.7% wounds (94 wounds) were successfully closed using non-surgical intervention. There was no evidence of wound infection during this study. The author concluded that Manuka honey was a safe and effective treatment option in this category of patients [19].

A study on seven patients with facial burns treated with Manuka honey measuring healing time, bacterial growth, patient satisfaction, and cost was done. Healing time was consistent with, or better than standard treatment, a mean healing time of 8.1 days. None of the patients were given antibiotic treatment, with wound culture results yielding no abnormal bacterial growth and overall patient satisfaction was high, incurring a cost of $26.15 per patient. This study showed that Manuka medical-grade honey is a feasible option both clinically and economically for treatment of partial-thickness facial burns [20].

62.4 Tissue Growth

Honey promotes the formation of granulation and epithelial tissue within a wound following debridement by encouraging the creation of collagen and subsequent angiogenesis. The rapid appearance of granulation tissue has been supported by in vitro studies in animals [8] and has also been supported with clinical studies in patients with burns and other infected wound [21]. It is thought that the nutritional composite of honey provides sugar, amino acids, vitamins, and minerals to the cells, encouraging growth. Alternatively, it may be due to the acidic pH of honey which encourages the release of oxygen from haemoglobin to the tissues [22].

62.5 Deodorizing

An increase in wound odour is one clinical indication of wound infection. This can be embarrassing and distressing for a patient and also their relatives who have to live with this symptom. The reduction in malodour following the topical application of honey can in part be attributed to its antibacterial properties and its bactericidal effects on the anaerobic bacteria. Moreover, it has been suggested that the malodorous substances created by bacteria such as fatty acid, ammonia, and sulphur compounds from the metabolism of amino acid is stopped when the bacteria use the glucose obtained from honey in preference to the amino acids.

62.6 Anti-inflammatory Action

An anti-inflammatory effect has been attributed to honey, and this has been supported histologically by biopsies taken from superficial burn wounds [23]. By reducing the inflammation within a wound, vasodilatation can occur with a resultant reduction in wound exudate and oedema, along with a reduction in the level of pain [22]. It is unclear, however, how this anti-inflammatory effect occurs.

62.7 Contraindications

Honey dressings should be avoided in patients with a known history of allergy to either honey or bee venom. Patients with diabetes should also have their blood sugar monitored as they may be at higher risk of hyperglycaemia due to the sugar content of the honey. However, there appears to be little evidence on the use of honey in patients with diabetes, thus guidance in this area is poor, and further research is advocated.

62.8 Conclusion

The use of honey as a modern wound dressing is gradually becoming more widespread. The antimicrobial action of honey has proved its value in the treatment of wounds infected with MRSA, Pseudomonas and Enterococcus. The evidence indicates that honey dressing can increase the wound healing rate and the bacterial clearance rate. In addition, it can shorten wound debridement time, wound healing time and bacterial clearance time. Acceptability of honey dressings appears to be high among patients. The impact on factors such as pain reduction, odour control and exudate management has positive impact on quality of life. The properties of honey that plays role in wound healing are summarized in Fig. 62.1. While studies have been conducted in patients with a variety of wounds including burn, the majority of evidence continues to come from patient case studies or small-scale studies. Honey impregnated dressings have only relatively recently been developed and become available for wound care use hence, supportive evidence for its application, effectiveness and future potential are still warranted. However, the studies to date have successfully demonstrated a place for honey within modern wound care armamentarium.

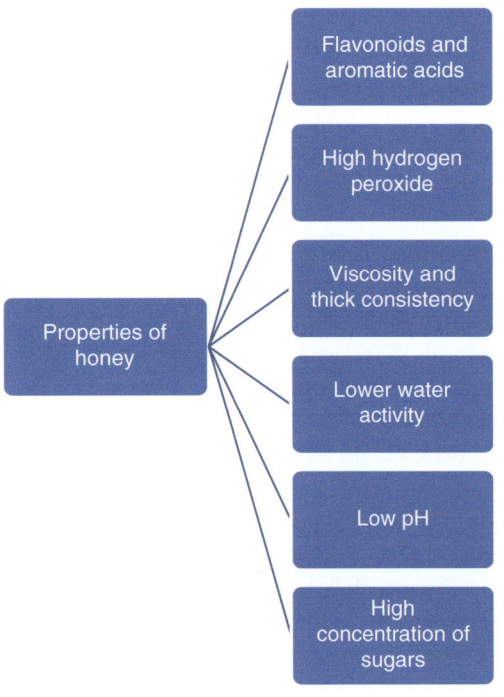

Fig. 62.1 Wound healing properties of Honey

References

1. Kus KJB, Ruiz ES. Wound dressings—a practical review. Curr Dermatol Rep. 2020;9:298–308.
2. Atkin L, Rippon M. Autolysis: mechanisms of action in the removal of devitalised tissue. Br J Nurs. 2016;25(20):S40–7.
3. Barrett S. Wound-bed preparation: a vital step in the healing process. Br J Nurs. 2017;26(12):S24–31.
4. Eteraf-Oskouei T, Najafi M. Traditional and modern uses of natural honey in human diseases: a review. Iran J Basic Med Sci. 2013;16(6):731–42.
5. Oryan A, Alemzadeh E, Moshiri A. Biological properties and therapeutic activities of honey in wound healing: a narrative review and meta-analysis. J Tissue Viability. 2016;25(2):98–118.
6. Hanaa T. Honey in wound healing: an updated review. Open Life Sci. 2021;16:1091–100.
7. Dunford C, Cooper R, Molan P, White. The use of honey in wound management. Nurs Standard. 2000;15(11):63–8.
8. Molan PC. The role of honey in the management of wounds. J Wound Care. 1999;8(8):415–8.
9. Roberts A, Brown HL, Jenkins R. On the antibacterial effects of manuka honey: mechanistic insights. Res Rep Biol. 2015;6:215–24.
10. Molan P, Cooper R, Molan P, White R. Honey in modern wound management. In: Why honey works, vol. 9. Aberdeen, UK: Wounds UK Ltd; 2009. p. 36–7.
11. Moore OA, Smith LA, Campbell F, Seers K, McQuay HJ, Moore RA. Systematic review of the use of honey as a wound dressing. BMC Complement Altern Med. 2001;1:2.
12. Gray D, White RJ, Cooper P, Kingsley AR. Understanding applied wound management. Wounds UK. 2005;1(1):62–8.
13. Blaser G, Santos K, Bode U, et al. Effect of medical honey on wounds colonised or infected in MRSA. J Wound Care. 2007;16(8):325–8.
14. Dunford CE, Hanano R. Acceptability to patients of a honey dressing for non-healing venous leg ulcers. J Wound Care. 2004;13(5):193–7.
15. Gethin G, Cowman S. Manuka honey vs hydrogel—a prospective, open label, multicentre, randomised controlled trial to compare desloughing efficacy and healing outcomes in venous ulcers. J Clin Nurs. 2009;18(3):466–74.
16. Biglari B, Linden PH, Simon A, Aytac S, Gerner HJ, Moghaddam A. Use of Medihoney as a non-surgical therapy for chronic pressure ulcers in patients with spinal cord injury. Spinal Cord. 2011;50(2):165–9.
17. Lloyd-Jones M. Case study: treating an infected wound of unknown aetiology. Br J Comm Nurs Suppl. 2012;17:S25–9.
18. Barcic M, Heasley D. Evaluation of a 100% Manuka honey (free of color additives and preservatives) in the debridement of diabetic foot ulcers versus a pharmaceutical chemical debrider and two other Manuka based products. Poster presentation symposium on advanced wound care (SAWC), Orlando, FL; 2014.
19. Amaya R. Safety and efficacy of active leptospermum honey in neonatal and paediatric wound debridement. J Wound Care. 2015;24(3):95–103.
20. Duncan CL, Enlow PT, Szabo MM, et al. A pilot study of the efficacy of active leptospermum honey for the treatment of partial-thickness facial burns. Adv Skin Wound Care. 2016;29(8):349–55.
21. Efem SEE. Clinical observations on the wound healing properties of honey. Br J Surg. 1988;75:679–81.
22. Molan P. Re-introducing honey in the management of wounds and ulcers—theory and practice. Ostomy Wound Manage. 2002;48(11):28–40.
23. Subrahmanyam M, Sahapure AG, Nagane NS, et al. Effects of topical application of honey on burn wound healing. Ann Burns Fire Disasters. 2001;15(3):143–5.

Open Access This chapter is licensed under the terms of the Creative Commons Attribution-NonCommercial-NoDerivatives 4.0 International License (http://creativecommons.org/licenses/by-nc-nd/4.0/), which permits any non-commercial use, sharing, distribution and reproduction in any medium or format, as long as you give appropriate credit to the original author(s) and the source, provide a link to the Creative Commons license and indicate if you modified the licensed material. You do not have permission under this license to share adapted material derived from this chapter or parts of it.

The images or other third party material in this chapter are included in the chapter's Creative Commons license, unless indicated otherwise in a credit line to the material. If material is not included in the chapter's Creative Commons license and your intended use is not permitted by statutory regulation or exceeds the permitted use, you will need to obtain permission directly from the copyright holder.

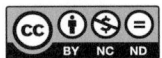

Recent Technologies in Necrosis Surgical Debridement

Luc Téot, Christian Herlin, and Sergiu Fluieraru

63.1 Introduction

This chapter describes the updated methods and respective indications of recent surgical debridement technologies applied for the management of necrotic tissues.

Their respective indications vary depending essentially on criteria like the hardness of the black cover and the extent of necrosis in depth and the extent of necrotic tissue over the skin.

Techniques using mechanical removal of a necrotic tissue have largely been diffused for many years; new techniques based on electrochemical removal of tissues using plasma technologies are now available and promising. Most of these technologies are not evidence based but are strongly defended by surgeons who aggressively clean the wound before getting a prepared wound bed prior to realizing a skin graft or a flap. A rapid and complete removal of undesired tissues from the wound, containing germs and biofilms, is the aim of any method of debridement [1, 2]. Successive technologies were proposed, from basic techniques using a scalpel to electrocautery, ultrasounds, lasers, high-power jets, and more recently plasma-based debriders.

L. Téot (✉) · C. Herlin · S. Fluieraru
Wound Healing Unit, Hôpital Lapeyronie,
Montpellier University Hospital, Montpellier, France
e-mail: l-teot@chu-montpellier.fr; s-fluieraru@chu-montpellier.fr

63.2 Description of Recently Developed Debridement Technologies

Scalpels and scissors were used by generations of surgeons, debridement being quickly and safely obtained within a short period of time. This technique used in trauma wounds is well defined, and, apart from necrosis, sloughy and fibrinous tissues should be removed, in order to minimize devascularization of the surrounding tissues.

1. Versajet™ (Smith and Nephew)

   - High-pressure hydrosurgery system of lavage by impulsions incrementing the debriding effect combined to an aspiration system linked to the Venturi effect may reach 850 bars [3].
   - Stationary and mobile use, the system includes an electrical power pad (pedal commanded) with a connection for saline perfusion and a single-use hose for saline perfusion connected to a trash collector to aspirate the debrided tissues [4, 5].
   - Allows to undermine, cut and excise, thanks to the high-speed liquid flow at the window level, with three different sizes (15°, 14 mm; 45°, 14 mm; 45°, 8 mm) (Fig. 63.1a–c).

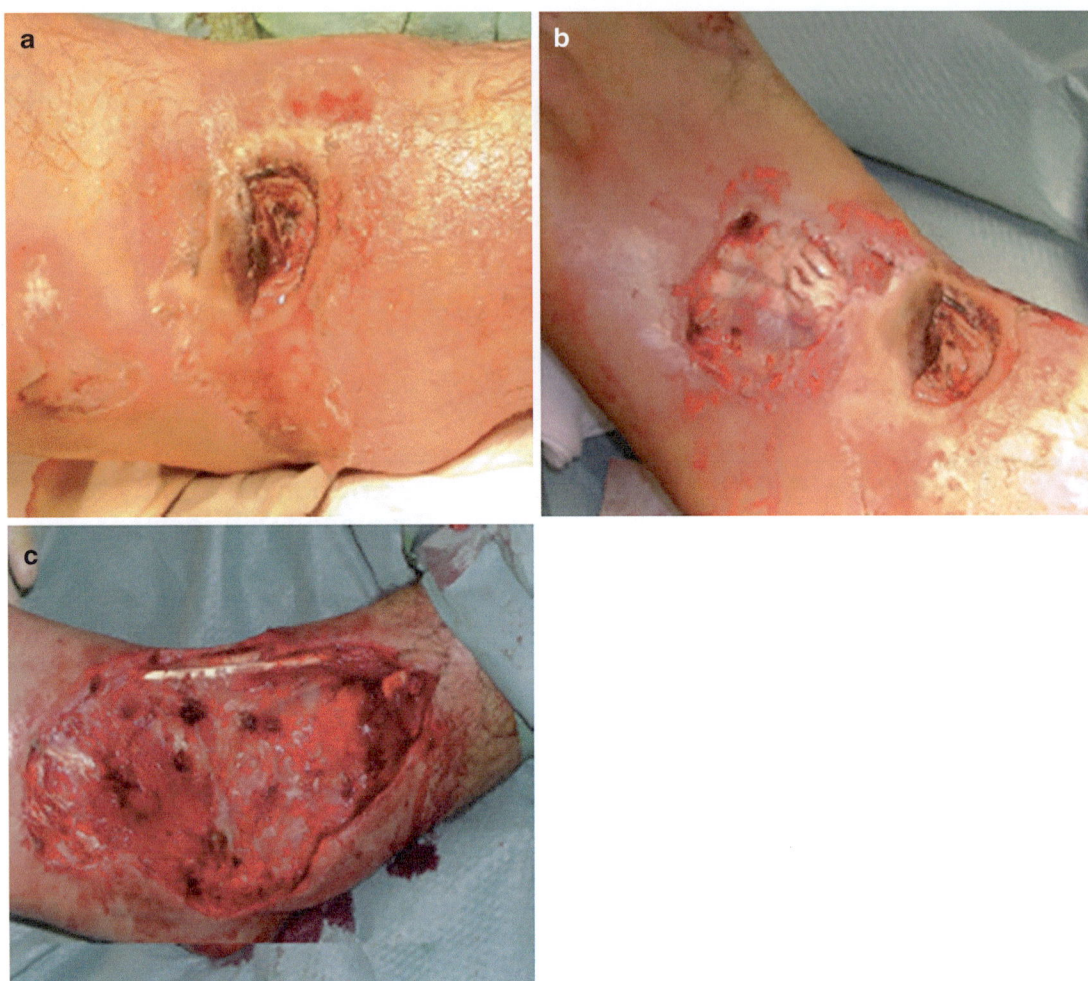

Fig. 63.1 (**a**) Electrical burns of the dorsal aspect of the foot. Extension of post burns necrotic tissue is hard to underline. (**b**) Starting debridement using Versajet$_{TM}$ exposes necrotic tendons. (**c**) Versajet$_{TM}$ has debrided step by step all devascularized structures, leaving the wound prepared for a skin graft

- Electrical burns: the extent in depth cannot be determined precisely.
- Using Versajet, hypodense necrotic structures will be destroyed and removed.
- Debridement completed: all remaining structures are living and ready to be covered using skin grafting.

2. **Instill Negative pressure Wound Therapy with vac cleanse choice (VCC) Foam**

    Recent improvement was proposed in the technology of NPWT including NPWT with instillation and dwell (NPWTi-d). NPWTi-d allows cleansing, irrigation, and nonexcisional debridement. Recent RCT have demonstrated that NPWTi-d decreases the time to complete wound healing and the length of hospitalization. NPWTi-d-using a reticulated open-cell foam dressing with "through" holes (ROCF-CC) facilitates solubilization, detachment, and elimination of infectious materials, such as slough and thick exudate. This technique is efficient and rapid (3–6 days max), limiting the time to get a drastic change of the wound surface in cases where surgical debridement is not an option [6, 7]. The combined action of the two superimposed layers, one perforated driving undesired tissues inside the holes and forming macrocolumns, the upper non-perforated ragging the top of these macrocolumns (Figs. 63.2 and 63.3).

3. **Cold Atmospheric Plasma**

Cold atmospheric plasma (CAP), a recent technology has been associated with benefits in wound infection and healing in different reports and randomized controlled trial of charged particles, free electrons and ions thermal, visible, and UV radiation and electrical fields, generate highly active species in the wound bed. These combined effects function as signaling or redox-reactive molecules. Ozone, hydroxyl radicals, superoxide, oxygen, and reactive nitrogen species, such as nitric oxide or peroxynitrite, are expected to act as active compounds [8].

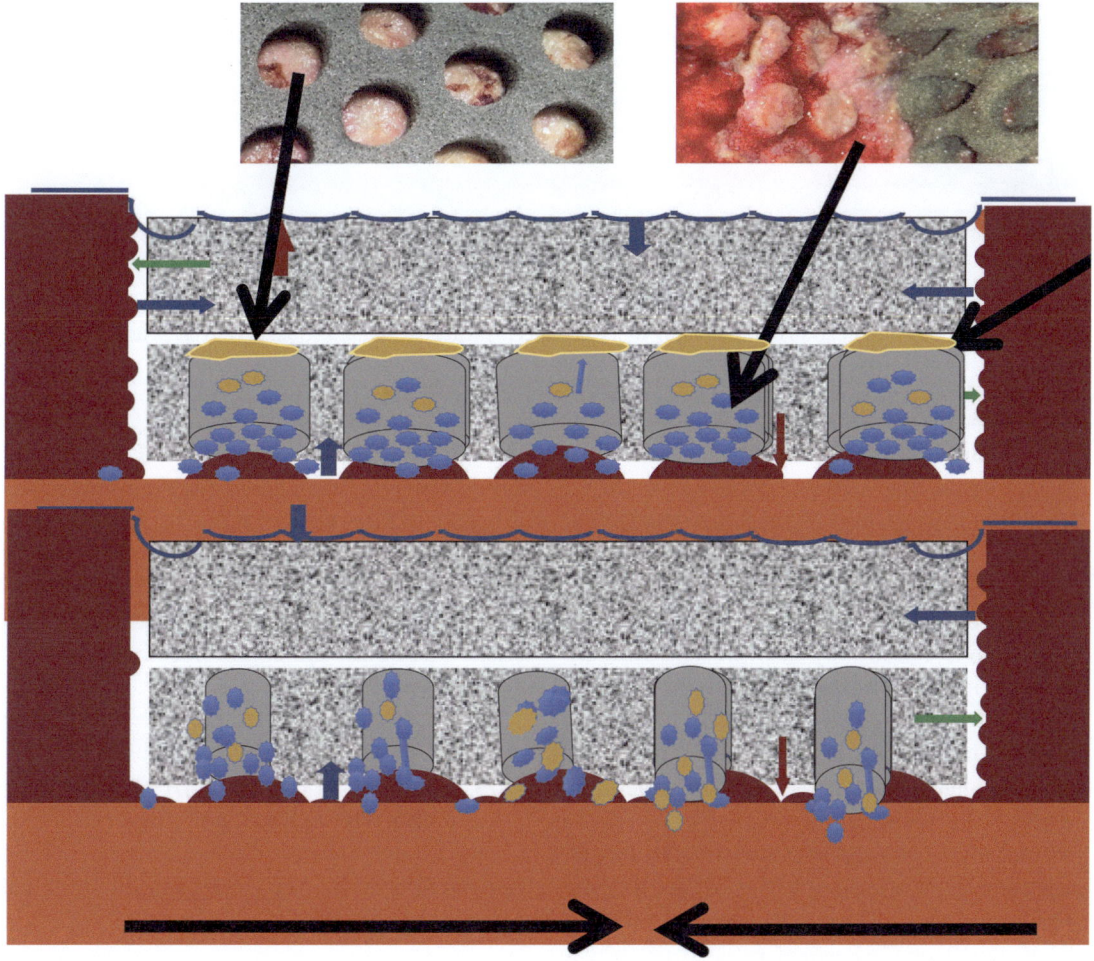

Fig. 63.2 The double mechanism of action of the through holes ROFC-CC foam is (&) a ragging effect on the wound seuface concentrating the undesired tissues in the holes, forming macrocolumns and (2) a ragging effect of the second non fenestrated layer over the top of the macrocolumns.

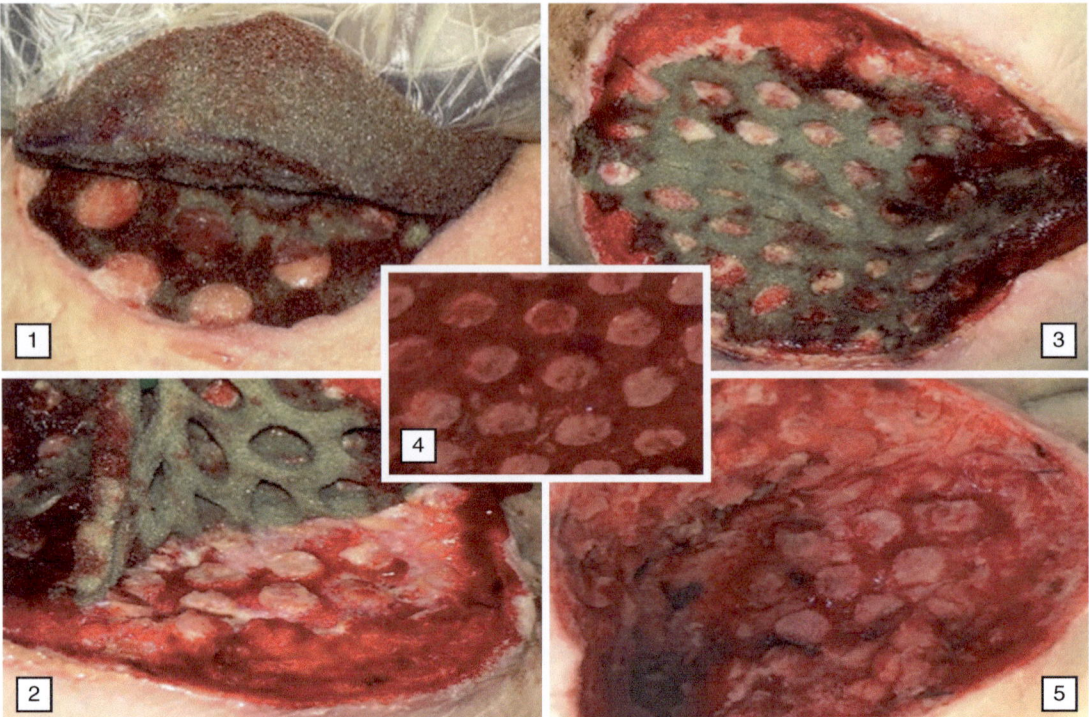

Fig. 63.3 (1,2,3,4,5): Extraction of the sloughy tissues by mechanical and solubilization. (1) day 3; (2 and 3) day 6; (4 and 5) day 9

63.3 Clinical Indications

The necrotic tissue density and the extent over the wound (uniform, sprayed, patches) and in the depth should be determined before using new expansive debridement techniques.

A necrotic tissue may also present different hardness, imposing different strategies in terms of management. In excessive bleeding observed in wound infection or in a patient under anticoagulation, haemorrhagic techniques should be limited. The need for saving blood during debridement is another important factor, having progressively restricted the use of sharp blade debridement to small wounds, preferring the use of Versajet™ or CAP when extensive debridement is needed over bleeding anatomical structures.

The interest of Versajet™ has been described in cavities and uneven wounds and the potential bacteriological long-term removal of germs when using the plasma technique. Debridement should minimize the wound edge devascularization and reduce the potential of renecrosis to minimum, using a good preoperative vascular check-up. Limits and contraindications of debridement are the poorly vascularized tissues where smooth nonaggressive technologies should be preferred.

63.3.1 Extent of Necrosis over the Wound Surface

The extent of a necrotic tissue may be presented under different aspects:

- Necrotic block: may form deep amount of necrotic tissues, extending in depth, with two separate parts, the superficial one, which looks hard and attached to the edges of the wound, and the deep one, which looks less dense,

formed by sloughy tissue. Encountered mainly in pressure ulcer but also after extensive hematomas of the leg
- Superficial uneven necrotic area: necrotic angiodermatitis may be covered with this type of necrotic tissue, unevenly spread over the ulcer surface, burns

63.3.2 Necrotic Tissues Vary Depending on the Aetiopathogeny of the Wound

- Burns

- Standard mechanical debridement using knives and/or scalpel is mostly used in this indication. However, local haemorrhage is the limiting factor, especially in extensive second-degree burns when tangential excision issues to excessive bleeding.

- The extent of the necrotic or sloughy tissues and the need to debride large areas should be analyzed before surgery, limiting the choice of the debriding operative technique. Time for surgical procedure and precise analysis of blood loss should help to choose the adapted technology. Most of the authors would agree not to exceed 10–15% of the body surface excision, plus harvesting the skin surface for skin grafts when necessary.

- In electrical burns, the extent of necrosis remains tricky to determine in the early stage as the complete necrosis will take 2 weeks before being obvious over the different impacted areas.
- Pressure ulcer cavity wounds
- Cavity wounds are difficult to debride, essentially at the cover level of undermined areas. This part has to be surgically removed to increase the granulation tissue formation coming from the lateral aspects and the deep part of the wound. Using NPWT with Instillation and the VCC foam, it is possible to get access to the whole cavity, after decaping the cover enough to allow to insert the foam inside the cavity and properly treat the edges.
- Necrotizing fasciitis

- The necrotic tissue is spread on an uneven manner, due to the heterogeneity of toxin repartition along the different tissues. The intensity of necrotic capacity is depending on the virulence of the germ.

63.4 Respective Indications of New Technologies

The JAC offers an adjunct to cleansing at home. This ambulatory technique has been proposed as capable of debriding small amount of tissues without the need for anaesthesia. The induced pain can easily be managed in the community or at home with simple measures.

Versajet offers the capacity of debriding localized hard necrotic tissue with a good precision, even if the window remains limited, creating a difficulty to uniformize the wound bed.

New cold atmospheric plasma replaces the previous laser techniques, offering a debridement leading to a germ-free wound bed well prepared for skin grafting. The action of plasma on germs has been demonstrated.

NPWT with Instillation and the new VCC foam is more adapted to large wounds with deep underminings in order to promote quickly a sterile granulation tissue and eliminate undesired tissues.

References

1. Téot L. Surgical debridement of wounds. Soins. 2011;752:36–7.
2. Granick M, Téot L. Surgical wound healing and management. 2nd ed. Informa Healthcare; 2012.
3. Bowling FL, Crews RT, Salgami E, Armstrong DG, Boulton AJ. The use of superoxidized aqueous solution versus saline as a replacement solution in the versajet lavage system in chronic diabetic foot ulcers: a pilot study. J Am Podiatr Med Assoc. 2011;101(2):124–6.
4. Fraccalvieri M, Serra R, Ruka E, Zingarelli E, Antoniotti U, Robbiano F, Viglione M, Frisicale L,

Bruschi S. Surgical debridement with Versajet: an analysis of bacteria load of the wound bed pre- and post-treatment and skin graft taken. A preliminary pilot study. Int Wound J. 2011;8(2):155–61.
5. Sainsbury DC. Evaluation of the quality and cost-effectiveness of Versajet hydrosurgery. Int Wound J. 2009;6(1):24–9. Review.
6. Téot L, Boissiere F, Fluieraru S. Novel foam dressing using negative pressure wound therapy with instillation to remove thick exudate. Int Wound J. 2017;14(5):842–8. https://doi.org/10.1111/iwj.12719. Epub 2017 Feb 28.
7. Rohrich RJ. The "soft-tissue wound management: current applications of negative-pressure wound therapy with instillation" supplement. Plast Reconstr Surg. 2021;147(1S-1):1S–2S. https://doi.org/10.1097/PRS.0000000000007629.
8. Stratmann B, Costea TC, Nolte C, Hiller J, Schmidt J, Reindel J, Masur K, Motz W, Timm J, Kerner W, Tschoepe D. Effect of cold atmospheric plasma therapy vs standard therapy placebo on wound healing in patients with diabetic foot ulcers: a randomized clinical trial. JAMA Netw Open. 2020;3(7):e2010411. https://doi.org/10.1001/jamanetworkopen.2020.10411.

Open Access This chapter is licensed under the terms of the Creative Commons Attribution-NonCommercial-NoDerivatives 4.0 International License (http://creativecommons.org/licenses/by-nc-nd/4.0/), which permits any non-commercial use, sharing, distribution and reproduction in any medium or format, as long as you give appropriate credit to the original author(s) and the source, provide a link to the Creative Commons license and indicate if you modified the licensed material. You do not have permission under this license to share adapted material derived from this chapter or parts of it.

The images or other third party material in this chapter are included in the chapter's Creative Commons license, unless indicated otherwise in a credit line to the material. If material is not included in the chapter's Creative Commons license and your intended use is not permitted by statutory regulation or exceeds the permitted use, you will need to obtain permission directly from the copyright holder.

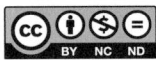

Part VIII

Skin Necrosis in Children

Introduction to Skin Necrosis Treatment in Young Age

Luc Téot

Skin in young age differs from adults, due to the physiological evolution from the immature skin present in the neonate to a highly inflammatory reactive skin, varying during the different stages of the child growth.

Neonatal skin acclimates rapidly to dry, aerobic conditions at birth, and skin function gradually matures throughout infancy. Three mechanisms are different from adults: oxygen tension-regulating angiogenesis and revascularization; transforming growth factor-β (TGF-β) kinetics controlling collagen deposition; and mechanical stretch stimulating cellular mitosis and extracellular matrix remodeling.

There is an increased systemic absorption of topics due to the skin fragility, and the tolerance of adhesives is limited in neonates and infants.

Wound types are more acute, like surgical wounds (extravasation and thermal injuries; chemical burns; pressure ulcers, iatrogenic intravascular injections) [1, 2] and wounds secondary to congenital conditions. Wound infection can lead to skin necrosis in highly contaminated situation like bite wounds which require special attention.

Radiations at high doses as well as drug injections may lead to severe skin lesions, including necrosis of the involved area [3, 4].

Deep wounds with suspected damage to nerves, tendons, and bones need general anesthetic to explore and assess the lesions. For instance, children and neonates very often receive intravenous therapy. There is a lack of systematic data on the incidence of extravasation injuries in children and neonates. Individual studies involving neonates receiving intravenous therapy on intensive care units report incidence rates of 18–46%. Serious complications, such as necrosis and ulceration, develop in 2.4–4% of cases, which in the long term can lead to contractures, deformities, and loss of limb function secondary to unfavorable scar formation [5]. There are no guidelines available to date on the management of pediatric extravasation injuries.

During childhood, hypertrophic scarring risk is increased, especially in persistent inflammatory periods like burns, or after surgical reconstruction of necrotic areas using skin grafting or flaps and have to be managed properly in proportion of the high risk of esthetic and psychological sequelae.

L. Téot (✉)
Department of Plastic Surgery, Burns and Wound Healing, Montpellier University Hospital, Hôpital La Colombière, CICAT Occitanie, Montpellier, France
e-mail: l-teot@chu-montpellier.fr

References

1. Koklu E, Ariguloglu AE, Koklu S. Foot Skin Ischemic Necrosis following Heel Prick in a Newborn. Case Rep Pediatr. 2013;2013:912876. https://doi.org/10.1155/2013/912876. Epub 2013 Oct 28.
2. Bakal Ü, Abeş M, Sarac M. Necrosis of the ventral penile skin flap: a complication of hypospadias surgery

in children. Adv Urol. 2015;2015:452870. https://doi.org/10.1155/2015/452870. Epub 2015 Apr 1.
3. Ravi M, Ridpath A, Audino AN, Guinipero T, Chung C. Fernandez faith E high-dose methotrexate-induced epidermal necrosis in two pediatric patients. Pediatr Dermatol. 2021;38(3):659–63. https://doi.org/10.1111/pde.14591. Epub 2021 Apr 7.
4. Brook I. Late side effects of radiation treatment for head and neck cancer. Radiat Oncol J. 2020;38(2):84–92. https://doi.org/10.3857/roj.2020.00213. Epub 2020 Jun 25.
5. Kostogloudis N, Demiri E, Tsimponis A, Dionyssiou D, Ioannidis S, Chatziioannidis I, Nikolaidis N. Severe extravasation injuries in neonates: a report of 34 cases. Pediatr Dermatol. 2015;32(6):830–5. https://doi.org/10.1111/pde.12664.

Open Access This chapter is licensed under the terms of the Creative Commons Attribution-NonCommercial-NoDerivatives 4.0 International License (http://creativecommons.org/licenses/by-nc-nd/4.0/), which permits any non-commercial use, sharing, distribution and reproduction in any medium or format, as long as you give appropriate credit to the original author(s) and the source, provide a link to the Creative Commons license and indicate if you modified the licensed material. You do not have permission under this license to share adapted material derived from this chapter or parts of it.

The images or other third party material in this chapter are included in the chapter's Creative Commons license, unless indicated otherwise in a credit line to the material. If material is not included in the chapter's Creative Commons license and your intended use is not permitted by statutory regulation or exceeds the permitted use, you will need to obtain permission directly from the copyright holder.

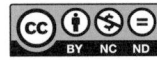

Skin Necrosis in Children: Physical and Infectious Causes

65

Guido Ciprandi

65.1 Introduction

When we talk about skin necrosis and the underlying soft tissues, we mean the death of a large number of cells, on the order of billions of cells, with consequent reworking of the tissues that can dehydrate and undergo decay. The final result is that of a brown, hard eschar, not removable, or a yellow, soft and sometimes soft eschar, with margins indistinguishable from surrounding healthy tissue. In both cases, the visible change on the surface represents only the tip of the iceberg, since the damage is first warped deeply, in the heart of the soft tissues, until it then reaches the size of a full-thickness damage that subsequently reaches the skin on the surface [1, 2].

In some situations, necrosis occurs secondary to the initial presence of bullous lesions (blistering early effect), and the child only after 48–72 h begins to manifest an ecchymotic and/or edematous skin area that is tinged more and more darkly. As a result, the necrosis proceeds and is much more evidenciating because of the last step of a direct substance-dependent damage or of an indirect damage following an arteriolar-capillary occlusion.

In the pediatric age, necrosis is very fast and whatever the cause that determines the blockage of arterial blood flow, locoregional hypo-oxygenation, or secondary damage to lymphatic-venous engorgement, a very rapid outcome in necrosis can be observed [3, 4].

This rapidity is noted for several reasons: on the one hand, the necrosis is due to the insufficient number of newly formed capillary beds and to an immaturity of growth and differentiation of the various layers of the skin. In this way, a small insult can already be very serious due to the poverty of the capillary networks and therefore cause serious damage with severe tissue loss.

From another perspective, the rapidity of necrosis can be attributed to the physiological edema observed in the neonatal period: the imbibition of the lining tissues, much richer in water than in later ages (85–90% in neonatal age and in infants 55–60% in senile ages), reduces the speed with which oxygen diffuses into the skin mantle. Normally, in fact, the oxygen comes out as ultrafiltered from the capillary bed of the dermis until it soaks the tissues of the dermoepidermal layer.

From the pathophysiological point of view, the occlusion pressure of the dermal capillaries, normally equal to 36–38 mmHg in adults, is very low in pediatric age and is equal to about 22–24 mmHg. Therefore, a much lower pressure is enough to occlude the dermal capillaries and this status is responsible, especially in patients with reduced mobility, for an early damage, often unexpected, with third degree necrotic pressure lesions that appear in less than 24 h. All the more reason, the reduction in thickness of the dermo-

G. Ciprandi (✉)
Division of Plastic and Maxillofacial Surgery, Bambino Gesu' Children's Hospital, Research Institute, Rome, Italy

epidermal complex which is observed from 0 to 36 months fails to adequately defend the host's tissues from the pressures exerted by the hospital materials.

Even the immaturity of the immune system of the youngest patients contributes to the rapid onset of a necrosis of the skin mantle, this time mostly on a septic basis. Poor immaturity is not only systemic in pediatric patients but also locoregional: especially the skin of the extremely preterm infant (LBW—Low Birth Weight, VLBW—Very Low Birth Weight) is structurally and functionally immature at birth [5].

Although there is rapid postnatal maturation, transient hypothermia, and reduced oxygen supply, manifesting fissures and skin breakdowns, with an increase in permeability toward toxins, pathogenic germs, are both responsible for inflammation and infection, first locoregional, and then systemic (Table 65.1).

Necrosis is the side effect, sometimes late effect of these crucial events.

Other than vascular occlusive disease, additional pediatric causes of necrosis include intrauterine epidermal necrosis, SSFTN, toxic epidermal necrolysis, severe and septic vasculitis (Neisseria meningitidis), drugs and injection extravasation (Arginine, Warfarin, Cysplatinum), necrosis resulting from bang bite and bike accidents or mainly due to inborn error of metabolism. But now let's go into the specifics of some single pathologies capable of inducing skin necrosis in neonatal and pediatric age and let's focus on these [6–10].

65.2 SSFTN (Skin and Subcutaneous Fat Necrosis of the Newborn: "Adiponecrosis Subcutanea Neonatorum")

65.2.1 General Aspects

This is a rare benign inflammatory condition which occurs in strictly neonatal age with firm and tense, well-circumscribed subcutaneous nodules (1–5 cm of largest diameter). Usually, the preferred sites of neonatal brown fat predominance (i.e., cheeks, neck, upper back or sacrococcygeal site, upper arm, thigh, buttocks) are much more affected by these injuries. The skin overlying these nodules looks like red purple induration plaque (sometimes very evident, sometimes quite invisible at the beginning) over the bone prominences, with which subsequently not infrequently undergoes necrosis with extensive ulceration and more often tends to a spontaneous resolution [11, 12].

The age at diagnosis is more often between 4 and 25 days, with a peak of incidence between 6 and 12 days. In most cases, the gestational age is normal, at term, the newborn weight is age-concordant but a severe perinatal hypoxia it's almost always part of the medical history: the fetal distress is reported in almost all cases and consequently an emergency cesarean section is required with a primary resuscitation needed, usually during the first 24–72 h of birth. In some cases, the hypoxic-ischemic encephalopathy could intervene [13]. This condition is mainly considered as a form of panniculitis, less severe than *sclerema neonatorum*, another condition causing hardened skin and limited necrosis during the neonatal period.

Table 65.1 Immature skin in different pediatric categories and topical impairment in host defense

Immature skin in different pediatric categories	
Premature/preterm	Born before 37 wg
Late preterm	Born between 34 and 36 wg
Moderate premature	Born between 32 and 34 wg
Very premature	Born before 32 wg
Micropreemie	Born at or before 26 wg

A micropreemie is a baby born weighing less than 800 g or before 26 weeks gestation

Topical impairment in host defense
1. Increased susceptibility to bacterial infections
2. 30% immature neutrophils (vs. 5–15% in childhood)
3. 30% storage pool (vs. 60% in childhood)
4. Severe reduction of myeloid progenitor stem cells
5. Severe impairment in adhesion of GN
6. Severely immature pseudopodal activities and phagocitosis

65.2.2 Predisposing Factors

There's neither a prevalent race nor a prevalent gender. However, some maternal predisposing factors have been studied and believed to be elements that may play a role in pathogenesis: preeclampsia, gestational type I diabetes, cocaine abuse, and use of calcium channel blockers during pregnancy have been all investigated and considered as predisposing to SSFTN.

On the other hand, they are believed to be specific neonatal factors in the development of neonatal adiponecrosis such as hypoxemia, hypothermia, rhesus incompatibility, birth asphyxia, meconium aspiration syndrome, hypoglycemia, and obstetric trauma (*perinatal asphyxia, therapeutic hypothermia*). The complex and often coincident set of these stressors results in reduced tissue perfusion, and the final hypoxemia leads to crystallization of free fatty acids in the subcutaneous fat tissue followed by tissue necrosis. Both the ischemia and the drastic inflammatory reaction that is activated consequently lead to an intense hyperemia and then to necrosis of the overlying skin, with local infection and often fistulization or confluence of skin areas of necrosis in the most serious and fortunately rare cases.

65.2.3 Laboratory Examinations

Serum albumin levels are usually normal, and serum calcium levels may be complicated by increased Ca++ or reduced Ca++ (manifesting with hypotonia and poor suking reflex). Whereas, vitamin D levels are normal and PTH is normal or slightly elevated. PLT–platelets showed a marked increase, low Mg and K blood levels.

65.2.4 Diagnosis

The anamnesis allows to highlight a previous fetal distress, associated with impaired calcium blood levels, subcutaneous nodules at various sites (clinical examination), and clearly evident during sonographic examinations: sometimes, if a colliquation has occurred, the ultrasound-guided fine-needle aspiration aspirates a thick liponecrotic liquid, otherwise drums of brownish yellow tissue are sent for histopathological examination. The histological pattern is as follows: some nodules are firm; others could become fluctuant as abscesses. Usually the fine-needle aspiration cytology revealed a dirty background with necrotic fat-containing characteristic, radially oriented, refractile, needle-shaped crystals [14, 15]. A tissue pattern-based approach to diagnosis shows clusters of adipocytes, histiocytes, fibroblasts, scanty lymphocytes, and numerous foreign body giant cells, granulomatous fat necrosis, and some calcification areas (Fig. 65.1). In a completely different way, sclerema neonatorum (SN) is characterized by hardening of the skin along with edema; histology shows a severe inflammatory infiltrate and edema in skin as well as in subcutaneous tissues. SN has a high case fatality rate, whereas SSFTN is a self-limiting condition and lesions resolve within a few weeks to months, when a skin necrosis is not part of the clinical pool of signs.

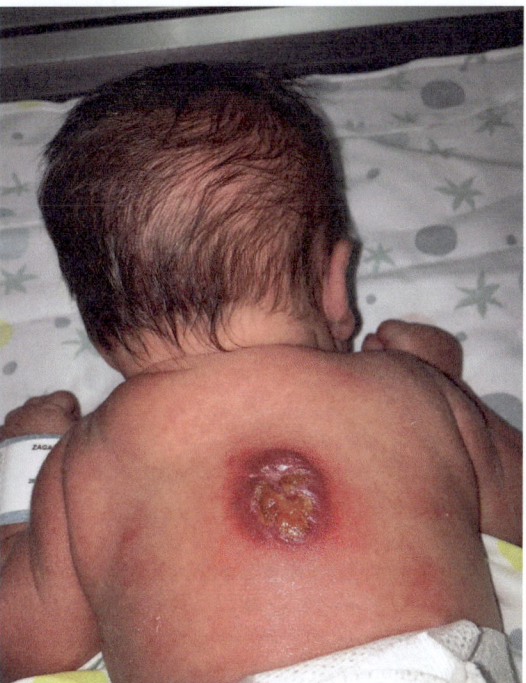

Fig. 65.1 Neonatal adiponecrosis in a 22-day-old patient: areas of skin necrosis overlying a large nodule of subcutaneous necrosis on the back. Other nodules without subcutaneous necrosis are present in the neck and right armpit

Table 65.2 Team of consultants and aetiopathogenetic steps

Team of consultants
Neonatologist
Neurologist
Cardiologist
Nephrologist
Dermatologist
Plastic surgeon
Aetiopathogenetic steps
1. Thrombocytosis
2. Lower blood perfusion
3. Hypoxia
4. Hypothermia
5. NSAdiponecrosis (transient panniculitis)

65.2.5 Course and Outcome

Diarrhea and vomiting are the most evident signs associated with the clinical picture, in a sort of self-limited course, with a spontaneous resolution occurring in the following 2 or 3 weeks up to 3 months. Specific therapies are not yet established and if something is required, this is limited to precise complications. In very few cases, low dose prednisone has been administered by mouth.

Among the systemic complication, we must mention hypercalcemia, hypocalcemia, hyperuricemia, hypoglycemia, hypertriglyceridemia, thrombocytopenia, resulting in morbidity and mortality, if not early detected and promptly cared.

Local complications are reported such as necrotic epidermal atrophy, ulceration, scarring, and/or local infection. At a discharge breast feeding is clearly advocate, and an oral Vit D supplementation (1.200 UI, each day) is introduced for at least 2–4 weeks [5] (Table 65.2).

65.3 Extravasation Injuries Necrosis

65.3.1 Introduction and Definition

Extravasation is the accidental release of one drug or a mixture of them from the veins used for the delivery of solutes and medicaments, into surrounding peri and paravascular connective tissue sheats. This phenomenon has an incidence ranging from 1 to 6%; however, the severity and type

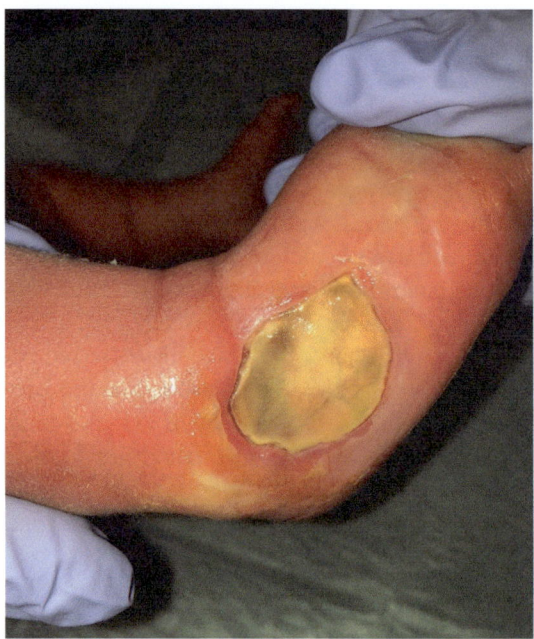

Fig. 65.2 Yellow necrosis due to extravasation of the saphenous right external to the malleolus in a 12-day-old infant. The necrosis area also affects the subcutaneous tissue and is due to extravasation of antibiotics

of treatment vary according to the type of extravasated fluid [16]. The outcomes of extravasation are related to the characteristics of the patient, his age, the state of the venous circulation, nutritional aspects, and various comorbidities. Pediatric patients most at risk are represented by premature (LBW, VLBW, micropreemies) and newborn for the characteristics of the fragile skin and because of a narrow and underdeveloped venous heritage. In first ages of life, the risk of extravasation and a subsequent necrosis are increased as well as the major late outcomes. The consequences can be of different severity: from local redness to deep tissue necrosis, which can involve tendons and ligaments, causing severe tissue damage and severe functional sequelae and disabilities including contractures, deformities, and loss of function of the limbs secondary to the formation of retracting and/or keloid scars [17, 18] (Figs. 65.2 and 65.3). Some studies conducted in infants admitted to intensive and subintensive care units report incidence rates of 18–46%. In 2.4–4% of these cases, serious complications develop and necrosis is the most unfa-

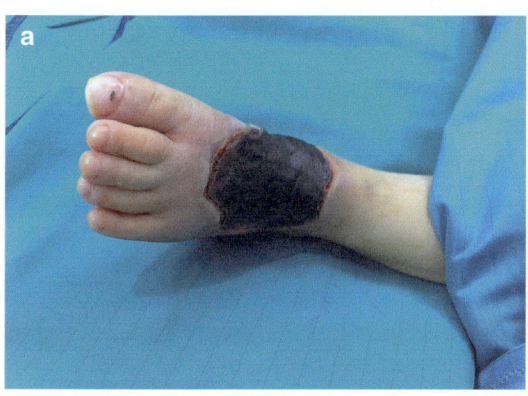 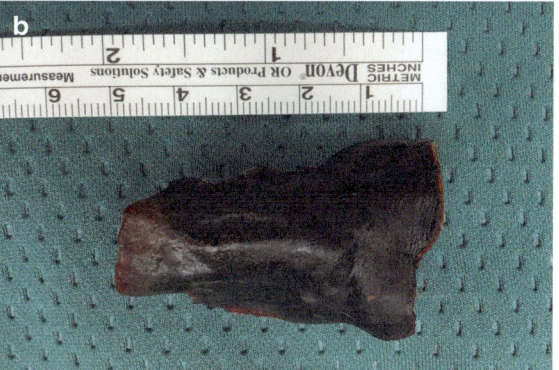

Fig. 65.3 (**a**, **b**) Brown eschar affecting the dorsum of the foot due to extravasation of hyperosmolar electrolytic agents after cannulation of the dorsal vein of the left foot. A large surface of about 5 cm is involved, as can be seen from the completely removed eschar, which also traces the convexity of the neck and back of the entire foot

vorable one, leading to permanent damages if not promptly surgically cared [19].

65.3.2 Actions and Injuries

Based on the potential tissue damage, various agents are recognized and then categorized on the basis of their ability to create the most evident necrotic effects with different mechanisms of action:

1. Transformations from **rapid tissue necrosis** are due to substances that produce immediate deep damage and, by binding to DNA, remain in the tissues for a long time causing progressive and worsening injuries, with severe necrotic ulcers or full-thickness necrosis which more often appear as real plaque of rigid, black or dark brown tissue, shaped on the anatomical site of the lesion. In these small patients, the plastic surgeon intervention is rapidly advocated. Severe pain and functional outcomes are always present if a surgical treatment is not instituted and sometimes even in an emergency regime.
2. **Blistering** substances that can cause deep tissue damage, as they are rapidly metabolized and cause severe or prolonged pain, they represent the second category of agents responsible for tissue necrosis, more often circumscribed and limited to small islands of skin that undergoes progressive and not immediate disintegration and exfoliation.

The mechanisms that determine necrosis resulting from extravasations are different:

- Some drugs bind to nucleic acids in DNA and are initially absorbed locally causing cell death. After endocytosis, the death of surrounding cells occurs through the release of the drug from dead cells. The repetitive nature of this process strongly delays the healing processes and can lead to progressive and chronic tissue damage, with deep scars.
- Other drugs do not bind to DNA but are metabolized, limiting the degree of tissue damage, and therefore are easier to pharmacologically neutralize.

65.3.3 Epidemiology

The incidence of extravasations in pediatric age ranges from 0.1 to 6.5% of children undergoing chemotherapy, in other estimates 11–28% in children admitted to a pediatric intensive care setting. A not recent UK-based survey of regional neonatal intensive care units published in 2004, estimated the incidence of extravasation injuries resulting in skin necrosis to be 38 per 1000 babies. Seventy percent of the cases occurred in preterm infants born before 27 weeks' gestation;

4% of infants leave the TIN with significant functional scars or lesions resulting from extravasation lesions [20, 21].

65.3.4 Distribution by Body Area and Care Setting

The incidence of necrotic injuries due to extravasation or drug infiltration and the deepness of tissue damage are related to various factors, including the infused agent, its concentration and volume, the duration of infiltration, the timing of diagnosis, the body site, and gestational age of the patient.

In the pediatric age, especially in the neonatal age, the areas chosen for finding venous accesses are the back of the hand, the forearm, the cubital fossa, the back of the foot, and the epicranial area. These areas are represented by a subcutis that allows easy retrieval of the vessels visible in transparency but, at the same time, they are more delicate and fragile. In situations perceived as more difficult, the positioning of the venous line is always ultrasound-guided, thus reducing possible risk for necrosis. No area of the body is exempt from the risk of extravasation. This is especially true for newborns and for those born preterm or low birth weight (LBW, VLBW, ELBW).

65.3.5 Care

When the first signs or symptoms of extravasation or infiltration occur, including, for example, redness or edema, the current infusion must be stopped immediately and the team involved. After stopping the infusion, the necessary antidote is administered through the same device within 1 h and then the device with the entire infusion line is removed. If the device was removed before administering the antidote, administer the antidote by subcutaneous injections in the area affected by the extravasation. The limb is then placed in unloading for at least 48 h to allow normal absorption and drainage of liquids. To facilitate the management of extravasation in "first aid," the Team has an antidote kit with the various procedures to be performed.

65.3.6 Physiology of Extravasation

In the human body, vascular lesions, oxidative stress, and inflammation are closely related. Infiltration and extravasation are both conditions responsible for vascular damage. When a vascular injury occurs, the release of free radicals is stimulated and the cells' ability to produce energy becomes dysfunctional due to damage to the mitochondria. This leads to limited energy production, and the balance between nitric oxide and superoxide is disrupted, increasing the damage. There is a continuous cycle of free radical production and endothelial apoptosis leading to damage to membranes and cell vessels.

Symptoms of this process include redness, swelling, and visible tissue lesions. The interaction of the biological response to chemical and non-chemical risk factors, when exposed to the extravasated drug, directly affects the healthy endothelium, leading to vascular lesions, starting from the vessel intima. Infiltration or extravasation can be caused by displacement of the intravenous catheter, puncture of the vein during insertion or handling of patients. The tolerance of the vein to an infusion is influenced by the osmolarity and pH of the blistering substance, the duration of exposure, and the irritation of the endothelial cells. An additional factor in causing the vein to rupture and leak is the pressure of the drug being infused.

65.3.7 Factors Affecting the Pathophysiology of Extravasation

- *The volume* of the drug infused; since, as is known, during extravasation there is a loss of fluids in the subcutis which impart pressure to the venous reticulum and then to the arterial one, present at the site of the extravasation, thus reducing the blood supply to others; therefore, depending on the volume of the extravasated drug, there will be more or less severe ischemic damage.
- *The local toxicity* of the drug, due to the chemical nature of the substance itself.

The *pH*, *osmolarity*, and *biological activity* as in the case of vasoactive substances or chemotherapeutic agents [22, 23].

65.3.8 Identification of Extravasation and Risk Factors

The Infusion Nurses Society adapted the scale to include guidelines for lesion size and suggesting that infiltrates involving blistering solutions, even if present in minimal quantities, should be considered as a stage 4 (Table 65.3). But the guidelines used to adults cannot be adapted to the pediatric patient; since lesions similar in size to those of adults are more severe in children due to the size of the body and the different skin structure. Suitable scales for pediatric and neonatal infiltrations were also created to account for the smaller surface area and different clinical presentations. The appearance of necrosis is clearly associated with poor prognosis and severe painful clinical symptoms.

65.3.9 Dangerous Substances

Intravenous drugs can be divided into three main categories:

1. *Not blistering or inert*.
2. *Irritants*: drugs capable of causing pain, swelling, venous irritation, and chemical phlebitis at the injection site.
3. *Blistering*: drugs that cause redness, pain, and blistering during infiltration and can progress to ulceration and tissue necrosis.

There are several characteristics of the drug that can affect potential tissue damage these include: osmolarity, pH, direct therapeutic effects, and solubility.

Osmolarity describes the number of particles that are suspended in solution. The normal serum osmolarity of a newborn is approximately 280 mOsm. When a solution has a higher osmolarity, it is considered hyperosmolar. The effects cause cells to shrink when a fluid moves from inside to the outside of the cell. This response occurs in order to

Table 65.3 PIV Scale (Peripheral Intravenous Extravasation Assessment scale): necrosis and clinical severe degrees (adapted from Cincinnati Children's Hospital Medical Center, February 2013)

Third degree: Severe extravasation (mild necrosis, limited small areas)	• Moderate swelling 25–50% of the insertion site • Cold skin • Whitening • Blistering
Fourth degree: Extreme extravasation (severe necrosis and large area, sometimes circumferential)	• Significant swelling, more than 50% around the insertion site • Infiltration of blistering and irritating products • Cold skin • wWhitening • Skin injury • >Blistering • Insertion site pain • Blood recirculation time greater than 4 s

increase the osmolarity within the cell to balance with the high osmolarity of the serum. The opposite of this effect would be a hyperosmolar solution. In this situation, the fluid would enter the cell in order to reduce the osmolarity of the cell to equal to the external one. In the extreme, this can result in cell lysis as the volume of the cell exceeds its capacity. Some preparations are classified as extremely hyperosmolar and one of them is the arginine hydrochloride, which is used in the evaluation of short stature and in the management of urea cycle disorders. The arginine extravasation rapidly induces necrosis and that is why it should be diluted to a 10% solution prior to infusion [24, 25].

Measuring the concentration of hydrogen ions and pH is another important consideration in assessing the risk of a drug, infiltration, or extravasation. A normal arterial blood pH is between 7.35 and 7.45. As the pH of drugs deviates from this normal range, the risk of tissue injury is higher. As the number of hydrogen ions increases, the solution will become more acidic. Most drugs have an acidic to neutral pH. Once medications move from 5 to 9 range, the risk of inflammation and vascular injury increases significantly. Drugs have a specific mechanism of action that can cause cell damage in case of infiltration or extravasation.

Vasoactive drugs, such as dopamine, have effects on alpha receptors. If this drug is introduced into the tissues, this alpha stimulation will result in constriction of the capillary beds, which will subsequently reduce local blood flow. Local tissue will be deprived of oxygen, and an ischemic injury will ensue. Another group of drugs that have direct effects on tissues are electrolytes. Calcium is needed for the depolarization and contraction of smooth muscle. If a concentrated calcium solution is infused into the tissue, this can cause capillary constriction, through stimulation of smooth muscle, resulting in ischemic damage to the hypoperfused tissue [26, 27].

The solubility of a drug can affect its contribution to local tissue damage. The more lipophilic a drug is, the less water soluble, thus rendering site washing impractical and leading to high concentrations of drugs located in relatively small areas of tissue which can lead to direct concentration-dependent tissue damage (Table 65.4).

65.3.10 Treatments

- *Topical Treatments*: Topical treatments are often used when talking about an open wound. These include nitroglycerin, silver sulfadiazine, and dimethyl sulfoxide (DMSO). These treatments promote a moist wound environment, which reduces healing times, the likelihood of infection and prevents scarring.
- *Antidotes*: Some blistering solutions may have a particular antidote which can be infused or injected into the affected area. This approach appears to be used most often for the treatment of chemotherapy extravasations.
- *Hyaluronidase*: Subcutaneous injections of hyaluronidase can be used in an attempt to break down the connective tissue and facilitate the absorption of extravasated fluid in the vascular and lymphatic circulation. Administration within 1 h of extravasation is recommended;

Table 65.4 Intravenous drugs

Not blistering or inert	Irritants	Blistering (with or without necrosis)	Necrotizing
Monoclonal antibodies	Bleomycin	Amsacrine	Daunomycin
Asparaginase	Carboplatin	Cisplatin	Doxorubicin
Cytarabine	Carmustine	Dacarbazine	Epirubicin
Cladribine	Cyclophosphamide	Dactinomycin	Idarubicin
Fludarabine	Cisplatin	Daunorubicin	Mitomycin
Methotrexate	Liposomal daunorubicin	Docetaxel	Vincristine
Thiotepa	Gemcitabine	Etoposide	Vindesine
	Ifofosfamide	Fluorouracil	Vinblastine
	Irinotecan	Mechlorethamine	Vinorelbine
	Streptozocin	Melphalan	Actinomycin D
	Topotecan	Mitoxantrone	Mechlorethamine
		Oxaliplatin	Liposomal doxorubicin
		Paclitaxel	
Blistering drugs that bind to DNA	• Alkylating agents: Maecloretamin • Anthracycline: Doxorubicin, epirubicin, idarubicin • Antibiotici antitumorali: Mitomicin; dactinomicin, mitoxantrone		
Blistering drugs that do not bind to DNA	Vinca alkaloids: Vinblastine, vincristine, vinorelbine, vindesine, texani, paclitaxel, docetaxel		
Irritating drugs	• Alkylating agents: Carmustine, dacarbazine, ifosfamide, melphalan, thiotepa • Platinum derivatives: Carboplatin, cisplatin, oxaliplatin • Inhibitors of topoisomerase II: Teniposide, etoposide • Anthracycline: Liposomal doxorubicin, liposomal daunorubicin • Inibitori della topoisomerasi I: Irinotecan, topotecan		

- *Saline flushing and liposuction*: Both saline flush-out and liposuction are administered in order to remove extravasated fluid before it can cause damage. As such, there is an implied requirement that these treatments be undertaken as soon as possible. Gault described both techniques, which can be administered alone or together, although various modifications to these techniques have also been reported [28].
- Saline lavage techniques generally involve skin incisions made in the extravasation lesion and syringe administration, injecting saline into each incision. The goal is for this process to clear the brew through the remaining incision points. The process is sometimes preceded by the injection of hyaluronidase to break down the hyaluronic acid in the connective tissues, thus favoring the dispersion of the infusion. The procedure is often performed under local anesthesia, although general anesthesia may sometimes be required, especially if liposuction is also to be performed.
- Liposuction is a minimally invasive surgical technique in which the cannula with side holes is inserted into the wound and subcutaneous fluid and fat are aspirated.
- *Surgery*: If less invasive treatments are unsuccessful and necrotic tissue is not resolved after a medium-/long-term period of treatment, the next step in the treatment pathway is surgical debridement (*sharp debridement*), plastic surgery minor/major interventions, or both. Hydrosurgery is another option easy to be used when necrosis shows irregular and indented contours which often can be quite difficult to debride with sharp methods. In newborn and small patients aged less than 3 years, this technique has some advantages such as a true tissue selectivity, great and safe handling in detaching the edges of the necrosis due to extravasation, handling in complex contours such as extravasation, and a possible preservation of the underlying adnexal [29].

The purpose of debridement is the removal of necrotic tissue (eschar), which accelerates wound healing. Typically it involves both a surgical technique (the use of sharp instruments to remove the eschar performed under general anesthesia) and an enzymatic debridement (which promotes the removal of the eschar tissue). When a topical anesthesia is not possible to be performed due to the age of the patient, all the procedures could be performed at one time in the operating room: escharotomy, wound bed preparation, and immediate or delayed graft (with or without interposition of a dermal substitute). We currently prefer the use of NPWT to accelerate direct or mediated adherence of the skin graft to the wound bed. If the appropriate timing of extravasation surgery is not yet clearly defined, and when it is not possible to ascertain with certainty the fluids and solutes responsible for extravasation, we advocate a "wait and see" conservative approach.

However, frequent patient follow-up is critical to identify early blisters or ulcers that require debridement or plastic surgery. Consultation by the plastic surgeon is recommended after extravasation of large volume vesicles, when a patient is in severe pain or if healing has not occurred within 1–3 weeks after extravasation. A conservative approach is not appropriate if the child has persistent pain, edema and erythema, blistering, and necrosis which may hide an ulcer covered with enlarged eschar. In case of delay in treatment, permanent functional damage can occur due to a prolonged tissue exposure. When a surgical procedure is not performed at the proper time repeated debridement are required, larger excision is usually necessary, and partial thickness skin grafting or flap reconstruction are mandatory actions. The complex of clinical manifestations related to an increase in tissue pressure within a non-compressible space such as that of the muscle lodges covered by their own fascia is called as compartment syndrome. Compartment pressure measurement is useful in evaluating questionable compartment syndrome or in patients who have sensory blunting or are under general anesthesia. Normal pressure in a muscle compartment is less than 10–20 mmHg.

Fasciotomy is recommended if pressure is greater than 30–45 mmHg; physiology studies show that a limb may be adequately perfused if the diastolic pressure is greater than 30 mmHg than the compartment. Therefore, the fasciotomy is indicated when the delta p between the diastolic pressure less that of the compartment varies between 20 and 30 mmHg. In children, diastolic pressure is low to easily bring a delta p less than 30 mmHg. Therefore, the average blood pressure is used in pediatric patients [30, 31].

An increase in specific Prevention Culture, Training of Pediatric Health Care Teams, Protocols and Related Kits (ETK), immediate and not delayed assistance following the Operational Guide (OG), prompt plastic surgeon consultation, close monitoring of pediatric patients are the main objectives to be pursued. The reduction of necrosis caused by infiltration and extravasation is based on the updating of the nursing and medical staff, on the positioning and on the management of a peripheral or central venous access. Difficult and complex patients (premature and newborn, patients with poor or fragile venous heritage) must be approached with ultrasound-guided positioning by expert anesthetists. In case of positioning a long-lasting CVC and choosing the type of catheter, the help of the interventional pediatric radiologist is essential.

Each hospital should draw up an updated procedure on the management of extravasation and compose a team of experienced and trained personnel who can manage this type of emergency and who can educate and sensitize the remaining health personnel. In our experience, both a skin care team and a wound prevention team are advocated because of the true experience with wounded children the components that deal with ES must have.

Immediate surgical management consists of two most frequently reported manoeuvers: post incisional washing and local debridement. However, signs of tissue and nervous ischemic damage and the rigidity of the limbs and extremities in griposis must be avoided promptly, since the cosmetic and functional sequelae arise very quickly. Fasciotomy is the only accepted treatment of compartment syndrome and should be performed quickly after the diagnosis is made. Outcomes after fasciotomy are best when there is no delay in treatment. In few words, all observational and decision-making activities must be taken with great timeliness and without time delays [32–34].

Currently, although there are numerous studies on severely staged necrosis due to extravasation syndromes. But there aren't available guidelines compiled on the basis of RCTs. This is due to the increase in the complexity of pediatric patients, the increase in survival related to prematurity, the implementation of the efforts of intensive and subintensive technological activities on patients at high risk of life. In addition, there is no doubt that necrosis occurring in these small and very small patients is challenging because of a multifactorial disease requiring a precision medicine approach [35].

65.4 SNSTIs (Severe Necrotizing Soft Tissue Infections)

65.4.1 Introduction

Severe necrotizing soft tissue infections (SNSTIs) are widespread and systemic bacterial infections.

In more details, these are highly thrombotic subtype of disseminated intravascular coagulation that can accompany severe bacterial, and more rarely, viral infections. Neisseria meningitidis is most commonly associated with SNSTIs, even if many other infectious etiologies have been identified and among these Haemophilus influenzae, Staphylococcus aureus, and Pneumococcus are described as responsible for necrotic skin damages.

Pediatric patients represent a fragile category also due to an immaturity of the immune system both of the surface and of the organ and organism. This, therefore, makes it easy to understand how necrosis occur quickly and are immediately rapidly progressive. Prevention and wound hygiene must be appropriate, a diagnosis must be early done, and treatments must be targeted immediately to minimize disabilities but also the hypothesis of mortality. Beyond treatment with antibiotics administered on the basis of an antibiogram and admission to neonatal and pediatric intensive care units for any resuscitation support, the surgical approach for debridement and a surgical toilet to be operated on are extremely important, to be performed in asepsis and in the operating room.

Although the death rate of NSTI appears to have decreased in recent decades, it remains very high in the first 3 years of life and at 5–20%.

It is evident that necrotic lesions are the largest ever considering all pediatric ages. Brown necrosis is often bilateral from the onset and affecting both lower limbs, reaching to include the root of the limbs, the external genitalia, and other sites rich in lymphatic vessels and innervation (Figs. 65.4 and 65.5).

Crucial points are represented not only by the extension per area of representation but also by the depth. The deeper necrosis is due not only to septic emboli, which induce mechanical vascular occlusion, but also to the effect of cytotropic toxins. Purpura fulminans is a severe subtype of disseminated intravascular coagulation associated in the majority of the cases with meningococcal septicemia in children. The patient's inflammatory response to meningococcal septicemia activates the coagulation pathway, resulting in the development of numerous superficial as well as visceral thromboses. Superficial thromboses of the skin produce pathognomonic or maculopapular rashes that progress into areas of full-thickness necrosis. Thrombus formation within the viscera can result in the development of multiorgan failure. Because of its severity, prompt diagnosis and treatment of purpura fulminans are vital for patient survival.

SNSTIs can be yet evident as a connatal syndrome in newborn with inherited deficit of protein-C due to homozygous or heterozygous mutations in the PROC or PROS1 genes.

65.4.2 Care

Frequently, plastic surgeons are consulted for the reconstruction of areas with full-thickness skin necrosis. The reconstructive process varies greatly based on soft tissues loss. Skin grafting, locoregional tissue transfer, and free tissue flaps are all potential reconstructive strategies to be used depending on the site, width, and depth of the defect.

When skin grafting is the best option, large full-thickness wounds in the pediatric population can be difficult to manage because of limited donor site options for autografts and shortcomings of many skin graft substitutes.

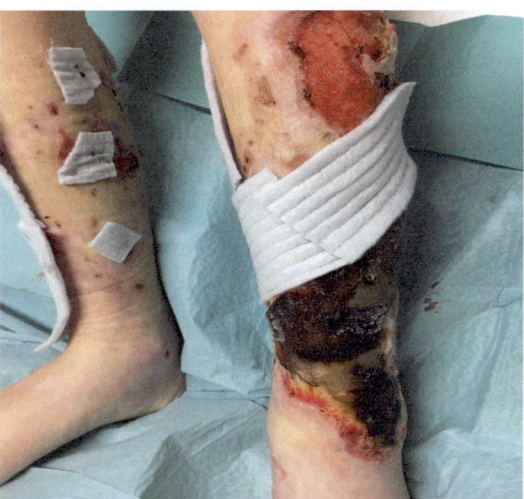

Fig. 65.4 Extensive multiple necrotic eschar affecting both lower limbs in a 9-year-old girl. The anterolateral surfaces of both the thigh and leg are affected

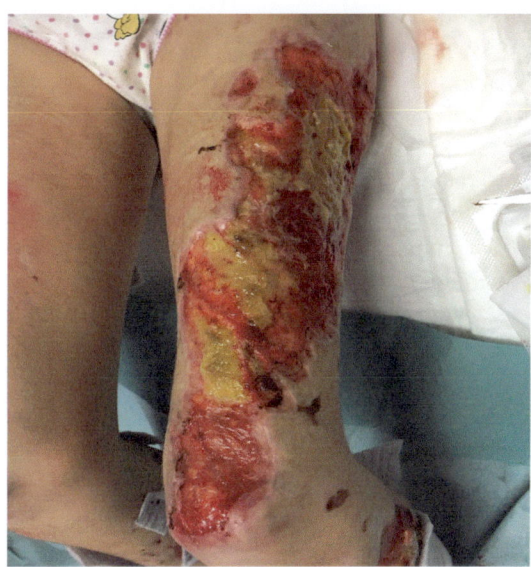

Fig. 65.5 The depth of damage after surgical necrosectomy is visible. Effect of both ischemic actions for vascular occlusion and for endotoxin damage from Neisseria meningitidis

Also of particular gravity are the plaques of necrosis near the junctional areas or the natural folds of the body (groin, axillary fold, ankle, popliteal cavity) and those that have aspects extended to the entire circumference of a limb, at the digital extremities (hands and feet).

The decrease in mortality results in an increase in the number of surviving children. When starting to treat infectious necrosis, it is always necessary to consider an approach with "tissue sparing procedure" techniques, since the procedures are all aimed at avoiding outcomes and severe distant sequelae that are often disabling. There are suggestions that a skin-sparing approach may result in a decreased need for skin transplants, which could potentially improve the quality of life in survivors [36].

The prognosis of a growing organism must always consider that children have in fact a fourth dimension (body growth) which drastically places the emphasis on how to promote a good prognosis quoad vitam but also how to pursue a good and future prognosis quoad valetudinem.

Improving the prognosis means performing targeted toilets, pursuing a debridement that is careful to spare otherwise healthy tissue, even when it may appear compromised by the infection [37].

All procedures are in fact guided by ultrasound aspects and MRI images. In pediatric age, it is preferable to perform more successive necrosectomy sessions under targeted antibiotic therapy rather than the removal of large tissue segments.

The improvement of necrosectomy techniques which in pediatric age is performed in many cases with microsurgical debridement technique (use of the operating microscope) can greatly benefit the prognosis of NSTI.

The first damage resulting from serious mutilations and disabling outcomes that may require long and repeated sessions of FKT as well as of tutorial tools and prosthetic aids are felt by the entire family. As a result, the child can experience psychological stress and pain, both of which are able of dangerously reducing the pain threshold.

An important factor that determines the extreme attention of the plastic surgeon in the removal of tissues is the consideration of possible future scarring events. Each removed tissue will in fact be filled with a volume of scar and harder tissues, they will be difficult to move later in the case of having to make local gliding flaps.

In other cases, post-necrosectomy scars are not only a cosmetic problem but also a functional one. When scar bands appear in the site of previous necrosis plaques, sometimes hypertrophic or keloid, the main enemy is the retraction that can prevent movements due to a marked retraction. In these cases, revision operations may require the completion of the removal of the necrosis bands, of the scarring, plastics with opposing flaps, grafts, local flaps, or transposition of flaps with microsurgical techniques [38].

References

1. Visscher MO, Narendran V. Newborn infant skin: anatomy, physiology and development. In: Ciprandi G, editor. Neonatal and pediatric wound care. Turin: Minerva Medica Publisher; 2022. p. 11–26.
2. Koster MI, Roop DR. Mechanisms regulating epithelial stratification. Annu Rev Cell Dev Biol. 2007;23:93–113.
3. Yosipovitch G, Maayan-Metzger A, Merlob P, et al. Skin barrier properties in different body areas in neonates. Pediatrics. 2000;106:105–8.
4. Nonato LB, Lund CH, Kalia YN, et al. Transepidermal water loss in 24 and 25 weeks gestational age infants. Acta Paediatr. 2000;89:747–8.
5. Onyiriuka AN, Utomi TE. Hypocalcemia associated with subcutaneous fat necrosis of the newborn: case report and literature review. Oman Med J. 2017;32(6):518–21.
6. Soua Y, Hamouda H, Njima M, et al. Subcutaneous fat necrosis of the newborn. Skinmed. 2021;19(5):392–4.
7. Patterson JW. Weedon's skin pathology. 5th ed. Elsevier Health; 2020.
8. Brown AS, Hoelzer DJ, Piercy SA. Skin necrosis from extravasation of intravenous fluids in children. Plast Reconstr Surg. 1979;64(2):145–50.
9. Day MK, Haub N, Betts H, Inwald D. Hyperglycemia is associated with morbidity in critically ill children with meningococcal sepsis. Pediatr Crit Care Med. 2008;9(6):636–40.
10. Fruchtman Y, Strauss T, Rubinstein M, et al. Skin necrosis and purpura fulminans in children with and without thrombophilia—a tertiary center's experience. Pediatr Hematol Oncol. 2015;32(7):505–10.
11. Fluhr JW, Darlenski R, Lachmann N, et al. Infant epidermal skin physiology:adaptation after birth. Br J Dermatol. 2012;166:483–90.
12. Sivanandan S, Rabi Y, Kamaluddeen M, et al. Subcutaneous fat necrosis as a complication of therapeutic hypothermia in a term neonate. Indian J Pediatr. 2012;79(5):664–6.
13. Llamas-Velasco M, Fernández-Figueras MT. A practical approach to the clinico-pathological diagnosis of panniculitis. Diagn Histopathol. 2021;27(1):34–41.
14. Nakalema G, Egesa WI, Kumbakulu PK, et al. Sclerema neonatorum in a term infant: a case report and literature review. Case Rep Pediatr. 2020;2020:8837064. https://doi.org/10.1155/2020/8837064.

15. Stefanko NS, Drolet BA. Subcutaneous fat necrosis of the newborn and associated hypercalcemia: a systematic review of the literature. Pediatr Dermatol. 2019;36(1):24–30.
16. Corbett M, Marshall D, Harden M, et al. Treatment of extravasation injuries in infants and young children: a scoping review and survey. Health Technol Assess. 2018;22(46):1–112.
17. Ching D, Wong KY. Pediatric extravasation injury management: a survey comparing 10 hospitals. Pediatr Neonatol. 2017;58(6):549–51.
18. Paquette V, McGloin R, Northway T, Dezorzi P, Singh A, Carr R. Describing intravenous extravasation in children (DIVE study). Can J Hosp Pharm. 2011;64:340–5.
19. Davies J, Gault D, Buchdahl R. Preventing the scars of neonatal intensive care. Arch Dis Child. 1994;70(1):F50–F5.
20. Yan YM, Gong M, Chen JL, et al. Incidence, risk factors and treatment outcomes of drug extravasation in pediatric patients in China. Turk J Pediatr. 2017;59(2):1621–168.
21. Harris PA, Bradley S, Moss AL. Limiting the damage of iatrogenic extravasation injury in neonates. Plast Reconstr Surg. 2001;107:893–4.
22. Ching DL, Wong KY, Milroy C. Paediatric extravasation injuries: a review of 69 consecutive patients. Int J Surg. 2014;12:1036–7.
23. Kishi C, Amano H, Shimizu A, Nagai Y, Ishikawa O. Cutaneous necrosis induced by extravasation of hydroxyzine. Eur J Dermatol. 2014;24:131–2.
24. Salameh Y, Shoufani A. Full thickness skin necrosis after arginine extravasation. A case report and review of literature. J Pediatr Surg. 2004;39:E9–11.
25. Abraham MB, van der Westhuizen J, Khanna V. Arginine extravasation leading to skin necrosis. J Paediatr Clin Health. 2012;48:E96–7.
26. Harrold K, Gould D, Drey N. The management of cytotoxic chemotherapy extravasation: a systematic review of the literature to evaluate the evidence underpinning contemporary practice. Eur J Cancer Care. 2015;24:771–800.
27. Boulanger J, Ducharme A, Dufour A, et al. Comité de l'évolution de la pratique des soins pharmaceutiques (CEPSP). Management of the extravasation of anti-neoplastic agents. Support Care Cancer. 2015;23:1459–71.
28. Onesti MG, Carella S, Maruccia M. The use of hyalomatrix PA in the treatment of extravasation affecting premature neonates. Plast Reconstr Surg. 2012;129:219e–21e.
29. Sivrioglu N, Irkoren S. Versajet hydrosurgery system in the debridement of skin necrosis after Ca++ gluconate extravasation. Report of nine infantile cases. Acta Orthop Traumatol Turc. 2014;48(1):6–9.
30. Broom A, Schur MD, Arkader A, Flynn J, Gornitzky A, Choi PD. Compartment syndrome in infants and toddlers. J Child Orthop. 2016;10:453–60.
31. Talbot SG, Rogers GF. Pediatric compartment syndrome caused by intravenous infiltration. Ann Plast Surg. 2011;67:531–3.
32. Little M, Dupré S, Wormald JCR, et al. Surgical intervention for paediatric infusion-related extravasation injury: a systematic review. BMJ Open. 2020;10(8):e034950. https://doi.org/10.1136/bmjopen-2019-034950.
33. Meszes A, Tálosi G, Máder K, Orvos H, Kemény L, Csoma ZR. Lesions requiring wound management in a central tertiary neonatal intensive care unit. World J Pediatr. 2017;13:165–72.
34. Ciprandi G. Quality of newly generated tissue in newborn using hyaluronic acid. In: EWMA fully virtual meeting 19 November, 2020. FIDIA symposium.
35. Weigelt MA, Lev-Tov HA, Tomic-Canic M, et al. Advanced wound diagnostics: toward transforming wound care into precision medicine. Adv Wound Care (New Rochelle). 2022;11(6):330–59.
36. Suijker J, Zheng KJ, Pijpe A, et al. The skin-sparing debridement technique in necrotizing soft-tissue infections: a systematic review. J Surg Res. 2021;264:296–308.
37. Chalmers E, Cooper P, Forman K, et al. Purpura fulminans: recognition, diagnosis and management. Arch Dis Child. 2011;96(11):1066–71.
38. Sarrami SM, Ferry AM, Buchanan EP, et al. Reconstructing severe lower extremity skin necrosis in a pediatric patient. Adv Skin Wound Care. 2021;34(7):1–6.

Open Access This chapter is licensed under the terms of the Creative Commons Attribution-NonCommercial-NoDerivatives 4.0 International License (http://creativecommons.org/licenses/by-nc-nd/4.0/), which permits any non-commercial use, sharing, distribution and reproduction in any medium or format, as long as you give appropriate credit to the original author(s) and the source, provide a link to the Creative Commons license and indicate if you modified the licensed material. You do not have permission under this license to share adapted material derived from this chapter or parts of it.

The images or other third party material in this chapter are included in the chapter's Creative Commons license, unless indicated otherwise in a credit line to the material. If material is not included in the chapter's Creative Commons license and your intended use is not permitted by statutory regulation or exceeds the permitted use, you will need to obtain permission directly from the copyright holder.

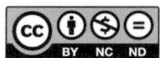

Neonatal Pressure Ulcer

Christian Herlin

66.1 Introduction

The structure of a premature newborn's skin is very different from that of the adult.

In the adult, the stratum corneum is composed of about 20 layers and has an important protective function. However, in the premature baby, this stratum is non-existent or minimal (0–3 layers). The thinness of these external layers is one of the principal sources of vulnerability (see Fig. 66.1).

The stratum corneum normally protects the body from toxins and infections, enables thermoregulation, and controls transepidermal water loss.

In the premature newborn, in addition to the thinness of the external layers, there is also a lack of collagen and elastin in the superficial dermal layers. This considerably increases the risk of pressure ulcers, with spontaneous oedema increasing the cutaneous ischaemia.

In the hospital environment, the incidence of neonatal pressure ulcers (NPUs) is significant, affecting one in four babies in the neonatal intensive care unit (NICU) [1, 2].

Four percent of babies who have been treated in a NICU are left with a scar [3]. In the majority of cases, these skin lesions are minor [4].

The significant incidence of NPUs in the NICU can be explained by the following risk factors [5]:

C. Herlin (✉)
Plastic and Reconstructive Surgery, Wond Healing Unit, Montpellier University, Montpellier, France
e-mail: c-herlin@chu-montpellier.fr

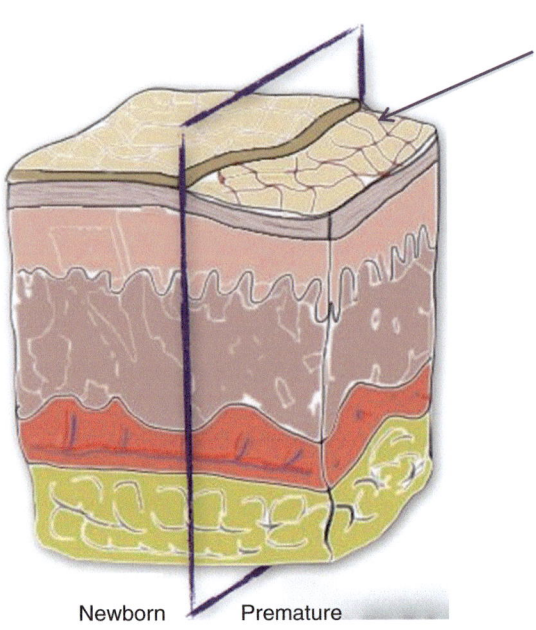

Fig. 66.1 Comparison of normal newborn and premature skin. The stratum corneum is absent or very underdeveloped in the premature skin

The majority of the stratum corneum layers are missing; they normally have a protective role.

- The immaturity of the skin
- The restriction of the baby's voluntary movements (e.g. due to a central venous line, mechanical ventilation, etc.)
- The hot and humid environment
- The use or not of invasive ventilation

This chapter describes the main sources of pressure ulcers in the newborn and premature baby, their characteristic features, the therapeutic principles, and the potential sequelae.

66.2 Risk Assessment Scales

There are many different types of risk assessment scales, most of which have not been tested on a large scale. The Braden Q Scale [1] and the Neonatal Skin Risk Assessment Scale [6] seem to be reliable tools in terms of sensitivity and specificity.

66.3 Principles of Treatment

66.3.1 Topic Treatment

For Stage 2 pressure ulcers, the use of hydrocolloids seems to us to be appropriate in the majority of cases.

For Stage 3 and 4 pressure ulcers, treatment is very similar to that of the adult, but the possibilities available in terms of wound cleaning are often reduced as the baby cannot be moved.

Throughout the liquefactive necrotic stage, the use of silver sulphadiazine as an alternative to hydrogels seems to us to be a possibility. The dressings need to be substantial, thus allowing for additional discharge.

66.3.2 Surgical Treatment

It is reserved for severe cases. It uses the classic reconstruction ladder (skin graft, local and distant flaps). Taking account of the healing capacity of the newborn, the flap realization is often performed in a second step during infant growth.

66.4 Main Areas Affected

66.4.1 The Nose

The nose is the main area affected, representing half of all NPUs [5]. This has been seen since the 1980s, with the development of nasal continuous positive airway pressure (NCPAP).

According to different studies, nasal lesion incidence is between 20% and 60% in premature treated with NCPAP [7, 8]. The majority of occurrence is due to the technique being incorrectly used and/or poor monitoring of skin tolerance [9].

The pressure ulcer most often involves the philtrum, the tip of the nose, the soft triangle, or the nasal septum.

A deformation or a change in function results, which is usually temporary. However, cases have unfortunately been reported in which columellar necrosis has led to a significant disorder in growth.

Figure 66.2 shows a typical lesion due to excessive pressure from an endotracheal tube, which, in bending the soft triangle, has resulted in ischaemia.

Figures 66.3 and 66.4 show two similar cases of columellar necrosis, at different ages. In Fig. 66.4, note the asymmetrical character of the lesion and the consequences on the development of the tip of the nose.

66.4.2 The Foot and Leg

Here, the lesions are genuine pressure ulcers as seen in the bedridden or the paralysed. The main areas affected are the malleoli and the heels.

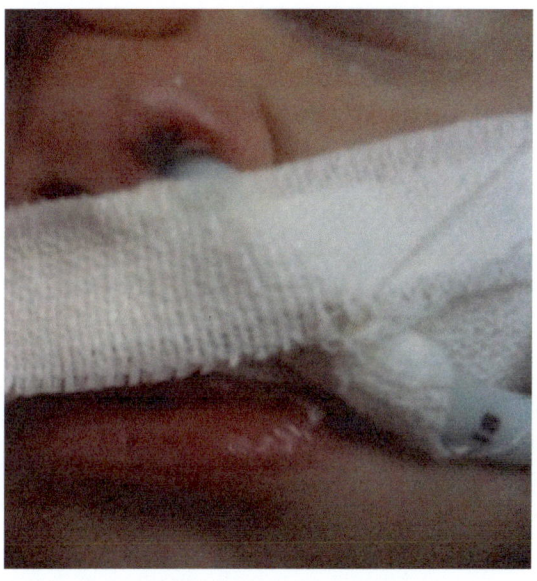

Fig. 66.2 Soft triangle pressure ulcer caused by excessive pressure from the endotracheal tube

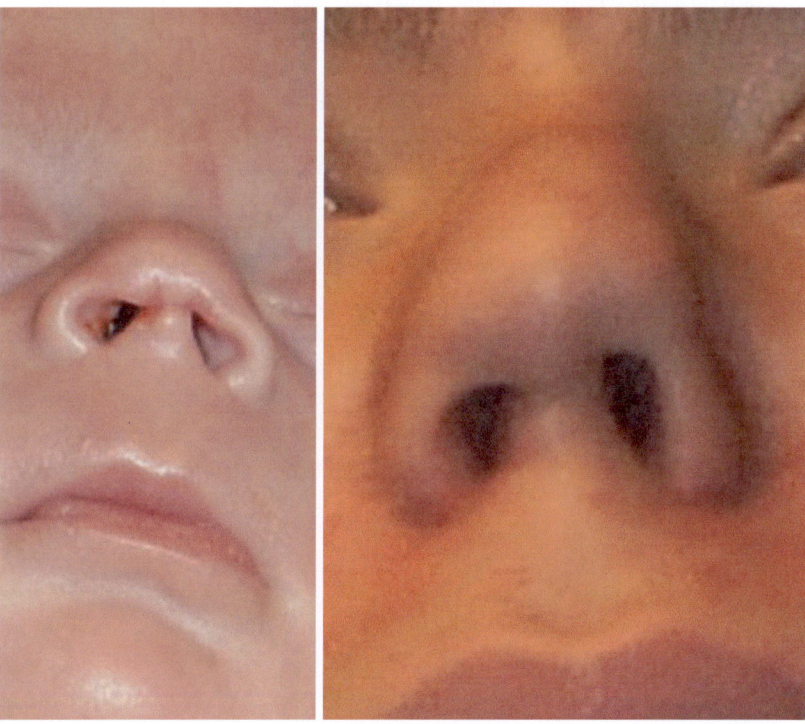

Figs. 66.3 and 66.4 Lesions linked to excessive pressure during NCPAP. The pressure ulcer especially affects the junction of the columella and the apex

Pressure ulcers have also been reported on the toes, due to the use of oximetry sensors. On the legs, they are often due to the premature use of postural splints.

These ulcers usually improve in a few days after removal of the pressure source and after mechanical or chemical debridement.

66.4.3 The Scalp and Back

The two main causes of scalp NPUs are birth trauma and excessive pressure on the occiput.

Scalp injuries are present in around 15% of babies born using ventouse or forceps [7]. The lesions are often deep and semicircular, leaving a visible area of scarred alopecia.

Figure 66.5 shows a case of scalp lesion secondary to ventouse extraction, which affected a ¾-circular area. Wound healing was obtained after 3 weeks of closely supervised healing by secondary intention and involved additional surgical intervention.

Wound healing is usually attained in a few weeks under such supervision. Dressings need to be changed daily and use silver sulphadiazine or hydrogel.

There are other rare locations, which are nevertheless worth mentioning. The use of EEG monitoring equipment can cause pressure on the forehead; this can be a source of ulcers, which are sometimes deep. Figure 66.6 shows an example of lesions seen in intensive care which caused visible scarring.

In a recent study [5], pressure ulcers on the back of the head were found to represent 14% of all NPUs.

Excessive pressure can cause occipital ulcers, which are sometimes extensive. They affect children in intensive care or recovery. Catastrophic situations can result from the combined risk factors of mechanical ventilation, sedation, a central venous line, humidity, the warmth of the incubator, and the baby's state of shock (see Fig. 66.7).

In the baby seen in Fig. 66.7, the pressure ulcer was due to prolonged excessive pressure in the context of major cardiac surgery, with prolonged low cardiac output. The child had not been turned because of its haemodynamic instability. Healing was obtained after surgical debridement in the intensive care bed, dressings using negative pressure therapy, followed by skin graft on a thin one-layer artificial dermis (Matriderm®). One part was closed without tension.

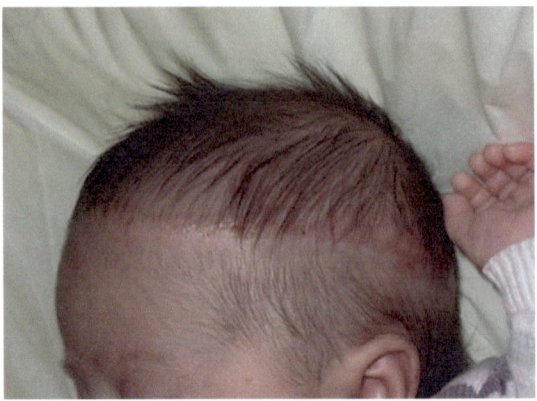

Fig. 66.5 Circular lesion caused by ventouse extraction

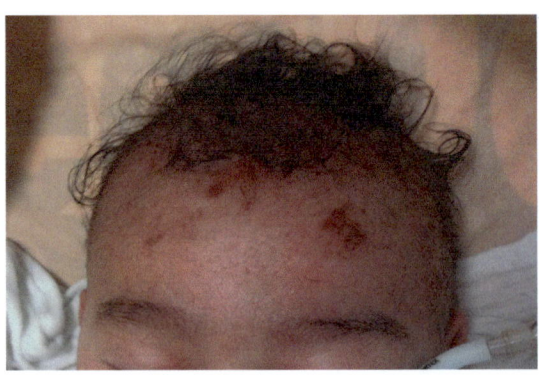

Fig. 66.6 Pressure ulcers on the forehead caused by EEG electrodes

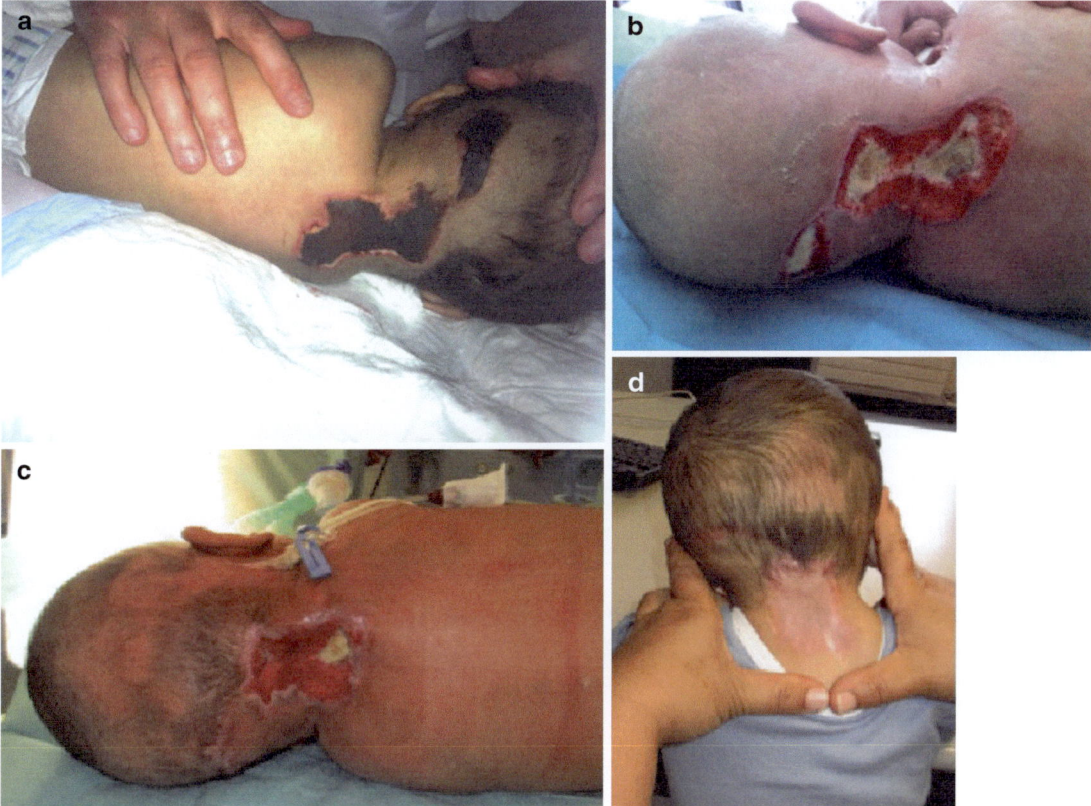

Fig. 66.7 (**a**) Extensive and deep pressure ulcer of the occipital and upper cervical region. (**b**) Result obtained after debridement and initiation of negative pressure therapy. The muscles and aponeurosis have been affected, with contact involving the cervical spine processes. (**c**) Closure of the superior area and repeated debridement (×5). (**d**) Results at 5 months after placement of artificial dermis and thin skin graft taken from the adjacent scalp

The result was not perfect (see Fig. 66.7d), but it enabled rapid coverage, without adhesion.

66.5 Conclusion

Neonatal pressure ulcers are specific entities which require special attention from neonatal care teams. The thinness of the stratum corneum makes the skin of the premature and nursing baby particularly vulnerable to pressure. During the critical maturation phase, care teams must remain alert to the possibility of pressure ulcer formation, especially in an environment which can encourage such ulcer development.

References

1. Curley MA, Quigley SM, Lin M. Pressure ulcers in pediatric intensive care: incidence and associated factors. Pediatr Crit Care Med. 2003;4(3):284–90.
2. Ligi I, Arnaud F, Jouve E, Tardieu S, Sambuc R, Simeoni U. Iatrogenic events in admitted neonates: a prospective cohort study. Lancet. 2008;371(9610):404–10.

3. Cartlidge PH, Fox PE, Rutter N. The scars of newborn intensive care. Early Hum Dev. 1990;21(1):1–10.
4. Zollo MB, Gostisha ML, Berens RJ, Schmidt JE, Weigle CG. Altered skin integrity in children admitted to a pediatric intensive care unit. J Nurs Care Qual. 1996;11(2):62–7.
5. Fujii K, Sugama J, Okuwa M, Sanada H, Mizokami Y. Incidence and risk factors of pressure ulcers in seven neonatal intensive care units in Japan: a multisite prospective cohort study. Int Wound J. 2010;7(5):323–8.
6. Huffines B, Logsdon MC. The Neonatal Skin Risk Assessment Scale for predicting skin breakdown in neonates. Issues Compr Pediatr Nurs. 1997;20(2):103–14.
7. Sardesai SR, Kornacka MK, Walas W, Ramanathan R. Iatrogenic skin injury in the neonatal intensive care unit. J Matern Fetal Neonatal Med. 2011;24(2):197–203.
8. Jatana KR, Oplatek A, Stein M, Phillips G, Kang DR, Elmaraghy CA. Effects of nasal continuous positive airway pressure and cannula use in the neonatal intensive care unit setting. Arch Otolaryngol Neck Head Surg. 2010;136(3):287–91.
9. Shanmugananda K, Rawal J. Nasal trauma due to nasal continuous positive airway pressure in newborns. Arch Dis Child Fetal Neonatal Ed. 2007;92(1):F18.

Open Access This chapter is licensed under the terms of the Creative Commons Attribution-NonCommercial-NoDerivatives 4.0 International License (http://creativecommons.org/licenses/by-nc-nd/4.0/), which permits any non-commercial use, sharing, distribution and reproduction in any medium or format, as long as you give appropriate credit to the original author(s) and the source, provide a link to the Creative Commons license and indicate if you modified the licensed material. You do not have permission under this license to share adapted material derived from this chapter or parts of it.

The images or other third party material in this chapter are included in the chapter's Creative Commons license, unless indicated otherwise in a credit line to the material. If material is not included in the chapter's Creative Commons license and your intended use is not permitted by statutory regulation or exceeds the permitted use, you will need to obtain permission directly from the copyright holder.

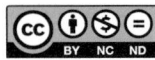

67. Skin Necrosis in Children: Genodermatosis

Cristina Has and Agnes Schwieger-Briel

67.1 Introduction

The term genodermatosis comprises a large group of dermatoses caused by genetic defects, including monogenic and mosaic disorders. From the physiopathogenic point of view, various compartments of the skin can be disturbed, such as intraepidermal or epidermal-dermal adhesion, cornification, DNA repair, the vascular system, etc. The onset of clinical symptoms is most commonly at birth or during early childhood, and the clinical course is progressive, without spontaneous healing or remission.

Cutaneous necrosis is a primary manifestation of several disorders reviewed in this chapter. Even though more common in the context of acquired inflammatory conditions predisposing to infectious or ischemic necrosis, it can also be a characteristic sign of genetic diseases.

C. Has (✉)
Department of Dermatology, Medical Center—University of Freiburg, Freiburg, Germany
e-mail: cristina.has@uniklinik-freiburg.de

A. Schwieger-Briel
Department of Dermatology, Medical Center—University of Freiburg, Freiburg, Germany

Pediatric Skin Center, Dermatology, University Children's Hospital Zurich, Zurich, Switzerland

67.2 Genodermatoses that Manifest with Cutaneous Necrosis as a Lead Symptom

67.2.1 Progeroid Syndromes

67.2.1.1 Hutchinson–Gilford Progeria Syndrome and Mandibuloacral Dysplasia

Hutchinson–Gilford progeria syndrome (HGPS, OMIM#176670) and mandibuloacral dysplasia with type A lipodystrophy (MADA, OMIM#248370) are allelic disorders that belong to the premature aging syndromes (syn. progeroid syndromes, laminopathies). They are caused by pathogenic variants in the gene for lamin A/C (LMNA), an essential structural component of the nuclear envelope. HGPS is extremely rare occurring in one per 20 million newborns due to a de novo mutation. MADA is an autosomal recessive condition.

1. Physiopathogeny and biology:
   In HGPS, a recurrent de novo monoallelic variant (c.1824C>T) leads to formation of a truncated prelamin A protein, called progerin, which cannot undergo normal processing to mature lamin A [1]. Normal prelamin A processing comprises four posttranslational modification steps. Mature lamin A is an intermediate filament protein that is incorporated into the nuclear lamina filament mesh-

work, where it interacts with many proteins important for nuclear structure integrity [1]. In HGPS, progerin accumulates as a farnesylated and methylated intermediate in the nuclear envelope where it is toxic and causes nuclear shape abnormalities and senescence. This is the molecular basis for the polymorphic disease manifestations in different organs in HGPS.

2. Diagnosis

The diagnosis is based on clinical features and genetic testing. Clinical manifestations are present in early childhood. Life expectancy is limited to the second decade of life in HGPS.

Medical context and semiology:

HGPS

(a) Cutaneous features include atrophic, scleroderma-like skin with progressive loss of subcutaneous fatty tissue, cigarette paper-like appearance, clearly visible venous network. Additional manifestations:

(b) Sparse hair, nail anomalies, delayed and abnormal dentition

(c) Progeroid features: 'bird' facies with sharp, thin nose and micrognathia

(d) Absent sexual secondary characteristics, high-pitched voice

(e) Growth failure, skeletal anomalies, aseptic necrosis of bones reported, acro-osteolysis and osteoporosis

(f) Cardiovascular anomalies (rapidly progressive atherosclerosis, early myocardial infarction and strokes, hypertension, congestive heart failure)

MADA

(a) Cutaneous features include pigmentary skin changes and lipodystrophy, characterized by a marked acral loss of fatty tissue with normal or increased fatty tissue in the neck and trunk.

(b) Inconstant progeroid features

(c) Growth retardation, mandibular hypoplasia, skeletal abnormalities with progressive osteolysis of the distal phalanges and clavicles

(d) Metabolic complications can arise due to insulin resistance and diabetes.

On the background of tissue atrophy and vascular changes, skin necrosis and ulcers can occur in both conditions in particular on acral and on bony surfaces.

3. Treatment:

There is no cure for these rare disorders, although many experimental strategies are under research [1]. They include genetic approaches or targeting the level and the post-translational modifications of progerin. The treatment of necrosis is symptomatic, aiming at controlling infections, saving tissue, and managing wounds. Prevention measures should include careful skin care with moisturizers and avoidance of mechanical pressure and trauma.

67.2.2 Vascular Anomalies

67.2.2.1 Cutis Marmorata Telangiectatica Congenita (Syn. Congenital Generalized Phlebectasia, Naevus Vascularis Reticularis, Congenital Phlebectasia, Congenital Livedo Reticularis and van Lohuizen Syndrome)

Cutis marmorata telangiectatica congenita (CMTC) is an uncommon congenital vascular anomaly with features including erythematous-to-violaceous, reticulated, net-like or marbled-appearing patches of skin phlebectasias, and cutaneous and subcutaneous atrophy [2]. It can mimic physiological cutis marmorata (CM) but does not disappear with warming. CMTC may be present in some disorders such as Adams–Oliver syndrome, phakomatosis pigmentovascularis type 5A, and neonatal lupus erythematosus [3]. CMTC is a slow-flow vascular lesion that affects capillaries and venules.

1. Physiopathogeny and biology:

CMTC is a mosaic disorder caused by *GNA11* mutations found in skin biopsies from

CMTC-affected skin areas. The mutation is either not detectable or found at a low level of 0.3% in blood [4].
2. Diagnosis:
    CMTC is a clinical diagnosis. When suspicion of CMTC is raised, it is recommended to perform a careful evaluation of the patient for associated anomalies, in cases with extensive findings, ideally in a multidisciplinary team with a pediatrician, dermatologist, ophthalmologist and, if needed, orthopedic surgeon [5].
    Medical context and semiology:
    The most important cutaneous manifestation of CMTC, the reticulate marbled vascular presentation. CMTC can be localized, segmental or widespread. Atrophy or skin ulceration and lipoatrophy at the sites of vascular discoloration, as well as prominent veins, telangiectasias and hyperkeratosis may be present. Association with limb asymmetry, glaucoma, intellectual disability, patent ductus arteriosus, and arterial stenosis have been reported [2, 3]. A review of the literature found extracutaneous anomalies in 42.5% of patients, predominantly body asymmetry and neurological defects like seizure and developmental delay. Fewer patients (10.1%) had ophthalmological defects, usually glaucoma [5].
3. Treatment:
    Some reports described effective laser therapy for erythema and ulceration, while other reports stated no effect of laser treatment [5–7]. PDL therapy for this condition shows a variable response, often disappointing. The skin lesions tend to fade with age. The only exception is a capillary malformation of the upper lip, often a feature of this condition, which can respond well to laser treatment [3].

67.2.3 Metabolic Disorders

67.2.3.1 Prolidase Deficiency
Prolidase deficiency (OMIM#170100) is an inborn metabolic multisystemic disease characterized by skin lesions, recurrent infections, dysmorphic facial features, variable intellectual disability, and organomegaly with elevated liver enzymes. Skeletal anomalies, chronic pulmonary disease, anemia, thrombocytopenia, hypergammaglobulinemia, and hypocomplementemia are inconstant features [8]. Prolidase deficiency is one of the rare causes of leg ulcers in children [9].

1. Physiopathogeny and biology:
    Biallelic pathogenic variants in the gene encoding prolidase are found in affected individuals. Prolidase is an enzyme that cleaves di- and tripeptides containing carboxyl-terminal proline or hydroxyproline [10]. It is a homodimer, with each subunit binding two manganese ions that are required for enzymatic activity. The enzyme is required in the final catabolic steps of endogenous and dietary proteins, rich in proline and hydroxyproline, such as collagen. The deficiency of prolidase leads to accumulation of imidodipeptides, or peptides with two amino acids, with a C-terminal proline or hydroxyproline [8].
2. Diagnosis:
    The diagnosis can be established based on characteristic clinical findings and imidodipeptiduria or reduced prolidase enzyme activity. Genetic testing identifies biallelic pathogenic variants in *PEPD*, the gene coding for prolidase.
    Medical context and semiology:
    (a) Typically severe, chronic, recalcitrant, and painful skin ulcers of the lower extremities (Fig. 67.1) and telangiectasias of the face and hands. A review of the literature identified skin ulcers in 61% of the reviewed cases. The ulcerations may appear on the dorsal part of the foot and on the sole and extend all over the legs, sometimes leading to tendon lesions and severe skin infections. No underlying vascular anomalies were described [11].
    (b) Infections of the skin and respiratory tract
    (c) Splenomegaly and inconstant hepatomegaly
3. *Treatment:*
    Skin ulcers require treatment by a wound care specialist; topical proline (often 5%) or

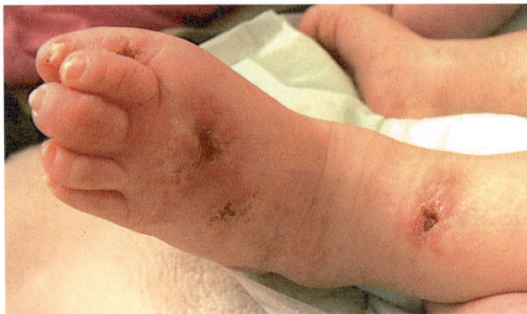

Fig. 67.1 Prolidase deficiency

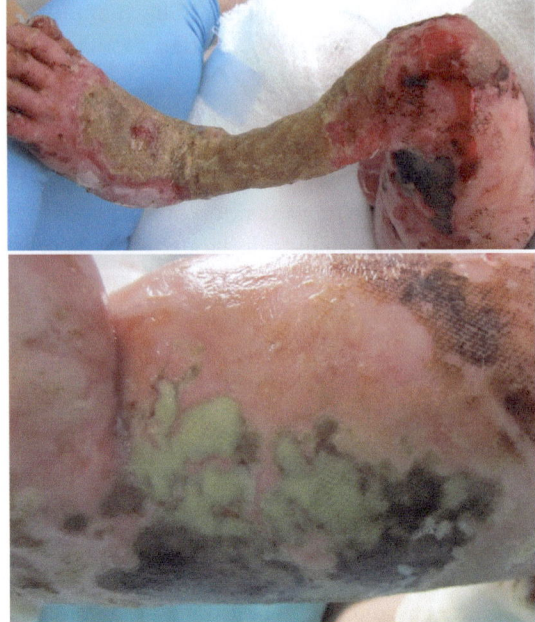

Fig. 67.2 Ecthyma gangrenosum in EBS (kindly provided by Dr. L. Weibel)

topical 5% proline-5% glycerine ointment applied with dressing changes has been successful in some affected individuals [12]. Standard treatment should be employed for developmental delay/intellectual disability, seizures, infections, reactive airways disease/pulmonary hypertension, respectively. One group reported improvement of skin findings with the use of anticoagulants [13].

67.2.4 Genodermatosis with Cutaneous Necrosis as a Possible Complication

67.2.4.1 Inherited Epidermolysis Bullosa

Epidermolysis bullosa (EB) encompasses genetic disorders characterized by skin fragility and blistering with a broad range of clinical severity. The main EB types are EB simplex, junctional EB, dystrophic EB, and Kindler EB. Skin necrosis is not a typical feature of EB but may occur in wounded areas in the context of infections (Fig. 67.2) [14].

1. Physiopathogeny and biology:

    EB is caused by loss of function pathogenic variants in genes encoding structural proteins assuring the mechanical stability of the skin, such as keratins, integrins, collagens, or laminins [15]. Consequently, keratin intermediate filaments, hemidesmosomes, focal adhesions, or anchoring fibrils are weakened. Blistering can be intraepidermal, junctional, dermal, or mixed and results in erosions, ulcerations, or chronic wounds. Congenital absence of the skin is relatively common on lower legs and can be a feature of any type of EB. There is an alteration in the cutaneous microbiome in EB, with loss of species diversity and abundance of Staphylococcus [16].

2. Diagnosis:

    The diagnosis of EB is clinically suspected based on mechanically induced blistering of the skin and additional cutaneous features as described in detail before [17]. Immunofluorescence mapping and genetic testing determine the type and subtype of EB [18].

    Medical context and semiology:
    (a) Blisters, erosions, ulcerations, and wounds, depending on the type of EB
    (b) Scarring is a main feature of dystrophic and Kindler EB

(c) Nail dystrophy is common in junctional and dystrophic EB
(d) Mucosal membranes are fragile leading to inflammation and scarring, in particular, in dystrophic and Kindler EB
(e) Extracutaneous organ involvement may occur primary in syndromic EB subtypes or secondary as a complication of severe EB

3. Treatment:

Blisters should be lanced; antiseptics should be used as well as proper wound dressings in order to assure uncomplicated healing of the wounds. Mechanical pressure should be avoided in particular on bony body areas. Various cell therapies (e.g., fibroblasts, mesenchymal stem cells) administered topically to epidermolysis bullosa wounds in small clinical trials, showed positive effect on wound healing [19–23].

Recently, Oleogel-S10 (containing birch triterpenes, Filsuvez®) [24] was approved by EMA and FDA for the treatment of wounds in junctional and dystrophic epidermolysis bullosa. Beremagene geperpavec (B-VEC, Vyjuvek®) is the first gene therapy approved by the FDA for the treatment of cutaneous wounds in patients with dystrophic epidermolysis bullosa. This represents a significant progress for the treatment of this devastating disease. It is based on non-replicative (nr) recombinant HSV-1 vector containing two copies of the *COL7A1* gene [25, 26].

67.2.5 Harlequin Ichthyosis

Harlequin ichthyosis (OMIM#242500) is one of the most severe types of congenital ichthyosis that manifests at birth with tight horny plaques that cover the entire body (harlequin-baby). There is no primary extracutaneous involvement, but skin contractions lead to ectropion, eclabion, ear deformities, and deformities of the hands and feet. Complications occur frequently in infants and include respiratory distress, dehydration, electrolyte imbalance, temperature instability, feeding problems, and bacterial infections, often with fatal consequences. Constriction bands may cause skin necrosis.

1. Physiopathogeny and biology:

Harlequin ichthyosis is caused by biallelic loss of function pathogenic variants in *ABCA12,* the gene that codes for ATP binding cassette subfamily A Member 12, a glucosylceramide transporter.

2. Diagnosis:

Medical context and semiology:
(a) Harlequin-baby at birth
(b) Erythroderma and generalized large lamellar scales
(c) Ectropion, eclabion, ear deformities
(d) Severe palmoplantar keratoderma
(e) Digital autoamputation [27]
(f) Respiratory distress, dehydration, electrolyte imbalance, temperature instability, feeding problems, and bacterial infections

3. *Treatment*

Early administration of oral retinoids (acitretin 1 mg/kg) is effective in shedding and softening of the large scales, reducing the risk of constrictive bands and skin necrosis. In addition, the use of skin moisturizers is mandatory (such as petrolatum).

67.2.6 Olmsted Syndrome

Olmsted syndrome (OS OMIM#614594, #619208, #300918) is a rare genodermatosis classically characterized by the combination of bilateral mutilating transgradient palmoplantar keratoderma (PPK) and periorificial keratotic plaques, but which shows considerable clinical heterogeneity. The disease starts usually at birth or in early childhood. Less than 100 cases have been reported worldwide [28].

1. Physiopathogeny and biology:

OS is genetically heterogeneous, being caused by pathogenic variants in three distinct genes *TRPV3* (transient receptor potential cat-

ion channel subfamily V member 3), *PERP* (TP53 apoptosis effector), or *MBTPS2* (membrane bound transcription factor peptidase, Site 2). TRPV3 is a thermosensible cation non selective channel, activated by temperature and several chemical ligands, predominately expressed in keratinocytes, and in sensory neurons. MBTPS2 is a zinc metalloprotease essential for cholesterol homeostasis and endoplasmic reticulum stress response [28].
2. Diagnosis:
   Medical context and semiology:
   (a) Bilateral mutilating transgradient palmoplantar keratoderma. Progression of the keratoderma may lead to flexion deformities, constrictions of digital bands, and even spontaneous digit amputations.
   (b) Periorificial keratotic plaques (mouth, nose, eyes, genital, anal, ears, navel)
   (c) Other features may be nonperiorificial keratotic lesions involving the thighs, arms, elbows, knees, and intertriginous folds; hyperkeratotic linear streaks, follicular keratosis, pachyderma, cheilitis, ichthyotic lesions, or chronic blepharitis.
   (d) High clinical variability and a wide range of inconsistent clinical manifestations have been reported [28]
3. *Treatment*
   (a) Symptomatic treatments of hyperkeratosis include emollients, keratolytics, retinoids, or corticosteroids, either topical or systemic
   (b) Recently, targeted inhibition of the epidermal growth factor receptor and mammalian target of rapamycin signaling pathways demonstrated significant improvement of clinical manifestations of OS [29, 30].

67.2.7 Leucocyte Adhesion Deficiency Type I

Leukocyte adhesion deficiency type 1 (LAD-I) (OMIM#116920) includes three types, of which type I is the most common.

1. Physiopathogeny and biology:
   Patients are lacking the β2-integrin chain CD18 (ITGB2) of the leukocyte cell adhesion molecule, essential for cell–cell and cell–extracellular matrix interactions. Consequently, the function of granulocytes, monocytes, and lymphocytes is impaired.
2. Diagnosis:
   Medical context and semiology:
   Newborns often suffer from navel infections with Pseudomonas aeruginosa, leading to severe skin necrosis. Skin manifestations consist of abscesses, mucosal ulcers, and wound healing defects.
   (a) Recurrent, life-threatening bacterial infections of the skin, mouth, and respiratory tract
   (b) Periodontitis and tooth loss
3. *Treatment*
   (a) Control of infections with antibiotics.
   (b) Hematopoietic cell transplantation represents the only cure for LAD-I.

67.2.8 Other Genetic Diseases

Skin necrosis may be a complication of various disorders:

- Autoinflammatory disorders who can have vasculopathies
- Interferonopathies
- Hematologic diseases such as sickle cell anemia cause severe ulcerations
- Genetic primary lymphedema
- Klinefelter syndrome

67.3 Conclusion/Take Home Messages

Skin necrosis is rare in children and may be a manifestation of a serious genodermatosis. The diagnosis should be made based on clinical manifestations and genetic testing. Although specific therapies are lacking, intensive symptomatic management of skin lesions should be the main focus.

References

1. Chen X, Yao H, Andrés V, et al. Status of treatment strategies for Hutchinson-Gilford progeria syndrome with a focus on prelamin: a posttranslational modification. Basic Clin Pharmacol Toxicol. 2022;131:217. https://doi.org/10.1111/bcpt.13770.
2. Lee B-B, Gloviczki P, Blei F, Markovic JN. Capilar malformations. In: Vascular malformations. CRC Press. Kindle-Version; 2020.
3. Hoeger P, Kinsler V, Yan A, Harper J, Oranje A, Bodemer C, Larralde M, Luk D, Mendiratta V, Purvis D, editors. Harper's textbook of pediatric dermatology. 4th ed. Wiley; 2020. p. 2019.
4. Schuart C, Bassi A, Kapp F, et al. Cutis marmorata telangiectatica congenita being caused by postzygotic GNA11 mutations. Eur J Med Genet. 2022;65:104472.
5. Bui TNPT, Corap A, Bygum A. Cutis marmorata telangiectatica congenita: a literature review. Orphanet J Rare Dis. 2019;14:283.
6. Tracey EH, Eversman A, Knabel D, Irfan M. Cutis marmorata telangiectatica congenita successfully treated with intense pulsed light and pulse dyed laser therapy: a case report. J Cosmet Laser Ther. 2020;22:177–9.
7. Deshpande AJ. Cutis mormorata telangiectatica congenital successfully treated with intense pulsed light therapy: a case report. J Cosmet Laser Ther. 2018;20:145–7.
8. Rossignol F, Wang H, Ferreira C. Prolidase Deficiency. In: Adam MP, Everman DB, Mirzaa GM, et al., editors. GeneReviews®. Seattle, WA: University of Washington, Seattle; 1993. http://www.ncbi.nlm.nih.gov/books/NBK299584/. Accessed 30 Sep 2022.
9. Say M, Tella E, Boccara O, et al. Leg ulcers in childhood: a multicenter study in France. Ann Dermatol Venereol. 2022;149:51–5.
10. Misiura M, Miltyk W. Current understanding of the emerging role of prolidase in cellular metabolism. Int J Mol Sci. 2020;21:E5906.
11. Spodenkiewicz M, Spodenkiewicz M, Cleary M, et al. Clinical genetics of prolidase deficiency: an updated review. Biology (Basel). 2020;9:E108.
12. Cathcart C, Hanley T, Gossan N, et al. Obstinate leg ulceration secondary to prolidase deficiency, treated with 5% topical proline. Clin Exp Dermatol. 2022;47:1010–2.
13. Süßmuth K, Metze D, Muresan A-M, et al. Ulceration in prolidase deficiency: successful treatment with anticoagulants. Acta Derm Venereol. 2020;100:adv00002.
14. Schlueer A-B, Schwieger-Briel A, Theiler M, et al. Negative pressure wound treatment in a neonate with epidermolysis bullosa simplex severe generalized: a case report. Pediatr Dermatol. 2020;37:1218–20.
15. Baradaran-Heravi A, Balgi AD, Hosseini-Farahabadi S, et al. Effect of small molecule eRF3 degraders on premature termination codon readthrough. Nucleic Acids Res. 2021;49:3692–708.
16. Reimer-Taschenbrecker A, Künstner A, Hirose M, et al. Predominance of staphylococcus correlates with wound burden and disease activity in dystrophic epidermolysis bullosa: a prospective case-control study. J Invest Dermatol. 2022;142:2117–2127.e8.
17. Has C, Bauer JW, Bodemer C, et al. Consensus reclassification of inherited epidermolysis bullosa and other disorders with skin fragility. Br J Dermatol. 2020;183:614–27.
18. Has C, Liu L, Bolling MC, et al. Clinical practice guidelines for laboratory diagnosis of epidermolysis bullosa. Br J Dermatol. 2020;182:574–92.
19. Niebergall-Roth E, Dieter K, Daniele C, et al. Kinetics of wound development and healing suggests a skin-stabilizing effect of allogeneic ABCB5+ mesenchymal stromal cell treatment in recessive dystrophic epidermolysis bullosa. Cells. 2023;12:1468.
20. Petrof G, Lwin SM, Martinez-Queipo M, et al. Potential of systemic allogeneic mesenchymal stromal cell therapy for children with recessive dystrophic epidermolysis bullosa. J Invest Dermatol. 2015;135:2319–21.
21. Kikuchi Y, Tamakoshi T, Ishida R, et al. Gene-modified blister fluid-derived mesenchymal stromal cells for treating recessive dystrophic epidermolysis bullosa. J Invest Dermatol. 2023;143:2447–2455.e8.
22. Petrova A, Georgiadis C, Fleck RA, et al. Human mesenchymal stromal cells engineered to express collagen VII can restore anchoring fibrils in recessive dystrophic epidermolysis bullosa skin graft chimeras. J Invest Dermatol. 2020;140:121–131.e6.
23. Lwin SM, Syed F, Di W-L, et al. Safety and early efficacy outcomes for lentiviral fibroblast gene therapy in recessive dystrophic epidermolysis bullosa. JCI Insight. 2019;4 https://doi.org/10.1172/jci.insight.126243.
24. Kern JS, Sprecher E, Fernandez MF, et al. Efficacy and safety of Oleogel-S10 (birch triterpenes) for epidermolysis bullosa: results from the phase III randomized double-blind phase of the EASE study. Br J Dermatol. 2023;188:12–21.
25. Gurevich I, Agarwal P, Zhang P, et al. In vivo topical gene therapy for recessive dystrophic epidermolysis bullosa: a phase 1 and 2 trial. Nat Med. 2022;28:780–8.
26. Guide SV, Gonzalez ME, Bağcı IS, et al. Trial of beremagene geperpavec (B-VEC) for dystrophic epidermolysis bullosa. N Engl J Med. 2022;387:2211–9.
27. Tanahashi K, Sugiura K, Sato T, Akiyama M. Noteworthy clinical findings of harlequin ichthyosis: digital autoamputation caused by cutaneous constriction bands in a case with novel ABCA12 mutations. Br J Dermatol. 2016;174:689–91.
28. Duchatelet S, Hovnanian A. Olmsted syndrome: clinical, molecular and therapeutic aspects. Orphanet J Rare Dis. 2015;10:33.
29. Greco C, Leclerc-Mercier S, Chaumon S, et al. Use of epidermal growth factor receptor inhibitor erlo-

tinib to treat palmoplantar keratoderma in patients with olmsted syndrome caused by TRPV3 mutations. JAMA Dermatol. 2020;156:191–5.
30. Zhang A, Duchatelet S, Lakdawala N, et al. Targeted inhibition of the epidermal growth factor receptor and mammalian target of rapamycin signaling pathways in olmsted syndrome. JAMA Dermatol. 2020;156:196–200.

Open Access This chapter is licensed under the terms of the Creative Commons Attribution-NonCommercial-NoDerivatives 4.0 International License (http://creativecommons.org/licenses/by-nc-nd/4.0/), which permits any non-commercial use, sharing, distribution and reproduction in any medium or format, as long as you give appropriate credit to the original author(s) and the source, provide a link to the Creative Commons license and indicate if you modified the licensed material. You do not have permission under this license to share adapted material derived from this chapter or parts of it.

The images or other third party material in this chapter are included in the chapter's Creative Commons license, unless indicated otherwise in a credit line to the material. If material is not included in the chapter's Creative Commons license and your intended use is not permitted by statutory regulation or exceeds the permitted use, you will need to obtain permission directly from the copyright holder.

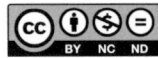

Skin Necrosis in Children: Vascular Causes and Angioma

Laurence M. Boon, Valérie Dekeuleneer, and Julien Coulie

68.1 Ulcerated Infantile Hemangioma

Infantile hemangiomas (IH) are the most common vascular tumors during infancy (5% of infants) [1, 2]. They appear during the first weeks of life and have typically an early rapid proliferation phase, followed by stabilization and finally a progressive spontaneous regression. Complications can be seen in 10–15% of cases [3, 4]. Ulceration is the most common complication (up to 15% of IH) [5]. These ulcerations are painful, with a risk of bleeding (mainly mild and benign), infection, and persistent scarring due to skin necrosis.

68.1.1 Physiopathology

– Pathogeny of IH is not yet fully elucidated. The trigger factor of endothelial cells proliferation seems to be hypoxic stress, leading to overproduction of angiogenic factors through lowered VEGFR1 expression [5, 6].

68.1.2 Clinical Presentation

– Ulcerations appear most of the time during the proliferation phase of IH with the highest risk between the age of 4 and 6 months (median age of 4 months).
– Ulcerations usually start with a central gray coloration appearing on the IH. This can be triggered by a local trauma.
– IH with ulcerations are more likely large, superficial/mixed or segmental and localized on lower lip, neck/ head, or anogenital area (Fig. 68.1a–c).
– All ulcerated IH will lead to significant scarring due to wound healing process.
– Moisture, maceration, and friction seem also to have a role in the appearance of these ulcerations [7–10].

68.1.3 Diagnosis

– The diagnosis of IH is mostly clinical [10, 11].
– In atypical subcutaneous IHs, a doppler ultrasonography (US) by a radiologist experienced in vascular anomalies, can help confirming the diagnosis. Doppler US during the proliferation phase shows hyper vascular high flow tumor, with a stromal or tumoral component. In some cases, a magnetic resonance imaging is needed, especially to delimit the extent of the IH. A skin biopsy showing GLUT-1 staining gives a definite diagnosis.

L. M. Boon (✉) · V. Dekeuleneer · J. Coulie
Division of Plastic Surgery, Center for Vascular Anomalies, Cliniques Universitaires Saint Luc, UCLouvain, Brussels, Belgium
e-mail: laurence.boon@uclouvain.be; valerie.dekeuleneer@saintluc.uclouvain.be; julien.coulie@saintluc.uclouvain.be

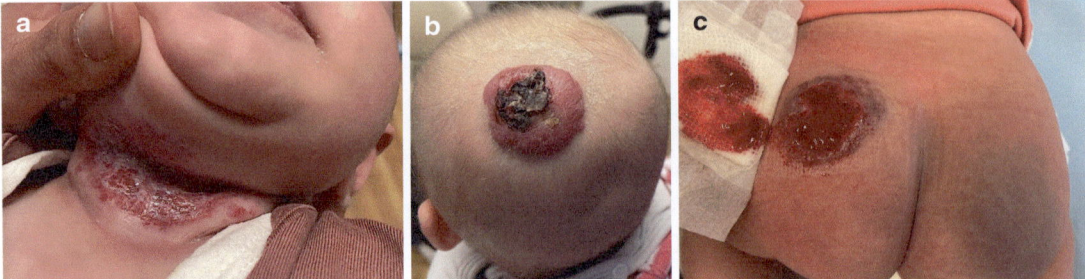

Fig. 68.1 (**a**) Cervical ulcerated infantile hemangioma. (**b**) Ulcerated infantile hemangioma with necrosis of the vertex. (**c**) Ulcerated infantile hemangioma of the genital area with bleeding

Fig. 68.2 (**a**) Ulcerated infantile hemangioma of the trunk. (**b**) Eight days after propranolol initiation (2 mg/kg/days)

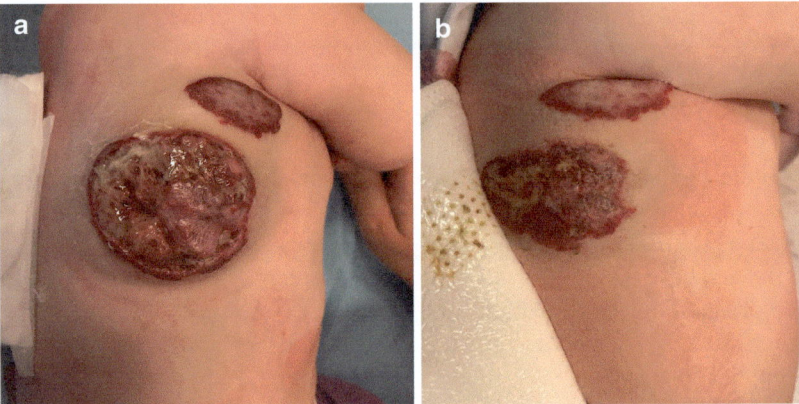

68.1.4 Treatment

- **Wound care** is central in the treatment of ulcerated infantile hemangioma [12]. It should be adapted to the type, localization, and size of ulceration. The wound should be protected and covered with atraumatic dressing to enhance the healing process and reduce the pain.
- If infection is suspected, local antibiotic can be applied.
- If the ulceration bleeds, hemostatic dressing can be used.
- **Pain control** with paracetamol should be considered.
- **Oral propranolol**: As for all complicated IH, oral propranolol is the first choice of treatment as it shortens the proliferation phase [4, 13] (Fig. 68.2a, b). Usually, it is administered at 2–3 mg/kg/day in 2 or 3 intakes [14, 15]. Some authors suggest that propranolol at this dose could induce or precipitate ulceration through vasoconstriction [16–18]. They propose to consider a lower dosage (up to 1 mg/kg/day or less) of oral propranolol if the IH is ulcerated (as it is used to treat segmental IH seen with PHACE syndrome). Topical timolol is not recommended due to the risk of systemic resorption [17].
- Pulsed dye laser can be used but its efficacy is variable and the procedure is painful [12].
- Early surgical resection can be proposed for strawberry-like ulcerated IH, knowing that they will leave sequalae after involution [19, 20]

68.2 Ulcerated Congenital Hemangiomas

Congenital hemangioma (CH) are rare, benign, vascular tumors fully developed at birth. There are three subtypes with common features: unique red or purple lesion, covered with telangiectasia with surrounding pallor. Rapidly Involuting Congenital

Hemangiomas (RICH) looks typically at birth as a large exophytic firm tumor with rapid regression during the first months of life (7–14 months) [21]. One third do not completely regress and are named Partially Involuting Congenital Hemangiomas (PICH) [22]. Ulceration is frequent in PICH. The third type of CH is called Non Involuting Congenital Hemangioma (NICH) which are usually flat at birth and do not regress [2].

68.2.1 Physiopathology

The pathophysiology of CH remains unclear. Histological features resemble pyogenic granulomas (PG) suggesting that an in-utero local vascular accident could trigger an abnormal vascular reparative process, as seen in PG [23]. The same missense mutations in *GNAQ* and *GNA11* are found in the three subtypes of CH suggesting that another post-natal phenomenon could induce spontaneous involution [6].

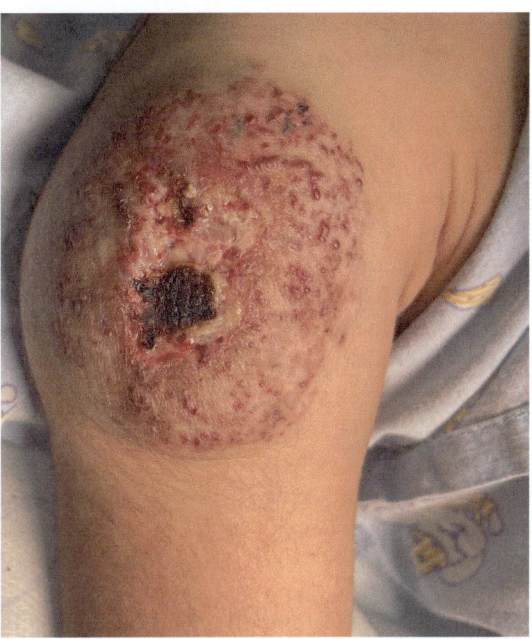

Fig. 68.3 Ulcerated congenital hemangioma of the shoulder

68.2.2 Clinical Presentation

– CH and especially RICH are hyper vascularized lesions. Ulceration is a possible complication. Severe and life-threatening bleeding are rare but described, sometimes needing radiological embolization. The cause of ulceration can be secondary to the erosion of large superficial vessel sometimes seen in CH. Ulceration can be a predictor for incomplete involution in RICH [24, 25].
– Heart failure, transient thrombocytopenia, and coagulopathy are also described [26, 27]. Associated thrombocytopenia can be a diagnostic challenge with sometimes a difficult differential diagnosis with a Kasabach-Merritt Phenomenon (KMP) as seen in Kaposiform Hemangioendotheliomas (KHE).

68.2.3 Diagnosis

– Unlike IH, CH are present and fully grown at birth. The diagnosis can be suspected during antenatal ultrasonography. Clinical presentation differs from an IH and is usually sufficient to make the diagnosis (Fig. 68.3).
– Doppler US (and in some atypical cases, magnetic resonance imagining) can be used to confirm the diagnosis and to evaluate the size and depth of the lesion. CH are highly vascularized tumors with many enlarged veins and arteries [24, 25].
– Differential diagnosis includes infantile fibrosarcomas, KHE, or tufted angioma (TA). A skin biopsy can help make the correct diagnosis if needed. Histopathological findings are similar in the three subtypes: capillary lobules and extralobular abnormal large superficial vessels (veins or lymphatic vessels), surrounded by fibrous tissue [28]. Endothelial cells from CH are negative for GLUT-1 immunostaining.

68.2.4 Treatment

In case of ulceration or severe hemorrhage, selective vascular embolization and/or surgical excision are recommended [24, 25]. Oral beta-blockers do not seem to be effective.

68.3 Arteriovenous Malformations

Arteriovenous malformations (AVMs) are congenital vascular anomalies, characterized by an abnormal connection between arteries and veins without the usual capillary network. This abnormal connection, known as the nidus, creates a direct pathway for blood flow between the high-pressure arteries and low-pressure veins. Those congenital lesions evolve over time with a progressive aggravation and invasion of surrounding healthy tissues [2, 29]. There seems to be a hormonal influence as some cases appeared or aggravated during pregnancy. Aggravation of the AVM is more frequent during adolescence, supporting the theory of hormonal influence [29].

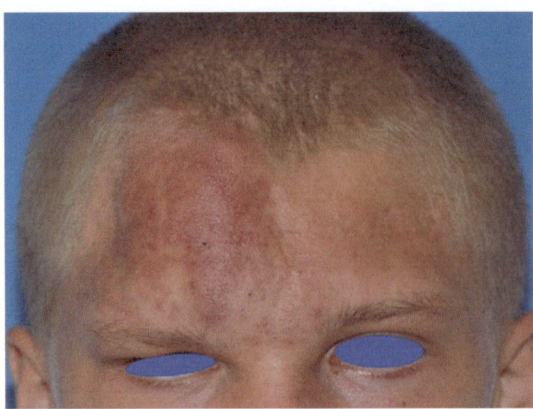

Fig. 68.4 Arteriovenous malformation (AVM) of the forehead presenting as a red, warm mass with abnormal palpated arteries and a local thrill

68.3.1 Physiopathology

The precise underlying physiopathology is not known. AVMs seem to result from a hyperactivation of the RAS/RAF/MEK/ERK pathway [6]. Mutations involving the MAPK-pathway causing sporadic AVMs are published in the literature [30, 31]. There seems to be a genotype–phenotype correlation showing that *KRAS* mutated AVMs cause more diffuse and extended facial AVMs [32].

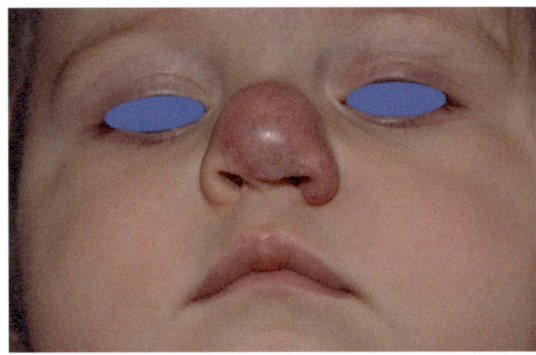

Fig. 68.5 Arteriovenous malformation (AVM) of the nose sends to our center for vascular anomalies with an initial diagnosis of infantile hemangioma (IH)

68.3.2 Clinical Presentation

AVMs present as a red warm lesion (Fig. 68.4). Clinical examination can reveal abnormal palpated arteries or a thrill. Although congenital, AVMs tend to evolve over time and become only visible during childhood or later in life. Local aggravation can be triggered by hormonal changes, local trauma, incomplete embolization, or surgery. If present at birth or in early childhood, differential diagnosis with CH or IH is not always easy (Fig. 68.5). Clinical presentation can be very similar, consisting of a red-violaceous warm lesion, that can grow over time and cause local ulcerations (Fig. 68.6), although ulceration will more likely appear later during childhood or adolescence, as opposed to IH. AVM presenting initially as a red mass with ulceration in early

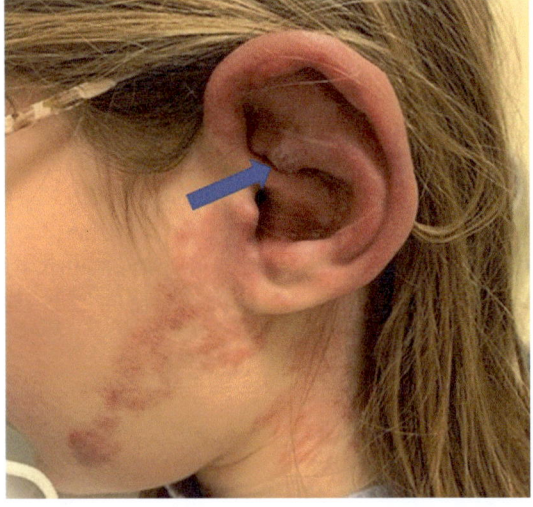

Fig. 68.6 Arteriovenous malformation (AVM) of the left ear. Blue arrow pointing at the ulceration site

childhood is very rare, but must be part of a differential diagnosis of an ulcerated vascular anomaly in pediatric patients.

68.3.3 Diagnosis

- Diagnosis can be clinical, with a red warm lesion or swelling associated with abnormally palpable arteries surrounding the lesion. Drainage veins will have a high blood flow velocity due to the vascular shunting and can cause a thrill that can be palpated.
- It can be confirmed with doppler US that will show high blood flow velocities, with lowered vascular resistance and very few or absent stromal tissue, as opposed to hemangiomas.
- Arteriography is essential to identify the afferent arteries and efferent veins before considering invasive treatments. It will show hypertrophic or abnormal arteries, rapid venous opacification, and a local blush which is consistent with the nidus.

68.3.4 Treatment

The only effective treatment is complete surgical excision with oncological-like margins to avoid local recurrence. Surgical excision can be associated with selective radiological embolization.

Embolization only is used in palliative cases if surgical resection is not an option. The long-term efficacy of embolization alone in AVMs is still under debate as late local recurrence can occur (up to 5 years).

Antiangiogenic treatments are becoming more and more used in adult patients. Thalidomide and trametinib seem to be the most promising medications [33, 34], although clinical pediatric trials are still lacking.

References

1. Krowchuk DP, Frieden I, Mancini AJ, Darrow DH, Blei F, Greene AK, Annam A, Baker CN, Frommelt PC, Hodak A, Pate BM, Pelletier JL, Sandrock D, Weinberg ST, Whelan MA, Subcommittee on the Management of Infantile Hemangiomas. Clinical practice guideline for the management of infantile hemangiomas. Pediatrics. 2019;143(1):e20183475.
2. Wassef M, Blei F, Adams D, Alomari A, Baselga E, Berenstein A, Burrows P, Frieden IJ, Garzon MC, Lopez-Gutierrez JC, Lord DJ, Mitchel S, Powell J, Prendiville J, Vikkula M, ISSVA Board and Scientific Committee. Vascular anomalies classification: recommendations from the International Society for the Study of Vascular Anomalies. Pediatrics. 2015;136(1):e203–14.
3. Luu M, Frieden IJ. Haemangioma: clinical course, complications and management. Br J Dermatol. 2013;169(1):20–30.
4. Léauté-Labrèze C, Harper JI, Hoeger PH. Infantile haemangioma. Lancet. 2017;390(10089):85–94.
5. Leaute-Labreze C, Prey S, Ezzedine K. Infantile haemangioma: part I. Pathophysiology, epidemiology, clinical features, life cycle and associated structural abnormalities. J Eur Acad Dermatol Venereol. 2011;25(11):1245–53.
6. Coulie J, Boon L, Vikkula M. Molecular pathways and possible therapies for head and neck vascular anomalies. J Oral Pathol Med. 2022;51:878–87.
7. Chamlin SL, et al. Multicenter prospective study of ulcerated hemangiomas. J Pediatr. 2007;151(6):684–9, 689 e1.
8. Hermans DJ, et al. Differences between ulcerated and non-ulcerated hemangiomas, a retrospective study of 465 cases. Eur J Dermatol. 2009;19(2):152–6.
9. Haggstrom AN, et al. Prospective study of infantile hemangiomas: clinical characteristics predicting complications and treatment. Pediatrics. 2006;118(3):882–7.
10. Maguiness SM, et al. Early white discoloration of infantile hemangioma: a sign of impending ulceration. Arch Dermatol. 2010;146(11):1235–9.
11. Andrea Diociaiuti et al. The VASCERN-VASCA working group diagnostic and management pathways for severe and/or rare infantile hemangiomas. EUropean J Med Genetics. 2022;65:104517.
12. Wang JY, et al. Medical, surgical, and wound care management of ulcerated infantile hemangiomas: a systematic review [Formula: see text]. J Cutan Med Surg. 2018;22(5):495–504.
13. Hoeger PH, Harper JI, Baselga E, Bonnet D, Boon LM, Atti MCD, el Hachem M, Oranje AP, Rubin AT, Weibel LL´eaut´e-Labr`eze, C. Treatment of infantile haemangiomas: recommendations of a European expert group. Eur. J. Pediatr. 2015.
14. Tiwari P, et al. Role of propranolol in ulcerated haemangioma of head and neck: a prospective comparative study. Oral Maxillofac Surg. 2016;20(1):73–7.
15. Saint-Jean M, et al. Propranolol for treatment of ulcerated infantile hemangiomas. J Am Acad Dermatol. 2011;64(5):827–32.
16. Fernandez Faith E, et al. Clinical features, prognostic factors, and treatment interventions for ulceration in patients with infantile hemangioma. JAMA Dermatol. 2021;157(5):566–72.

17. Colmant C, Powell J. Medical management of infantile hemangiomas: an update. Paediatr Drugs. 2022;24(1):29–43.
18. Metry D, et al. Propranolol use in PHACE syndrome with cervical and intracranial arterial anomalies: collective experience in 32 infants. Pediatr Dermatol. 2013;30(1):71–89.
19. Baselga E, et al. Risk factors for degree and type of sequelae after involution of untreated hemangiomas of infancy. JAMA Dermatol. 2016;152(11):1239–43.
20. Coulie J, Coyette M, Moniotte S, Bataille AC, Boon LM. Has propranolol eradicated the need for surgery in the management of infantile hemangioma? Plast Reconstr Surg. 2015;136:154.
21. Boon LM, Enjolras O, Mulliken JB. Congenital hemangioma: evidence of accelerated involution. J Pediatr. 1996;128(3):329–35.
22. Nasseri E, et al. Partially involuting congenital hemangiomas: a report of 8 cases and review of the literature. J Am Acad Dermatol. 2014;70(1):75–9.
23. North PE. Classification and pathology of congenital and perinatal vascular anomalies of the head and neck. Otolaryngol Clin North Am. 2018;51(1):1–39.
24. Braun V, et al. Congenital haemangiomas: a single-centre retrospective review. BMJ Paediatr Open. 2020;4(1):e000816.
25. Vildy S, et al. Life-threatening hemorrhaging in neonatal ulcerated congenital hemangioma: two case reports. JAMA Dermatol. 2015;151(4):422–5.
26. Weitz NA, et al. Congenital cutaneous hemangioma causing cardiac failure: a case report and review of the literature. Pediatr Dermatol. 2013;30(6):e180–90.
27. Baselga E, et al. Rapidly involuting congenital haemangioma associated with transient thrombocytopenia and coagulopathy: a case series. Br J Dermatol. 2008;158(6):1363–70.
28. El Zein L, et al. The histopathology of congenital haemangioma and its clinical correlations: a long-term follow-up study of 55 cases. Histopathology. 2020;77(2):275–83.
29. Liu AS, et al. Extracranial arteriovenous malformations: natural progression and recurrence after treatment. Plast Reconstr Surg. 2010;125(4):1185–94.
30. Couto JA, et al. Somatic MAP2K1 mutations are associated with extracranial arteriovenous malformation. Am J Hum Genet. 2017;100(3):546–54.
31. Al-Olabi L, et al. Mosaic RAS/MAPK variants cause sporadic vascular malformations which respond to targeted therapy. J Clin Invest. 2018;128(4):1496–508.
32. El Sissy FN, et al. Somatic mutational landscape of extracranial arteriovenous malformations and phenotypic correlations. J Eur Acad Dermatol Venereol. 2022;36(6):905–12.
33. Boon LM, et al. Case report study of thalidomide therapy in 18 patients with severe arteriovenous malformations. Nat Cardiovasc Res. 2022;1(6):562–7.
34. Coulie Julien, Dekeuleneer Valérie, Hammer Frank, Roelandts Fabienne, Vikkula Miikka, Boon Laurence M. Monocentric pilot trial evaluating the safety and efficacy of trametinib in arteriovenous malformations that are refractory to standard care. ISSVA World Congress 2022, Oral presentation, May 2022.

Open Access This chapter is licensed under the terms of the Creative Commons Attribution-NonCommercial-NoDerivatives 4.0 International License (http://creativecommons.org/licenses/by-nc-nd/4.0/), which permits any non-commercial use, sharing, distribution and reproduction in any medium or format, as long as you give appropriate credit to the original author(s) and the source, provide a link to the Creative Commons license and indicate if you modified the licensed material. You do not have permission under this license to share adapted material derived from this chapter or parts of it.

The images or other third party material in this chapter are included in the chapter's Creative Commons license, unless indicated otherwise in a credit line to the material. If material is not included in the chapter's Creative Commons license and your intended use is not permitted by statutory regulation or exceeds the permitted use, you will need to obtain permission directly from the copyright holder.

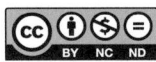

Part IX

Skin Necrosis in the Elderly

Introduction: Skin Necrosis in the Elderly

Sylvie Meaume

Several causes of necrosis are observed in the elderly. Some are specific to this population such as **deep dissecting hematomas** which are one of the complications of dermatoporosis in patients who receive anticoagulation more and more frequently for heart rhythm disorders or arterial or venous thrombosis problems. The cover of deep dissecting hematomas which is no longer vascularized becomes necrotic and requires surgical intervention, the urgency of which is often relative. The use of negative pressure therapy and skin grafts has led to an improvement in care and a reduction in the length of hospitalization.

Skin tears linked to the skin fragility of dermatoporosis also lead to necrosis in certain cases of the flap which is poorly vascularized and/or repositioned late.

Lesions of **incontinence associated dermatitis** (IAD) are sometimes associated with pressure or friction or shear forces and become difficult to distinguish from **pressure ulcers** which are generally deeper lesions in front of bone like sacrum. In the older population, it remains complicated to have sufficient off-loading of pressure ulcers and stop fecal incontinence is mandatory to obtain wound healing of the superficial lesions of IAD (Fig. 69.1).

Arterial disease in the lower limbs (**chronic obliterating arteriopathy**) is a classic cause of necrosis in this population. It is frequently underestimated because it is frequently asymptomatic (no intermittent claudication in this population who often no longer walks much). The systematic search for pulses and the measurement of ankle brachial pressure index (ABBPI) make it possible to diagnose this component in the case of wounds to the lower limbs: mixed leg ulcers for which the compression must be adapted, foots wounds which sometimes do not heal except after angioplasty associated with off-loading (Fig. 69.2).

Rarer causes of necrosis are discussed in the other chapters but often concerns the elderly: **necrotic angiodermatitis** which will require a rapid graft to reduce pain, **pyoderma gan-**

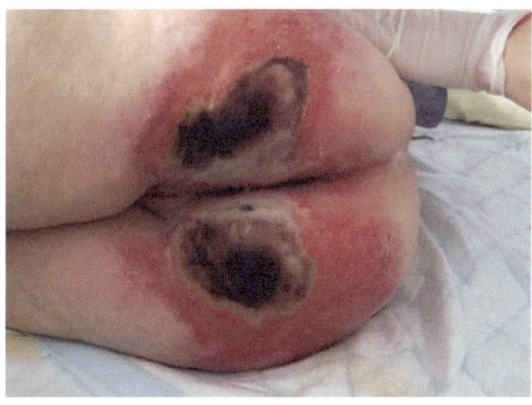

Fig. 69.1 Aspect of IAD on incontinent elderly patient

S. Meaume (✉)
Head of Geriatric and wound care department, Rothschild University Hospital, Assistance Publique Hôpitaux de Paris, Sorbonne Université, France
e-mail: sylvie.meaume@aphp.fr

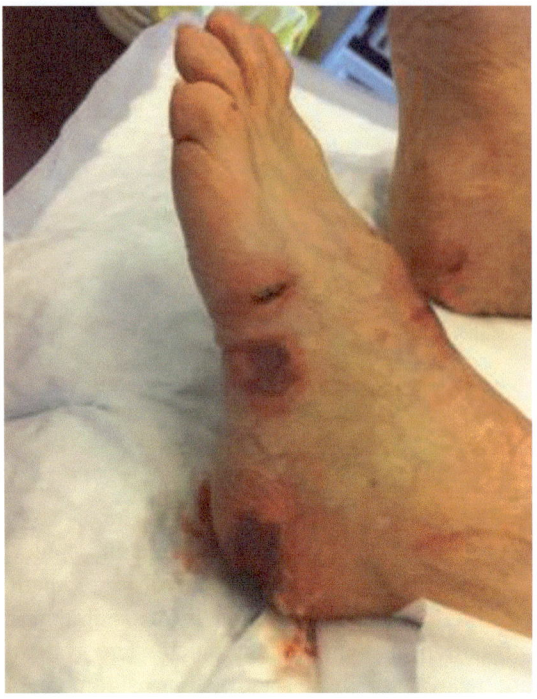

Fig. 69.2 Pressure ulcer of the heel and edge of the foot aggravated by severe arteriopathy of the lower limbs

grenosum whose treatment will sometimes have to be adapted with regard to biotherapies and the doses of general corticosteroids, **calciphylaxis** in the case of end-stage renal failure has a very poor prognosis in this population, **drug necrosis** with hydroxyurea is frequent with the increase in this population of essential thrombocythemia and polycythemia treated with this molecule generally well tolerated. **Infectious necrosis** also exists in this population and will require antibiotic therapy adapted to the often impaired renal function in these patients (Fig. 69.3).

Necrosis in the elderly is always worrying. The risk of amputation in the event of a wound to the lower limbs often poses an ethical problem in this population to be discussed with trained teams: wearing a suitable prosthesis is often not possible, and walking is rarely regained. We have to remember that less than 50% of elderly people survive more than a year after a major amputation.

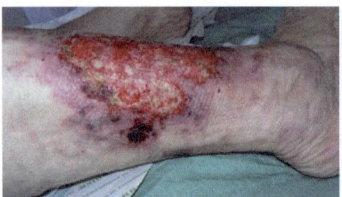 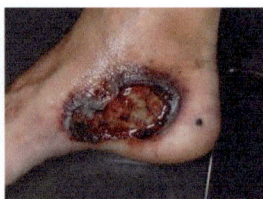 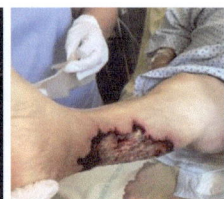 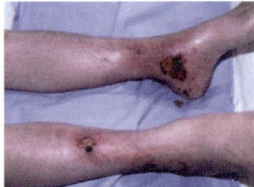

Fig. 69.3 Martorell ulcer, pyoderma gangrenosum, calciphylaxis, and hydroxyurea ulcer

Open Access This chapter is licensed under the terms of the Creative Commons Attribution-NonCommercial-NoDerivatives 4.0 International License (http://creativecommons.org/licenses/by-nc-nd/4.0/), which permits any non-commercial use, sharing, distribution and reproduction in any medium or format, as long as you give appropriate credit to the original author(s) and the source, provide a link to the Creative Commons license and indicate if you modified the licensed material. You do not have permission under this license to share adapted material derived from this chapter or parts of it.

The images or other third party material in this chapter are included in the chapter's Creative Commons license, unless indicated otherwise in a credit line to the material. If material is not included in the chapter's Creative Commons license and your intended use is not permitted by statutory regulation or exceeds the permitted use, you will need to obtain permission directly from the copyright holder.

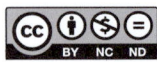

Pressure Necrosis in Geriatric Patients

Joyce Black

70.1 Background

The elderly remains one of the highest at-risk populations for pressure ulcers. A systematic review reported that on average, the incidence of pressure injury is 12% in all persons [1]. However, the highest reported rates were in elders with fractured hips; 70% of them developed pressure ulcers [2]. The incidence of pressure ulcers in elderly population varies by care setting, but evidence on risk factors indicates that age will increase the probability of pressure ulcers, particularly in patients with limited mobility. Chronic medical conditions are also more prevalent in older adults. Long-term care patients have the highest rate of PU development associated with higher frequency of mortality and advanced severe chronic conditions. The common age-related chronic diseases are identified as cardiovascular, diabetes, lung, renal, musculoskeletal, and neurodegenerative diseases. Progression of these diseases is often seen as impaired motor, sensory, immune, and hormonal systems and lead to frailty, disability, geriatric syndromes, and isolation. The significance of comorbidity risk factors in the pathogenesis of PU requires further investigation, recognizing the insolvability of PU prevention solely with external relief devices [3].

J. Black (✉)
University of Nebraska Medical Center, College of Nursing, Omaha, NE, USA
e-mail: jblack@unmc.edu

70.2 Etiology/Pathophysiology

Pressure ulcers are aptly named because they develop due to pressure. Pressure is a static, direct compressive force on tissue leading to hypoxia of the skin and soft tissue by restricting blood flow. When pressure reaches magnitudes that deform cells, the resulting injury is classified today as deep tissue injury, in that the pressure was applied to the deep tissues (muscle, fascia) and deformed the cells leading to their death [4, 5]. Pressure of less magnitude and of long duration creates tissue ischemia. Ischemia of tissue also leads to necrosis, but the mechanism is due to depletion of oxygen and glucose and accumulation of lactic acid [6, 7].

The time needed to create ischemia in soft tissue and skin which leads to necrosis is elusive. In an ischemic animal model, 70% of cell viability remained for over 22 h. In contrast, cell deformation which would lead to deep tissue injury was evident within the hour [8] (see Fig. 70.1). Of the various tissues that are at risk of death due to pressure, muscle tissue is damaged first, likely because of its increased need for oxygen and higher metabolic requirements. By the time ulceration is visible in the skin, significant damage of underlying muscle may already have occurred. The tissue fed by the vertical perforators through the muscle remains viable for a while; a series of cases showed the first sign of skin injury from intense pressure was apparent 48 h after the pressure was applied [9]. An addi-

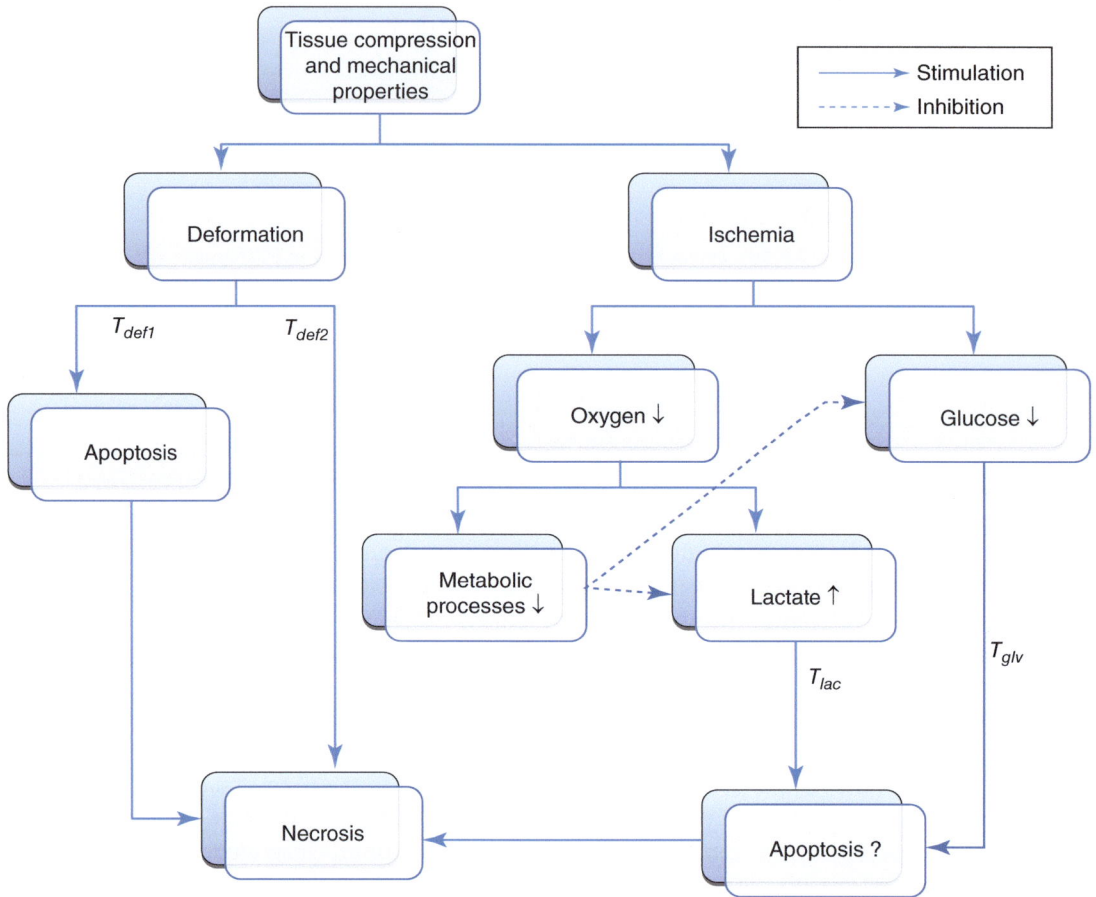

Fig. 70.1 Model of proposed sequence of events leads to necrosis of tissue. Deformation of tissue leads to damage when the threshold is met (T def 1), and cells will start a programmed cell death leading to necrosis. If the deformation of the cell exceeds its tolerance, the cells will die immediately from necrosis. Cells can also be injured from ischemia, reducing the metabolic substrates needed and leading to anaerobic metabolism and accumulation of lactic acid. Both cellular starvation and acidification lead to apoptosis and cellular necrosis (From Stekelenburg [10])

tional finding from this case series is that patients who sustained deep tissue injury were not aware of the ischemia; they were unconscious.

Restoration of blood flow to an ischemic area of tissue, or reperfusion injury, causes more damage to the injured area, causing a pressure ulcer to enlarge or fail to heal. Reperfusion of blood causing cellular edema, tissue damage, and overproduction of reactive oxygen species trigger a process termed oxidative stress, which may cause the accumulation of unfolded proteins in the endoplasmic reticulum [11].

Shear is also a cause of pressure ulcers and undermining in existing ulcers. Shear is a tangential (angular) force associated with movement, for example, sliding down in bed or being pulled over to the side of the bed. Shear forces distort blood vessels in the skin, making the effect of pressure more deleterious because the tissue is already hypoxic. Research has shown that positioning a patient at 45° head of bed elevation leads to the most detrimental combination of pressure and shear on the sacrum, because the shear stresses combined with pressure cause greater obstruction and distortion of capillaries in skeletal muscle around bony prominences than does pressure alone [7].

Microclimate, the moisture and heat of the skin, increases the risk for pressure ulcers because the moisture macerates the skin. The boggy skin does not glide against bed sheets and leads to superficial tissue injury. Skin exposure to urine or stool also injures the skin and increases risk of tissue damage from pressure and shear. Gefen [12] has provided a theoretical explanation of the ways in which a changing microclimate may influence the development of superficial pressure ulcers. From a mathematical model, Gefen postulated that four microclimate changes may influence pressure ulcer development—increasing skin temperature, increasing ambient temperature, increasing relative humidity, and decreasing the permeability of sheets or clothing.

The tolerance of the skin and soft tissue for pressure and shear is also crucial to understand how pressure ulcers develop. Atherosclerosis is a common disease of the elderly. As the disease progresses blood flow to distal areas, such as the lower leg is significantly reduced. The reduced perfusion limits the ability of the soft tissue to be reperfused following a pressure loading event. A lack of sensation, due to stroke or peripheral neuropathy especially from diabetes creates an unawareness of pressure on the heel in a bedridden patient. When these comorbid states are combined with a traumatic event, such as a fall with hip fracture, the risk is much greater. Heel ulcer development in hip fracture patients with underlying diabetes and peripheral vascular disease is not only common, but is also very slow to heal due to the same processes.

In part due to the chronic conditions, many patients will experience dysphagia or anorexia and as a result lose weight. Sarcopenia leads to decreased strength of the lower extremities, frailty, and often of immobility. Malnutrition also impairs immune and hormonal function, causes skin changes (epidermis, dermis), reduces subcutaneous tissue, and causes muscle atrophy, all increasing vulnerability to PU [13]. Finally, urinary and fecal incontinence reduce the tolerance of skin for pressure and shear as well as chemically damage the skin. Incontinence is one of the most common reasons for admission to long-term care. Efforts should be made to determine the causes such as urinary infection and reduce the continuous exposure to urine and diarrheal stool.

70.3 Presentation

Pressure necrosis appears on tissue that has been subjected to intense pressure in patients who cannot feel the pressure or respond to it and change positions. Pressure ulcers are categorized based on the amount of visible tissue in the wound bed.

Category/Stage 1: Nonblanchable erythema.
Category/Stage 2: Superficial loss of mid dermis. Appears bright red if ulcer is in the papillary dermis and off-white if in the reticular dermis.
Category/Stage 3: Loss of dermis with exposed fat when not on a bony prominence. Granulation tissue present when healing.
Category/Stage 4: Loss of dermis with exposure of muscle, tendon, bone, cartilage. Granulation tissue present when healing.
Unstageable: wound bed obscured with slough or eschar so that true extent of the ulcer cannot be described. If the ulcer is debrided, it is then staged.
Deep tissue pressure injury: initially purple or maroon intact skin. Within 48 h, epidermis slough occurs, which looks like a broken blister. As the ulcer evolves, it should be classified as noted above almost all of these wounds are stage 4.

High-risk patients and the common locations for pressure necrosis are as follows. It is important to identify the location of the patient at the time the pressure injury started, so that position is avoided. Continued pressure on a pressure ulcer will increase the ischemia in the issue and lead to significant deterioration.

Position	Common location of pressure necrosis	Example pressure necrosis leading to deep tissue injury
Flat in supine position (e.g., during surgery, hypotensive)	Buttocks tissue, unless patient is quite thin, with no buttocks tissue Necrosis appears bilaterally	
Supine with head of bed elevated 30–45° or slouching in a chair	Sacrum and adjacent buttocks tissue	
Sitting erect in chair	Ischial tuberosities	

Position	Common location of pressure necrosis	Example pressure necrosis leading to deep tissue injury
Supine with heels on the bed	Posterior heel in patients with immobile legs, neuropathic legs, or peripheral vascular disease	
Wearing medical devices that are tight	Bridge of the nose from noninvasive positive pressure masks, behind the ears from oxygen tubing, shin, top of foot, and along Achilles tendon from stockings	

70.4 Differential Diagnosis [14]

- Abscess
- Arterial leg ulcer
- Bruising
- Calciphylaxis
- Cellulitis
- Critical limb ischemia
- Cutaneous malignancy
- Diabetic foot ulcer
- Fournier's gangrene
- Hematoma/Morel–Lavellée lesions
- Incontinence-associated dermatitis/moisture-associated skin damage
- Ischemia of the skin beneath tightly wrapped dressings
- Necrotizing fasciitis
- Skin tear
- Venous leg ulcer
- Warfarin-induced necrosis
- Wound dehiscence

70.5 Prevention

Reducing the duration and magnitude of pressure is paramount. The duration of pressure is reduced by turning the patient off of high-risk areas. Most pressure necrosis develops on the sacrum, and therefore immobile patients should be turned to the side to relieve pressure. The frequency of turning can be every 3 h as long as the patient is on a quality mattress [15]. The magnitude of pressure can also be reduced by placing the patient on a support surface with adequate envelopment and immersion. High-density foam mattresses have been shown to be effective in reducing pressure injury as long as the patient is moved about in bed. For very high-risk patients, alternating pressure mattress helps prevent tissue damage; however, the patient still must be moved on these support surfaces. No support surface replaces turning the patient to reduce duration of pressure. Use mattress of 4 inches (10 cm) of viscoelastic foam during times when patients cannot be moved, such as surgical cases over 3 h cardiopulmonary bypass cases, and in the emergency department [16]. For bedbound patients, the use of signaling devices to notify staff when the patient should be turned have been shown to reduce pressure injury rates [17]. Turn teams have also been able to reduce pressure injury rates [18].

Heels should be elevated from the bed in high-risk patients. Heel elevation can be done with a pillow placed under the calf of the leg in order to "float" the heel from the bed. Pressure-relieving boots can be used when patients do not stay in place on pillows; however, boots themselves can create pressure points. Therefore, boots need to be removed 2–3 times daily to assess for early signs of pressure injury.

Medical devices should be removed 2–3 times a day, if only long enough to inspect for signs of pressure on the skin [19]. High-risk areas, such as the bridge of the nose and face, should be padded with thin foam dressings prior to the use of non-invasive positive pressure masks [20]. Oxygen tubing should be padded to reduce the intensity of pressure behind the ear.

Multilayer foam dressings have been shown to reduce sacral and heel pressure injury in the critically ill patient, the general hospitalized patient, and even patients in long-term care. These dressings can reduce the intensity of pressure and shear on the soft tissues [18].

Nutrition is paramount to prevent pressure injury. Patients who are catabolic cannot repair injured tissue. In addition, the lack of subcutaneous tissue in frail patients places more body areas at risk for pressure injury [13].

70.6 Treatment

Pressure necrosis of the sacrum, buttocks, and ischia will need debridement to viable tissue if healing is the goal for the patient (Fig. 70.2a, b). During the healing process, pressure on the wound must be limited to 1 h 3 times a day (for

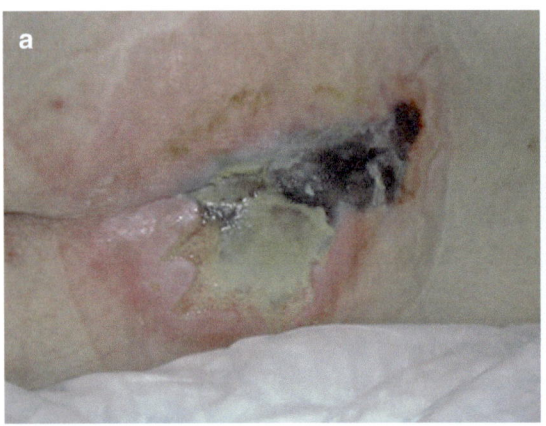 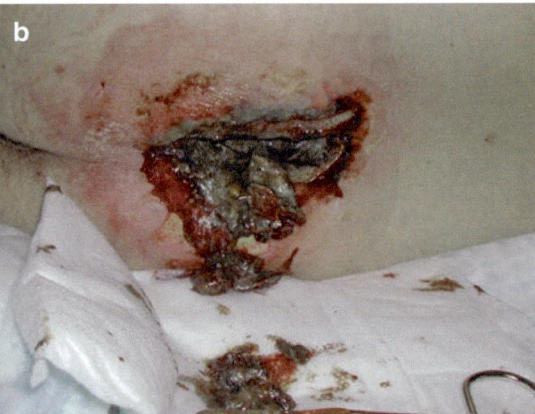

Fig. 70.2 (a) This patient is a 65-year-old male who refused to move from his bed at home for several days. When admitted to the hospital, he was septic. Cellulitis and frank necrosis are visible on the sacrum and buttocks. (b) His wound was debrided at bedside in the ICU due to the wound being the cause of the sepsis

meals). Caution must be used to avoid placing patients in chairs for multiple hours at a time. Nutrition must also be adequate to promote healing and reduce the risk of infection. Biofilm quickly develops in these wounds, so debridement is needed along with biofilm-resistant antiseptics should be used (silver, cadexomer iodine, honey, polyhexanide) [21]. An excellent review of biofilm is provided by Vererosa [22].

Pressure necrosis of the heel should not be debrided in patients with ischemic limbs. As long as the eschar remains stable, local wound care with topical iodine is recommended. The eschar will lift from the edges and should be trimmed to prevent it from snagging on clothing. If the eschar cap is removed from the wound, or the eschar cap is softened, infection rapidly develops. The poor inherent blood flow in the limb reduces the likelihood of healing and often leads to amputation due to critical limb ischemia [14].

Pressure ulcers from medical devices continue to occur. They are due to several factors: the plastic used to create the device is firm, the sizes are limited and often need to be forced to fit, the devices are monitoring life altering disease and cannot be moved, the device is providing lifesaving treatment and cannot be moved. However, many medical devices can and should be removed or moved twice daily, to inspect the skin and pad the skin beneath the device.

The use of bundles of care has improved pressure injury rates for many facilities. The National Pressure Injury Advisory Panel has created a bundle for the critically ill. Others are being developed.

References

1. Borojeny LA, Albatineh AN, Dehkordi AH, Gheshlagh RG. The incidence of pressure ulcers and its associations in different wards of the hospital: a systematic review and meta-analysis. Int J Prev Med. 2020;11:171.
2. Donnelly J, Winder J, Kernohan W, Stevenson M. An RCT to determine the effect of a heel elevation device in pressure ulcer prevention post-hip fracture. J Wound Care. 2011;20:309–18.
3. Jaul E, Barron J, Rosenzweig JP, Menczel J. An overview of co-morbidities and the development of pressure ulcers among older adults. BMC Geriatr. 2018;18(305) https://doi.org/10.1186/s12877-018-0997-7.
4. Gefen A. The etiology of pressure injuries. In: Emily Haesler editor, European Pressure Ulcer Advisory Panel, National Pressure Injury Advisory Panel and Pan Pacific Pressure Injury Alliance. Prevention and Treatment of Pressure Ulcers/Injuries: Clinical Practice Guideline. EPUAP/NPIAP/PPPIA; 2019.
5. Gefen A. Reswick and Rogers pressure-time curve for pressure ulcer risk. Part 1. Nurs Stand. 2009;23(45):64–74.
6. Gefen A. Reswick and Rogers pressure-time curve for pressure ulcer risk. Part 2. Nurs Stand. 2009;23(46):40–4.
7. Linder-Ganz E, Gefen A. The effects of pressure and shear on capillary closure in the microstructure of skeletal muscles. Ann Biomed Eng. 2007;35(12):2095–107.
8. Gawlitta D, Li W, Oomens CW, Baaijens FP, Bader DL, Bouten CV. The relative contributions of compression and hypoxia to development of muscle tissue damage: an in vitro study. Ann Biomed Eng. 2007;35(2):273–84.
9. Black JM, Brindle CT, Honaker J. Deep tissue injury: diagnosis and differential diagnosis. Int Wound J. 2016;13:531–9.
10. Stekelenburg A. Understanding deep tissue injury. Arch Phys Med Rehabil. 2008;89:1411.
11. Tsuji S, Ichioka S, Sekiya N, Nakatsuka T. Analysis of ischemia-reperfusion injury in a microcirculatory model of pressure ulcers. Wound Repair Regen. 2005;13(2):209–15.
12. Gefen A. How do microclimate factors affect the risk for superficial pressure ulcers: a mathematical modeling study. J Tissue Viability. 2011;20(3):81–8.
13. Munoz N, Posthauer ME, Cereda E, Schols JMGA, Haesler E. The role of nutrition for pressure injury prevention and healing: the 2019 international clinical practice guideline recommendations. Adv Skin Wound Care. 2020;33(3):123–36.
14. Morton LM, Phillips TJ. Wound healing and treating wounds: differential diagnosis and evaluation of chronic wounds. J Am Acad Dermatol. 2016;74(4):589–605.
15. Yap TL, Kennerly SM, Horn SD, Bergstrom N, Datta S, Colon-Emeric C. TEAM-UP for quality: a cluster randomized controlled trial protocol focused on preventing pressure ulcers through repositioning frequency and precipitating factors. BMC Geriatr. 2018;18(1):540.
16. Gillespie BM, Walker RM, Latimer SL, Thalib L, Whitty JA, McInnes E, Lockwood I, Chaboyer WP. Repositioning for pressure injury prevention in adults: an abridged Cochrane systematic review and meta-analysis. Int J Nurs Stud. 2021;120:103976.
17. Yap TL, Kennerly SM, Ly K. J pressure injury prevention: outcomes and challenges to use of resident monitoring technology in a nursing home. J Wound Ostomy Continence Nurs. 2019;46(3):207–13.

18. Avsar P, Moore Z, Patton D, O'Connor T, Budri A, Nugent L. Repositioning for preventing pressure ulcers: a systematic review and meta-analysis. J Wound Care. 2020;29(9):496–508.
19. Pittman J, Gillespie C. Medical device-related pressure injuries. Crit Care Nurs Clin North Am. 2020;32(4):533–42.
20. Arundel L, Irani E, Barkema G. Reducing the incidence of medical device-related pressure injuries from use of CPAP/BiPAP masks: a quality improvement project. J Wound Ostomy Continence Nurs. 2021;48(2):108–14. https://doi.org/10.1097/WON.0000000000000742.
21. Alves PJ, Barreto RT, Barrois BM, Gryson LG, Meaume S, Monstrey SJ. Update on the role of antiseptics in the management of chronic wounds with critical colonisation and/or biofilm. Int Wound J. 2021;18(3):342–58. https://doi.org/10.1111/iwj.13537.
22. Verderosa AD, Totsika M, Fairfull-Smith KE. Bacterial biofilm eradication agents: a current review front. Chem. 2019;7 https://doi.org/10.3389/fchem.2019.00824.

Open Access This chapter is licensed under the terms of the Creative Commons Attribution-NonCommercial-NoDerivatives 4.0 International License (http://creativecommons.org/licenses/by-nc-nd/4.0/), which permits any non-commercial use, sharing, distribution and reproduction in any medium or format, as long as you give appropriate credit to the original author(s) and the source, provide a link to the Creative Commons license and indicate if you modified the licensed material. You do not have permission under this license to share adapted material derived from this chapter or parts of it.

The images or other third party material in this chapter are included in the chapter's Creative Commons license, unless indicated otherwise in a credit line to the material. If material is not included in the chapter's Creative Commons license and your intended use is not permitted by statutory regulation or exceeds the permitted use, you will need to obtain permission directly from the copyright holder.

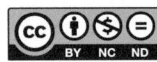

71

Deep Dissecting Haematoma: A Frequent Cause of Necrosis in Elderly Patient

Hester Colboc and Sylvie Meaume

Deep dissecting haematomas (DDH) are the result of bleeding, either spontaneous or following trauma [1, 2]. This collection of blood forms between the hypodermis and the muscular fascia [1–3], causing a dissection between these two subcutaneous layers. This dissection deprives the areas concerned of their blood supply and causes necrosis of the skin of the top of the haematoma.

It can be very voluminous and, in extreme cases, can have hemodynamic consequences that can even lead to death if the patient is not treated quickly and appropriately [4].

DDH are diagnosed clinically, but sometimes require at least a blood test to check for anaemia if the haematoma is large, and a standard X-ray to rule out an associated fracture in the event of a fall or trauma.

71.1 Pathophysiology

DDH is a little-known pathology, which has mainly been described in elderly people suffering from dermatoporosis and/or on anticoagulant or antiplatelet therapy (present in more than half of the patients concerned) [1, 2, 5].

The term dermatoporosis, by analogy with osteoporosis, was proposed by Saurat and Kaya in 2007 to define all the manifestations associated with skin ageing, leading to fragility and skin insufficiency [6]. It is characterised by a structural change in the skin, caused by a reduction in collagen and hyaluronic acid and the absence of the CD44 glycoprotein (differentiation cluster 44), which is usually present [7]. Traditionally, a distinction is made between two forms: primary and secondary [8].

The most common form is primary, combining intrinsic factors such as skin aging and extrinsic factors such as chronic sun exposure [9].

The secondary form is iatrogenic due to long-term treatment with topical and/or systemic corticosteroids [10].

There were no significant clinical differences between the two types of dermatoporosis.

Clinically, there are four progressive stages of dermatoporosis [3, 11–13]:

- Stage 1: thin skin, nearly translucent, revealing a prominence of the underlying veins and tendons, senile purpura (Bateman purpura) (Fig. 71.1a) and white pseudo scar classically describe as having a stellate configuration but can might be also linear or plaque-like (Fig. 71.1b) [1, 12, 14].
- Stage 2: manifestations of stage 1 and small, localised skin laceration resulting from a

H. Colboc (✉) · S. Meaume
Geriatric and Wound Care Department, Rothschild University Hospital, Assistance Publique Hôpitaux de Paris, Sorbonne Université, Paris, France
e-mail: hester.colboc@aphp.fr

© The Authors(s) 2024
L. Téot et al. (eds.), *Skin Necrosis*, https://doi.org/10.1007/978-3-031-60954-1_71

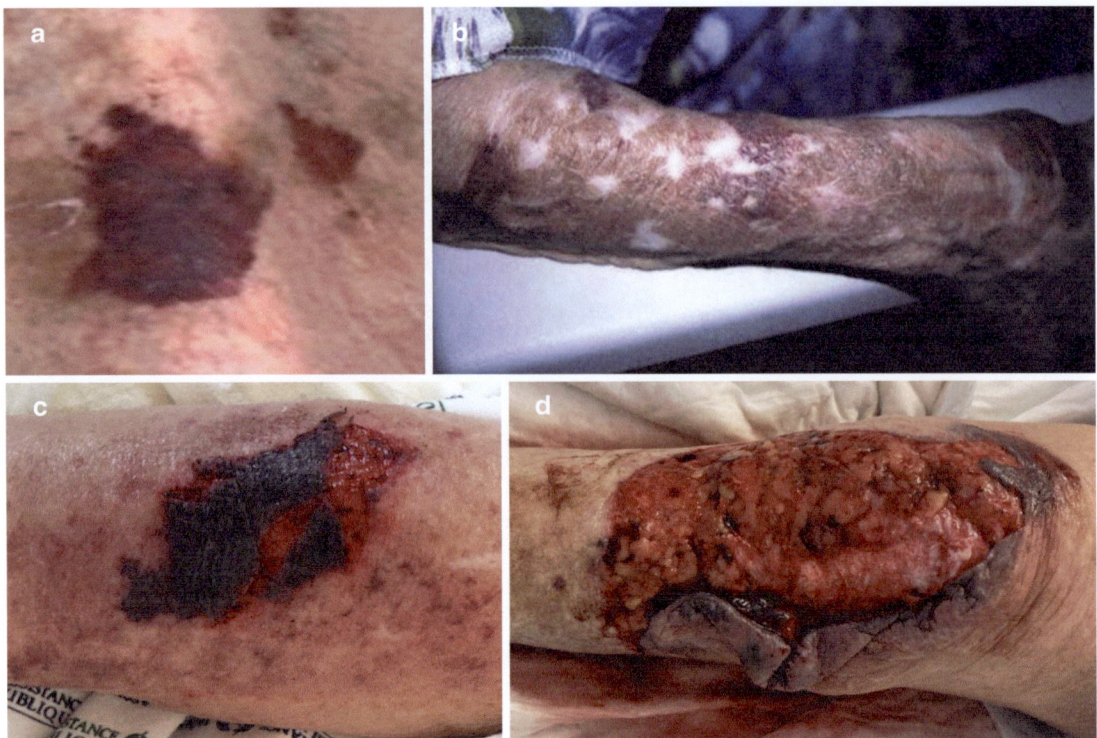

Fig. 71.1 Somes clinical aspect of dermatoporosis. (**a**) Bateman purpura characterized by hemorrhagic areas with confluent ecchymoses. (**b**) Typical aspect of dermatorosis: white stellar scar, fragile skin and Bateman purpura. (**c**) Small skin tear or laceration. (**d**) Large skin tear

cleavage between the dermis and the epidermis (Fig. 71.1c).
- Stage 3: more numerous and larger skin lacerations (Fig. 71.1d) with a significant delay in healing [15].
- Stage 4: progression of the lesions described above leads to the formation of DDH which may progress to skin necrosis [1, 12].

71.2 Epidemiology

The incidence of DDH is not well known.

An initial retrospective study, carried out in 2009 on 34 patients, revealed an average age of 81.7 years, with a predominance of women (5 women to 1 man) and advanced dermatoporosis in all patients [1].

Another prospective study was carried out in the geriatrics department. Out of 202 patients aged over 60, signs of dermatoporosis were present in 32% of hospitalised patients. There was a significant association ($p < 0.05$) with haematomas of the lower limbs, although the dissecting nature was not specified [16].

71.3 Clinical Signs

DDH is most often localised to the lower limbs [1, 3]. More rarely, it may be found on the face (forehead), occiput, trunk, or upper limbs [2].

It is manifested by aspecific clinical signs such as intense pain, and/or tension, and/or swelling, and/or erythema, which can lead to misdiagnosis. However, fever is not one of the clinical signs of

DDH [1, 3]. The lack of specificity of these clinical signs and the lack of knowledge about the disease frequently lead to delays in diagnosis and management.

There are several clinical forms, depending on the extent, age and whether or not the affected limb has been operated on [3]:

(a) Early closed form: swelling or tumefaction on the affected limb with normal skin coloration
(b) Advanced closed form: swelling or puckering, with changes in skin colour (erythema, purplish appearance) (Fig. 71.2)
(c) Advanced form with necrosis of the haematoma roof: appearance of an area of skin necrosis above the swelling or curvature (Fig. 71.3)
(d) Spontaneous open form or after surgery
(e) Lastly, there are forms of late revelation [17]

71.4 Differential Diagnosis

All the clinical signs and a lack of awareness of this common condition are the cause of many misdiagnoses, with a significant delay in treatment [3, 7].

The main differential diagnoses are as follows:

(a) The diagnosis of **erysipelas** (bacterial dermo-hypodermatitis) is often made in the first instance, mainly in the lower limb [1, 3, 10] (Fig. 71.4a). In the series by Kaya et al., almost half the patients had been treated for erysipelas before the DDH was diagnosed. The average delay between the onset of clinical signs and the diagnosis of cutaneous dissecting haematoma was 2 weeks [1]
(b) A **simple haematoma** appears as a more or less coloured bulge, without extension or necrosis. Drawing the outline of the bulge with a pen on the skin allows you to monitor its development and determine whether it is dissecting or not (Fig. 71.2)
(c) c] **Deep vein thrombosis (DVT)** is also sometimes suspected with a tense, painful calf and the presence of a Homans's sign ± an indurated cord. Doppler examination is used to rule out this diagnosis
(d) More rare, **Morel-Lavallée syndrome** occurs following violent trauma with shearing of the skin on the deep planes. It often occurs in young people practicing a violent

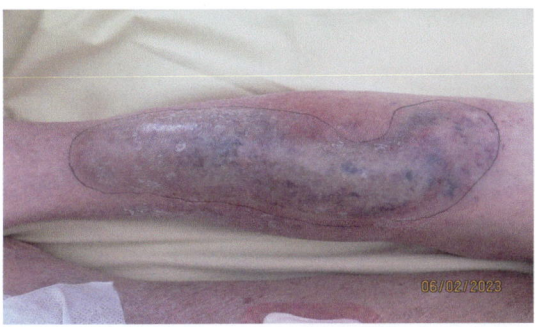

Fig. 71.2 Advanced closed form of DDH: tumefaction or swelling, with change in skin color (erythema, purplish appearance). Note pen mark to monitor evolution of the dissection

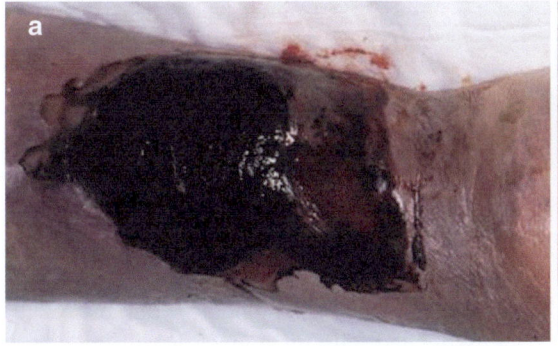 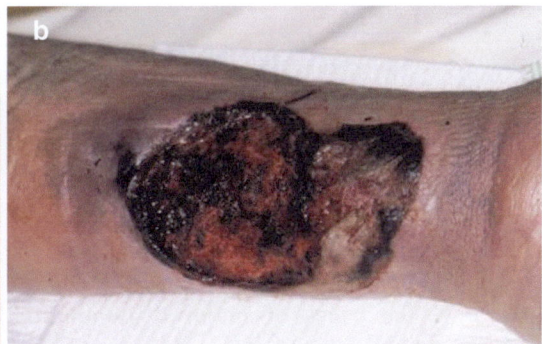

Fig. 71.3 Example of advanced DDH with complete moist necrosis of the skin cover (**a**) and appearance of the basement after partial mechanical debridement (**b**)

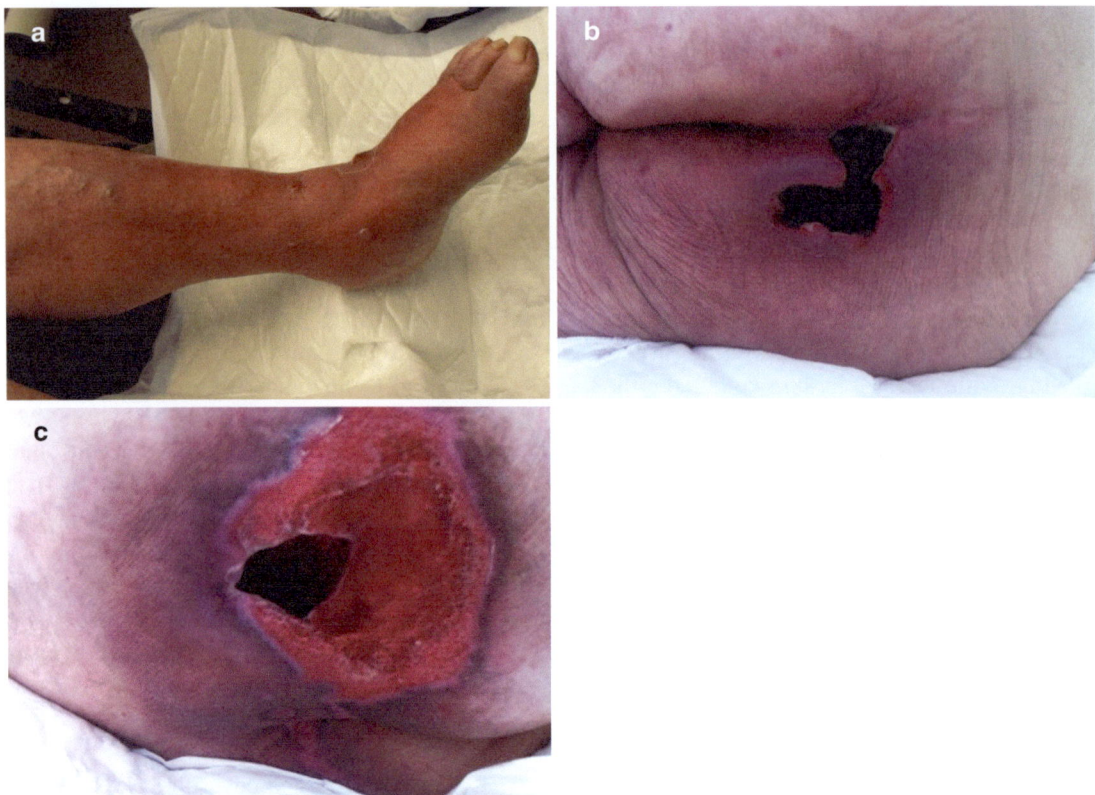

Fig. 71.4 Differential diagnosis. (**a**) Erysipelas in an elderly patient. (**b**, **c**) Necrosis and underlying cavity on Morel-Lavallée in an elderly patient

sport during a slip (motorbike, skiing, etc.). Diagnosis is usually late, often >1 year. Men are more often affected. They consult their doctor because of skin puckering and functional or cosmetic discomfort. The surrounding skin is rarely necrotic unless it occurs in an elderly person with atrophic skin (Fig. 71.4b, c).

71.5 Complications

(a) **Deglobulation** in DDH is a classic complication. In the vast majority of cases, patients receive at least one transfusion of red blood cells [2]. However, DDH is rarely the cause of major deglobulation during active bleeding, with hemorrhagic shock or hypovolemic shock leading to death [1, 3, 4]

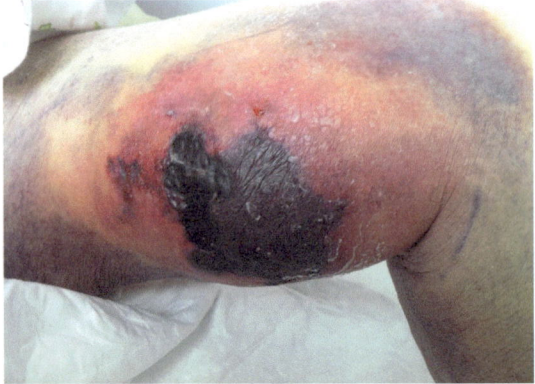

Fig. 71.5 DDH complicated by infection

(b) **Infection**, which can progress to severe sepsis, is also a possible complication. A cutaneous breach (spontaneous or provoked) associated with the collection of blood, constitutes a real "culture broth" often at the origin of the infection (Fig. 71.5). The infection

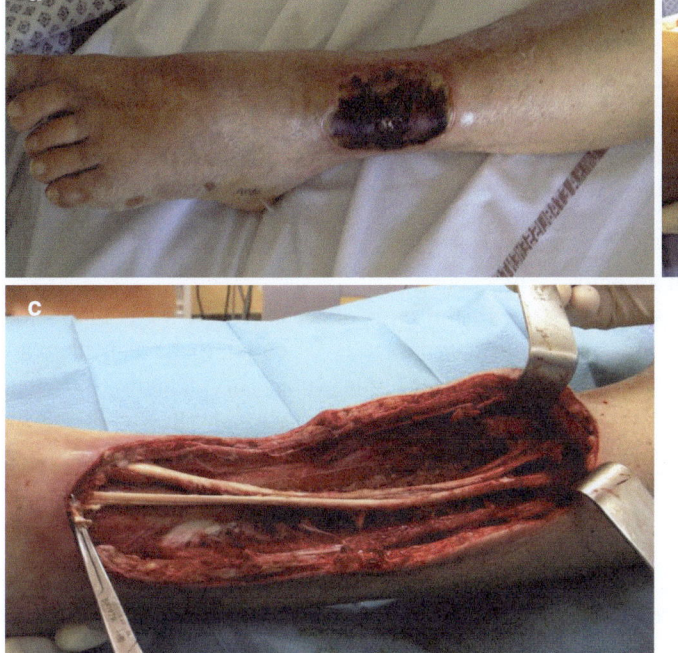

Fig. 71.6 Complicated DDH with compartment syndrome (**a**). But unfortunatly aponeurotomy will not (**b**, **c**) prevent amputation

may be acute, with the onset of erysipelas, manifested by erythema, skin heat, pain, fever with hyperleukocytosis, and the possible presence of adenopathy. It can also develop quietly, leading to endocarditis in the absence of rapid, appropriate antibiotic treatment.

(c) **Compartment syndrome** in the lower limb occurs when there is a large and often rapid increase in haematoma in a confined space, which interrupts the blood supply to the muscles. Clinically, it manifests itself as intense pain, resistant to morphine, with a persistent pedal pulse. MRI confirms muscle damage and treatment consists of emergency aponeurotomy, which does not always prevent amputation (Fig. 71.6a–c)

(d) **Delayed healing** of the flattened haematoma, in the case of DDH of the lower limbs, if associated with arterial disease or chronic venous insufficiency with delayed healing if the arterial disease (revascularisation) or venous disease (compression) is not treated.

71.6 Additional Examinations

They are not systematic, but are selected according to the terrain and the clinic.

1. A **blood sample** is often taken urgently in the event of DH in order to carry out a blood count, blood crase, AB0, and rhesus blood group to consider a blood transfusion if necessary [3].
2. Emergency **imaging** is necessary in cases of large and/or rapidly expanding DDH [3]. This confirms the diagnosis, clarifies the lesion status, and should not delay medical and surgical management.
   (a) Ultrasound of the soft tissues allows the haematoma to be located and the extent of the haematoma to be determined.
   (b) An angio-TDM or angio-MRI angiogram is used to determine whether or not there is active bleeding.
   (c) An X-ray can be used to check for associated fractures.

3. There is no indication for a skin biopsy; the diagnosis is made clinically and radiologically [3].

71.7 Medical and Surgical Management

71.7.1 Medical Management

While some DDH can be managed on an outpatient basis, serious or potentially serious haemorrhage requires hospital treatment.

If the patient is on anticoagulation, its continuation must be assessed on the basis of the benefit/risk balance and adapted in the event of overdose, which must be investigated [2].

A blood transfusion may be necessary if the patient develops deglobulation [1–3].

There is no place for antibiotics in the treatment of DDH, in the absence of fever or associated erysipelas.

71.7.2 Surgical Management

The indication for surgical management depends on the age and stage of the DH (see above) [1, 3] may be performed in the patient's bed or in the operating room [18].

In the first case, when the DDH is small and often old (dry necrosis), the procedure can be carried out by a nurse or doctor trained in the procedure.

In the case of an extensive or complicated haematoma, it is essential to have a team of experienced surgeons: orthopaedic surgeon, vascular surgeon, general surgeon, or plastic surgeon.

Necrotic tissue must be excised and debridement down to the muscle plane must be performed, often resulting in significant skin breakdown. In the presence of an old HD (redcurrant jelly appearance), debridement down to the healthy layer is carried out (Fig. 71.7a–c).

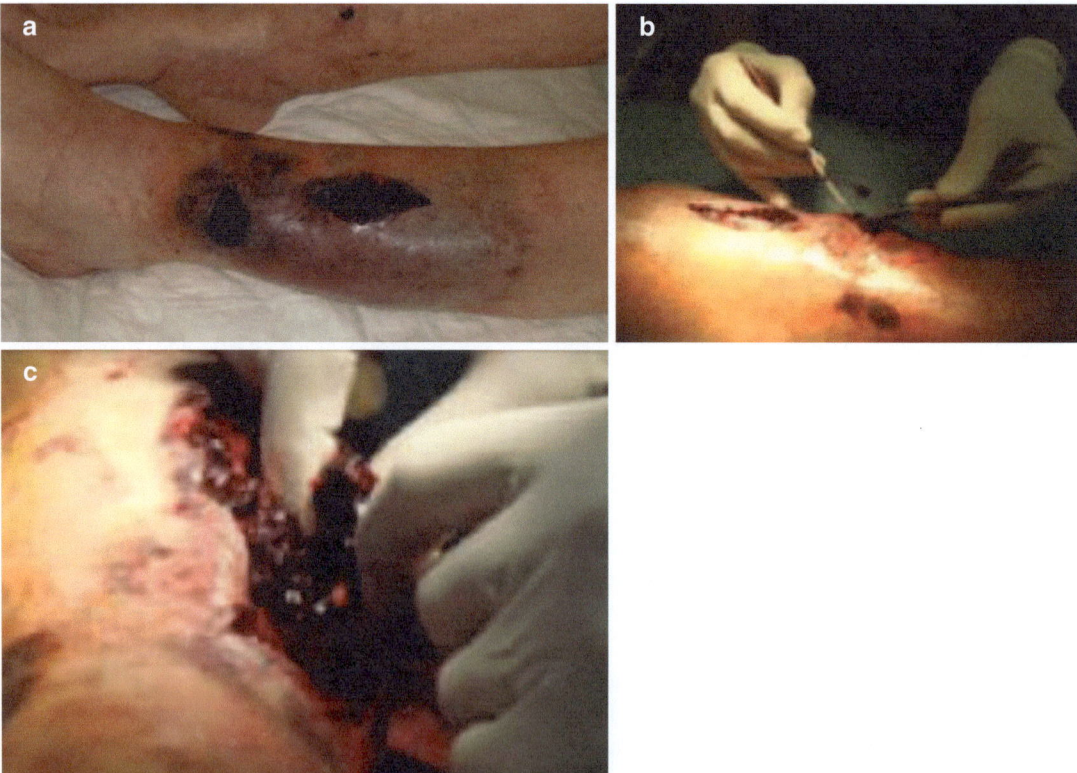

Fig. 71.7 Old DDH constituted: the necrotic tissue is excised (**a**) a declotting of the coagulated blood (appearance of currant jelly) until the healthy plan is carried out (**b, c**)

It should be noted that if DDH is diagnosed early and treated at an early stage, it will spread less and surgery will be less disruptive [3].

In general, the following management can be proposed, depending on the stage of the DDH:

- Early or advanced stage, closed, small: no surgery
- Advanced stage, large, extensive: experienced surgeon ± vascular surgeon
- Advanced stage with skin necrosis
  - Limited old dry necrosis: nurse at the bedside (Fig. 71.8a–d)
  - Extensive necrosis with large haematoma: experienced surgeon
- Open stage: experienced surgeon, major risk of infection

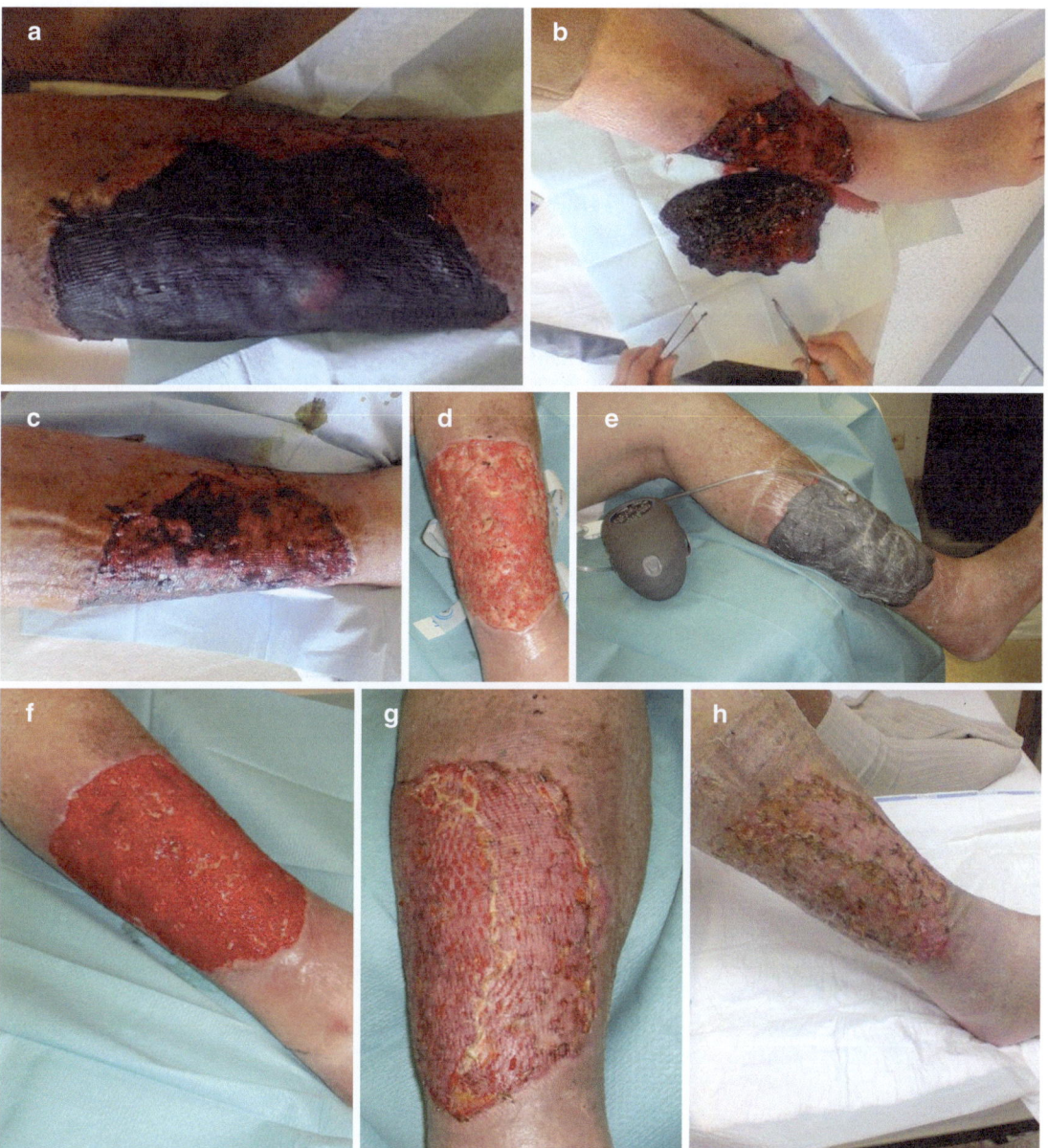

Fig. 71.8 Necrotic DDH (**a**) bedside clean (**b**, **c**, **d**) with NPWT placement (**e**), granulation tissue (**f**) then mesh graft (**g**) and complete healing (**h**)

There are no data in the literature on the benefits of limb compression or ice bag placement in the initial phase of DDH management.

71.7.3 Healing

The method chosen for healing the wound after flattening depends on the extent of the wound and the type of surgery (dislocating or not).

The use of Negative Pressure Wound Therapy (NPWT) is very effective in large wounds with significant loss of substance (Fig. 71.8e, f). After obtaining granulation tissue (Fig. 71.8g), it can be followed by a skin graft: often a mesh graft (Figs. 71.8h and 71.9a) or split skin graft (Fig. 71.9b) performed by a team of plastic surgeons, or else pinch grafts (Fig. 71.9c) in case of smaller wounds.

Wound healing can be obtained using advanced dressings (alginate, fibre dressing) in case of small wounds [18]. It is usually performed in geriatric wards to ensure comprehensive care for patients, who are often elderly and disabled.

However, despite careful management, healing is often slow and may be delayed by malnutrition or in patients with associated venous and/or arterial insufficiency. This difficulty in healing has been observed in half of all patients, and is associated with diabetes, venous insufficiency, and the presence of arterial disease [1–3].

71.8 Prevention

Care also involves prevention, particularly against minor trauma in people identified as being at risk of DDH. Education of nursing staff, protection of the lower limbs, prevention of the risk of falls by adapting home furnishings and correcting visual problems. Dosage of anticoagulant treatment must be adjusted in elderly patients, who are therefore at risk of renal failure and drug interactions.

Detection and management of dermatoporosis are also essential. Photoprotection is a key factor in preventing the worsening of dermatoporosis if it is applied early enough in life. The use of local retinoids thickens the epidermis and stimulates epidermal differentiation. The maximum effect is obtained after 6 months, but this topical often causes skin irritation, which limits its use.

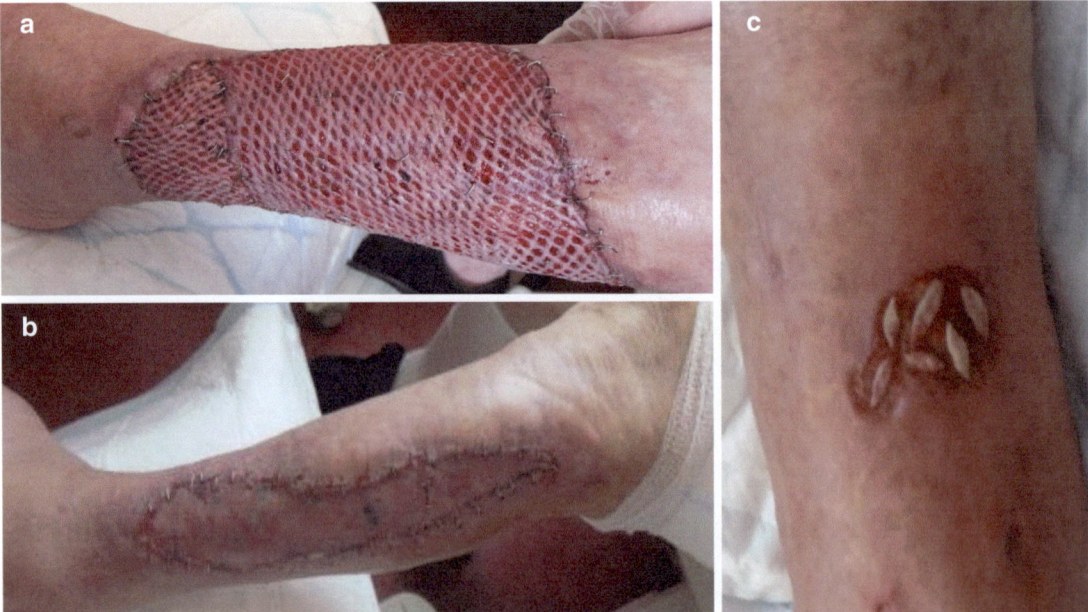

Fig. 71.9 Different types of grafts used to close DDH-related defects. Mesh graft (**a**) or split skin graft (**b**) for large DDH. Pinch graft (**c**) for small DDH

Conversely, dermocorticoid treatments that increase skin atrophy should be avoided wherever possible.

Kaya et al raised the possibility of using topical treatments comprising intermediate-sized hyaluronic acid fragments to correct the cutaneous atrophy of dermatoporosis by a CD44-dependent mechanism in elderly subjects [7]. The patients who respond best are those aged between 74 and 86 years [19].

A synergistic action has recently been shown in mice, and also in patients suffering from dermatoporosis, when retinaldehyde and intermediate-sized hyaluronic acid fragments are applied [20].

71.9 Conclusion

DDH is a serious and often overlooked complication of anticoagulant therapy. It most often occurs on the lower limbs of elderly subjects with skin fragility linked to dermatoporosis. It generally follows trauma, but this may be minimal or even absent in the case of spontaneous haematomas.

In extreme cases, it can lead to hemorrhagic shock and extensive skin necrosis around the haematoma.

Management should be as early as possible and is mainly surgical, with evacuation of the haematoma, debridement of necrotic tissue, granulation encouraged by NWPT.

Prevention is based on adjusting the dosage of anticoagulant treatments, preventing the risk of elderly people falling and limiting, as far as possible, the factors that aggravate dermatoporosis.

References

1. Kaya G, Jacobs F, Prins C, Viero D, Kaya A, Saurat JH. Deep dissecting hematoma: an emerging severe complication of dermatoporosis. Arch Dermatol. 2008;144:1303–8.
2. Toutous-Trellu L, Weiss L, Tarteaut MH, Kaya A, Cheretakis A, Kaya G. Deep dissecting hematoma: a plea for an early and specialized management. Eur Geriatr Med. 2010;1:228–30.
3. Fennira F, Colboc H, Meaume S. Dissecting haematoma, a frequent but little-known pathology. Revue Francophone de Cicatrisation. 2017;1(3):59–63.
4. Wollina U, Heinig B, Langner D. Chronic expanding organized hematoma of the lower leg: a rare cause for nonhealing leg ulcers. Int J Low Extrem Wounds. 2015;14(3):295–8.
5. Thomson WL, Pujol-Nicolas A, Tahir A, et al. A kick in the shins: the financial impact of uncontrolled warfarin use in pre-tibial haematomas. Injury. 2014;45(1):250–2.
6. Saurat JH. Dermatoporosis. The functional side of skin aging. Dermatology. 2007;215:271–2.
7. Kaya G, Tran C, Sorg O, Hotz R, Grand D, Carraux P, Didierjean L, Stamenkovic I, Saurat JH. Hyaluronate fragments reverse skin atrophy by a CD44-dependent mechanism. PLoS Med. 2006;3:e493.
8. Farage MA, Miller KW, Elsner P, Maibach HI. Intrinsic and extrinsic factors in skin ageing: a review. Int J Cosmet Sci. 2008;30(2):87–95.
9. Tagami H. Functional characteristics of the stratum corneum in photoaged skin in comparison with those found in intrinsic aging. Arch Dermatol Res. 2008;300(S1):1–6.
10. Schoepe S, Schacke H, May E, Asadullah K. Glucocorticoid therapy-induced skin atrophy. Exp Dermatol. 2006;15(6):406–20.
11. Kaya G. Dermatoporosis: an emerging syndrome. Rev Med Suisse. 2008;4(155):1078–9.
12. Kaya G, Saurat JH. Dermatoporosis: a chronic cutaneous insufficiency/fragility syndrome. Clinicopathological features, mechanisms, prevention and potential treatments. Dermatology. 2007;215:284–94.
13. Gamo R, Vicente J, Calzado L, Sanz H, Lopez-Estebaranz JL. Hematoma profundo disecante o estadio lv de dermatoporosis; 2010.
14. Bateman T. Abbildungen von Hautkrankheiten, wodurch die characteristischen Erscheinungen der Gattungen und Arten nach der Willan'schen Classification dargestellt werden. Weimar: Großherzoglichen Sächsischen Privilegirten Landes-Industrie-Comptoirs; 1830.
15. LeBlanc K, Baranoski S, Skin Tear Consensus Panel Members. Skin tears: state of the science: consensus statements for the prevention, prediction, assessment, and treatment of skin tears. Adv Skin Wound Care. 2011;24(9):2–15.
16. Mengeaud V, Dautezac-Vieu C, Josse G, Vellas B, Schmitt AM. Prevalence of dermatoporosis in elderly French hospital in-patients: a cross-sectional study. Br J Dermatol. 2012;166:442–3.

17. Hamadan R, Zwetyenga N, Macheboeuf Y, Ray R. Rapidly spreading deep dissecting hematoma occurring 1 month after a minor trauma: a case report. SAGE Open Med Case Rep. 2022;10:2050313X221135257.
18. Vanzi V, Toma E. Deep dissecting haematoma in patients with dermatoporosis: implications for home nursing. Br J Community Nurs. 2021;26(Suppl. 3):S6–S13.
19. Kaya G. New therapeutic targets in dermatoporosis. J Nutr Health Aging. 2012;16(4):285–8.
20. Nikolic DS, Ziori C, Kostaki M, Fontao L, Saurat J-H, Kaya G. Hyalurosome gene regulation and dose dependent restoration of skin atrophy by retinaldehyde and defined-size hyaluronate fragments in dermatoporosis. Dermatol Basel Switz. 2014;229(2):110–5.

Open Access This chapter is licensed under the terms of the Creative Commons Attribution-NonCommercial-NoDerivatives 4.0 International License (http://creativecommons.org/licenses/by-nc-nd/4.0/), which permits any non-commercial use, sharing, distribution and reproduction in any medium or format, as long as you give appropriate credit to the original author(s) and the source, provide a link to the Creative Commons license and indicate if you modified the licensed material. You do not have permission under this license to share adapted material derived from this chapter or parts of it.

The images or other third party material in this chapter are included in the chapter's Creative Commons license, unless indicated otherwise in a credit line to the material. If material is not included in the chapter's Creative Commons license and your intended use is not permitted by statutory regulation or exceeds the permitted use, you will need to obtain permission directly from the copyright holder.

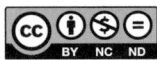

Part X

Education on Debridement

Introduction

Sebastian Probst

In recent years, a range of wound care courses, study days, and conferences have been developed in an attempt to update health care professionals about advances in wound management. One of the knowledge and skills that have to be acquired are the techniques of the debridement. Debridement is an important element of the wound bed preparation paradigm [1] and describes any method by which devitalized tissues/necrosis are removed [2]. In addition, tissue necrosis in the wound bed serves as an area ideal for bacterial overgrowth and infection; it can contribute to protein losses in wound exudate and often delays healing [3]. They also form a barrier to prevent angiogenesis, the formation of granulation tissue or the extracellular matrix, as well as the re-epithelialization [4]. Necrotic tissue may inhibit the direct contact of agents applied in the wound bed and hamper the clinician from making a proper assessment, for example, in masking a possible underlying infection [2]. There is a growing body of evidence and agreement among wound clinicians and scientists that debridement represents a necessary process in reducing bacteria, infection, and a biofilm within a wound and promotes a stimulatory environment for healing [5].

The main methods of debridement are autolytic, chemical/enzymatic, mechanical/sharp/hydro-surgery, and bio-surgery. In the following, the different methods are outlined:

- **Autolytic debridement** is widely used in clinical practice. Wound dressings such as hydrogels, alginates, or hydrocolloids support the maintenance of moisture and provide optimal conditions to activate the wound debridement [6].
- When using a **chemical debridement,** exogenous enzymes such as fibrinolytic enzymes or collagenase are applied the wound bed. Enzymatic debridement is part of the chemical debridement and is a selective method for debridement of necrotic tissue [7].
- **Mechanical debridement** method includes wet-to-dry dressing, irrigation (high-pressure irrigation and pulsatile high-pressure lavage), whirlpool, and wound scrubbing [6]. **Sharp debridement** is considered as a surgical wound debridement. It is the most aggressive type of debridement [2], but is generally considered to be the most rapid and effective method even though there is a risk of injury of the healthy tissue [7]. **Hydro-surgery**

S. Probst (✉)
HES-SO University of Applied Sciences and Arts Western Switzerland, Geneva, Switzerland

University Hospital Geneva, Geneva, Switzerland

University of Geneva, Geneva, Switzerland

University of Galway, Galway, Ireland

Monash University, Melbourne, Australia
e-mail: sebastian.probst@hesge.ch

debridement is a debridement where devitalized tissue is removed with a jet of water used as a dissecting tool [8, 9].
- **Bio-surgery** called also larval or maggot therapy is a debridement where live Lucilia sericata larvae are applied to the wound either directly or contained within a sealed bag [10]. Lucilia sericata larvae ingest necrotic tissue and kill ingested bacteria [2].

This chapter will highlight the different aspects of debridement taught and regulatory facts.

References

1. Sibbald RG, Elliott JA, Persaud-Jaimangal R, Goodman L, Armstrong DG, Harley C, et al. Wound bed preparation 2021. Adv Skin Wound Care. 2021;34(4):183–95.
2. Probst S. Wound care nursing—a person-centred approach. 3rd ed. London: Elsevier; 2021.
3. Strohal R, Dissemond J, Jordan O'Brien J, Piaggesi A, Rimdeika R, Young T, et al. EWMA document: debridement. An updated overview and clarification of the principle role of debridement. J Wound Care. 2013;22(1):5.
4. Eriksson E, Liu PY, Schultz GS, Martins-Green MM, Tanaka R, Weir D, et al. Chronic wounds: treatment consensus. Wound Repair Regen. 2022;30(2):156–71.
5. Swanson T, Angel D, Sussman G, Cooper R, Haesler E, Ousey K, et al. Wound infection in clinical practice: principles of best practice. 3rd ed. International Wound Infection Institute; 2022.
6. Choo J, Nixon J, Nelson A, McGinnis E. Autolytic debridement for pressure ulcers. Cochrane Database Syst Rev. 2019;2019(6)
7. Thomas DC, Tsu CL, Nain RA, Arsat N, Fun SS, Lah SN, NA. The role of debridement in wound bed preparation in chronic wound: a narrative review. Ann Med Surg (Lond). 2021;71:102876.
8. Matsumine H, Giatsidis G, Takagi M, Kamei W, Shimizu M, Takeuchi M. Hydrosurgical debridement allows effective wound bed preparation of pressure injuries: a prospective case series. Plast Reconstr Surg Glob Open. 2020;8(6):e2921.
9. Wormald JC, Wade RG, Dunne JA, Collins DP, Jain A. Hydrosurgical debridement versus conventional surgical debridement for acute partial-thickness burns. Cochrane Database Syst Rev. 2020;9(9):Cd012826.
10. Romeyke T. Maggot therapy as a part of a holistic approach in the treatment of multimorbid patients with chronic ulcer. Clin Pract. 2021;11(2):347–57.

Open Access This chapter is licensed under the terms of the Creative Commons Attribution-NonCommercial-NoDerivatives 4.0 International License (http://creativecommons.org/licenses/by-nc-nd/4.0/), which permits any non-commercial use, sharing, distribution and reproduction in any medium or format, as long as you give appropriate credit to the original author(s) and the source, provide a link to the Creative Commons license and indicate if you modified the licensed material. You do not have permission under this license to share adapted material derived from this chapter or parts of it.

The images or other third party material in this chapter are included in the chapter's Creative Commons license, unless indicated otherwise in a credit line to the material. If material is not included in the chapter's Creative Commons license and your intended use is not permitted by statutory regulation or exceeds the permitted use, you will need to obtain permission directly from the copyright holder.

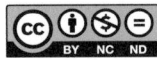

Education on Debridement: Non-specialized Nurses and Debridement

Paul Bobbink

Taking care of people living with chronic wounds is central to nursing practice [1] and research [2]. Due to the high prevalence of chronic wounds [3] and the allocation of healthcare expenses, non-specialized nurses regularly treat people across hospital wards, nursing homes, or homecare. Therefore, non-specialized nurses should have basic knowledge and understanding of clinical assessment and wound bed preparation, which includes debridement.

For years, best practices recommendations have included debridement to remove devitalized tissue [4, 5] or biofilm [6, 7] to enhance healing. Although evidence to support wound debridement in some types of chronic wounds remains limited [8], this intervention is recommended by multiple guidelines [9–11] and can be repeated frequently, especially for diabetic foot ulcers [12].

In light of variations in nursing education across the world, depending on regulations, healthcare systems, and scope of nursing practice, this chapter aims to provide a basis of knowledge of what a non-specialized nurse should know on wound debridement.

73.1 Nurses Should Be Able to Assess a Person Living with a Chronic Wound

Prior to debridement, nurses should be able to provide a holistic assessment of people living with chronic wounds to identify contraindications and expected benefits of wound debridement. This first step enables a patient-centred care approach [13] and includes previous patient experiences of wound debridement. Due to the complexity and negative consequences of living with a chronic wound [1] and as patients' needs are frequently overlooked [14], a nurse should have special skills in communication based on interpersonal relationship frameworks and use specific assessment tools like TIMERS [4] or the wound prevention and management circle [15].

73.2 Nurses Should Have Knowledge on Basic Wound Aetiology and Wound Bed Evaluation

Clarifying and confirming a wound's aetiology are part of nurses' clinical practice, as they are regularly involved in dressing changes or follow-up of patients with wounds [16]. During this step, registered nurses should be able to identify the cause of the principal wounds to implement the best clinical guidelines according to aetiology. For example, pressure ulcers (PUs) result from

P. Bobbink (✉)
Geneva School of Health Sciences, HES-SO University of Applied Sciences and Arts, Geneva, Switzerland
e-mail: paul.bobbink@hesge.ch

pressure or pressure and shearing forces applied to soft tissues [17] and need discharge to promote healing. Regarding this aetiology, stable heel eschars should not be debrided [10]. Furthermore, clinical signs and symptoms are indicators of whether or not to perform wound debridement. In clinical practice, intermittent claudication or rest pain indicates peripheral arterial disease (PAD) resulting from poor blood flow. PAD is a contraindication for sharp wound debridement [4, 18] as wound healing needs sufficient blood flow. Regarding diabetic foot ulcers (DFUs), they are defined as a wound localized under the ankle in persons living with diabetes and usually with a diagnosis of neuropathy and/or PAD [19]. DFUs are typically localized in the plantar area, the side of the foot, or the toes, and it is estimated that around half of patients with a DFU also have an ischemic aetiology [20]. Therefore, in this specific population, debridement should be provided after a complete assessment by a multidisciplinary team.

Finally, the nurse must be competent in wound bed evaluation/assessment and should be able to differentiate tissue in the wound bed, for example, granulation, epithelialization, or devitalized tissue like necrosis or slough (see Fig. 73.1). Healthy granulation tissue is red/pink in colour, whereas a friable or bleeding granulation tissue could be an indicator of wound infection [21]. Devitalized tissue such as an eschar or necrotic tissue is generally black or dark brown, usually dry/thick and firmly attached to the wound bed. Slough is also devitalized tissue, yellow-green or brown in colour that is loosely attached to the wound bed and usually moist [22, 23]. Nurses should also be able to identify structures such as bones or tendons in the wound bed, as shown in Fig. 73.2.

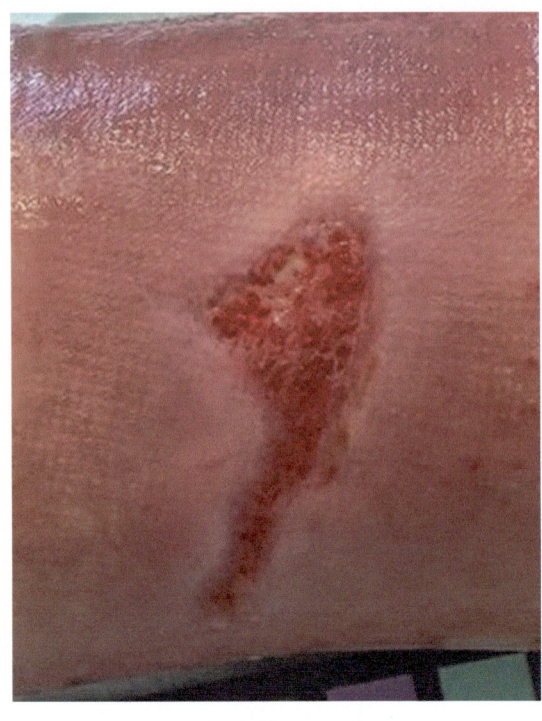

Fig. 73.1 Wound with granulation, epithelialization, and few devitalized tissue

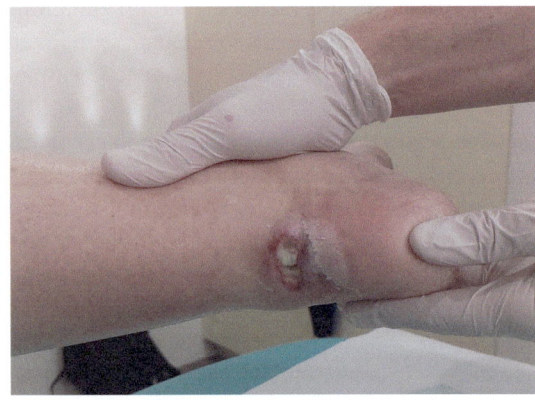

Fig. 73.2 Wound with an exposed tendon

73.3 Nurses Should Be Aware of Types of Debridement

In practice, wound cleansing refers to superficial removal of dead tissue, bacteria, or contaminants [24, 25]; debridement refers to deep removal of adherent, devitalized, contaminated or necrotic tissue, including senescent cells, bacteria, and biofilms, that may delay wound healing [26, 27]. Debridement can be mechanical, autolytic, enzymatic, biological, sharp or surgical [26, 27] and may have the aim of promoting healing, preventing infection and odour, or promoting patient wellbeing by removing excess devitalized tissue [28].

Registered nurses can use autolytic debridement, mechanical debridement, and sometimes sharp debridement, depending on local regulations, scopes of practice, and the contextual situation. As it is recommended that the initial debridement be aggressive [18], it is important to differentiate initial/first wound debridement, which should be practiced by experts, from conservative and repetitive debridement, which can be provided by registered nurses. To make meaningful clinical decisions, nurses should be able to differentiate existing methods of wound debridement and support patient decisions by providing clear explanations of the methods.

Autolytic debridement occurs if a wound is vascularized and moisture balance is present in the wound to rehydrate tissues so that the body's natural enzymes will soften and partially digest devitalized tissue [22]. Depending on wound exudate, various dressings may be applied. For example, hydrogels should be applied in a layer of at least 5 mm thick on wounds with no or small quantities of exudates, whereas dressings like alginates could be combined with secondary dressings to absorb significant amounts of exudates [27]. Autolytic debridement takes place over time and requires frequent dressing changes; therefore, it is recommended for small quantities of slough. Moreover, this is not a painful procedure [22, 27], and therefore it is commonly used for wound bed preparation.

Mechanical debridement is defined as a physical removal of devitalized tissue with gauzes, tulles, or monofilament fibre pads [27]. Mechanical debridement is the most common method [27] used in wound care. Over the last year, the development and use of debridement pads have increased in clinical practice. These pads are easy to use, will not harm the underlying tissue [27], and are effective for removing biofilm and slough [29]. However, these devices are not recommended for dry eschars [30]. Due to the time necessary for wound debridement, mechanical debridement is one of the most expensive approaches [31]. Therefore, other approaches to mechanical debridement like hydro jets or low frequency ultrasound have been developed, but they require a highly specialized approach.

Sharp debridement is defined as a minor surgical bedside procedure involving cutting away tissue with a scalpel or scissors [27]. It should be used when there is a thick and adherent layer of slough or necrotic tissue. Conservative sharp debridement usually stops above the level of viable tissue. It can be practiced by nurses, but as clinical risks increase with the use of scalpels, sharp debridement is usually part of specialized practice. However, in practice, the amount of remaining devitalized tissue can be greater when an untrained nurse performs the procedure, which limits risks of harm to patients. Sharp debridement, especially with scalpels, requires some mentoring and training.

Surgical, biological, and enzymatic debridement are usually part of specialized nursing practice or other disciplines as they require specific skills, knowledge, and equipment. Nevertheless, registered nurses should know of their existence to refer patients to the right clinicians. For example, nurses should have positive knowledge about maggot therapy, used as biological debridement, to refer patients quickly to a specific team [32]. In all cases, debridement should be performed after the provision of medical advice and fit the scope of practice of local legislation.

73.4 Nurses Should Be Able to Select the Most Suitable Type of Debridement

Selection of the appropriate debridement method should be based on clinical indication or contraindication of debridement, patients' preferences, including their previous experiences, the nurses' knowledge and skills, the legal aspects of debridement, cost-effectiveness, and contextual resources. Nurses' skills developed during undergraduate education vary across countries, and therefore autolytic and mechanical debridement may be the best solution for nurses without specific training, even if the process is more time-consuming than sharp debridement [28]. Due to discrepancies in undergraduate training, it is of utmost importance that nurses be able to identify their own limits before they engage in wound debridement. Debridement is sometimes an emergency treatment, and therefore nurses should know why, when, and how to refer a patient quickly to an interdisciplinary wound care team. Box 73.1 provides some questions which should be answered prior to wound debridement.

> **Box 73.1 Skills and Assessment Checklist Prior to Debridement**
> - Does this wound need debridement?
> - Does the patient agree to debridement?
> - Which type of debridement should be used?
> - Does this type of debridement fit my skills and scope of practice?
> - If I have not received education in this field, have I undergone a training programme or clinical supervision on wound debridement?
> - Have I received medical agreement to proceed with debridement?
> - If complications of debridement appear, can I refer this patient urgently?
> - Is it reasonable to undertake wound debridement in this setting and condition?

Legal aspects of debridement for nurses vary across countries and institutions [33], and nurses should refer to local guidance, taking the context into consideration, before engaging in debridement procedures. Costs related to wound care interventions are important when implementing clinical recommendations. In a cost analysis in Canada, taking into consideration health care personnel costs, materials, transportation, and frequency of visits, Woo et al. [31] found that, among the debridement methods discussed in this chapter that registered nurses can perform, conservative sharp costs approximately $1120, whereas autolytic debridement costs $1500, and mechanical debridement, up to $1840.

73.5 Nurses Should Have an Understanding of Moist Wound Healing to Implement an Effective After-Debridement Care Plan

Understanding wound healing phases and, more specifically, the benefit of moist wound healing makes it possible to identify the best method for wound bed preparation, including wound cleansing and debridement, and implement an effective 'after-debridement' care plan. The dressing selected after debridement should promote moisture balance [28], prevent complications, or continue to debride with an autolytic approach. Thus, debridement should not be used as an isolated intervention but should be integrated into a global care plan to promote wound healing and patient well-being. Table 73.1 provides an overview of wound types, their characteristics and suggestion for type of debridement selection.

Take-Home Message
One can learn the theoretical aspects of debridement through online or face-to-face education. However, debriding a wound requires psychomotor skills that can only be developed by training, first on specific materials like oranges, pigs' feet or simulators and then by mentoring during clinical practice. The EWMA curricula for nurses Levels 4 [34] and 5 [35] can provide guidance for developing further nursing education and improving congruence in nursing practice.

Table 73.1 Wound type, characteristics, and type of debridement

Wound type	Usual site and characteristics	Type of debridement	Details
Pressure ulcer	Sacrum, heel, trochanter	Sharp, mechanical and autolytic	PUs on the heel should not be debrided. Eschar debridement on PUs could quickly extend the wound size.
Venous leg ulcer	Gaiter area of the leg	Autolytic and mechanical. Sharp debridement may be used depending on patients' experience of pain	When using conservative sharp debridement, implement an effective pain management plan to reduce procedural pain.
Mixed leg ulcer	Characteristics of both venous and arterial leg ulcers	Various approaches may be used. Refer to a specialized wound care team	
Arterial leg ulcer	Toes, heels or ankle	No debridement for non-specialized wound care team.	Evaluate the possibility of revascularization prior to debridement.
Diabetic foot ulcer	Lateral foot, plantar or toe	Plantar: sharp debridement of hyperkeratosis followed by autolytic debridement for the wound bed may be used. Toe: No debridement for non-specialized wound care team	High risk of infection. Ensure correct blood flow to promote healing.
Acute wound		Wound cleansing using tap water or saline No debridement for non-specialized wound care team	
Malignant fungating wound		Use autolytic dressing for comfortable debridement. No aggressive debridement for non-specialized wound care team.	High risks of bleeding

NB Absence of patient consent or a patient with bleeding disorders or contact sensitization to dressing contents are person-related contraindications

Ischemic, infected, bleeding or undiagnosed (atypical, malignant) wounds, specific localisation such as the genital area, head, neck, extremities or near vessels, nerves are wound-related contraindications to debridement by non-specialised nurses

These wounds should **not be debrided** by nurses and should be referred to a multidisciplinary wound care team to implement the best care plan with a patient-centred approach

References

1. Lindholm C, Searle R. Wound management for the 21st century: combining effectiveness and efficiency. Int Wound J. 2016;13(Suppl 2):5–15. https://doi.org/10.1111/iwj.12623.
2. Gethin G, Probst S, Weller C, Kottner J, Beeckman D. Nurses are research leaders in skin and wound care. Int Wound J. 2020b;17(6):2005–9. https://doi.org/10.1111/iwj.13492.
3. Olsson M, Jarbrink K, Divakar U, Bajpai R, Upton Z, Schmidtchen A, Car J. The humanistic and economic burden of chronic wounds: a systematic review. Wound Repair Regen. 2019;27(1):114–25. https://doi.org/10.1111/wrr.12683.
4. Atkin L, Bucko Z, Conde Montero E, Cutting K, Moffatt C, Probst A, Romanelli M, Schultz GS, Tettelbach W. Implementing TIMERS: the race against hard-to-heal wounds. J Wound Care. 2019;23(Sup3a):S1–S50. https://doi.org/10.12968/jowc.2019.28.Sup3a.S1.
5. Schultz GS, Sibbald RG, Falanga V, Ayello EA, Dowsett C, Harding K, Romanelli M, Stacey MC, Teot L, Vanscheidt W. Wound bed preparation: a systematic approach to wound management. Wound Repair Regen. 2003;11(Suppl 1):S1–28. https://doi.org/10.1046/j.1524-475x.11.s2.1.x.
6. Bianchi T, Wolcott RD, Peghetti A, Leaper D, Cutting K, Polignano R, Rosa Rita Z, Moscatelli A, Greco A, Romanelli M, Pancani S, Bellingeri A, Ruggeri V, Postacchini L, Tedesco S, Manfredi L, Camerlingo M, Rowan S, Gabrielli A, Pomponio G. Recommendations for the management of biofilm: a consensus document. J Wound Care. 2016;25(6):305–17. https://doi.org/10.12968/jowc.2016.25.6.305.
7. Schultz G, Bjarnsholt T, James GA, Leaper DJ, McBain AJ, Malone M, Stoodley P, Swanson T,

Tachi M, Wolcott RD, Global Wound Biofilm Expert P. Consensus guidelines for the identification and treatment of biofilms in chronic nonhealing wounds. Wound Repair Regen. 2017;25(5):744–57. https://doi.org/10.1111/wrr.12590.

8. Gethin G, Cowman S, Kolbach DN. Debridement for venous leg ulcers. Cochrane Database Syst Rev. 2015;2015(9):CD008599. https://doi.org/10.1002/14651858.CD008599.pub2.

9. Franks PJ, Barker J, Collier M, Gethin G, Haesler E, Jawien A, Laeuchli S, Mosti G, Probst S, Weller C. Management of patients with venous leg ulcers: challenges and current best practice. J Wound Care. 2016;25(Suppl 6):S1–S67. https://doi.org/10.12968/jowc.2016.25.Sup6.S1.

10. Kottner J, Cuddigan J, Carville K, et al. European Pressure Ulcer Advisory Panel, National Pressure Injury Advisory Panel and Pan Pacific Pressure Injury Alliance. Prevention and Treatment of Pressure Ulcers/Injuries: Clinical Practice Guideline. The International Guideline. Emily Haesler (Ed.). EPUAP/NPIAP/PPPIA: 2019. https://internationalguideline.com/.

11. Rayman G, Prashant V, Dhatariya V, et al.. IWGDF Guideline on interventions to enhance healing of foot ulcers in persons with diabetes; 2019. www.iwgdfguidelines.org

12. Nube VL, Alison JA, Twigg SM. Frequency of sharp wound debridement in the management of diabetes-related foot ulcers: exploring current practice. J Foot Ankle Res. 2021;14(1):52. https://doi.org/10.1186/s13047-021-00489-1.

13. Gethin G, Probst S, Stryja J, Christiansen N, Price P. Evidence for person-centred care in chronic wound care: a systematic review and recommendations for practice. J Wound Care. 2020a;29(Sup9b):S1–S22. https://doi.org/10.12968/jowc.2020.29.Sup9b.S1.

14. Green J, Jester R, McKinley R, Pooler A. Nurse-patient consultations in primary care: do patients disclose their concerns? J Wound Care. 2013;22(10):534–6, 538–539. https://doi.org/10.12968/jowc.2013.22.10.534.

15. Orsted H, Keast D, Forest-Laland L, Kuhnke J, O'Sullivan-Drombolis D, Jin S. Best practice recommendations for the prevention and management of wounds. In: Woundscanada.ca, editor, Foundations of best practice for skin and wound management; 2017. https://www.woundscanada.ca/docman/public/health-care-professional/bpr-workshop/165-wc-bpr-prevention-and-management-of-wounds/file

16. Guest JF, Fuller GW, Vowden P. Cohort study evaluating the burden of wounds to the UK's National Health Service in 2017/2018: update from 2012/2013. BMJ Open. 2020;10(12):e045253. https://doi.org/10.1136/bmjopen-2020-045253.

17. Gefen A, Brienza DM, Cuddigan J, Haesler E, Kottner J. Our contemporary understanding of the aetiology of pressure ulcers/pressure injuries. Int Wound J. 2022;19(3):692–704. https://doi.org/10.1111/iwj.13667.

18. Eriksson E, Liu PY, Schultz GS, Martins-Green MM, Tanaka R, Weir D, Gould LJ, Armstrong DG, Gibbons GW, Wolcott R, Olutoye OO, Kirsner RS, Gurtner GC. Chronic wounds: treatment consensus. Wound Repair Regen. 2022;30(2):156–71. https://doi.org/10.1111/wrr.12994.

19. van Netten JJ, Bus SA, Apelqvist J, Lipsky BA, Hinchliffe RJ, Game F, Rayman G, Lazzarini PA, Forsythe RO, Peters EJG, Senneville E, Vas P, Monteiro-Soares M, Schaper NC, International Working Group on the Diabetic F. Definitions and criteria for diabetic foot disease. Diabetes Metab Res Rev. 2020;36(Suppl 1):e3268. https://doi.org/10.1002/dmrr.3268.

20. Prompers L, Huijberts M, Apelqvist J, Jude E, Piaggesi A, Bakker K, Edmonds M, Holstein P, Jirkovska A, Mauricio D, Ragnarson Tennvall G, Reike H, Spraul M, Uccioli L, Urbancic V, Van Acker K, van Baal J, van Merode F, Schaper N. High prevalence of ischaemia, infection and serious comorbidity in patients with diabetic foot disease in Europe. Baseline results from the Eurodiale study. Diabetologia. 2007;50(1):18–25. https://doi.org/10.1007/s00125-006-0491-1.

21. Swanson T, Ousey K, Haesler E, Bjarnsholt T, Carville K, Idensohn P, Kalan L, Keast DH, Larsen D, Percival S, Schultz G, Sussman G, Waters N, Weir D. IWII wound infection in clinical practice consensus document: 2022 update. J Wound Care. 2022;31(Sup12):S10–S21. https://doi.org/10.12968/jowc.2022.31.Sup12.S10.

22. Atkin L, Rippon M. Autolysis: mechanisms of action in the removal of devitalised tissue. Br J Nurs. 2016;25(20 Suppl):S40–7. https://doi.org/10.12968/bjon.2016.25.20.S40.

23. Grey JE, Enoch S, Harding KG. Wound assessment. BMJ. 2006;332(7536):285–8. https://doi.org/10.1136/bmj.332.7536.285.

24. McLain NE, Moore ZE, Avsar P. Wound cleansing for treating venous leg ulcers. Cochrane Database Syst Rev. 2021;3:CD011675. https://doi.org/10.1002/14651858.CD011675.pub2.

25. Weir D, Swanson T. Ten top tips: wound cleansing. Wounds Int. 2019;10(4). www.woundsinternational.com

26. Niederstatter IM, Schiefer JL, Fuchs PC. Surgical strategies to promote cutaneous healing. Med Sci (Basel). 2021;9(2) https://doi.org/10.3390/medsci9020045.

27. Strohal R, Dissemond J, Jordan O'Brien J, Piaggesi A, Rimdeika R, Young T, Apelqvist J. EWMA document: debridement. An updated overview and clarification of the principle role of debridement. J Wound Care. 2013;22(1):5. https://doi.org/10.12968/jowc.2013.22.Sup1.S1.

28. Sibbald RG, Elliott JA, Persaud-Jaimangal R, Goodman L, Armstrong DG, Harley C, Coelho S, Xi N, Evans R, Mayer DO, Zhao X, Heil J, Kotru B, Delmore B, LeBlanc K, Ayello EA, Smart H, Tariq G, Alavi A, Somayaji R. Wound bed preparation 2021.

Adv Skin Wound Care. 2021;34(4):183–95. https://doi.org/10.1097/01.ASW.0000733724.87630.d6.
29. Schultz GS, Woo K, Weir D, Yang Q. Effectiveness of a monofilament wound debridement pad at removing biofilm and slough: ex vivo and clinical performance. J Wound Care. 2018;27(2):80–90. https://doi.org/10.12968/jowc.2018.27.2.80.
30. Atkin L. A guide to wound debridement. Ind Nurs. 2016;2:20. https://doi.org/10.12968/indn.2016.2.20.
31. Woo KY, Keast D, Parsons N, Sibbald RG, Mittmann N. The cost of wound debridement: a Canadian perspective. Int Wound J. 2015;12(4):402–7. https://doi.org/10.1111/iwj.12122.
32. Bazalinski D, Przybek Mita J, Scislo L, Wiech P. Perception and readiness to undertake maggot debridement therapy with the use of Lucilia sericata larvae in the group of nurses. Int J Environ Res Public Health. 2022;19(5) https://doi.org/10.3390/ijerph19052895.
33. Rodd-Nielsen E, Harris CL. Conservative sharp wound debridement: an overview of Canadian education, practice, risk, and policy. J Wound Ostomy Continence Nurs. 2013;40(6):594–601. https://doi.org/10.1097/WON.0b013e3182a9ae8c.
34. Lindhal E, Holloway S, Bobbink P, Gryson L, Pokorna A, Ousey K, Samuriwo R, Pancorbo Hidalgo P. Wound curriculum for student nurses: European Qualification Framework Level 4. J Wound Manag. 2021;22(3). https://viewer.ipaper.io/jowm/1035279jowm202110/supp01/
35. Pokorna A, Holloway S, Strohal R, Verheyen-Cronau I. Wound curriculum for nurses. J Wound Care. 2017;26(Sup12):S1–S27. https://doi.org/10.12968/jowc.2017.28.Sup12.S1.

Open Access This chapter is licensed under the terms of the Creative Commons Attribution-NonCommercial-NoDerivatives 4.0 International License (http://creativecommons.org/licenses/by-nc-nd/4.0/), which permits any non-commercial use, sharing, distribution and reproduction in any medium or format, as long as you give appropriate credit to the original author(s) and the source, provide a link to the Creative Commons license and indicate if you modified the licensed material. You do not have permission under this license to share adapted material derived from this chapter or parts of it.

The images or other third party material in this chapter are included in the chapter's Creative Commons license, unless indicated otherwise in a credit line to the material. If material is not included in the chapter's Creative Commons license and your intended use is not permitted by statutory regulation or exceeds the permitted use, you will need to obtain permission directly from the copyright holder.

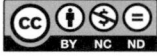

How to Become an Expert in Debridement: Nurse Perspective

74

Georgina Gethin

74.1 Introduction

In its simplest form, debridement can be seen as the process of removal of necrotic tissue from a wound. This book has provided a comprehensive description of debridement and the pathophysiology underpinning it, together with an overview of the methods of debridement and thus will not be revisited in this chapter. Instead, this chapter will look at the evolving role of the nurse in advanced practice and the contributions they have made to patient care and service delivery. It will map the role of the advanced practice nurse and that of an expert in debridement to the various types of debridement and the model of 'Novice to Expert' as first described by Benner in 1982. This chapter will show that debridement should not simply been seen as the 'removal of necrotic tissue' but should be seen as a treatment that is appropriately delivered within an overall episode and system of care by a person with the appropriate knowledge, skills, and understanding to do so.

G. Gethin (✉)
School of Nursing and Midwifery, University of Galway, Galway, Ireland
e-mail: georgina.gethin@nuigalway.ie

74.2 The Nurse in Advanced Practice

There are varied titles, roles, and levels of practice included under the Advanced Nurse Practitioner (ANP) umbrella, and this variation in titles can limit cross-border comparisons, standardisation, and dialogue [1]. The advanced practice nurse possesses the critical thinking skills, expanded clinical knowledge, and analytical skills together with increased confidence, improved decision making skills, and use of more evidence-based approaches to care [1]. These improved decision making skills are associated with improvements in critical analysis of care, clinical judgement, autonomous practice, application of evidence-based care with changing patient conditions and faster patient-related responses [1].

As the titles used to describe advanced practice vary globally, so too do education requirements and education attainment. A national survey of nurses in Australia sought to investigate the relationship between level of education and nursing domain practice scores of nurses in advanced practice [1]. Five domains were assessed: clinical care, optimising health systems; education; research; and leadership. Results compared the influence of education on each domain mean score for advanced practice nurses who held higher degrees (masters or doctoral level degrees) with those who did not. The differences were significant for optimising health systems and education domains ($p < 0.05$), highly significant for both research and leadership domains ($p < 0.001$) but not significant for clinical care ($p = 0.12$).

Nurses working in advanced practice are considered as 'knowledge brokers' where they promote the uptake of knowledge and evidence-based practice. APNs are also involved in facilitating change through collaboration and consultation with health care providers and decision-makers. Those with doctoral and master level degrees have shown higher scores in clinical care and other practice domains (such as research, leadership, optimising health systems) than APNs with less education [1]. This describes practice at an advanced level based on layers of knowledge and clinical engagement that is grounded in academic preparation. APNs function at a higher level of 'care coordination' looking after populations with high complexity health care needs with many holding individual caseloads. APNs also add to the wider system as they have the capacity to improve the efficiency of care, improve access to care, reduce costs, and improve quality of life [1]. Research has shown the impact of specialist and advanced practice roles and identified strong positive contributions across a range of domains. The impact of specialist and advanced practice roles may seem similar, but additional contributions are evident from advanced practitioners particularly in the areas of research activities, the development of guidelines for national distribution, and the development of their scope of practice for more complex care provision including the total journey of care up to discharge [2]. In addition, specialist nurses and advanced practice nurses have full prescribing authority in some jurisdictions, a factor that is supportive of sharp debridement as it facilitates appropriate pain management. Specialist and advanced practitioners also enable timely, seamless and integrated multidisciplinary care by making the right care intervention and referrals at the right time while brokering care between healthcare professionals and other organisations.

In 2020, the European Wound Management Association (EWMA) document on *Wound Curriculum for Nurses: post-registration qualification wound management European qualification framework Level 7*, set out the learning goals, outcomes, and estimated hours to develop knowledge in all areas related to wound management, including that of debridement [3]. Nurses working at level 7 will hold a Master's degree qualification and thus are well-aligned with that of Advanced Practice Nurses and in some cases Clinical Nurse Specialists. Their document is mapped against the European Qualifications Framework (EQF) and sees those at level 7 as having highly specialised knowledge and critical awareness of knowledge issues in a field and at the interface between different fields; they will have attained the skills of specialised problem solving that are required in research and/or innovation in order to develop new knowledge and procedures and to integrate knowledge from different fields; and they will have the responsibility and autonomy to manage and transform work or study context that are complex, unpredictable and require new strategic approaches and take responsibility for contributing to professional knowledge and practice and/or for reviewing the strategic performance of teams [3].

The competencies of the nurse working at an advanced level have recently been examined in the context of Australian Advanced Nursing Practice, resulting in an agreed set of standards under six areas of health care [4]. Wound care could fall within many domains but perhaps is best aligned with the chronic and complex care domain under which 14 standards are identified. These standards are similar to those in the advanced practice policy document from the Department of Health in Ireland (2019) who similarly referred to standards from other jurisdictions. The wordings of 'standards' in both documents are similar and when taken in the context of considering wound assessment, wound management, and specifically wound debridement, it is easy to see that advanced knowledge, skills, and competencies are required to accurately deliver on this care. Examples include:

> *undertakes a comprehensive and expert assessment of person with chronic and/or complex ill-*

ness, including rehabilitation needs and potential for self-management

ensures provision of timely and appropriate access to treatment for the person with chronic or complex illness, demonstrating high level of clinical confidence and proficiency

The seminal work of Patricia Benner (1982) proposed a theory of the stages of proficiency moving from novice to expert, that represents a systematic way of understanding how a learner, a student, new or seasoned nurse develops skills and understanding of a practice situation or event over time [5] (see Table 74.1). The theory proposes that moving from novice to expert across five stages is not a strict linear one but one that may see the learner move in a cyclical way as they reflect on their practice and learn additional knowledge and skills. The model moves from the novice such as, for example, a new student nurse, to the expert, for example, the advanced nurse practitioner. The advanced nurse practitioner has an extensive knowledge of situations that allow for confidence and an intuitive grasp of complex patients situations, rules, guidelines or maxims are no longer relied upon during the expert stage because the individual is able to grasp the situation and understand what needs to be accomplished at this point [5]. The nurse at all stages of the framework should be cognisant of and supportive of a patient-centred approach, so that all treatments are aligned with patient goals [6]. The five stages proposed in Benner's model have been mapped here against the different types of debridement and represented schematically in Fig. 74.1.

To commemorate 2020 as the International Year of the Nurse and Midwife, a systematic review of the contribution of nurses as leaders in research in the field of wound care was completed [7]. This report clearly demonstrated the increasing profile of nurses in the contribution to research in the field with the strongest contributions in the area of cohort studies, systematic reviews and critically appraising the literature, further supporting the domains of competence of those in advance practice nursing. The authors argue that nurse-led research seems to particularly support the work of nurses as frontline caregivers. Nurse research leadership in the field of

Table 74.1 Stages of proficiency. Adapted from Benner (1982)

Stage	Definition	Potential strategies for skills and knowledge acquisition
Novice	The learner has had no previous experience making them struggle to decide which tasks are more relevant to accomplish	Teach simple, objective concepts/attributes that are easily identified
Advanced beginner	The learner has enough real-world situations that the recurrent component is easily identified when it is related to rules and guidelines	Increase assistance and support in setting priorities to clients' needs by providing guidelines for recognising patterns
Competent	The learner has been on the job 2 or 3 years and is able to see actions in terms of goals or plans and works in an efficient and organised manner	Offer in-service education or opportunities
Proficient	The learner performs by using pieces of evidence that provide direction to see a situation as a whole	Use case studies to stimulate critical thinking especially in situations which principles or rule that are contradictory
Expert	The learner grasps the situation and understand what needs to be accomplished beyond rules, guidelines, and maxims	Provide opportunities for experts to share their skills and knowledge and also their analytical abilities to solve new situations

skin and wound care over the last 20 years has led >40% of the highest level of evidence publications in this time [7]. This is a significant achievement when one considers the short time frame within which nursing has moved to university led degree programmes and the establishment of advanced practice roles internationally.

It is argued that skills acquisition such as, for example, sharp debridement is a more important predictor of competency than time in role [8]. This

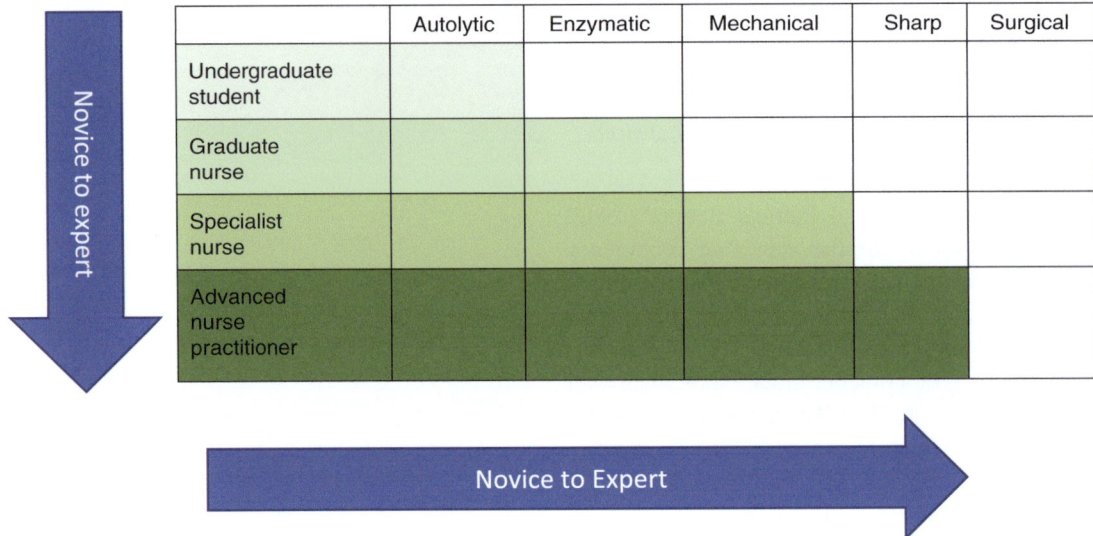

Fig. 74.1 Novice to expert in nursing practice and debridement

is important because when an individual is in a position for a length of time, others may view the person as competent or proficient, but the reality may be the opposite. Competent and proficient nurses will not approach or solve problems in the same way due to past experiences [5]. Thus, the expert nurse can perform the skills of debridement but importantly has the knowledge and understanding to assess the situation and make decisions as to the appropriateness of debridement and the choice of debridement method.

It can be reasonably seen that the student nurse as the novice has no prior knowledge or experience of wound care, wound assessment, or wound debridement. However, autolytic debridement is the body's own method to remove sloughy or devitalised tissue and can be facilitated by the application of wound dressings such as hydrogels. This can be taught easily and performed under supervision by the novice. As one moves across the continuum of debridement methods, an increasing level of skill and knowledge as to the appropriateness of each method is required (see Fig. 74.1). This is achieved through further education, learning from others and as proposed by Benner, being increasingly exposed to the situation at hand. The 'expert' nurse, most often seen as the tissue viability specialist, has this advanced knowledge and is well positioned to make a judgement on the type of debridement that is necessary and aligned with patient and treatment goals. It should be noted that as shown in Fig. 74.1, the nurse does not perform surgical debridement as this is beyond their scope of practice.

74.3 Conclusion

The decision to initiate wound debridement and the choice of method depends on patient and treatment goals, available resources, and the knowledge, skills, and expertise of the attending clinician. The nurse, working at an advanced level of practice is fully competent and proficient to make such decisions and initiate treatment in consultation with the patient. Nurses as expert clinicians significantly impact on patient care and improve patient outcomes.

References

1. Duffield C, et al. Does education level influence the practice profile of advanced practice nursing? Collegian. 2021;28:255–60.
2. Begley C, et al. An evaluation of clinical nurse and midwife specialist and advanced nurse and midwife practitioner roles in Ireland (SCAPE). Dublin: National Council for the professional development of nursing and midwifery in Ireland; 2010.

3. Holloway S, et al. Wound curriculum for nurses: post-registration qualification wound management- European qualification framework level 7. J Wound Care. 2020;29:S1.
4. Gardner A, et al. Development of nurse practitioner metaspecialty clinical practice standards: a national sequential mixed methods study. J Adv Nurs. 2021;77(3):1453–64.
5. Benner P. From novice to expert. Am J Nurs. 1982;82(3):402–7.
6. Gethin G, et al. Evidence for person-centred care in chronic wound care: a systematic review and recommendations for practice. J Wound Care. 2020;29(Sup9b):S1–S22.
7. Gethin G, et al. Nurses are research leaders in skin and wound care. Int Wound J. 2020;17(6):2005–9.
8. Shirey MR. Competencies and tips for effective leadership: from novice to expert. J Nurs Adm. 2007;37(4):167–70.

Open Access This chapter is licensed under the terms of the Creative Commons Attribution-NonCommercial-NoDerivatives 4.0 International License (http://creativecommons.org/licenses/by-nc-nd/4.0/), which permits any non-commercial use, sharing, distribution and reproduction in any medium or format, as long as you give appropriate credit to the original author(s) and the source, provide a link to the Creative Commons license and indicate if you modified the licensed material. You do not have permission under this license to share adapted material derived from this chapter or parts of it.

The images or other third party material in this chapter are included in the chapter's Creative Commons license, unless indicated otherwise in a credit line to the material. If material is not included in the chapter's Creative Commons license and your intended use is not permitted by statutory regulation or exceeds the permitted use, you will need to obtain permission directly from the copyright holder.

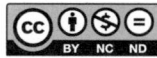

How to Become an Expert in Debridement? Physician Perspective

75

Kirsi Isoherranen and Virve Koljonen

75.1 Introduction

Debridement means removal of nonviable, i.e., necrotic, damaged, infected tissue or foreign bodies to enhance healthy tissue healing. Wounds with necrotic tissue will not heal until all the necrotic tissue is removed. Debridement also provides an opportunity to take a deep tissue sample as a bacterial swab. Early and aggressive debridement in wounds is claimed to be a cornerstone of wound care, and failure to use the optimal debridement method may lead to patient suffering and increased costs of care [1, 2].

Instead of becoming expert only in the debridement technical skills, you need to become expert in determining different types of tissues, to know what to remove and what to leave. Nonviable tissues in (chronic) wounds include slough, eschar, and macerated tissues. Viable tissues include granulation tissue, subcutaneous tissue, muscle, bone, tendon, and vascular structures.

Wounds with different etiologies need different and often personalized treatment regimens. Atypical wounds, such as pyoderma gangrenosum and vasculitic wounds, exhibit pathergy when debrided with sharp instruments [3]. Arterial wounds should not be debrided until comprehensive arterial evaluation by a vascular surgeon has been conducted [4]. Surgical debridement may not be needed if the wound is not healable, e.g., in palliative care and wounds of non-adherent patients. It must be noted that distinctive circumstances such as systemic infection with wound infection as focus may need on-call intervention. In patients with diabetes or receiving immunosuppressive therapy, signs of infection may be reduced or less obvious, and these patients need a thorough and proper assessment in order to exclude infection [5, 6]. Further, dark skin color may hamper detection of redness in the skin. Therefore, other signs of infection should be carefully monitored, and diagnosis of infection should be based on thorough examination of the patient.

Thorough understanding of anatomy together with proper tissue and instrument handling on wounds that benefit from debridement guarantee a successful outcome. Importantly, attention should be paid to wound edges and peri-wound skin and they should be debrided as well if needed [7]. There is no universal agreement on when and how to debride or how much tissue to take [1]. The skills of debridement increase by exercise, and to become an expert in wound debridement, you only need to practice, practice, and practice and to monitor the effect of your debridement. Surgical debridement requires skills and training in the operating room with a senior surgeon.

K. Isoherranen (✉)
Helsinki University Central Hospital and Helsinki University, Wound Healing Centre and Dermatology Clinic, Helsinki, Finland
e-mail: kirsi.isoherranen@hus.fi

V. Koljonen
Department of Plastic Surgery, Töölö Hospital, University of Helsinki, Helsinki, Finland

75.2 How to Debride

Before debridement, a comprehensive and holistic patient assessment is mandatory. This includes the diagnosis of the wound or skin necrosis to be debrided. The patient should be informed carefully about the debridement process, and optimally an informed consent is obtained. Information should include the benefits and risks of debridement and alternatives to treatment [7].

An expert in debridement knows the advantages and disadvantages of different debridement methods (Table 75.1) and can choose the optimal debridement method for each situation.

75.2.1 Autolytic Debridement

Autolytic debridement means the process in which the wound bed clears itself by utilizing phagocytic cells and proteolytic enzymes, such as collagenase, elastase, and lysozymes. This process can be promoted by maintaining a moist wound environment by hydrogels, honey and by using occlusive dressings. Autolytic debridement is the easiest form of debridement, and it is natural, selective, and usually painless. Autolytic debridement does not damage healthy tissue and is claimed to promote the formation of granulation tissue and epithelialization. However, it is a slow process and is contraindicated in infected wounds [1, 2, 7] (Table 75.1).

75.2.2 Enzymatic Debridement

Enzymatic debridement contains the use of proteolytic enzymes that are able to digest cellular debris of the wound bed. It can be a useful method when mechanical debridement is contraindicated, for example, in patients with bleeding problems (Table 75.1). Side effects include pain, burning sensation, and irritation of the periwound skin [1, 2, 7].

Table 75.1 Methods of debridement

Method of debridement	Advantages	Disadvantages
Autolytic debridement	Easy to perform, does not require special skills Safe and selective for necrotic tissue, does not damage surrounding tissues	Slow process Contraindicated in infected wounds May promote anaerobic growth if used with occlusive dressings
Enzymatic debridement	Easy to perform Works faster than autolytic debridement and is also selective for necrotic tissue	Fairly expensive May cause wound pain and burning sensation Need to cross-hatch eschar prior to application of the product
Biologic debridement	Highly selective and safe Works well in wounds exhibiting pathergy phenomenon	Expensive Not recommended in wounds colonized with pseudomonas Can not be used with compression therapy
Mechanical debridement	Easy to perform, no special skills needed Relatively quick and painless Faster than autolytic and chemical debridement	Not suitable in wounds with hard eschar Nonselective Risk of damage to viable tissue
Hydrosurgery	Preserves as much as possible healthy tissues Especially feasible in burns	Disposable handpieces and tubing, thus increasing the carbon footprint
Ultrasonic-assisted debridement	High precision with little risk of damaging viable tissue	Risk of cross-contamination Requires analgesia
Surgical debridement	The fastest method to obtain a clean wound bed Works well in wounds with large amount of necrotic material and exudate	Requires skilled clinician May cause bleeding and pain may require general anesthesia

75.2.3 Mechanical Debridement

The use of wet-to-dry, plain, and paraffin tulle gauzes has been replaced by the newer and more sensitive techniques such as the monofilament fiber pad. A potential disadvantage of mechanical debridement is that it is nonselective and can remove viable tissue along with necrotic material [7] (Table 75.1).

75.2.4 Biological Debridement

Biological debridement or biosurgery includes the use of larvae in the removal of devitalized tissue. In addition to debridement, the action of larvae is antimicrobial. Larval therapy can be administered by "free range" maggots or by using a biobag. Before applying the larvae into the wound bed, they should be checked for activity. One of the major advantages of larval therapy is the selectivity of maggots to separate the necrotic tissue from live tissue (Table 75.1). This allows an easier surgical debridement. Contraindications include usage near eyes, upper gastrointestinal tract and upper respiratory tract, and allergy to fly larvae, brewer's yeast, or soybean protein. Wounds with exposed blood vessels and malignant wounds are not suitable for larval therapy [7].

75.2.5 Surgical or Sharp Debridement

Surgical debridement into viable tissue is the most effective method of wound debridement. It is a common practice to use surgical debridement at the first or second visits followed by enzymatic or autolytic debridement [4]. This debridement is performed in the operating room in general regional or sedation anesthesia using surgical instruments, such as scalpel, Goulian or Humby knife. Pros of this procedure include possibility of large tissue removal when required, readiness to take tissue samples from different tissues, and option to reconstruct the defect simultaneously. In those easy to bleed situations, such as infection or wound with vascular structures exposed, controlling hemorrhage and bleeding is feasible and safe in the operation room setting. Surgical debridement is valuable in identifying osteomyelitis. Infected bone appears soft and does not bleed as much as healthy bone. Debridement of infected bone should be performed until the bone appears solid and bleeds until biopsies [1].

Cons of the procedure include special resources, surgical specialist training with specific knowledge.

Conservative sharp wound debridement uses curettage, scissors, or scalpel to remove only nonviable tissue and wound debris (Fig. 75.1). Pros include conservative sharp wound debridement which can be performed at outpatient clinic or bedside (Figs. 75.2 and 75.3). Bleeding after debridement can be controlled through direct pressure, cauterization by silver nitrate, electrocautery or by hemostatic agents such as hydrogen peroxide, thrombin, or oxidized cellulose [1].

Hydrosurgery [8], a high-pressure, water-based jet system for debridement was designed for accurate debridement for preserving as much as possible healthy tissues. However, despite the intuitive advantages, the use of a hydrosurgery system has been recommended for tangential excision in burns or large wounds with a thin layer of nonviable tissue [9]. Cons are disposable handpieces and tubing, thus increasing the carbon footprint.

Ultrasonic or ultrasound debridement is a method of removing nonviable tissue through microstreaming and cavitational effects [10]. Recent studies show that ultrasound may be a real alternative for surgical debridement when a patient is not fit for anesthesia. Pros include that ultrasound debridement can be performed in an outpatient setting.

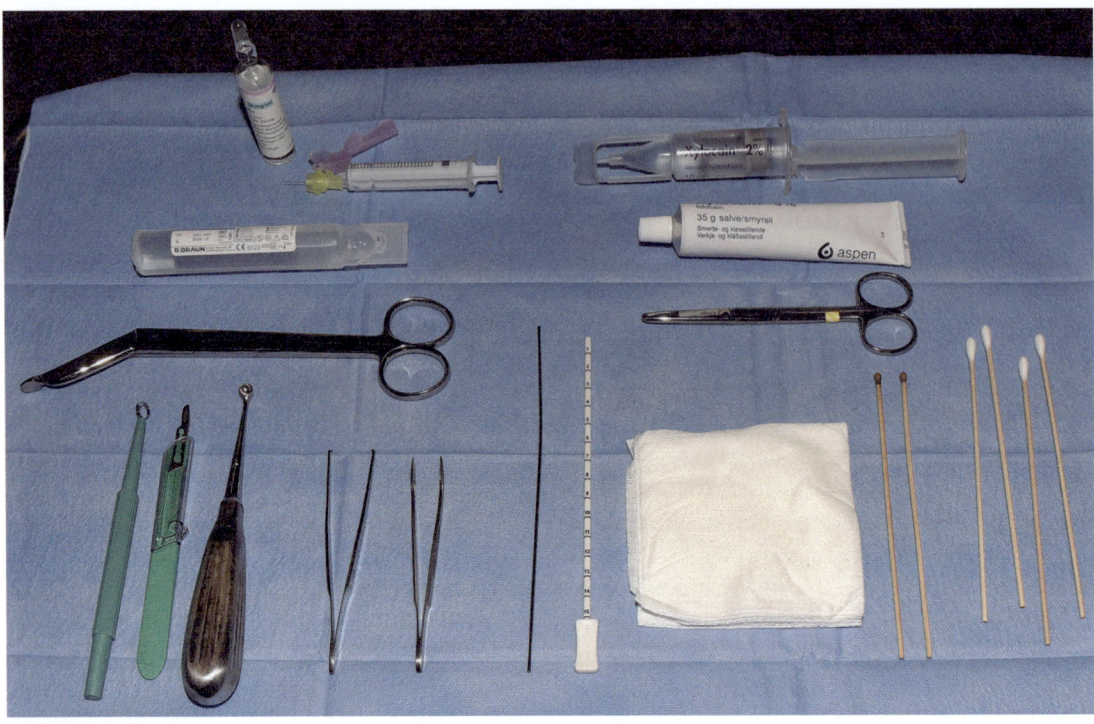

Fig. 75.1 Instruments and agents needed for sharp debridement

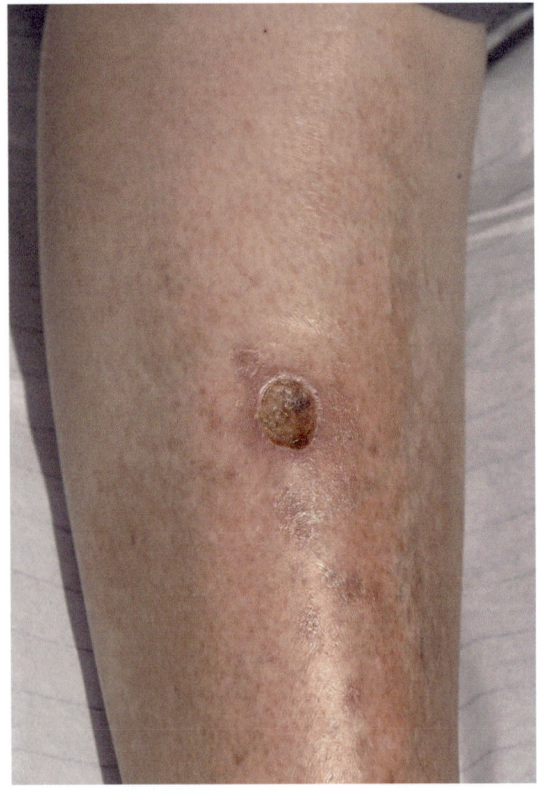

Fig. 75.2 A non-healing, traumatic ulcer in a patient suffering from rheumatoid arthritis

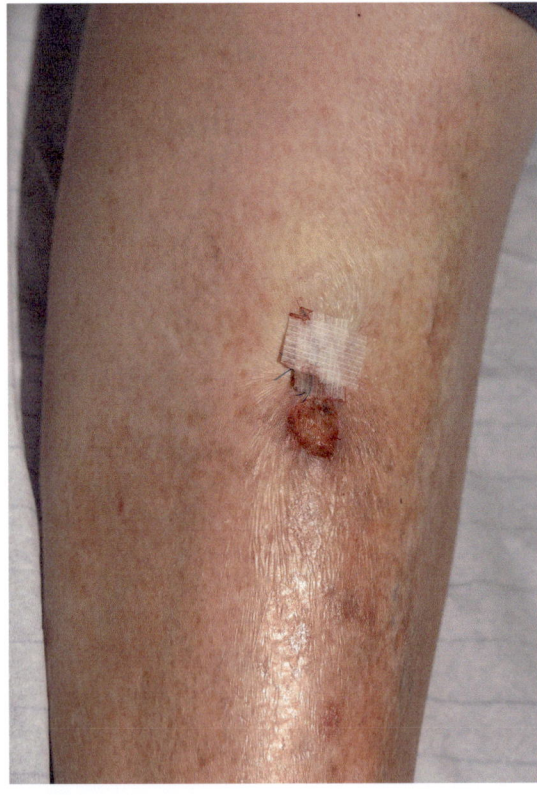

Fig. 75.3 The ulcer after local anesthesia, biopsy, and sharp debridement with curettage

75.3 When NOT to Debride?

In order to be skillful you need to recognize situations when surgical or other forms of debridement would worsen the healing process. When the wound is covered by a dry, black eschar, it does not have to be debrided in every case. Ischemic wounds before vascular assessment and intervention belong to this category. If the eschar is firmly adherent, the patient is afebrile and there is no drainage from the wound, the dry eschar does not have to be removed [1]. Atypical wounds in the active inflammatory process are wounds that worsen by sharp or surgical debridement [3].

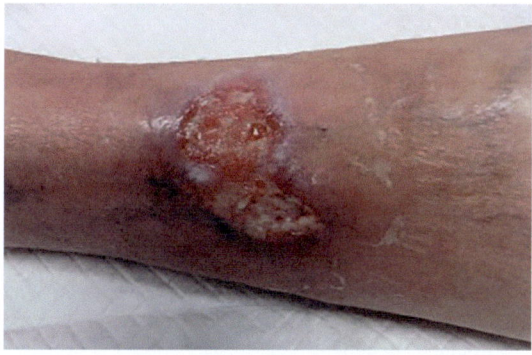

Fig. 75.5 The Martorell ulcer after local anesthesia and sharp debridement with curettage. Debridement continued with autolytic debridement

75.4 Debridement in Atypical Wounds

Atypical wounds need a specialized approach in debridement (Figs. 75.4 and 75.5). Pyoderma gangrenosum and vasculitic wounds exhibit pathergy, i.e., worsening by trauma, and sharp debridement leads to deterioration and enlarging of the wound [3]. Recommended debridement techniques in these wounds are autolytic and biologic treatment. The advantages of biologic treatment include specificity; maggots ingest only dead tissue, not the viable one, and the pathergy reaction is minimal. Conservative sharp and surgical debridement can be performed when inflammation has been reduced by an immunosuppressant, e.g., prednisolone, and this usually takes 2–3 weeks. The clinical evaluation of the stage of the inflammatory reaction needs training, so the decision of the right timing of debridement should be done by a trained dermatologist.

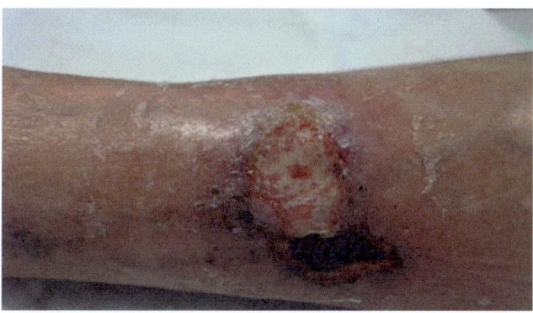

Fig. 75.4 A Martorell hypertensive ulcer

75.5 Pain Treatment During Debridement

Expertise in debridement includes adequate analgesia during treatment. Dead tissue does not feel pain, and sometimes debridement can be performed feasible without analgesia. However, many wound types are very painful, and adequate analgesia must be planned beforehand. Talking through the procedure and explaining the efforts employed to minimize pain, reduces the experienced pain. A skillful physician uses "verbal" anesthesia frequently. If systemic analgesics or topical local analgesics are used, they should be applied 30–60 min before debridement [1, 7]. As procedural pain can be very intense, it is acceptable to go directly to opioids (e.g., oxycodone) without following the three-step approach to pain treatment recommended by WHO. Adequate anesthesia can usually be achieved through direct infiltration of the anesthetic agent locally into the wound bed. In this process, the needle is directed from healthy tissue to the wound bed to avoid microbial contamination.

75.5.1 The Future of Debridement

Future aspects include imaging devices that could determine the amount of tissue to be removed, and the depth of debridement and one promising technology is optical coherence tomography [11]. There is also a clear need for technology that assists the clinician in identifying viable tissue from nonviable one [4, 12].

References

1. Steed DL. Debridement. Am J Surg. 2004;187:71S–4S.
2. Falabella AF. Debridement and wound bed preparation. Dermatol Ther. 2006;19:317–25.
3. Isoherranen K, O'Brien JJ, Barker J, Dissemond J, Hafner J, GBE J, Kamarachev J, Läuchli S, Monetro EC, Nobbe S, Sunderkötter C, Velasco ML. Atypical wounds. Best clinical practice and challenges. J Wound Care. 2019;28(Sup6):S1–S92.
4. Eriksson E, Liu PY, Schultz GS, Martins-Green MM, Tanaka R, Weir D, Gould LJ, et al. Chronic wounds: treatment consensus. Wound Rep Reg. 2022;30:156–71.
5. Schultz G, Bjarnsholt T, James GA, Leaper DJ, McBain AJ, Malone M, et al. Consensus guidelines for the identification and treatment of biofilms in chronic nonhealing wounds. Wound Repair Regen. 2017;25(5):744–57.
6. Malone M, Schultz G. Challenges in the diagnosis and management of wound infection. Br J Dermatol. 2022:1–8.
7. Strohal R, Dissemond J, O'Brien JJ, Piaggesi A, Rimdeika R, Young T, Apelqvist J. EWMA document: debridement. An updated overview and clarification of the principle role of debridement; 2013
8. Ferrer-Sola M, Sureda-Vidal H, Altimiras-Roset J, Fontsere-Candell E, Gonzalez-Martinez V, Espaulella-Panicot J, et al. Hydrosurgery as a safe and efficient debridement method in a clinical wound unit. J Wound Care. 2017;26(10):593–9.
9. Hurd T, Kirsner RS, Sancho-Insenser JJ, Fumarola S, Garten A, Patel M, et al. International consensus panel recommendations for the optimization of traditional and single-use negative pressure wound therapy in the treatment of acute and chronic wounds. Wounds. 2021;33(suppl 2):S1–S11.
10. Flores-Escobar S, Alvaro-Afonso FJ, Garcia-Alvarez Y, Lopez-Moral M, Lazaro-Martinez JL, Garcia-Morales E. Ultrasound-Assisted Wound (UAW) debridement in the treatment of diabetic foot ulcer: a systematic review and meta-analysis. J Clin Med. 2022;11(7):1911.
11. Tsai M-T, Yang C-H, Shen S-C, Lee Y-J, Chang F-Y, Feng C-S. Monitoring of wound healing process of human skin after fractional laser treatments with optical coherence tomography. Biomed. Opt Express. 2013;4(11):2362–75.
12. Falanga V, Brem H, Ennis WJ, Wolcott R, Gould LJ, Ayello EA. Maintenance debridement in the treatment of difficult-hard-to-heal chronic wounds. Recommendations of an expert panel. Ostomy Wound Manage. 2008;(Suppl):2–13.

Open Access This chapter is licensed under the terms of the Creative Commons Attribution-NonCommercial-NoDerivatives 4.0 International License (http://creativecommons.org/licenses/by-nc-nd/4.0/), which permits any non-commercial use, sharing, distribution and reproduction in any medium or format, as long as you give appropriate credit to the original author(s) and the source, provide a link to the Creative Commons license and indicate if you modified the licensed material. You do not have permission under this license to share adapted material derived from this chapter or parts of it.

The images or other third party material in this chapter are included in the chapter's Creative Commons license, unless indicated otherwise in a credit line to the material. If material is not included in the chapter's Creative Commons license and your intended use is not permitted by statutory regulation or exceeds the permitted use, you will need to obtain permission directly from the copyright holder.

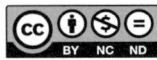

Regulations for Conservative Sharp Debridement for Nurses in Europe

76

Sebastian Probst

76.1 Introduction

In Europe, different levels of nursing educations with a different level of competences exist. The RN4CAST, for example, demonstrates how vast the nursing education as well as their conditions of service, their regulations and policies within Europe are [1]. The report demonstrates that each European country has their own definitions, regulations, and policies about the nursing profession. This can, in clinical practice, easily lead to confusion. As a result of this confusion, specialized knowledge, skills, and competencies are required to initiate, direct, and perform safe and effective debridement [2]. These skills have to be acquired during the nursing education and have to be practiced in different workshops and in clinical practice.

When performing wound debridement, nurses should always work within their scope of practice and local policy and procedures [3, 4]. This chapter will overview regulations for sharp debridement for nurses in Europe and will show when to debride and what are the requirements of nurses to debride a wound.

S. Probst (✉)
HES-SO University of Applied Sciences and Arts Western Switzerland, Geneva, Switzerland

University Hospital Geneva, Geneva, Switzerland

University of Geneva, Geneva, Switzerland

University of Galway, Galway, Ireland

Monash University, Melbourne, Australia
e-mail: sebastian.probst@hesge.ch

76.2 Regulations for Conservative Sharp Debridement for Nurses in Europe

Performing a bed-side conservative sharp debridement may be independently restricted either by safety factors regarding the physical setting or by the legislation that governs a health care sector. In most European countries, it is a physician delegated task. However, conducting a debridement by a nurse in clinical practice requires a certain level of education. For example, the Ashford and St. Peter Hospital in the UK [5] require that only registered nurse with a wound care specializations having completed an education program in wound debridement, that includes conservative sharp debridement, recognized by a University and at a minimum of level 6 and/or endorsed and approved by the European Wound Management Association [6]. Initial and continued competency shall be required and documented for all registered nurse with a wound care specializations performing debridement. Competency is not only a skill demonstration, but also includes assessment contributing to a nursing diagnosis with the development and application of a plan of care, evaluation, and reassessment. The registered nurse performing wound debridement ensures that an assessment of the total patient care requirements before, during, and after wound debridement has been completed by a registered nurse. The registered nurse has to recognize potential complications of wound debridement and if so has to apply universal precautions and other measures to prevent bleeding or infection and contamination.

76.3 When to Debride?

The type of tissue found in the wound bed often provides a clear indication as to whether debridement is required or not [7]. In addition, factors such as bio-burden, wound edges, and condition of peri-wound skin can also influence the decision of whether debridement is required [8]. Nurses performing a debridement need to have a clear understanding of the underlying cause. In certain circumstances, a wound debridement may not be beneficial or may be contraindicated. This is the case, for example, for persons with peripheral arterial disease (PAD) who develop distal gangrene. In this case, the dry gangrene should be treated without any moist dressing and not with debridement. A debridement may develop levels of moisture at the wound bed leading to a greater risk of infection with the risk of amputation [9].

76.4 Who Can Debride?

It is recommended that a conservative sharp wound debridement may be provided by only those registered nurses with advanced preparation in the wound debridement processes [10]. Nurses have to be aware about local policies and guidelines related to wound management and in most European countries have to get approval from their employer to perform the extended role.

76.5 What Is the Procedure of a Sharp Debridement?

Before a specialized nurse is undertaking the procedure, it is important to be informed about the differential diagnosis as well as the prescribed medication. Diabetes, for example, is associated with small and large vessel disease, resulting in an increased risk of infection and poor healing. When debriding an ulcer on the food, be aware of there may be an underlying neuropathy (Charcot's joints/foot). Patients need careful assessment with control of their diabetes and infection. Repeated appropriate debridement can avoid the need for proximal amputation with the attendant huge drain on resources for rehabilitation. Additionally, when taking consent, it is important that the patient understands what should be achieved. Be aware that to try and to undertake too much at once may reduce the confidence between the patient and the nurse. The following procedure is recommended:

76.6 Assess

- What is the nature of the necrotic/devitalized tissue and what is the best adapted method of debridement?
- Is there a risk of spreading infection?
- Is there a possibility of underlying disease processes?
- Is there an extent of existing ischemia (check skin color and pulse)?
- Where is the location of the wound in relation to the surrounding anatomy?

76.7 Pain Relief

- Is there any pain medication prescribed targeting the nociceptive and/or the neuropathic pain?
- Is it necessary and what form should it take?

76.8 Question, What Can Be Possible Complications When Doing a Sharp Debridement

- Conservative sharp debridement is a surgical procedure and may involve some bleeding.
- Bleeding can be stopped with local pressure with a finger.
- The application of successive layers of gauzes can hide considerable hemorrhage and is ineffective.

- Stop the procedure when the anatomy of the wound and surrounding area is unclear or a structure cannot be identified or bleeding is excessive or the source is unclear.

The debridement method with sharp instruments is subdivided into 3 levels. Level 1 is defined as sharp debridement using scissors and forceps, level 2 is the conservative sharp debridement, and level 3 is defined as sharp surgical debridement. Table 76.1 will outline the mechanism of action, the advantages and disadvantages, and the level of nursing education required to perform this task.

Table 76.1 Levels of debridement with sharp instruments

Method	Mechanism of action	Advantages	Disadvantages	Level of nursing education
Level 1 Sharp debridement Using tweezers, forceps, scissors	Use of tweezers, forceps, and scissors to remove loose avascular tissue Scalpels are **not** used No tissue is removed below level of dermis	Produces immediate debridement Is selective removing necrotic tissue	Requires additional education	Nurses with a Bachelor in Nursing Science (EWMA curriculum for nurses' level 5 [11])
Level 2 Conservative sharp wound debridement	Use of a sharp instrument (scalpel, curette or scissors) to remove of non-viable tissue to the level of but not into viable tissue	Produces immediate debridement Selective in removing necrotic tissue Very effective on heavily exudating wounds Should not cause pain but may cause minor amounts of bleeding	Requires additional education for nurses as carries a higher degree of clinical risk than other debridement methods Requires appropriate setting and equipment Use caution with painful wounds or for patients taking anticoagulants Not indicated for wounds in which demarcation between viable and non-viable tissue is not clear	Nurses with a Bachelor in Nursing Science and a postgraduate education in wound care (EWMA curriculum for nurses' level 6 [6])
Level 3 Sharp surgical debridement	Done by an advanced practice nurse in collaboration with a surgeon in a suitable environment Goes below the level of non-viable tissue, i.e., wound edge so can cause pain and bleeding	Produces immediate debridement Turns a chronic wound into an acute wound, thereby promoting more rapid wound healing	Non-selective- viable tissue is removed Painful	Advanced practice nurse in wound care (EWMA curriculum for nurses' level 7 [12])

76.9 Debridement Methods with Sharp Instruments

In the following, an adapted version of a step by step procedure of the conservative sharp wound debridement by the British Colombia College of Nurses and Midwifes [13] is outlined.

Step	Key points
1. Explain the procedure to the patient and obtain verbal consent to carry out the procedure from patient and/or family	
2. Wash hands	
3. Set up dressing tray, add instruments to the sterile field; apply clean gloves, remove dressing, and cleanse wound and surrounding area with body temperature normal saline or antiseptic	To ensure a clean environment prior to carrying out debridement
4. Do wound assessment including measurements; remove gloves. If camera is available take a photo prior to debridementWash hands	Provides a baseline assessment prior to debridement
5. Put on sterile or clean gloves as indicated based on the patient assessment	
6. Always remove necrotic tissue in layers. Working from either the edge or the base of the wound, grasp the edges of the necrotic tissue (eschar) with tissue forceps, lift the necrotic tissue and begin removing necrotic tissue using one or more of the following techniques	Lifting the necrotic tissue will help to identify adherence between necrotic and viable tissues. Tissue forceps 1 × 2 teeth provide a good grasp without applying excessive pressure
7. Scalpel technique: Hold the scalpel like a pen, 3–4 cm away from the handle/blade joint; the belly of the blade is sharpest and should be used to cut necrotic tissue. Lift the necrotic tissue with the forceps and carefully cut away necrotic tissue with the scalpel parallel to or angled away from the wound bed. Movement of the scalpel should follow the tissue planes	This minimizes pain and avoids damage to healthy tissue
8. Scissor technique: Lift the necrotic tissue with the forceps; hold the scissors using a tripod grip technique and use the tip of the scissors to carefully cut away necrotic tissue	Tripod grip—Place the thumb and ring fingers through the scissor handles and rest the index finger on the area of the scissors distal the screw (fulcrum). This 3-finger grip is safer as a 2-finger grip allows the cut to wander. Scissors cut flaccid, loose tissue more effectively than a scalpel, providing better control of depth. Cutting is more precise when tissue is closer to the scissor tip than the fulcrum
9. Blunt dissection technique: Insert the closed blunt tips of scissors or arterial forceps into the non-viable tissue and gently open the instrument. This safely separates the tissue, allowing non-viable tissue to be more easily debrided with scissors	Blunt dissection technique gently separates the tissue allowing for identification of viable and non-viable tissue which will decrease the risk of injury to healthy tissue and nearby structures, e.g., blood vessels, tendons
10. Ring curette technique: Hold the curette like a pen at a 10–200 angles toward the area to be debrided; stretch the skin-wound base with the non-dominant hand, and move the curette toward yourself scraping away loose, non-viable tissue	Ring curettes are suitable for scooping out loose and lightly loose non-viable tissue and to remove biofilm from the base
11. If bleeding occurs stop debridement: Apply pressure with a sterile gauze or cotton tip applicator for 5 min to stop the bleeding. If bleeding continues, identify the specific bleeding site and apply a sliver nitrate stick to the site Use absorbable gelatin/plant cellulose sponges to control small amounts of oozing blood	For small amounts of bleeding, direct pressure can achieve hemostasis without other interventions. Silver nitrate sticks release silver ions that bind to tissue proteins producing a thin eschar that obstructs small bleeding vessels

Step	Key points
12. If pain occurs, stop debridement: Offer the patient an analgesic and resume debridement once the analgesic has taken effect If necessary, complete the debridement at another time	Encourage the patient to request a "time-out" if the procedure is painful. It is not necessary to remove all necrotic tissue at one time
13. Once debridement is completed, flush the wound bed with body temperature normal saline using an irrigation tip catheter and a 30–35 cc syringe	When irrigating the wound, use personal protective equipment to protect from back-splash Irrigation removes loose bits of necrotic tissue

76.10 Conclusions

Due to the different regulations within Europe, the procedure of a conservative sharp debridement should only be undertaken by specialists be it specialist nurses in tissue viability or physicians who have successfully completed a validated educational program in wound debridement or a minimum of degree level including assessment of competency in practice.

References

1. Rafferty A, Busse R, Zander-Jentsch B, Sermeus W, Bruyneel L. Strengthening health systems through nursing: evidence from 14 European countries. Copenhagen: World Health Organization; 2019. p. 163.
2. Rajhathy EM, Chaplain V, Hill MC, Woo KY, Parslow NE. Executive summary: debridement: Canadian best practice recommendations for nurses developed by nurses specialized in wound, ostomy and continence Canada (NSWOCC). J Wound Ostomy Continence Nurs. 2021;48(6):516–22.
3. Harris C. Creating a conservative sharp wound debridement (CSWD) education program for frontline nurses. Wound Care Canada. 2013;11(2):18–24.
4. Swanson T, Angel D, Sussman G, Cooper R, Haesler E, Ousey K, et al. Wound infection in clinical practice: principles of best practice. 3rd ed; 2022.
5. Harris S, Williams A. Procedure for conservative sharp debridement of wounds. Ashfort and St. Peter Hospital: NHS Foundation Trust; 2020. p. 10.
6. Probst S, Holloway S, Rowan S, Pokornà A. Wound curriculum for nurses: post-registration qualification wound management—European qualification framework level 6. J Wound Care. 2019;28(Sup2a):S1–s33.
7. Probst S. Wound care nursing—a person-centred approach. 3rd ed. London: Elsevier; 2021.
8. Strohal R, Dissemond J, Jordan O'Brien J, Piaggesi A, Rimdeika R, Young T, et al. EWMA document: debridement. An updated overview and clarification of the principle role of debridement. J Wound Care. 2013;22(1):5.
9. Olivieri B, Yates TE, Vianna S, Adenikinju O, Beasley RE, Houseworth J. On the cutting edge: wound care for the endovascular specialist. Semin Intervent Radiol. 2018;35(5):406–26.
10. Gordon B. Conservative sharp wound debridement: state boards of nursing positions. J Wound Ostomy Continence Nurs. 1996;23(3):137–43.
11. Pokorná A, Holloway S, Strohal R, Verheyen-Cronau I. Wound curriculum for nurses. J Wound Care. 2017;26(Sup12):S1–s27.
12. Holloway S, Pokorná A, Janssen A, Ousey K, Probst S. Wound curriculum for nurses: post-registration qualification wound management-European qualification framework level 7. J Wound Care. 2020;29(Sup7a):S1–s39.
13. British Colombia College of Nurses and Midwifes. Scope of practice for registred nurses, standards, limits, conditions; 2022.

Open Access This chapter is licensed under the terms of the Creative Commons Attribution-NonCommercial-NoDerivatives 4.0 International License (http://creativecommons.org/licenses/by-nc-nd/4.0/), which permits any non-commercial use, sharing, distribution and reproduction in any medium or format, as long as you give appropriate credit to the original author(s) and the source, provide a link to the Creative Commons license and indicate if you modified the licensed material. You do not have permission under this license to share adapted material derived from this chapter or parts of it.

The images or other third party material in this chapter are included in the chapter's Creative Commons license, unless indicated otherwise in a credit line to the material. If material is not included in the chapter's Creative Commons license and your intended use is not permitted by statutory regulation or exceeds the permitted use, you will need to obtain permission directly from the copyright holder.

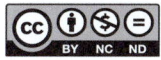

Regulations for Conservative Debridement for Nurses in North America

77

Maryse Beaumier

77.1 Introduction

There is a growing body of evidence and agreement among wound clinicians and scientists that debridement represents a necessary process in reducing bacteria, infection, and a biofilm within a wound and promotes a stimulatory environment for healing [1]. The selection of a debridement method should be based on the clinical context, goals of care, the clinician's expertise, and local resources. Despite the fact that the cost savings demonstrated when conservative sharp debridement (CSD) is part of a best practice plan of care for wounds, many community nursing agencies are not able to provide CSD as part of their care delivery, or they may not be aware of what their nurses are doing [2]. As a result of this confusion, specialized knowledge, skills, and competencies are required to initiate, direct, and perform safe and effective debridement [3]. When performing wound debridement, clinicians should always work within their scope of practice and local policies and procedures [1, 4]. This chapter will briefly overview regulations for CSD for nurses in North America after review on debridement type and clinical decisions for debridement's use.

77.2 The Precision of Debridement Types

Often, in the literature, it states that all forms of debridement can carry high risk when initiated inappropriately; however, CSD is considered higher risk [5]. Performed at the bedside or in the clinic setting, CSD is considered the most aggressive form of debridement performed by nursing [4]. It is referred to as a conventional debridement using a scalpel blade (Fig. 77.1) or scissors to remove necrotic tissue with limited pain or bleeding [6]. It can be also performed in a clinic by a skilled clinician with wound specialist training [6]. Clinicians must distinguish tissue types and understand anatomy as the procedure carries the risk of damage to blood vessels, nerves, and tendons.

The notion of danger to the patient for debridement is more with CSD that nurses should possess, and too often, the dangers of this type of debridement are confused with the dangers of surgical sharp debridement made by physicians. But this danger is poorly defined in the literature. This danger can often be associated with failure to assess the arterial blood flow of the wound prior to debridement as stated by national and international guidelines [7–9] and failure to recognize the anatomy of the tissue, where wet

M. Beaumier (✉)
Health Science Department, Université du Québec à Rimouski, campus de Lévis, Lévis, Québec, Canada

Research Center CISSS Chaudière-Appalaches, Lévis, QC, Canada
e-mail: maryse_beaumier@uqar.ca

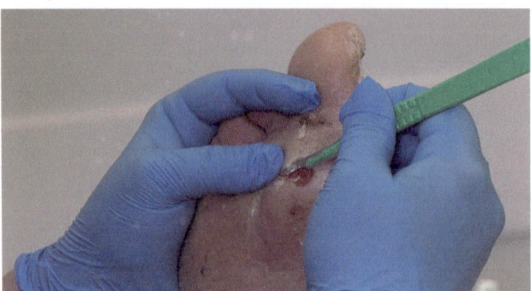

Fig. 77.1 Scalpel (authorized by Maryse Beaumier)

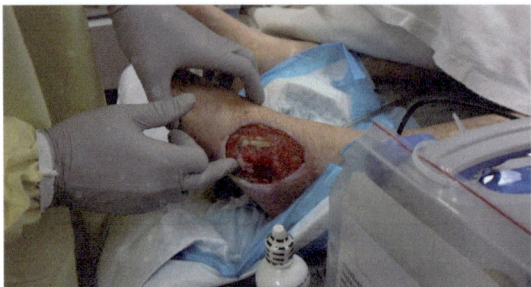

Fig. 77.2 Bone and tendon (authorized by Maryse Beaumier)

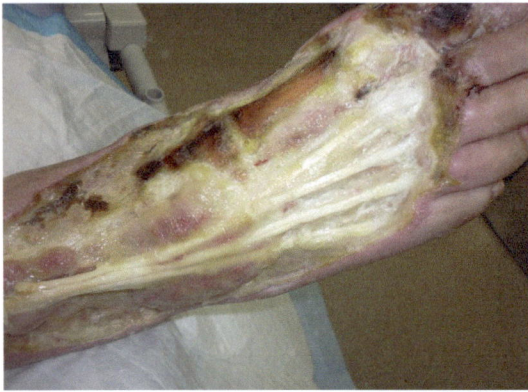

Fig. 77.3 Tendons (authorized by Maryse Beaumier)

necrosis may be mistaken for tendon and the ligaments, for example, or exaggerated depth of contact with bone that can lead to osteitis (Figs. 77.2 and 77.3).

Surgical sharp debridement, on its side, is the *gold standard* of wound debridement, conducted in a strict sterility environment in the operation area by a surgeon [10–12]. The outcome is rapid, and the patient underwent this type of debridement requiring adequate pain management, similar to post-operative nursing care [6]. The main quality of these two types of surgical debridement is the rapid removal of necrotic tissue and microorganisms from the wound bed [1]. It is known that one primary justification to use the rapidity of CSD is that the evidence that biofilms can reside deep within the extracellular matrix of the slough, debris, necrotic, and other tissues provides a rationale for removing non-viable tissue via rapid debridement methods to reduce them [1, 13]. For the other types of debridement, without any education, the nurses are already doing them as, for example: a nurse who uses an interactive dressing such as a hydrofiber or alginate or a product such as a cadexomer proceeds with an autolytic debridement. If a nurse uses a dry dressing such as a cotton pad on a granulation wound bed, she will perform a mechanical wet-to-dry debridement (mechanical) and finally, if she uses a wound cleaning pressure greater than 15 psi for irrigation, she does mechanical debridement. Is these three type of debridement are so much harmful for the patient? It will be important in the future to distinguish between the types of debridement and their associated risks before developing specialized debridement courses so as not to delay the transfer of knowledge into practice. Rather, it is important to emphasize the contraindications to initiating any debridement, i.e., poor blood flow to the wound.

Unfortunately, even legislation framing nurses' clinical practice does not consider the specifics of the types of debridement that can contribute to harm in patients when it is well documented that necrotic tissue left in place in a wound bed with healing potential can easily lead to wound infection by inhibiting oxygen delivery [1].

77.3 The Clinical Decision for Debridement's Use

Applying the best practice in wound assessment and management promotes the maintenance of a healthy wound bed; it always involves therapeutic wound cleansing and debridement, which aims to disrupt biofilm, prevent its reformation, and facilitate removal of necrotic, non-viable or infected tissue. Distinguishing the healable wound, maintenance wound, and the non-healable wound is critical before initiating any type of debridement and especially CSD [5, 6]. To eliminate one of the main dangers associated with conservative surgical debridement is to disseminate to all nurses the first recommendation for best practice in wound care, which is to assess, prior to any intervention on the wound bed, the healing potential of the wound by measuring the blood flow at the wound [7, 9]. Without sufficient blood flow, any type of debridement is always contraindicated [7–9]. Furthermore, best practices recommend cleaning and debridement before sampling for wound culture [14]. Thus, it is more than essential that clinical practice guidelines and regulations be transferred in knowledge to nurses.

Based on *Debridement: Canadian Best Practice Recommendations for Nurses* and in nursing law of the province of Quebec in Canada, prior to initiating any method of debridement, the nurse must be knowledgeable about the different methods of debridement and the level of skill and training required to perform each type; be aware of their attitudes, limitations, skills, and competency; recognize and understand the indications, precautions, and contraindications for the various debridement methods; evaluate the patient's health status; solicit patient preferences and wishes; review wound assessment findings and wound healing potential to determine if decisions about debridement can be made independently, or in consultation with the interprofessional team is warranted [5, 15–17] and be able to identify, manage, and mitigate potential complications and adverse events including, but not limited to, bleeding, pain, anxiety, or damage to underlying structures [5].

77.4 Regulations

In Canada and the United States, several levels of nursing education exist and can lead to confusion in roles by regulations for the clinical practice of debridement. Furthermore, there is an even more significant distinction between French and English training in Canada. Nonetheless, the three categories of nurses in North America that are considered for the regulation are registered nurse (RN), nurse practitioner (NP), and registered/licensed practical nurse (RPN/LPN) [5, 18]. The Canadian and United States precisions can, respectively, be found in Table 6 of the NSWOCC (2021) document and Tomaselli (2015) chapter in the previous edition of this book.

In the USA, regulations for conservative sharp debridement vary from state to state, and each state's *Nurse Practice Act or Board of Nursing* dictates specific regulations for this procedure (Tomaselli, 2015). Tomaselli (2015) dressed a precise list of contact information for each state nursing board in the previous edition of this book. This list can also be found at the following link: https://www.allnursingschools.com/how-to-become-a-nurse/nursing-license/ [19].

In Canada, the provincial/territorial governments delegate the power to regulate all categories of nurses to the provincial/territorial nursing regulatory bodies [5]. Each provincial or territorial regulatory body for nursing in Canada has an individual scope of practice, too [4, 5]. Some allow the performance of CSD provided the nurse has the knowledge, skill, and judgment necessary to assess the individual situation for risks and benefits [4]. Some do not. NSWOCC published in 2021 the results of a scoping review to edit the *Debridement: Canadian best practices recommendations for nurses*. This document can be found on the website https://www.nswoc.ca/bpr?lang=fr. This document further informs the regulation of debridement in nursing practice generally and specifically for each province. The first recommendation states:

> All classes of nurses, including RN, RPN/LPN, and NP must work within the controls of federal and provincial/territorial legislation, regulatory bodies, organizational policies and individual competency. For debridement of wounds, this includes having the knowledge, skills, judgment, and authority to perform all forms of debridement. Nurses are accountable for knowing their national code of ethics and expectations, respective provin-

cial/territorial practice standards and guidelines, employer's policies, procedures, and operational guidelines, and own competence and limitations for all methods of debridement (NSWOCC, 2021, p. 10).

They add that each employer has the ability to restrict further a nurse's ability to perform an act, and ultimately, the nurse is accountable for ensuring they possess the knowledge, skills, judgment, experience, and authorization before initiating or performing debridement [5]. However, other regulations in each province may prevent nurses from performing CSD even when the college of nurses allows it [4]. For example, some hospital and long-term care acts may prevent a nurse from performing CSD in their employing organization without a medical delegation or transfer of function [4]. Even in those employment situations where CSD by nurses is allowed, high-level support and clear organizational policies and procedures that outline the educational and practice requirements for anyone performing CSD must be present [4].

As in the other provinces, in the province of Quebec, the regulations for debridement are clear theoretically but not in clinical practice because the last authorization comes from the organizational management even if it goes against best practices. Sadly, they do not authorize it even if the nurse's professional order mentions that:

> In the presence of a wound and before intervening, the nurse must make an appropriate assessment of the patient's clinical situation, health condition and the wound (possible etiology, type of wound and characteristics) and ensure the wound's healing potential. In the case of a lower extremity wound, she should obtain a measurement of the ankle-arm systolic pressure. Then, she can decide to proceed with wound debridement, foreign body removal or removal of loose tissue and debris, determine the frequency and method of the patient's health condition and the purpose of the treatment; decide whether to perform scarification of an eschar to accelerate debridement autolytic or enzymatic debridement (OIIQ, 2016, p. 50).

In addition, an interdisciplinary consensus on regulations is clear between nurses, occupational therapist (OT), and physiotherapists for a known contribution to debridement for nurses and a complementary contribution for OT and physiotherapists [20]. But the problem remains the same, namely that the regulations on debridement are on all types of debridement. Even if no education program exists, the nurses still promote autolytic, mechanic, and chemically debridement by, respectively, using interactive dressing, irrigation cleaning and cadexomer without using scalpel, scissors, and pliers.

In *Debridement: Canadian Best recommendations for Nurses,* the primary objective of these recommendations is to positively influence patient outcomes and enhance safety [3, 5]. The 12 recommendations place the safety of the patient and nurse at the forefront and highlight the educational, competency, certification, preceptor/mentorship, and legal requirements for nurses to initiate, direct, and perform all methods of debridement. These recommendations were designed to be circulated and implemented widely by nurses of various professional levels across the continuum of care and advocate for organizations and government agencies to clearly define debridement in their policies and legislative regulations [3].

77.5 Conclusion

Debridement should be considered an integral part of the process of caring for a patient with a wound. For practitioners to best care for their patients, they must be equipped with the knowledge to be able to consider accelerating healing through debridement and must understand the debridement options available, and how and why they are undertaken [16]. With a higher level of evidence, NSWOCC (2021) suggests prior to initiating or performing debridement, successful completion of a rigorous curriculum-based wound management program followed by a separate competency-based education program for debridement is highly recommended for all nurses. According to NSWOCC (2021), debridement education program should include theoretical and clinical preceptorship components.

To follow the best practices for the patient in his wound healing process and to harmonize the regulations and the clinical practice, the educational institutions in nursing will have to introduce the notions of all types of debridement in the teaching in theoretical and practical way, emphasizing CSD for the safety of the patient and to avoid all infections and biofilms in chronic wounds. Regulations may change in time, so the nurse who wants to practice CSD is responsible for contacting the individual state practice act before performing this procedure (Tomaselli, 2015).

Take Home Messages

- Debridement is an essential component for wound healing; knowledge have to follow nurses skills [5].
- Education, knowledge, technical skills, experience, critical thinking, and judgment have to go in the same way as debridement regulations for the healing wound process for the best quality of life for our patients.
- Teaching debridement should be a mandatory part of nursing curricula for optimal care of patients with wounds.

References

1. Swanson T, Angel D, Sussman G, Cooper R, Haesler E, Ousey K, et al. Wound infection in clinical practice: principles of best practice. 3rd ed; 2022.
2. Shannon R, Harris C, Harley C, Kozell K, Woo K, Alavi A, et al. The importance of sharp debridement in foot ulcer care in the community. Wound Care Canada. 2007;5(Suppl 1):S51–S2.
3. Rajhathy EM, Chaplain V, Hill MC, Woo KY, Parslow NE. Executive summary: debridement: Canadian best practice recommendations for nurses developed by nurses specialized in wound, ostomy and continence Canada (NSWOCC). J Wound Ostomy Continence Nurs. 2021;48(6):516–22.
4. Harris C. Creating a conservative sharp wound debridement (CSWD) education program for frontline nurses. Wound Care Canada. 2013;11(2):18–24.
5. Nurses specialized in wound ostomy and continence Canada (NSWOCC). Debridement: Canadian best practices recommendations for nurses; 2021.
6. Thomas DC, Tsu CL, Nain RA, Arsat N, Fun SS, Lah NASN. The role of debridement in wound bed preparation in chronic wound: a narrative review. Ann Med Surg. 2021;71:102876.
7. Sibbald RG, Elliott JA, Persaud-Jaimangal R, Goodman L, Armstrong DG, Harley C, et al. Wound bed preparation 2021. Adv Skin Wound Care. 2021;34(4):183.
8. Conte MS, Bradbury AW, Kolh P, White JV, Dick F, Fitridge R, et al. Global vascular guidelines on the management of chronic limb-threatening ischemia. Eur J Vasc Endovasc Surg. 2019;58(1):S1–S109. e33
9. Beaumier M, Murray BA, Despatis M-A, Patry J, Murphy C, Jin S, et al. Best practice recommendations for the prevention and management of peripheral arterial ulcers. In: Foundations of best practice for skin and wound management a supplement of wound care Canada; 2020.
10. Falcone M, De Angelis B, Pea F, Scalise A, Stefani S, Tasinato R, et al. Challenges in the management of chronic wound infections. J Glob Antimicrob Resist. 2021;26:140–7.
11. Madhok BM, Vowden K, Vowden P. New techniques for wound debridement. Int Wound J. 2013;10(3):247–51.
12. Vowden KR, Vowden P. Debridement made easy. https://www.wounds-uk.com/resources/details/debridement-made-easy. Wounds UK; 2011;7(4 Nov):1–4.
13. Schultz G, Bjarnsholt T, James GA, Leaper DJ, McBain AJ, Malone M, et al. Consensus guidelines for the identification and treatment of biofilms in chronic nonhealing wounds. Wound Repair Regen. 2017;25(5):744–57.
14. Institut national d'excellence en santé et services sociaux (INESSS). La culture de plaie: pertinence et indications. Avis rédigé par Anne Bergeron. Québec, Qc: INESSS2020. 198 p.
15. Gray D, Acton C, Chadwick P, Fumarola S, Leaper D, Morris C, et al. Consensus guidance for the use of debridement techniques in the UK: Wounds UK; 2010.
16. Wounds U. Effective debridement in a changing NHS. A UK Consensus Document; 2013.
17. OIIQ. Le champ d'exercice et les activités réservées des infirmières, 3e Éd; 2016.
18. Tomaselli N. Regulations for conservative sharp debridement for nurses in the USA. In: Téot L, Meaume S, Akita S, Ennis WJ, del Marmol V, editors. Skin necrosis. Vienna: Springer Vienna; 2015. p. 283–5.
19. All Nursing School. 2022. https://www.allnursingschools.com/how-to-become-a-nurse/nursing-license/
20. OEQ, OIIQ, OPPQ. Une action concertée pour optimiser le traitement des plaies chroniques et complexes: Cadre de collaboration interprofessionnelle pour les ergothérapeutes, les infirmières et les professionnels physiothérapeutes; 2014.

Open Access This chapter is licensed under the terms of the Creative Commons Attribution-NonCommercial-NoDerivatives 4.0 International License (http://creativecommons.org/licenses/by-nc-nd/4.0/), which permits any non-commercial use, sharing, distribution and reproduction in any medium or format, as long as you give appropriate credit to the original author(s) and the source, provide a link to the Creative Commons license and indicate if you modified the licensed material. You do not have permission under this license to share adapted material derived from this chapter or parts of it.

The images or other third party material in this chapter are included in the chapter's Creative Commons license, unless indicated otherwise in a credit line to the material. If material is not included in the chapter's Creative Commons license and your intended use is not permitted by statutory regulation or exceeds the permitted use, you will need to obtain permission directly from the copyright holder.

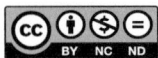

Distance Skin Necrosis Management

Chloé Geri

78.1 Introduction

In 2013, EWMA [1] defined debridement as the "Elimination of necrotic, devitalised, infected tissue, hyperkeratosis, hematomas, foreign bodies, debris, bone splinters or any other type of element." The purpose of removing the necrosis is both to make the diagnosis (e.g., evaluation of the stage of a pressure ulcer after debridement), but also to avoid infection by reducing the bacterial load present in the wound bed.

However, it is essential not only to have eliminated the contraindications beforehand (AOMI, cancerous etiology, undernutrition, ttt, etc.), but also to have the right tools at your disposal and to have acquired the right gestures. The training and support of caregivers are the keystone of a proper debridement and therefore of an optimization of the healing prognosis.

In order to best support local caregivers, telemedicine has become in a few years an essential tool in the therapeutic arsenal [2, 3].

As a reminder, the public health code [4] specifies that teleconsultation is a synchronous act, which "aims to allow a medical professional to give a remote consultation to a patient. A healthcare professional may be present with the patient and, if necessary, assist the medical professional during the teleconsultation." It therefore allows the wound and healing expert to intervene as close as possible to the patient's living environment [5].

But a simple remote opinion is not always enough and the primary care givers are sometimes in difficulty when it comes to perform technical or unusual gestures in everyday practice. Moreover, it is not always easy or even possible for a patient to go to the expert to benefit from this procedure. Tele-assistance will then allow the expert to guide the local care giver in complete safety, as specified in the public health code [4] since its "aim is to allow a medical professional to assist a another healthcare professional during the performance of an act."

By bringing together the local caregiver and the healing expert synchronously around the patient, remote assistance will make it possible to manage necrosis remotely in specific medical indications, at the appropriate time and according to a defined regulatory framework.

78.2 Who Is Concerned?

78.2.1 The Patients

The patient remains at the center of the problem. Indeed, the EWMA stresses the need for access to expertise to optimize wound healing: "Access to care and referral to clinicians whose knowledge, skills and resources are up to date are essential if the 'we want to make the diagnosis quickly, initi-

C. Geri (✉)
CICAT-Occitanie, Montpellier, France
e-mail: c-geri@chu-montpellier.fr

ate the appropriate treatment as soon as possible and avoid complications." [6].

However, access to expertise is sometimes difficult: the patient is not always close to an expert center because the creation of healing centers was done spontaneously on the territory. and we are currently witnessing a significant heterogeneity of resources [7].

A face-to-face consultation is therefore not always possible: some patients are very far from these centers [8] and very fragile or institutionalized patients do not have the possibility of traveling to the expert [9, 10].

In addition, we emphasize the importance of the health context which, during the COVID pandemic, justified the closure of outpatient consultations, depriving the most vulnerable patients of access to care considered non-emergency.

Not only are these patients, given their multiple comorbidities, the most at risk of a serious form in the event of Covid19 infection, but their frequent visits and hospitalizations expose them to a greater risk of contact with Covid 19 and other communicable diseases [11, 12].

Finally, several studies underline the interest of the telemedicine tool in improving the prognosis of chronic diseases and in particular diabetes [13].

For all patients, the telemedical tool is therefore now a natural part of the healthcare access offer, regardless of geographical location.

78.2.2 Local or First-Line Caregivers

In a survey [14] of 711 medical residents, training in wound healing was considered insufficient by 94% of students. The support that telemedicine, and more specifically tele-assistance, can provide, is an essential response to the lack of initial training of primary caregivers, whether nurses or physicians.

The first-line pair most often made up of the attending physician and the nurse will thus be accompanied for the management of wound care [15].

The nurse will be able to be reassured as to the quality of the gesture and guided to carry out unusual or more advanced care than in his daily practice. A nurse without specific training in wounds and healing will probably not dare perform the trimming of extensive necrosis alone at home, but teleconsultation will allow the presence of an expert, directly at the patient's bedside during treatment [16].

78.2.3 The Experts

Healing experts, for their part, also need to be reassured about the correct understanding of the instructions, compliance with their recommendations and safety when carrying out specific or technical procedures at home.

During a "classic" consultation in a healing center, it is very rare for the expert to be able to discuss directly with the local caregiver at the time of treatment to jointly define the most appropriate strategy for the home. And the situation is all the more complex when the patient is fragile, demented, or even sometimes non-communicative. In the majority of situations, only a letter will make the link between the expert center and the care giver at home or in a community.

As early as 2018, a medico-economic study [17] compared follow-up in consultation in an expert center, follow-up at home with travel by the expert, and follow-up at home by telemedicine and did not note any significant difference between the three groups of patients on complete healing. Only the decrease in transportation costs was significant.

Without replacing the consultation by an expert, tele-assistance is naturally positioned as the most adapted to a particular health context or to the accompaniment of very specific gestures for the management of necrosis. We can cite, for example, the remote accompaniment of debridement by larva therapy, this technique not usually being used at home [18].

78.3 Why to Choose Tele-Assistance?

Telemedicine has shown its interest in the management of chronic wounds, whether in relation to diabetic foot wounds [19], leg ulcers [20], or pressure ulcers at the end of life [21].

This accompaniment will allow the realization of unusual technical gestures: for example, cleaning the necrosis (Figs. 78.1, 78.2, 78.3), evacuating and flattening of an aged hematoma (Figs. 78.4,

78 Distance Skin Necrosis Management

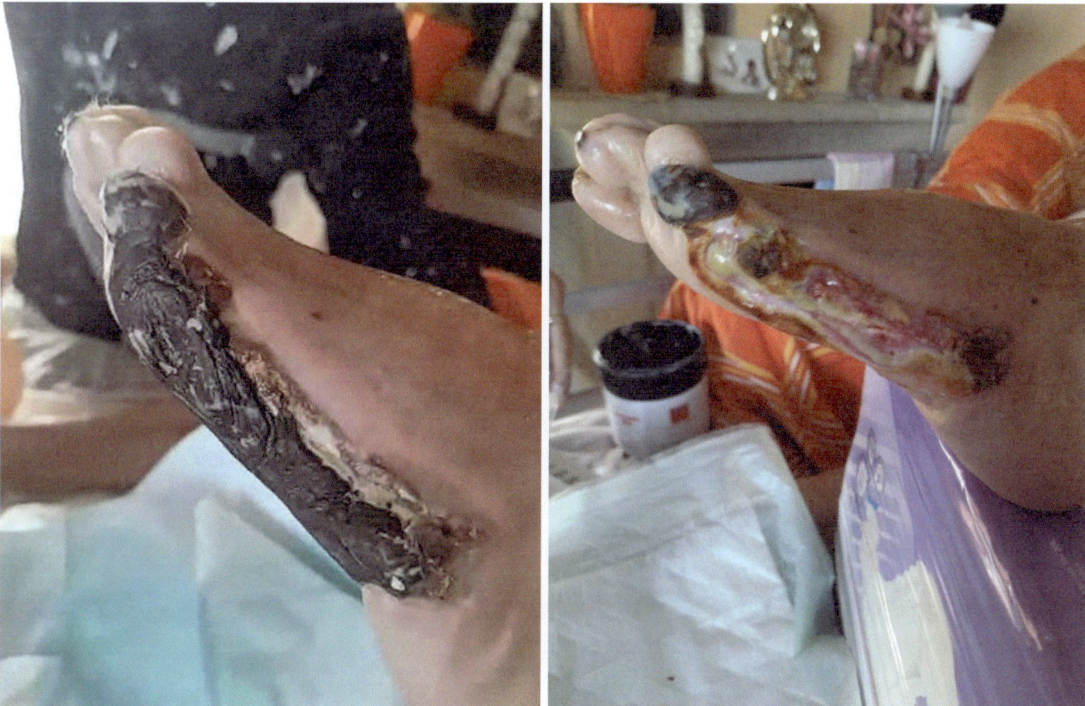

Figs. 78.1 and 78.2 Debridement during tele-assistance

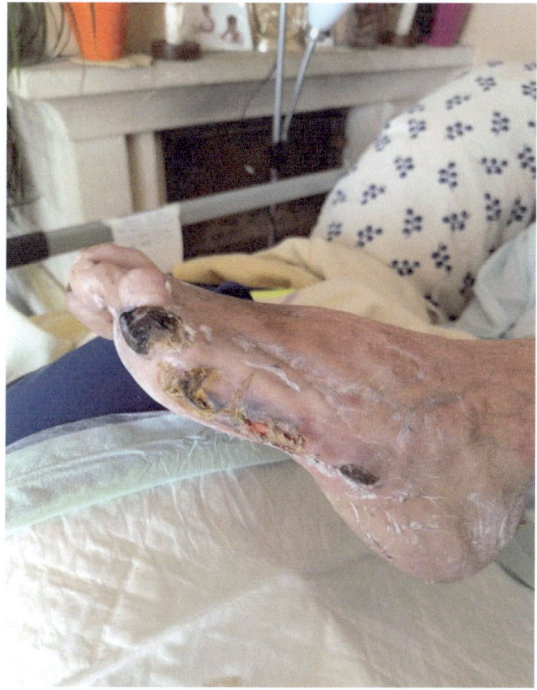

Fig. 78.3 Follow-up at 3 months after necrosectomy

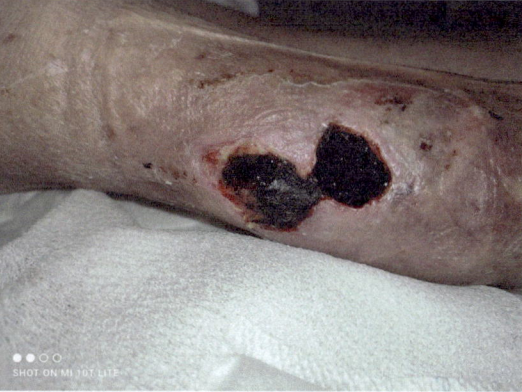

Fig. 78.4 Assessment during teleconsultation

78.5, 78.6, 78.9, 78.10, 78.11, and 78.12), arthrectomy (Figs. 78.7, 78.8) or amputation of toe after mummification.

In some situations, debridement is not indicated as first-line treatment and care is temporarily or permanently directed toward stabilizing the necrosis whether waiting for the surgical moment or in a palliative context. This stabilization requires close monitoring but does not justify frequent transportation of a fragile patient.

In addition, several studies underline the satisfaction of patients and caregivers during remote monitoring [22, 23] which will not only make it possible to avoid unnecessary travel but also to better target the indications, and better organize

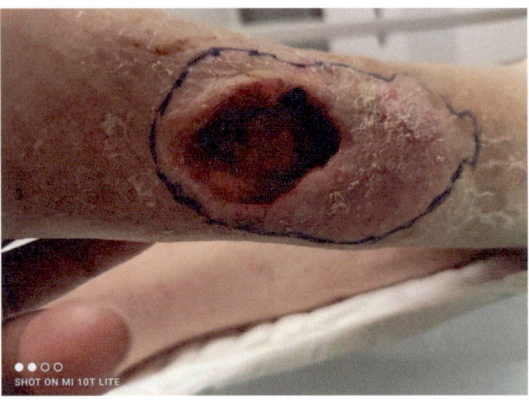

Fig. 78.5 Removing the haematoma and explore the wound using tele-assistance

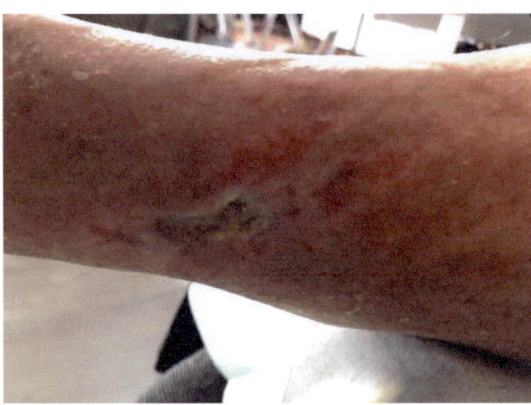

Fig. 78.6 Follow-up at 2 months

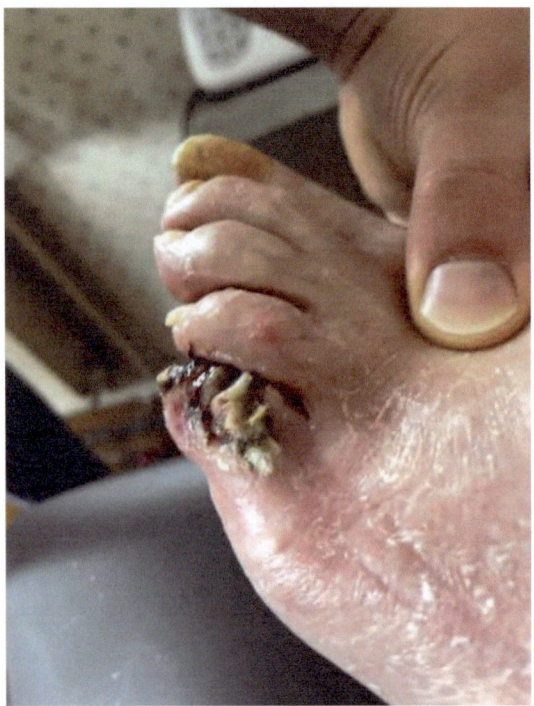

Fig. 78.7 Assessment using TLC

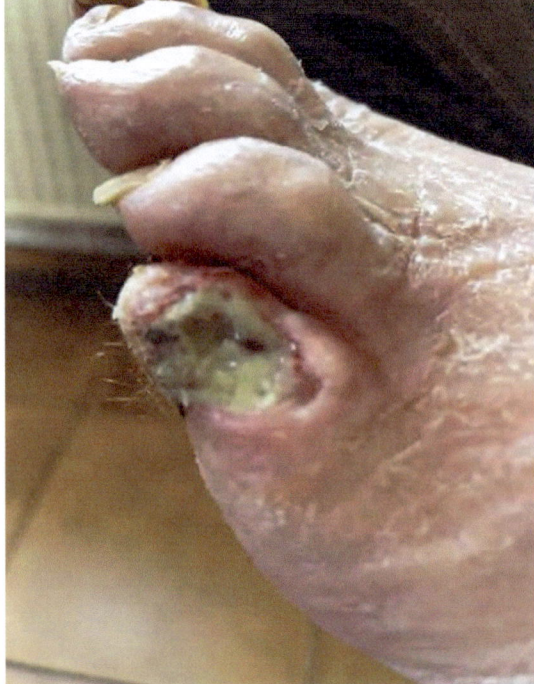

Fig. 78.8 After arthrectomy using tele-assistance

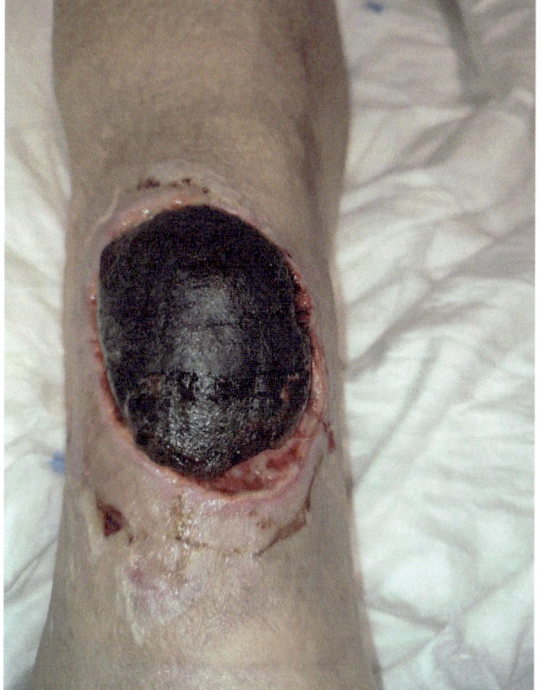

Fig. 78.9 100 years old patient with haematoma

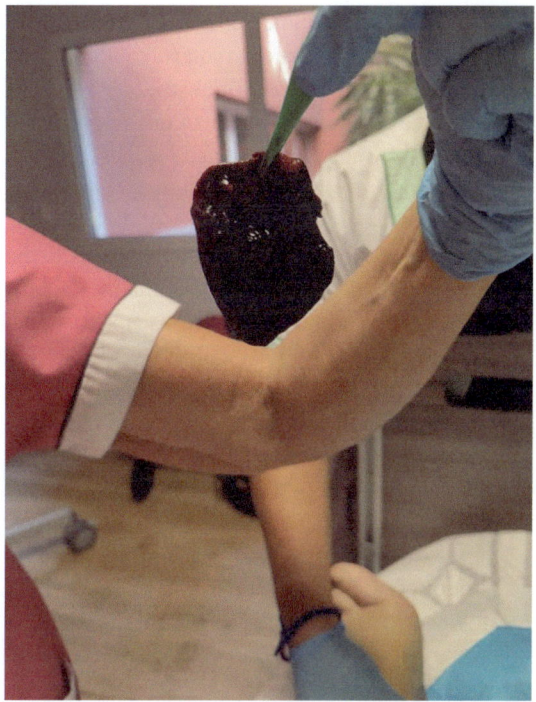

Fig. 78.10 Remove the necrosis by the nurse using tele-assistance

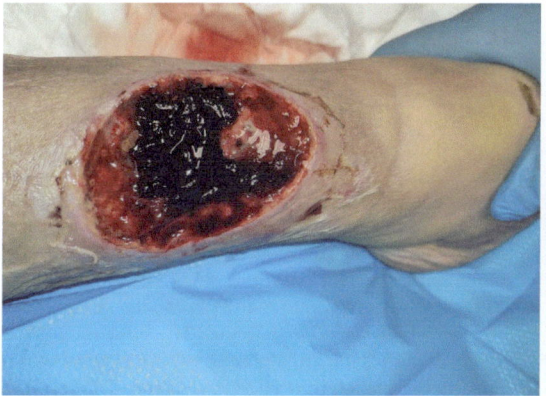
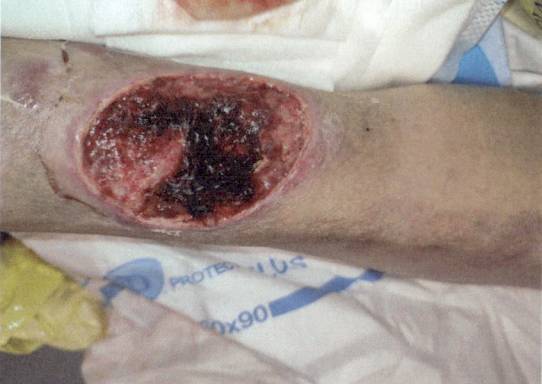

Figs. 78.11 and 78.12 Removing the haematoma and cleaning the wound using tele-assistance

the management in healing center when displacement is necessary.

A support network for caregivers operating in telemedicine and also providing assistance in the coordination of the course could therefore be the most complete response to the management of complex wounds at home [24].

78.4 When? How? 'OR' What?

In the vast majority of cases, remote assistance takes place during a teleconsultation and allows local caregivers to benefit from real-time care support, but also to improve their training in contact with experts. In some situations, a dedicated time is scheduled for the remote assistance of a technical gesture so that the material and the time are available without additional stress.

In any case, improvisation is not appropriate and meetings must be planned so that all the actors can be fully available and act in complete safety [25].

Prior to teleconsultation or tele-assistance, the legal and financial aspects, as well as the technical aspects will be addressed so as not to be an obstacle to remote support [26]:

- The consent of the patient, and the cooperation of his entourage are essential.
- The tool must also be adapted to the patient's place of residence, and the local caregiver must become familiar with the medium (smartphone, tablet, etc.), software, or app. However, it is currently difficult to conclude on the superiority of one device over the others [27].
- Similarly, the quality and security of the transmission of health data must be verified in order to correspond to the legislation in force in the country.

78.5 Conclusion

Telemedicine now appears to be a real companion tool: teleconsultation offers "theoretical" support to local caregivers, and complete tele-assistance by a "practical" support; the local caregiver becoming the arm of the expert.

By allowing in particular the management of necrosis remotely, the latter makes it possible to carry out technical gestures in complete safety. Bedside cleaning can be performed in a quasi-surgical way if the caregiver and the patient are well supported.

Coordinated care network operation and the use of telemedicine tools now offer care teams the possibility of offering their patients with wounds a tailor-made solution where equity replaces equal access to care.

References

1. Strohal R, Apelqvist J, Dissemond J, et al. EWMA Document: Debridement. J Wound Care. 2013;22(Suppl. 1):S1–S52.
2. Shannon RJ. Telemedicine in wound healing. Int Wound J. 2005;2(3):239–40. https://doi.org/10.1111/j.1742-4801.2005.0124b.x.
3. Blanchére JP, Dompmartin A. Quoi de neuf en télémédecine appliquée aux plaies? [The latest developments in telemedicine applied to wound care]. Soins Gerontol. 2013;(101):38–40. French.
4. Code de la santé publique. Article R6316-1. Modifié par décret n°2021-707 du 3 juin 2021-Art.1.
5. Ablaza V, Fisher J. Telemedicine and wound care management. Home Care Provid. 1998;3(4):206–11; quiz 212–3. https://doi.org/10.1016/s1084-628x(98)90132-0.
6. European Wound Management Association. Position document. Hard to heal wounds: a holistic approach. London: MEP Ltd; 2008.
7. Groupe de travail SFFPC « centres de cicatrisation » sous la direction du Dr P. Leger. http://www.sffpc.org/centres-de-cicatrisation
8. Clegg A, Brown T, Engels D, Griffin P, Simonds D. Telemedicine in a rural community hospital for remote wound care consultations. J Wound Ostomy Continence Nurs. 2011;38(3):301–4. https://doi.org/10.1097/WON.0b013e3182164214.
9. Sparsa A, Doffoel-Hantz V, Bonnetblanc JM. Une expérience de télé-expertise en établissement d'hébergement de personnes âgées dépendantes (EHPAD) [Assessment of tele-expertise among elderly subjects in retirement homes]. Ann Dermatol Venereol. 2013;140(3):165–9. https://doi.org/10.1016/j.annder.2012.11.008. French. Epub 2013 Jan 16.
10. Vowden K, Vowden P. A pilot study on the potential of remote support to enhance wound care for nursing-home patients. J Wound Care. 2013;22(9):481–8. https://doi.org/10.12968/jowc.2013.22.9.481.
11. The Novel Coronavirus Pneumonia Emergency Response Epidemiology Team. The epidemiological characteristics of an outbreak of 2019 novel coronavirus diseases (COVID-19)—China. China CDC Weekly. 2020;2(8):113–23.
12. Rogers LC, Lavery LA, Joseph WS, Armstrong DG. All feet on deck-the role of podiatry during the COVID-19 pandemic: preventing hospitalizations in an overburdened healthcare system, reducing amputation and death in people with diabetes. J Am Podiatr Med Assoc. 2020;113:20-051. https://doi.org/10.7547/20-051.
13. Su D, Zhou J, Kelley MS, Michaud TL, Siahpush M, Kim J, Wilson F, Stimpson JP, Pagán JA. Does telemedicine improve treatment outcomes for diabetes?

A meta-analysis of results from 55 randomized controlled trials. Diabetes Res Clin Pract. 2016;116:136. Epub 2016 Apr 26.
14. Lupona V, Turrian U, Malloizel-Delaunay J, Bura-Rivière A, Grolleaud J. Internes en médecine et cicatrisation des plaies: une étude descriptive multicentrique entre février et avril 2018 Medical residents and wound healing: a French national survey. JMV-Journal de Médecine Vasculaire. 2019;44(5):324–30.
15. Rasmussen BS, Jensen LK, Froekjaer J, Kidholm K, Kensing F, Yderstraede KB. A qualitative study of the key factors in implementing telemedical monitoring of diabetic foot ulcer patients. Int J Med Inform. 2015;84(10):799–807. https://doi.org/10.1016/j.ijmedinf.2015.05.012. Epub 2015 May 29.
16. Gagnon MP, Breton E, Courcy F, Quirion S, Côté J, Paré J. The influence of a wound care teleassistance service on nursing practice: a case study in Quebec. Telemed J E Health. 2014;20(6):593–600. https://doi.org/10.1089/tmj.2013.0287. Epub 2014 Apr 2.
17. Le Goff-Pronost M, Mourgeon B, Blanchere JP, Teot L, Benateau H, Dompmartin A. Real-world clinical evaluation and costs of telemedicine for chronic wounds management. Int J Technol Assess Health Care. 2018;34(6):567–75. https://doi.org/10.1017/S0266462318000685. Epub 2018 Oct 29.
18. Armstrong DG, Rowe VL, D'Huyvetter K, Sherman RA. Telehealth-guided home-based maggot debridement therapy for chronic complex wounds: peri- and post-pandemic potential. Int Wound J 2020;17:1490–1495.
19. Tchero H, Noubou L, Becsangele B, Mukisi-Mukaza M, Retali GR, Rusch E. Telemedicine in diabetic foot care: a systematic literature review of interventions and meta-analysis of controlled trials. Int J Low Extrem Wounds. 2017;16(4):274–83. https://doi.org/10.1177/1534734617739195. Epub 2017 Nov 23.
20. Nordheim LV, Haavind MT, Iversen MM. Effect of telemedicine follow-up care of leg and foot ulcers: a systematic review. BMC Health Serv Res. 2014;14:565. https://doi.org/10.1186/s12913-014-0565-6.
21. Barateau M, Salles N. L'apport de la télémédecine dans la prise en charge des escarres en soins palliatifs [The contribution of telemedicine in the management of pressure ulcers in palliative care]. Soins. 2015;(792):46–8. French.
22. Institut de recherche et documentation en économie de la santé (IRDES). La télémédecine. L'expérience des patients et des professionnels de santé en télésurveillance. Juillet 2019.
23. Foong HF, Kyaw BM, Upton Z, Tudor CL. Facilitators and barriers of using digital technology for the management of diabetic foot ulcers: a qualitative systematic review. Int Wound J. 2020;17(5):1266–81. https://doi.org/10.1111/iwj.13396. Epub 2020 May 10.
24. Téot L, Geri C, Lano J, Cabrol M, Linet C, Mercier G. Complex wound healing outcomes for outpatients receiving care via telemedicine, home health, or wound clinic: a randomized controlled trial. Int J Low Extrem Wounds. 2020;19(2):197–204. https://doi.org/10.1177/1534734619894485. Epub 2019 Dec 18.
25. Collectif e-santé Plaies et cicatrisation. Livre blanc. www.sffpc.org
26. Paul B. Impact d'interventions personnalisées de sensibilisation aux téléconsultations: cas du réseau Cicat-Occitanie pour les professionnels de santé des EHPAD lozériens. Thèses d'exercice et mémoires—UFR de Médecine Montpellier-Nîmes.
27. Ting JJ, Garnett A. E-health decision support Technologies in the prevention and management of pressure ulcers: a systematic review. Comput Inform Nurs. 2021;39(12):955–73. https://doi.org/10.1097/CIN.0000000000000780.

Open Access This chapter is licensed under the terms of the Creative Commons Attribution-NonCommercial-NoDerivatives 4.0 International License (http://creativecommons.org/licenses/by-nc-nd/4.0/), which permits any non-commercial use, sharing, distribution and reproduction in any medium or format, as long as you give appropriate credit to the original author(s) and the source, provide a link to the Creative Commons license and indicate if you modified the licensed material. You do not have permission under this license to share adapted material derived from this chapter or parts of it.

The images or other third party material in this chapter are included in the chapter's Creative Commons license, unless indicated otherwise in a credit line to the material. If material is not included in the chapter's Creative Commons license and your intended use is not permitted by statutory regulation or exceeds the permitted use, you will need to obtain permission directly from the copyright holder.

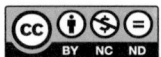

Index

A

Abdominal hyperpressure, 117
Ablative CO_2 laser, 195
Ablative lasers, 312
Abrasion ring, 94
Absorbent dressings, 379
Acellular matrices, 333
    dermal matrices, 334
Achilles tendon, 139
Acinetobacter baumannii, 265, 266
Acral necrosis, 122, 123
Acute compartment syndrome, 17, 18
Acute coronary syndrome (ACS), 42
Acute radiation injury, 109
Adiponecrosis subcutanea neonatorum, 416–418
Adjunctive hyperbaric oxygen therapy, 232
Advanced glycation end products (AGEs), 43
Advanced Nurse Practitioner (ANP), 483
Advanced practice, 483–485
Advanced Trauma Life Support (ATLS®) protocol, 93
Aesthetic medicine, 311, 314
After-debridement care plan, 478
Alginates, 379
Amezinium methylsulfate, 139
Amputation, 3
Amputation-free survival, 322
Anagrelide, 137
Angiodermatitis, 8, 9
Angioplasty, 330
Angiotensin converting enzyme (ACEI), 55
Angiotensin receptor blocker (ARB), 55
Ankle brachial pressure index (ABI), 42, 46, 64–66, 305, 307, 349
Ankle joint dysfunction, 180
Anterior tibial artery recanalization, 326
Anterolateral thigh flap, 350
    artery, 350
Antibiotic prophylaxis, 318
Antibiotic therapy, 162
Antidotes, 423
Antiphospholipid antibody syndrome, 227
Anti-TNF-α agents, 237
Aorto-bifemoral bypass, 324
Aorto-bi-iliac extensive occlusion, 324
Apoptosis, 83, 169, 171

dermal cells, 83
Arginine, 416
Arterial disease, 451
Arterial Doppler ultrasound, 64
Arterial hypertension, 140
Arterial insufficiency, 181
Arterial leg ulcers, 64–66, 392
    causes, 305
    clinical findings, 306
    diagnosis, 307
    epidemiology, 305
    Fontaine classification, 306
    noninvasive vascular tests, 308
    treatment, 308, 309
Arterial vascular complications, 312
Arteriography, 65, 308
Arteriovenous malformations (AVMs), 23–27, 446
    antiangiogenic treatments, 447
    clinical presentation, 446–447
    diagnosis, 447
    physiopathology, 446
Artificial dermis, 284, 285, 356
Atherosclerosis, 43, 46, 366, 455
Atherothrombosis, 61
Atrophie blanche, 235, 237
Atypical wounds, 493
Audiovisual communication system, 122
Australian Advanced Nursing Practice, 484
Autoamputation, 250
Autoimmune thyroiditis, 215
Autologous adipose-derived regenerative cells (ADRCs), 111
Autolytic debridement, 11, 381, 473, 477, 490

B

Bacteria, 265
Bacterial polymerase chain reaction, 220
Behcet's syndrome, 182
Best practices, 503, 504
BEST-CLI group, 328
Bilayered three dimensional porous matrix, 334
Biochemical imbalance, 341
Biofilm, 501–503, 505
Biological debridement, 491

Bio-surgery, 474
Birth asphyxia, 417
Blades and scissors, 405
Blastomycetes dermatitidis, 267
Blastomycosis, 267
Blisters, 168, 419
Blunt dissection technique, 498
Blunt trauma, 385
Bone fragment, 95, 96
Breast cancer, 113
Brown eschar, 419
Buerger's disease, 394
Bullet wipe, 94
Burns, 409
Buruli ulcer, 266
Bypass surgery, 324
Bypass versus Angioplasty in Severe Ischemia of the Leg (BASIL) study, 325

C
Calcified uraemic arteritis (CUA), 227
Calciphylaxis, 118, 121, 122, 177, 201, 227, 228, 231
 clinical manifestation, 231
 diagnosis, 232
 pathophysiology, 232
 risk factor, 231
 treatment, 232, 233
Calciphylaxy, 452
Calcium alginate, 96
Calcium channel blocker, 55
Canada, 503
Candida infection, 268
Carbon dioxide arteriography (CO_2 arteriography), 49
Cardiac catheterization, 109, 112
Caregivers, 507, 508, 510–512
Catheter arteriography, 48, 50, 54, 56
Caustic wounds, 258
Cavity wounds, 409
CD45RO immunoreactivity, 169, 171
Cerium nitrate, 12
Cervical ulcerated infantile hemangioma, 444
CHAP regimen, 237
Charcot-foot, 45
Charcot's joints/foot, 496
Chemical debridement, 473
Chronic hepatitis C infection, 267
Chronic hyperglycemias, 45
Chronic inflammatory skin disease, 193
Chronic insulin resistance, 339
Chronic limb threatening ischemia (CLTI), 41, 42, 45, 47, 48, 50, 52, 54, 55, 321–326, 328, 330, 342
Chronic myelogenous leukemia, 135
Chronic obliterating arteriopathy, 451
Chronic ulcerations, 237
Chronic venous insufficiency, 61, 63, 235, 307
Chronic wounds, 475
Churg-Strauss syndrome, 209
Citrobacter freundii, 265
Clindamycin, 276

Clinical Nurse Specialists, 484
Clotting disorders, 366
Coagulation pathway, 223
Coefficient of friction (COF), 74
Cold atmospheric plasma (CAP), 407
Coma blisters, 167
 case examination, 168
 description, 167
 features of, 170, 171
 immunohistochemical examinations, 168
Coma-induced blisters, 127
Compartment syndrome, 89, 90, 96, 360
Competency, 485
Compression bandage, 153
Compression therapy, 66, 142
Computed tomographic angiography (CTA), 46
Computed tomographic arteriography, 49, 50, 54
Congenital hemangioma (CH)
 clinical presentation, 445
 diagnosis, 445
 pathophysiology of, 445
 treatment, 445
Connective tissue diseases, 181–183, 236
Conservative sharp wound debridement (CSD), 491, 501
Contemporary negative pressure wound therapy systems, 79
Contrast induced nephropathy (CIN), 49, 51
Conventional plain X-rays, 24
Corticosteroids, 203
 therapy, 181
Cosmetic medicine
 ablative lasers, 312
 cryolipolysis, 314
 epidermal peels, 314
 Erbium-YAG laser, 312
 filling products, 311, 312
 HIFU (High Intensity Focused Ultrasound), 314
 infectious, 315
 inflammation, 314
 LEDs, 314
 lifting effect or collagen stimulation by threads, 312
 medium and deep dermal peels, 314
 mesotherapy, 314
 non-ablative lasers, 312
 pigmentation, 314
 pigment lasers, 313
 radiofrequency, 313
 scars, 315
 vascular lasers, 313
Coumarins, 137
COVID-19 pandemic, 76, 267, 508
Critical Leg ischemia Prevention Study (CLIPS) group, 55
Critical limb ischemia (CLI), 41, 305–307, 346
Cryoglobulin, 177
Cryoglobulinemia (CR)
 biology, 244
 histology, 244
 laboratory diagnosis, 243
 local treatment, 245

physiopathology, 243
semiology, 244
systemic treatment, 244
Cryoglobulinemia vasculitis, 209, 268
Cryolipolysis, 314
Cutaneous lesions, 258
Cutaneous vasculitis, 205
    approach to the diagnosis of, 207, 210
    classification, 210
    clinical manifestations, 208, 209
    clinical pathologic correlation, 208
    diagnosis of, 205, 206
    management, 211
Cutaneous wound healing, 77
Cutis marmorata telangiectatica congenita (CMTC), 436, 437
Cyclophosphamide, 245
Cysplatinum, 416

D

Dangerous substances, 421–423
Debridement, 110, 111, 347–348, 375, 400
    'after-debridement' care plan, 478
    algorithm of, 9
    atypical wounds, 493
    autolytic debridement, 477, 490
    biological debridement, 491
    clinical decision for, 502, 503
    definition, 477, 489, 507
    dissecting haematomas, 9
    enzymatic debridement, 490
    evidence-based medicine, 8
    future of, 493
    indications and contraindications of, 8
    levels of, 497
    mechanical debridement, 477, 491
    nurses selection, 477
    pain treatment, 493
    precision, 501, 502
    progressive autolytic debridement, 11, 12
    recommendations, 475
    sharp debridement, 477
    with sharp instruments, 498–499
    skills and assessment checklist, 478
    surgical or sharp debridement, 491
    type of, 479
Deep dissecting hematomas (DDH), 451
    additional examinations, 465–466
    clinical signs, 462–463
    complications, 464–465
    differential diagnoses, 463
    healing, 468
    incidence of, 462
    medical management, 466
    pathophysiology, 461–462
    prevention, 468–469
    surgical management, 466–468
Deep infection, 293, 294, 296
Deep partial thickness burns, 83

Deep skin and soft tissue infections, 281
Deep vein thrombosis (DVT), 463
Degenerated sweat glands, 169–171
Delayed skin necrosis, 296
Delay wound healing, 93, 96
Delta pressure, 18
Dermal fibroblasts, 77
Dermal necrosis, 8
Dermal regeneration template, 334
Dermatomyositis, 182
Dermatoporosis, 461
Devitalized tissue, 476
Diabetes mellitus, 274, 496
Diabetic foot abcess, 118, 119
Diabetic foot infection (DFI), 45
Diabetic foot ulcers (DFUs), 46, 289, 386–388, 393, 476
    debridement, 347–348
    detecting early change, 345–346
    reconstruction, 347–351
        using free flaps, 349–351
    risk factors for, 345
    treatment, 347–351
    vascular intervention, 348–349
    wet necrosis, 346
Diarrhea, 418
Diffuse erythroderma, 146
Digital ischemia, 248
    clinical presentation of, 249
    diagnosis, 249, 250
    management, 250
Digital necrosis
    etiologies, 248
    mechanisms, 247
    vascularization, 247
Digital subtraction angiography (DSA), 48–49
Digital ulceration, 249
Diltiazem, 140
Direct immunofluorescence examination (DIF), 205
Direct revascularisation (DR), 321
Disease-modifying antirheumatic drugs (DMARDs), 183
Dissecting hematomas, 9, 11, 117
Disseminated intravascular coagulation, 219
Distal anastomosis, 324
Distal arterial necrosis, 306, 307
Distal gangrene, 249
Distal necrosis, 289, 393
Doppler ankle-brachial ratio, 307
Doppler ultrasonography (US), 443
Doppler waveform analysis, 47
Dressings containing salts, 380–381
Drug coated balloon angioplasty, 330
Drug necrosis, 452
Dry bites, 152
Dry necrosis, 7, 111, 249, 250, 346–347
Duplex ultrasonography, 24

E

Early ischemic stage, 250
Ecthyma gangrenosum (EG), 265

Edematous tissues, 386
Electrical burns, 406
   buccal mucosa damage, 89
   deep damage, 89
   global management, 91
   Joule effect, 87
   medical management, 89–90
   muscle injury, 88–89
   myocardial damage, 89
   nerve damage, 89
   prevention, 91–92
   surgical management, 90–91
Electrostimulation, 203
End stage renal disease (ESRD), 231, 232
End stage renal insufficiency, 225
Endotracheal tube, 431
Endovascular-first strategy/endovascular-first approach, 54
Endovascular revascularisation, 323–326, 328–330
Enterostomal therapy nurses, 122
Entonox®, 162
Enzymatic debridement, 308, 490
Eosinophilic homogenization, 169
Epidermal atrophy, 236
Epidermal cells, 77
Epidermal-dermal necrosis, 8
Epidermal growth factor receptor (EGFR), 383
Epidermal peels, 314
Epidermis, 73
Epidermolysis bullosa (EB), 438
Erysipelas, 463
Escherichia coli, 265
E-selectin, 389
Estimated glomerular filtration rate (eGFR), 49, 51
Europe, 495, 496, 499
European Qualifications Framework (EQF), 484
European Society for Dermatology and Psychiatry, 255
European Society for Vascular Surgery (ESVS), 42
European Wound Management Association (EWMA), 484, 495
Extracellular matrix (ECM), 73
Extravasation injuries necrosis
   care, 420
   definition, 418–419
   distribution, 420
   epidemiology, 420
   pathophysiology of, 421
   physiology of, 420–421
   rapid tissue necrosis, 419
   risk factors, 421
   treatments, 423–424

F
Face-to-face consultation, 508
Factitious disorders (Pathomimia), 257
   adolescence, 258
   caustic wounds/burning, 258
   classification, 255
   communication between patient and health care providers, 258
   communication between physician and health-care teams, 259
   communication between physician, patient's relatives and his/her general practitioner, 259
   comorbidities, 258
   diagnosis, 257
   prognostic aspects, 259
   specific therapeutic options, 259
   young girl, 257
Fascia, 389
Fasciotomy, 153, 424
Femoro-popliteal bypass, 324
Femoro-tibial bypass, 324
Fiber dressings, 380
Fibroblasts, 73, 77, 78
Fibronectin, 77
Filling products, 311, 312
Finger necrosis, 180
Fish derived acellular matrix, 335
Flammacerium®, 12, 391, 395, 396
Flap failure
   causes of, 364
   etiology, 363–364
   free flap procedure, 368
   intraoperative flap handling, 364–365
   microsurgical technique, 364–365
   non-microsurgical therapy, 368–370
   pathogenesis, 363–364
   postoperative management, 365
   reconstructive goals, 366–370
Flaps, 356
Flesh-eating disease, *see* Necrotizing fasciitis
Fluorodeoxyglucose (FDG), 37, 38
Focal asymmetry, 34
Foot necrosis
   clincal presentation, 129
   follow-up, 133
   resuscitation, 132
   surgical intervention, 132
   therapeutic decision, 129, 130
Forensic autopsy, 167
Fournier gangrene
   diagnosis of, 275
   frozen biopsy, 276
   history, 273
   imaging, 275
   mortality rate, 273
   nonspecific signs, 275
   pathophysiology of, 274
   physiopathogeny, 274
   prevalence, 273
   reconstructive process, 278
   subcutaneous emphysema, 275
   treatment, 276
   ultrasonography, 276
Free flaps, 131–133, 295
Freeze-Thaw-Refreeze injury, 101

Frostbite
    acute frostbite management, 102–104
    aetiological factors, 100
    classification of, 99–100
    early surgical debridement, 105
    examination, 101–102
    extracellular effects, 101
    history, 101
    intracellular effects, 100
    long-term sequelae, 101
    management of blisters, 104–105
    pharmacological support, 103–104
    physiotherapy protocols, 105
    radiological investigations, 102
Fungal infections, 267
Fusarium solani, 271

G
Gadolinium contrast medium, 36
Gangrene, 209
Gastroschisis, 117
Genital herpes, 267
Genodermatosis
    DNA repair, 435
    epidermal-dermal adhesion, 435
    HGPS, 436
    MADA, 436
    physiopathogeny, 435
    vascular anomalies, 436–437
Giant cell arteritis
    ACR classification criteria, 188
    diagnosis, 187–189
    glucocorticosteroids, 189
    methotrexate, 189
    physiopathology, 187
    tocilizumab, 189
    treatment, 189
Global limb Anatomic Staging System (GLASS), 323
Glucocorticoids, 181
Glucocorticosteroids, 189
Glycolic acid, 314
Granuloma, 209
Graves' disease, 140
Group A streptococcus (GAS), 281
Gunshot wounds (GSWs), 93
    characteristics of
        abrasion ring, 94
        bullet wipe, 94
        cavity, 94
        crush and laceration, 94
        retained foreign materials, 95
        secondary shock wave, 94
        skin burn, 94
        smudging, 95
        tattooing, 95
    etiopathogeny, 93
    with hematoma, 95
    management
        arm or leg, 96
        dressing and closure, 96
        face, 96
        head, 96
        initial dressing, 95
        irrigation and debridement, 95
        wound surgery, 95
    principles of
        local wound care to prevent infection, 95
        save life, 95

H
Haematoma, 227
Haemodialysis, 10
Haemophilus influenzae, 425
Harlequin ichthyosis, 439
Healing, 501–504
Heel pressure ulcer, 393
Hemodialysis, 231, 233
Heparin, 138
Hepatitis C virus (HCV) infection, 243
Herpes simplex type 1, 267
Herpes zoster, 267
Herpetic infections, 315
Heterotopic ossifications, 118
Hidradenitis suppurativa, 274
    adjuvant therapy, 196
    description, 193
    diagnosis, 193, 194
    pathophysiology, 194
    treatment, 195
HIFU (high intensity focused ultrasound), 314
High-pressure hydrosurgery, 95
Hirudotherapy, 318
HMG-CoA reductase inhibitors, 55
Holistic limb preservation program, 343
Honey dressings, 399
Horton's disease, *see* Giant cell arteritis
Hot-water technique, 162
Hutchinson–Gilford progeria syndrome (HGPS), 435
Hyaluronan (HA), 341
Hyaluronidase, 423
Hybrid revascularisation, 323, 325
Hydralazine, 139
Hydrating dressings, 377–378
HydroClean Plus, 378
Hydrocolloids, 378–379
    dressings, 164
Hydrofiber, 380
    dressings, 96
Hydrofiber technology, 380
Hydrogel-like devices, 378
Hydrogels, 11, 96, 377, 486, 490
Hydrojets, 11
Hydrosurgery, 423, 491
Hydro-surgery debridement, 474
Hydroxycarbamide, 135
Hydroxyurea, 135, 136

ulcer, 452
Hygiene, 381
Hyperabsorbent dressings, 375
Hyperbaric oxygen (HBO), 277
Hyperbaric oxygen therapy (HBOT), 96, 162
Hyperglycemia, 43, 45, 339, 340, 342
Hypertrophic scarring, 84
Hypodermal fat necrosis
    computed tomography (CT), 37
    magnetic resonance imaging, 36
    positron emission tomography (PET), 37, 38
    ultrasound, 34, 35
    X-ray mammography, 33
Hypoechoic halo, 34
Hypoglycemia, 417
Hypothermia, 102, 417
Hypoxemia, 417

I
Immobilization, 353, 355
Immune cells, 77
Immunomodulators, 239, 240
Incontinence associated dermatitis (IAD), 451
Indigo carmine, 53
Indocyanine green (ICG), 52
Infantile hemangiomas (IHs), 23
    clinical presentation, 443
    diagnosis of, 443
    physiopathology, 443
    treatment, 444
Infection, 263, 501, 502, 505
Infectious necrosis, 452
Inflammation, 83, 314
Inflammatory bowel disease, 215, 239, 240
Inflammatory nodules, 193
Insulin resistance, 43
Intense pain, 160, 161, 163
Intercellular adhesion molecule-1 (ICAM-1), 389
Intermittent claudication (IC), 42
International Year of the Nurse and Midwife, 485
Intralesional sodium thiosulfate, 233
Intramuscular acidosis, 16
Intraoperative flap handling, 364–365
Intravascular hemolysis, 151
Intravenous drugs, 421
Intravenous immunoglobulin (IVIG), 149, 277, 284
Ionizing radiation, 109
Irrigo-absorbent dressings, 378
Ischaemia, 7, 8
Ischaemic limbs, 3
Ischemia/Reperfusion Injury (IRI)
    acute compartment syndrome, 17
    definition, 15
    future research, 19
    pathophysiology, 15–17
    prevention, 19
    tissue edema, 17
    tissue necrosis, 18
    treatment, 18

Ischemic wounds, 493
Itching, 225

J
Janus kinases inhibitors, 237
Japanese viper, 154, 155

K
Kaposiform hemangioendotheliomas (KHE), 23, 445
Kasabach-Merritt phenomenon (KMP), 445
Klippel-Trénaunay syndrome, 24
Knowledge, 501–505

L
Laboratory Risk Indicator for Necrotizing Fasciitis
    (LRINEC) score, 284
Laceration, 94
Large haematomas, 359
    anatomical lesions, 359
    clinical signs, 359
    complementary exams, 360
    surgical management, 360–361
Larval therapy, 491
Laser, 312
    angiography, 52
Laser-assisted fluorescence angiography (LAFA), 52
Laser Doppler flowmetry, 51
Laser speckle contrast imaging (LSCI), 53
Late necrotic stage, 250
Latissimus dorsi muscle, 131, 132
Law, 503
LEDs, *see* Light-emitting diode (LED)
Leeches
    clinical indications, 318
    conservation and use, 317
    mode of action, 317
Leflunomide, 139
Left iliac artery recanalization, 325
Leg ulcers, 140, 388–389
    ankle brachial pressure index (ABI), 64
    arterial Doppler ultrasound, 64
    arterial ulcers, 63
    incidence, 61
    metabolic origin, 61
    mixed ulcers, 64
    mixed ulcers associated with venous insufficiency, 62
    PAD related to atherothrombosis, 61
    TCPO2, 65
    toe brachial index (TBI), 65
    treatment, 65
    vascular imaging, 65
    venous Doppler ultrasound, 64
Leishmaniasis, 268
Leprosy, 266
Lesion site, 240
Leukocyte adhesion deficiency type 1 (LAD-I), 440
Leukocytoclastic vasculitis, 243, 244

Leukopenia, 392
Levamisole, 140
Lifting effect or collagen stimulation by threads, 312
Light-emitting diode (LED), 314
Limb salvage, 129, 321, 322, 324–326, 328
Limb staging, 53
Liposuction, 423
Livedoid vasculitis (LV), 177, 235
    diagnosis, 236
    general management, 236
    histology, 235
    location, 236
    pathogenesis, 235
    possible associated conditions, 236
    signs and symptoms, 235
    therapeutic modalities, 236
    treatment, 236
    ulceration, 237
Livedo reticularis, 243
Live interactive systems, 122
Livid erythema, 136
Local/first-line caregivers, 508
Localization of necrosis, 251
Locoregional anaesthesia, 162
Low-molecular-weight heparins, 162
Low to medium income countries (LMIC), 42

M
Major adverse cardiovascular events (MACE), 42
Major adverse limb events (MALE), 43
Malignant wound, 394
Malingering, 255, 257
Malperfusion, 363
Manuka honey, 401
Martorell hypertensive ischemic ulcer, 177, 199, 452
    clinical diagnosis, 199
    differential diagnosis, 201
    epidemiology, 199
    etiopathogenesis, 199
    evolution, 202
    histopathology, 200
    leg ulcers, 305
    treatment, 202
Maximal walking distance (MWD), 55
Mechanical debridement, 10, 12, 473, 477, 491
Mechanobiology of human skin
    biomechanics on tissue scale, 74–76
    cell-scale, 77
Meconium aspiration syndrome, 417
Medial arterial calcification (MAC), 343
Medical honey dressings, 381
Medications responsible for skin necrosis and ulcers, 135
    amezinium methylsulfate, 139
    anagrelide, 137
    coumarins, 137
    diltiazem, 140
    heparin, 138
    hydralazine, 139
    hydroxyurea, 135

    leflunomide, 139
    levamisole, 140
    methotrexate, 138
    nicorandil, 140
    pentazocine, 141
    propylthiouracil, 140
    tyrosine kinase inhibitors, 141
Medium and deep dermal peels, 314
Menstrual TSS, 145
Mesotherapy, 314
Metabolic abnormalities, 233
Methemoglobinemia, 12, 392
Methicillin-resistant Staphylococcus aureus (MRSA), 284, 400
Methicillin-susceptible Staphylococcus aureus (MSSA), 284
Methotrexate, 138, 189
Microangiopathy, 45
Microarray analysis, 383
Microclimate, 454
Micro-lightguide spectrophotometry (O_2C), 53
Microsurgical technique, 364–365
Microvascular free tissue, 317
Midtarsal amputation, 12
Mitochondrial permeability transitional pores (mPTPs), 16
Mixed cryoglobulinemia, 243, 244, 267
Mixed leg ulcer, 61, 63–66
Modern dressings, 377
Moist wound healing, 478
Mönckeberg mediacalcinosis, 308
Monoclonal gammopathy, 215
Monoclonal immunoglobulin, 243
Morel-Lavallée syndrome, 463
Multiple comorbidities, 395
Munchausen syndrome, 257
Mycobacteria, 266
Mycobacterium leprae, 266
Mycobacterium ulcerans, 266
Mycophenolate mofetil, 217
Myocutaneous flaps, 117

N
Nasal continuous positive airway pressure (NCPAP), 430
National Pressure Ulcer Advisory Panel (NPUAP) classification, 7
Near infrared spectroscopy (NIRS), 53
Neck radiation-induced injury, 114
Necrobiosis lipoidica
    and diabetes mellitus, 215
    clinical findings and complications, 215, 216
    description, 215
    epidemiology, 215
    pathogenesis and histology, 215
    treatment, 216
Necrosis, 452
    physiopathology, 3
    vascular investigations, 3

Necrotic angiodermatitis, 177, 451, *see* Martorell hypertensive ischemic ulcer
Necrotic burns
    inflammation, 83
    limit cell apoptosis, 82
    origination of, 82
    pathophysiology of, 81–83
    primary necrosis, 83–84
    secondary necrosis, 84
    tertiary necrosis, 84
Necrotic diabetic foot, 350
Necrotic tissue, 466
Necrotic ulcerated skin tumor, 121
Necrotizing angiodermatitis, 394
Necrotizing fasciitis, 8, 9, 265, 273–275, 409
    clinical course, 282
    epidemiology, 281
    incidence, 281
    LRINEC score, 284
    medical therapy, 284
    physical diagnosis, 283
    surgical therapy, 284
    symptom, 282
    treatment, 284
Necrotizing infection, 273–275, 279
    soft tissue, 273
Negative pressure therapy, 203, 333, 360
Negative pressure wound therapy (NPWT), 11, 12, 356, 375, 385, 406, 468
    devices, 278
Neonatal adiponecrosis, 417, 418
Neonatal intensive care unit (NICU), 429
Neonatal pressure ulcer
    risk assessment scales, 430
    surgical treatment, 430
    topic treatment, 430
Neonatal skin, 413
Nephrogenic dermal fibrosis (NDF), 225, 226
Neuro-osteoarthropathy, 45
Neuropathic analgesic treatments, 202
Neuropathic foot, 345
Neutrophilic dermatoses, 180
Nicorandil, 140
Non-ablative lasers, 312
Non-Hodgkin's lymphoma, 138
Non-involuting congenital hemangioma (NICH), 23
Nonmenstrual TSS, 145
Non-specialized nurses, 475
Novice to Expert, 483, 485, 486
NPWTi system, 294
Nuclear factor kappa B (NF-κB), 43
Nuclear imaging modality, 37
Nurse practitioner (NP), 503
Nurses
    in advanced practice, 483
    debridement and, 477, 478
Nurses in North America
    clinical decision for debridement's use, 502
    precision of debridement types, 501, 502
    regulations, 503, 504

Nursing law, 503
Nutrition, 458

O

Objective Performance Goals (OPGs), 43
Obstetric trauma, 417
Occlusive dressings, 183
Occupational therapist (OT), 504
Olmsted syndrome (OS), 439, 440
Oncosis, 83
Open fracture, 293–295
Open vascular bypass procedure, 48, 54
Oral propranolol, 444
Orthopox virus, 267
Osmolarity, 421
Osteosynthetic material, 293, 294, 296
Oxygen tubing, 458

P

Pain medication, 496
Palpable purpura, 208, 243, 244
Panniculitis, 209
Paralytic ileus, 89
Paraosteoarthropathy, 118
Parasites, 268
Parkes Weber syndrome, 24
Partially involuting congenital hemangioma (PICH), 23
Pathogens, 268
Pathological SISL, 255
Pathomimicry, 257
Patient, Limb and ANatomy (PLAN), 323
Pediatric extravasation injuries, 413
Pentazocine, 141
Peripheral arterial disease (PAD), 476, 496
    anatomic location, 41
    atherosclerosis, 43
    biological therapy, 55
    diabetic foot, 45
    effects of diabetes on, 45
    epidemiology, 41
    macrovascular assessment of tissue viability, 46–51
    microvascular assessments of tissue viability, 51–53
    morbidity and mortality, 42
    non-operative treatment, 55
    pathophysiology of, 43
    revascularization procedure, 54
    risk factors, 42
    symptomatology, 44
    treatment strategy for limb salvage, 53
    wound care, 54
Peripheral arterial occlusive disease (PAOD), 305–308
Peripheral artery disease (PAD), 339
Peroneal artery recanalization, 325
Phenol, 314
Phenprocoumon coumarins, 137
Phosphodiesterase III inhibitor, 55
Physical injuries, 71
Physiotherapists, 504

Pigment lasers, 313
Pigmentary disorders, 225
Pigmentation, 314
Plain old balloon angioplasty (POBA), 330
Plantar thermography (PT), 53
Plasma-based debriders, 405
Plasma technologies, 405
Pneumococcus, 425
Polyacrylate fiber dressing, 381
Polyarteritis nodosa, 236
Polymorphonuclear cells, 268
Polytrauma, 263
Porcine origin matrix, 335
Posterior acoustic enhancement, 34
Postoperative skin necrosis
    alternatives to flap cover, 296
    debridement, 293
    hardware removal, 294
    NPWT system, 294
    soft-tissue reconstruction, 294, 296
Pressure immobilization, 153
Pressure necrosis
    categories, 455
    differential diagnosis, 457
    etiology, 453–455
    pathophysiology, 453–455
    prevention, 457–458
    treatment, 458–459
Pressure ulcers (PUs), 7, 8, 10, 118, 385, 432, 451, 453, 475
Primary necrosis, 83–84
Probe-to-bone (PTB) test, 342
Proficiency, 485
Progressive autolytic debridement, 11
Progressive necrosis, 8, 10
Prolidase deficiency, 437
Prophylactic antibiotherapy, 318
Propylthiouracil, 140
Protein C deficiency, 219, 221
    diagnosis, 223, 224
    physiopathology, 223
    treatment, 224
Protein kinase C (PKC) activation, 43
Protein S deficiency
    diagnosis, 223, 224
    physiopathology, 223
    treatment, 224
P-selectin, 389
P-selectin glycoprotein ligand-1 (PSGL-1), 389
Pseudocysts, 34
Pseudomonas aeruginosa, 265, 391
Pseudonodules, 34–38
Psoralen plus ultraviolet A (PUVA) therapy, 216
PTFE strengthened prosthesis, 324
Public health code, 507
Pulpaire necrosis, 163
Pulse volume recorder (PVR), 47
Purpura fulminans, 219, 223
    clinical presentation, 220
    differential diagnosis, 220
    long-term sequelae of, 220
    management, 220
    pathogenesis, 219
    subtypes, 219
Pyoderma gangrenosum (PG), 177, 180, 185, 194, 201, 305, 452, 489
    causes of ulcers mimicking, 239, 240
    clinical manifestation, 239
    etiopathogeny, 239
    incidence, 239
    treatment, 240, 241

R

Radiation therapy, 109, 111
Radiation ulcers, 110
    debridement, 110
    management of, 110, 111
    stem cell therapy, 111
    surgical treatment, 110
    wound closure methods, 110, 111
Radical ablation, 154
Radiofrequency, 313
Radio-isotope methods, 51
Radionecrosis, 394
Rapidly involuting congenital hemangioma (RICH), 23
Rapid tissue necrosis, 419
Raynaud's phenomenon, 209
Reepithelialization, 83
Refractory radiation ulcers, 110
Registered/licensed practical nurse (RPN/LPN), 503
Registered nurse (RN), 477, 495, 496, 503
Regulations, 495, 499, 503–504
Removal of necrotic tissue, 483
Renal insufficiency
    causes, 227
    co morbidity, 226
    differential diagnosis in necrotic lesion, 228
    exacerbation, 227
    KDOQI classification, 226
    treatment, 228
Renecrosis, 3
Residual tension stresses, 73
Resuscitation, 130, 132
Retained foreign materials, 95
Retiform purpura, 208
Revascularization, 61, 65, 66
Rheological therapy concepts, 142
Rhesus incompatibility, 417
Rheumatoid arthritis, 139, 141, 179
    prevention of recurrence, 186
    several adjuvant devices, 183
    surgical wound closure, 184
    systemic treatment approach, 182
    topical wound treatment, 183
    ulcer development, 179
        arterial insufficiency, 181
        corticosteroid therapy, 181
        neutrophilic dermatoses, 180

vasculitis, 179
venous stasis, 180
Right leg ulcer, 240
Ring curette technique, 498
Rituximab, 212, 245

S

Saline lavage techniques, 423
Scalpel technique, 498
Scars, 315
Scissor technique, 498
Sclerema neonatorum (SN), 417
Scleroderma, 182, 394
Scuba diver, 160, 161
Secondary bacterial infection, 240
Secondary necrosis, 84
Secondary shock wave, 94
Selective stenting, 330
Self-inflicted skin lesions (SISLs), 255, 257
Self-ischaemia, 359
Septicaemia, 359
Serum sickness-type reactions, 153
Severe acute respiratory syndrome coronavirus 2 (SARS-CoV-2), 267
Severe arteriopathy, 452
Severe necrotizing soft tissue infections (SNSTIs)
    care, 426
    PROC/PROS1 genes, 426
Severe perinatal hypoxia, 416
Severe tissue damage, 282, 283
Sharp debridement, 473, 477
    complications, 496
    for nurses in Europe, 495
    procedure of, 496
Shear, 454
Silver sulfadiazine, 12
Simple haematoma, 463
Simulation, 257
Single antiplatelet, 55
Sinus tracts, 193–195
Sjögren's syndrome, 182
Skin
    blood flow, 51
    burn, 94
    damage, 74
    exposure, 455
    functions, 73
    grafts, 202
    layers, 73
    mechanobiology (*see* Mechanobiology of the human skin)
Skin blood flow, 51
Skin burn, 94
Skin exposure, 455
Skin grafts, 202
Skin infection, 265
    bacteria, 265, 266
    COVID-19 pandemic, 267

    mycobacteria, 266
    parasites, 268
    pathological mechanisms, 268
    viruses, 267
    yeast, 267
Skin necrosis, 117, 123, 359
    acellular dermal matrix, 334
    arteriolar-capillary occlusion, 415
    bilayered three dimensional porous matrix, 334
    causes, 127
    course and outcome, 418
    dermal regeneration template, 334
    diagnosis of, 121, 417–418
    dimensional porous matrix, 334
    general anaesthesia, 375
    immaturity of immune system, 416
    laboratory examinations, 417
    non-invasive adsorbing dressings, 375
    origin, 177
    porcine origin matrix, 335
    post traumatic, 335, 336
    and telemedicine, 122
Skin substitute, 296
Skin tears, 451
Smudging, 95
Snakebites
    allergic reactions to antivenom, 153
    antivenom treatment, 153
    case reports, 154, 155
    debridement of fang marks, 154
    first aid, 153
    severity of, 152
    surgical treatment, 153
    systemic and local complications, 151
Society for Vascular Surgery (SVS), 42
Sodium thiosulfate, 228
Soft-tissue reconstruction, 294
SO_2 probes, 52
Split-skin grafting, 383
Split-thickness skin grafts, 278
Staphylococcal enterotoxins, 148
Staphylococcal TSS, 145–146
Staphylococcus aureus, 315, 391, 425
Statin therapy, 55
Steroids, 162
Stonefish
    habitat, 160
    identification, 159
    stings by, 160
        antibiotic therapy, 162
        circumstances, 160
        clinical cases, 163, 164
        clinical evidence, 160
        diagnosis, 161
        medical complications, 161
        severity of wound, 161
        steroids, 162
        treatment, 162
        wound location, 160

thorns and glands with venom, 160
Store and forward technology, 122
Streptococcal TSS, 146
Subcutaneous emphysema, 275
Subdermal necrosis, 7, 8
Subepidermal tissue degradation, 8
Subepidermal vesicles, 169
Succion effect, 318
Sufficient blood flow, 503
Sufficient Treatment of Peripheral Intervention by Cilostazol (STOP-IC) study, 55
Superantigens, 148
Superficial temporal arteries, 187
Surgeons, 289
Surgical debridement, 9–11, 273, 275–277, 279, 289
    acute and chronic wounds, 383
    burns, 383
    extensive scald burn, 384
    high-energy trauma wound, 385
    leg ulcer, 388–389
    mesh skin grafting, 384
    pressure ulcers, 385
    surgical equipment, 389
    wound bed preparation, 389
Surgical or sharp debridement, 491, 502
Surgical specialist training, 491
SVS Wound, Ischemia, and Foot infection (WIfI) classification, 47, 343
Sweat gland degeneration, 171
Symptomatology, 43
Synanceia verrucosa, 159
Syphilis, 266
Systemic collagenosis vasculitis, 179
    ulcers
        Behcet's syndrome, 182
        dermatomyositis, 182
        occlusive dressings, 183
        scleroderma, 182
        Sjögren's syndrome, 182
        SLE, 181
        systemic sclerosis, 182
Systemic disease, 239, 240, 366
Systemic lupus erythematosus (SLE), 241
Systemic sclerosis, 182

T
Target artery pathway (TAP), 323
Tattooing, 95
Technology, 122
Tele-assistance, 123, 507, 508, 510–512
Teleconsultation, 507–509, 511, 512
Telemedicine, 122, 507, 508, 511, 512
Temporal arteritis, 187
Temporal artery biopsy, 188
Temporization, 395
TenderWet, 378
Tendon immobilization, 356
Tendon necrosis

artificial dermis, 356
burns, 356–357
flaps, 356
immobilization, 355
NPWT, 356
staging, 353–354
traumatic skin avulsion, 357
Tendon repair, 356
Tertiary necrosis, 84
Thalidomide, 447
Therapeutic strategy, 271
Threads, 312
Thrombolytic therapy, 103
Thrombosis, 232
Tissue diffuse necrosis, 224
Tissue edema, 17
Tissue infusion visualization technique, 52
Tissue necrosis, 15–19
Tissue plasminogen activator, 235, 236
Tissue viability, 51, 53
Tocilizumab, 189
Toe brachial index (TBI), 47, 64–66
Toe necrosis, 10
Topical corticosteroids, 211
Topical negative pressure therapy (TNP), 367
Topical p38 MAPK inhibition, 84
Topical therapy, 195
Toxic shock syndrome (TSS)
    antibiotic therapy, 148, 149
    epidemiology and clinical features, 145–147
    intravenous immune globulin, 149
    pathophysiology, 148
    surgical therapy, 149
Toxin, 263
Tranquillizers, 259
Trans Atlantic Society Consensus classification (TASC), 323
Transcutaneous oxygen measurement (TCOM), 46, 349
Transcutaneous oxygen tension (TcPO2), 46, 51
Traumatic skin avulsion, 357
Traumatic wounds, 385
Treponema pallidum, 266
Trichloroacetic acid, 314
Triple phase bone scan, 251
Tufted angioma (TA), 445
TUNEL method, 169, 171
Two-dimensional perfusion angiography (2D-PA), 53
Tyrosine kinase inhibitors, 141

U
Ulcerated congenital hemangioma, 445
Ulcerated infantile hemangioma, 444
Ulceration, 235, 237, 268
Ultrasonic duplex scanning, 308
Ultrasonic/ultrasound debridement, 491
Ultrasonography, 360
Unique Manuka factor (UMF) rating, 400
Urticaria, 208

V

Vacuum-assisted closure (VAC) devices, 277, 278
Vacuum-assisted therapy (VAC), 196
Vascular disease, 366
Vascular imaging, 65
Vascular injury, 364
Vascular insufficiency, 391
Vascularization, 247
Vascular lasers, 313
Vascular leg ulcers, 289
Vascular malformations, 23, 24
Vascular smooth muscle cells (VSMCs), 43
Vascular tumor, 23
Vasculitic wounds, 489
Vasculitis, 177, 179
Venomous animals, 160
Venous Doppler ultrasound, 65
Venous embolisms, 312
Venous insufficiency, 62–66, 235–236, 305
Venous malformation (VM), 23, 25
    AVM, 26
    computed tomography (CT), 25
    conventional plain X-rays, 24
    duplex ultrasonography, 24
    magnetic resonance imaging (MRI), 25
    vascular imaging, 25
Venous stasis ulcer, 181
Ventouse extraction, 432
Versajet™, 9, 405, 408, 409
Vitamin K supplementation, 233

W

Warfarin, 137, 416
Wet necrosis, 8, 13, 249, 250, 346
White side method, 18
WIFI classification, 322
Winkelmann granuloma, 206
Wolff-Parkinson-White (WPW) syndrome, 140
Wound aetiology, 475
Wound bed evaluation, 475–476
Wound care, 203, 444
Wound cleansing, 477, 478
Wound healing, 73, 77, 432, 468
    antibacterial properties, 399–400
    anti-inflammatory effect, 402
    chemical and honey debridement method, 401
    contraindications, 402
    debridement, 400
    deodorizing, 402
    tissue growth, 401

X

Xerosis, 225
X-ray mammography, 33

Y

Yeast, 267
Yellow necrosis, 419
Yellow orange, 216